FIFTH EDITION

CASE FILES®
Surgery

Eugene C. Toy, MD
Assistant Dean for Educational Programs
Director of Doctoring Courses Program
Director of the Scholarly Concentrations in
    Women's Health
Professor and Vice Chair of Medical Education
Department of Obstetrics and Gynecology
McGovern Medical School at University of
    Texas Health Science Center at Houston
    (UTHealth)
Houston, Texas

Terrence H. Liu, MD, MPH
Professor of Clinical Surgery
University of California San Francisco School
    of Medicine
San Francisco, California
Program Director
University of California, San Francisco East Bay
    Surgery Residency
San Francisco, California
Attending Surgeon, Alameda County Medical
    Center
Oakland, California

Andre R. Campbell, MD, FACS, FACP, FCCM
Professor of Surgery and Director
    Third Year Clerkship
University of California San Francisco
School of Medicine
Medical Director Surgical Intensive
    Care Unit and Attending Surgeon
San Francisco General Hospital
Director Surgical Critical Care Fellowship
UCSF School of Medicine
San Francisco, California

Barnard J. A. Palmer, MD, MEd
Assistant Clinical Professor and Associate
    Residency Program Director
Department of Surgery
University of California, San Francisco-East Bay
Oakland, California

New York   Chicago   San Francisco   Athens   London   Madrid
Mexico City   Milan   New Delhi   Singapore   Sydney   Toronto

This book was set in Adobe Jenson Pro by Cenveo® Publisher Services.
The editors were Catherine A. Johnson and Cindy Yoo.
The production supervisor was Catherine H. Saggese.
Project management was provided by Hardik Popli.
RR Donnelley was printer and binder.

This book is printed on acid-free paper.

Library of Congress Cataloging-in-Publication Data

Names: Toy, Eugene C., author. | Liu, Terrence H., author. | Campbell, Andre R., author. |
    Palmer, Barnard J. A., author.
Title: Case files. Surgery / Eugene C. Toy, Terrence H. Liu, Andre R. Campbell, Barnard J.A. Palmer.
Other titles: Surgery
Description: Fifth edition. | New York : McGraw-Hill Education, [2016] |
    Includes bibliographical references and index.
Identifiers: LCCN 2015050423| ISBN 9781259585227 (pbk.) | ISBN 1259585220 (pbk.)
Subjects: | MESH: Surgical Procedures, Operative—methods | Examination Questions | Case Reports
Classification: LCC RD34 | NLM WO 18.2 | DDC 617—dc23 LC record available at http://lccn.loc.gov/
    2015050423

DEDICATION

To my dear parents Chuck and Grace who taught me the importance of pursuing excellence and instilled in me a love for books; to my sister Nancy for her compassion and unselfishness, her husband Jason and their beautiful daughters Madison and Peyton; and to my brother Glen for his friendship and our fond memories growing up, his wife Linda, and their precious son Eric.

—ECT

To my wife Eileen for her love, friendship, support, and encouragement. To my parents George and Jackie for their constant loving support, and to my sons Andrew and Gabriel who show to me the importance of family values, every day. To all my teachers and mentors, who took the time and effort to teach and serve as role models.

—THL

I would like to dedicate this book to my lovely wife, Gillian, and our son, Andre Jr., who have allowed me to pursue my life's work and supported me my entire career as a trauma surgeon and educator.

—ARC

To the residents and students who continue to challenge and push the frontiers of medicine. And to my wife, Samantha, and daughter, Mieko, who have rekindled my appreciation for everything that is wonderful in life.

—BJAP

To the wonderful medical students of the McGovern Medical School at The University of Texas Health Science Center at Houston (UTHealth) for whom this curriculum was developed.

—THE AUTHORS

CONTENTS

Eileen T. Consorti, MD, MS
President of Medical Staff
Alta Bates Medical Center
Berkeley, California and
Medical Director of Carol Anne Read Breast Care Center
Oakland, California
Breast Cancer
Breast Cancer Risk and Surveillance
Nipple Discharge (Serosanguineous)

Vikas S. Gupta
Medical Student
McGovern Medical School at The University of Texas
    Health Science Center at Houston (UTHealth)
Houston, Texas
Manuscript Reviewer

Gregory P. Victorino, MD
Chief of Trauma
Professor of Clinical Surgery
University of California, San Francisco-East Bay
Oakland, California
Postoperative Acute Respiratory Insufficiency

We appreciate all the kind remarks and suggestions from the many medical students over the past four years. Your positive reception has been an incredible encouragement, especially in light of the short life of the *Case Files®* series. In this fifth edition of *Case Files®: Surgery*, the basic format of the book has been retained. Improvements were made by updating many of the chapters, with five completely rewritten cases: Breast Cancer Risk and Surveillance, Colon Cancer, Thyroid Mass, Pheochromocytoma, and Hemorrhage and Hypotension. We reviewed the clinical scenarios with the intent on improving them; however, we found that their real-life presentations patterned after actual clinical experience remained accurate and instructive. The multiple-choice questions have been carefully reviewed and rewritten to ensure that they comply with the National Board and USMLE formats. By reading this fifth edition, we hope that you will continue to enjoy learning surgical management through the simulated clinical cases. It is certainly a privilege to be a teacher for so many students, and it is with humility that we present this edition.

The Authors

ACKNOWLEDGMENTS

The curriculum that evolved into the ideas for this series was inspired by two talented and forthright students, Philbert Yao and Chuck Rosipal, who have since graduated from medical school. It has been a tremendous joy to work with my friend since medical school, Terry Liu, a brilliant surgeon. It has been rewarding to collaborate once again with Andre Campbell, who has deservedly advanced to have many educational and clinical leadership roles at the University of California, San Francisco. It has been a pleasure to have Barnard Palmer, a very astute surgeon and educator, to join our team. We also thank our excellent contributors. I am greatly indebted to my editor, Catherine Johnson, whose exuberance, experience, and vision helped to shape this series. I appreciate McGraw-Hill's believing in the concept of teaching through clinical cases. I am also grateful to Catherine Saggese for her excellent production expertise and Cindy Yoo for her wonderful editing. Hardik Popli deserves acknowledgement for his amazing patience and precision as project manager for this book. At McGovern Medical School, I appreciate the great support from Drs. Sean Blackwell, Patricia Butler, and John Riggs, without whom I would not have been able to complete this book. Most of all, I appreciate my loving wife, Terri, and my four wonderful children, Andy and his wife Anna, Michael, Allison, and Christina, for their patience, encouragement, and understanding.

Eugene C. Toy

Mastering the cognitive knowledge within a field such as general surgery is a formidable task. It is even more difficult to draw on that knowledge, procure and filter through the clinical and laboratory data, develop a differential diagnosis, and finally form a rational treatment plan. To gain these skills, the student often learns best at the bedside, guided and instructed by experienced teachers and inspired toward self-directed, diligent reading. Clearly, there is no replacement for education at the bedside. Unfortunately, clinical situations usually do not encompass the breadth of the specialty. Perhaps the best alternative is a carefully crafted patient case designed to stimulate the clinical approach and decision making. In an attempt to achieve this goal, we have constructed a collection of clinical vignettes to teach diagnostic or therapeutic approaches relevant to general surgery. Most importantly, the explanations for the cases emphasize the mechanisms and underlying principles rather than merely rote questions and answers.

This book is organized for versatility to allow the student "in a rush" to go quickly through the scenarios and check the corresponding answers, and to provide more detailed information for the student who wants thought-provoking explanations. The answers are arranged from simple to complex: a summary of the pertinent points, the bare answers, an analysis of the case, an approach to the topic, a comprehension test at the end for reinforcement and emphasis, and a list of resources for further reading. The clinical vignettes are purposely arranged randomly in order to simulate the way that real patients present to the practitioner. A listing of cases is included in Section III to aid the student who desires to test his or her knowledge of a certain area or to review a topic, including basic definitions. Finally, we intentionally did not primarily use a multiple-choice question format because clues (or distractions) are not available in the real world. Nevertheless, several multiple-choice questions are included at the end of each scenario to reinforce concepts or introduce related topics.

HOW TO GET THE MOST OUT OF THIS BOOK

Each case is designed to simulate a patient encounter and includes open-ended questions. At times, the patient's complaint differs from the issue of most concern, and sometimes extraneous information is given. The answers are organized into four different parts:

PART I

1. **Summary:** The salient aspects of the case are identified, filtering out the extraneous information. The student should formulate his or her summary from the case before looking at the answers. A comparison with the summation in the answer help to improve one's ability to focus on the important data while appropriately discarding irrelevant information, a fundamental skill required in clinical problem solving.

2. **A straightforward answer** is given to each open-ended question.
3. An **analysis of the case,** which consists of two parts:
   a. **Objectives:** A listing of the two or three main principles, which are crucial for a practitioner in treating a patient. Again, the student is challenged to make educated "guesses" about the objectives of the case after an initial review of the case scenario, which help to sharpen his or her clinical and analytical skills.
   b. **Considerations:** A discussion of the relevant points and a brief approach to a specific patient.

PART II

An **approach to the disease process,** consisting of two distinct parts:
   a. **Definitions:** Terminology pertinent to the disease process
   b. **Clinical Approach:** A discussion of the approach to the clinical problem in general, including tables, figures, and algorithms.

PART III

Comprehension Questions: Each case includes several multiple-choice questions, which reinforce the material or introduce new and related concepts. Questions about material not found in the text are explained in the answers.

PART IV

Clinical Pearls: A listing of several clinically important points, which are reiterated as a summation of the text and to allow for easy review, such as before an examination.

LISTING BY CASE NUMBER

LISTING BY DISORDER (ALPHABETICAL)

How to Approach Clinical Problems

Part 1. Approach to the Patient

The transition from textbook or journal article learning to an application of the information in a specific clinical situation is one of the most challenging tasks in medicine. It requires retention of information, organization of the facts, and recall of myriad data with precise application to the patient. The purpose of this text is to facilitate this process. The first step is gathering information, also known as establishing the database. This includes recording the patient's history; performing the physical examination; and obtaining selective laboratory examinations, special evaluations such as breast ductograms, and/or imaging tests. Of these, the historical examination is the most important and most useful. Sensitivity and respect should always be exercised during the interview of patients.

CLINICAL PEARL

▶ The history is usually the single most important tool in reaching a diagnosis. The art of obtaining this information in a nonjudgmental, sensitive, and thorough manner cannot be overemphasized.

HISTORY

1. **Basic information:**
   a. **Age:** Must be recorded because some conditions are more common at certain ages; for instance, age is one of the most important risk factors for the development of breast cancer.
   b. **Gender:** Some disorders are more common in or found exclusively in men such as prostatic hypertrophy and cancer. In contrast, women more commonly have autoimmune problems such as immune thrombocytopenia purpura and thyroid nodules. Also, the possibility of pregnancy must be considered in any woman of childbearing age.
   c. **Ethnicity:** Some disease processes are more common in certain ethnic groups (such as diabetes mellitus in the Hispanic population).

CLINICAL PEARL

▶ The possibility of pregnancy must be entertained in any woman of childbearing age.

2. **Chief complaint:** What is it that brought the patient into the hospital or office? Is it a scheduled appointment or an unexpected symptom such as abdominal pain or hematemesis? The duration and character of the complaint, associated symptoms, and exacerbating and/or relieving factors should be recorded. The chief complaint engenders a differential diagnosis, and the possible etiologies should be explored by further inquiry.

> ## CLINICAL PEARL

> ▸ The first line of any surgical presentation should include **age, ethnicity, gender,** and **chief complaint.** Example: A 32-year-old Caucasian man complains of lower abdominal pain over an 8-hour duration.

3. **Past medical history:**
   a. Major illnesses such as hypertension, diabetes, reactive airway disease, congestive heart failure, and angina should be detailed.
      i. Age of onset, severity, end-organ involvement.
      ii. Medications taken for a particular illness, including any recent change in medications and the reason for the change.
      iii. Last evaluation of the condition. (eg, When was the last echocardiogram performed in a patient with congestive heart failure?)
      iv. Which physician or clinic is following the patient for the disorder?
   b. Minor illnesses such as a recent upper respiratory tract infection may impact on the scheduling of elective surgery.
   c. Hospitalizations no matter how trivial should be detailed.

4. **Past surgical history:** Date , types, indications, and outcomes of procedures should be elicited. Laparoscopy versus laparotomy should be distinguished. Surgeon, hospital name, and location should be listed. This information should be correlated with the surgical scars on the patient's body. Any complications should be delineated, including anesthetic complications, difficult intubations, and so on.

5. **Allergies:** Reactions to medications should be recorded, including severity and temporal relationship to administration of medication. Immediate hypersensitivity should be distinguished from an adverse reaction.

6. **Medications:** A list of medications including dosage, route of administration and frequency, and duration of use should be developed. Prescription, over-the-counter, and herbal remedies are all relevant.

7. **Social history:** Marital status; family support; alcohol use, use or abuse of illicit drugs, and tobacco use; and tendencies toward depression or anxiety are important.

8. **Family history:** Major medical problems, genetically transmitted disorders such as breast cancer, and important reactions to anesthetic medications such as malignant hyperthermia (an autosomal dominant transmitted disorder) should be explored.

9. **Review of systems:** A system review should be performed focusing on the more common diseases. For example, in a young man with a testicular mass, trauma to the area, weight loss, neck masses, and lymphadenopathy are important. In an elderly woman, symptoms suggestive of cardiac disease should be elicited, such as chest pain, shortness of breath, fatigue, weaknesses, and palpitations.

> CLINICAL PEARL

> ▶ Malignant hyperthermia is a rare condition inherited in an autosomal dominant fashion. It is associated with a rapid rise in temperature up to 40.6°C (105°F), usually on induction by general anesthetic agents such as succinylcholine and halogenated inhalant gases. Prevention is the best treatment.

PHYSICAL EXAMINATION

1. **General appearance:** Note whether the patient is cachectic versus well nourished, anxious versus calm, alert versus obtunded.

2. **Vital signs:** Record the temperature, blood pressure, heart rate, and respiratory rate. Height and weight are often included here. For trauma patients, the Glasgow Coma Scale (GCS) is important.

3. **Head and neck examination:** Evidence of trauma, tumors, facial edema, goiter and thyroid nodules, and carotid bruits should be sought. With a closed-head injury, pupillary reflexes and unequal pupil sizes are important. Cervical and supraclavicular nodes should be palpated.

4. **Breast examination:** Perform an inspection for symmetry and for skin or nipple retraction with the patient's hands on her hips (to accentuate the pectoral muscles) and with her arms raised. With the patient supine, the breasts should be palpated systematically to assess for masses. The nipples should be assessed for discharge, and the axillary and supraclavicular regions should be examined for adenopathy.

5. **Cardiac examination:** The point of maximal impulse should be ascertained, and the heart auscultated at the apex as well as at the base. Heart sounds, murmurs, and clicks should be characterized. Systolic flow murmurs are fairly common in pregnant women because of the increased cardiac output, but significant diastolic murmurs are unusual.

6. **Pulmonary examination:** The lung fields should be examined systematically and thoroughly. Wheezes, rales, rhonchi, and bronchial breath sounds should be recorded.

7. **Abdominal examination:** The abdomen should be inspected for scars, distension, masses or organomegaly (ie, spleen or liver), and discoloration. For instance, the Grey Turner sign of discoloration on the flank areas may indicate an intra-abdominal or retroperitoneal hemorrhage. Auscultation should be performed to identify normal versus high-pitched, and hyperactive versus hypoactive, bowel sounds. The abdomen should be percussed for the presence of shifting dullness (indicating ascites). Careful palpation should begin initially away from the area of pain, involving one hand on top of the other, to assess for masses, tenderness, and peritoneal signs. Tenderness should be recorded on

a scale (eg, 1-4, where 4 is the most severe pain). Guarding and whether it is voluntary or involuntary should be noted.

8. **Back and spine examination:** The back should be assessed for symmetry, tenderness, or masses. The flank regions are particularly important in assessing for pain on percussion that may indicate renal disease.

9. **Genital examination:**

   a. **Female:** The external genitalia should be inspected, and the speculum then used to visualize the cervix and vagina. A bimanual examination should attempt to elicit cervical motion tenderness, uterine size, and ovarian masses or tenderness.

   b. **Male:** The penis should be examined for hypospadias, lesions, and infection. The scrotum should be palpated for masses and, if present, transillumination should be used to distinguish between solid and cystic masses. The groin region should be carefully palpated for bulging (hernias) on rest and on provocation (coughing). This procedure should optimally be repeated with the patient in different positions.

   c. **Rectal examination:** A rectal examination can reveal masses in the posterior pelvis and may identify occult blood in the stool. In females, nodularity and tenderness in the uterosacral ligament may be signs of endometriosis. The posterior uterus and palpable masses in the cul-de-sac may be identified by rectal examination. In the male, the prostate gland should be palpated for tenderness, nodularity, and enlargement.

10. **Extremities and skin:** The presence of joint effusions, tenderness, skin edema, and cyanosis should be recorded.

11. **Neurologic examination:** Patients who present with neurologic complaints usually require thorough assessments, including evaluation of the cranial nerves, strength, sensation, and reflexes.

CLINICAL PEARL

▶ A thorough understanding of anatomy is important to optimally interpret the physical examination findings.

---

12. Laboratory assessment depends on the circumstances.

   a. **A complete blood count:** To assess for anemia, leukocytosis (infection), and thrombocytopenia.

   b. **Urine culture or urinalysis:** To assess for infection or hematuria when ureteral stones, renal carcinoma, or trauma is suspected.

   c. **Tumor markers:** For example, in testicular cancer, β-human chorionic gonadotropin, α-fetoprotein, and lactate dehydrogenase values are often elevated.

    d. **Serum creatinine and serum urea nitrogen levels:** To assess renal function, and aspartate aminotransferase (AST) and alanine aminotransferase (ALT) values to assess liver function.

13. **Imaging procedures:**
    a. An ultrasound examination is the most commonly used imaging procedure to distinguish a pelvic process in female patients, such as pelvic inflammatory disease. It is also very useful in diagnosing gallstones and measuring the caliber of the common bile duct. It can also help discern solid versus cystic masses.
    b. Computed tomography (CT) is extremely useful in assessing fluid and abscess collections in the abdomen and pelvis. It can also help determine the size of lymph nodes in the retroperitoneal space.
    c. Magnetic resonance imaging identifies soft tissue planes and may assist in assessing prolapsed lumbar nucleus pulposus and various orthopedic injuries.
    d. Intravenous pyelography uses dye to assess the concentrating ability of the kidneys, the patency of the ureters, and the integrity of the bladder. It is also useful in detecting hydronephrosis, ureteral stones, and ureteral obstructions.

Part 2. Approach to Clinical Problem Solving

There are typically four distinct steps that a clinician takes to systematically solve most clinical problems:

1. Making the diagnosis

2. Assessing the severity or stage of the disease

3. Proposing a treatment based on the stage of the disease

4. Following the patient's response to the treatment

MAKING THE DIAGNOSIS

A diagnosis is made by a careful evaluation of the database, analyzing the information, assessing the risk factors, and developing the list of possibilities (the differential diagnosis). Experience and knowledge help the physician "key in" on the most important possibilities. A good clinician also knows how to ask the same question in several different ways and use different terminology. For example, a patient may deny having been treated for "cholelithiasis" but answer affirmatively when asked if he has been hospitalized for "gallstones." Reaching a diagnosis may be achieved by systematically reading about each possible cause and disease.

    Usually a long list of possible diagnoses can be pared down to two or three that are the most likely, based on selective laboratory or imaging tests. For example, a patient who complains of upper abdominal pain *and* has a history of nonsteroidal anti-inflammatory drug use may have peptic ulcer disease; another patient who has abdominal pain, fatty food intolerance, and abdominal bloating may have cholelithiasis. Yet another individual with a 1-day history of periumbilical pain localizing to the right lower quadrant may have acute appendicitis.

> ### CLINICAL PEARL
>
> ▶ The first step in clinical problem solving is **making the diagnosis.**

ASSESSING THE SEVERITY OF THE DISEASE

After establishing the diagnosis, the next step is to characterize the severity of the disease process. in other words, describing "how bad" a disease is. With malignancy, this is done formally by staging the cancer. Most cancers are categorized from stage I (least severe) to stage IV (most severe). With some diseases, such as with head trauma, there is a formal scale (the GCS) based on the patient's eye-opening response, verbal response, and motor response.

> ### CLINICAL PEARL
>
> ▶ The second step in clinical problem solving is to **establish the severity or stage of the disease.** There is usually prognostic or treatment significance based on the stage.

TREATING BASED ON THE STAGE

Many illnesses are stratified according to severity because the prognosis and treatment often vary based on the severity. If neither the prognosis nor the treatment were affected by the stage of the disease process, there would be no reason to subcategorize the illness as mild or severe. For example, obesity is subcategorized as moderate (body mass index [BMI] 35 to 40 kg/m^2) or severe (BMI > 40 kg/m^2), with different prognoses and recommended interventions. Surgical procedures for obesity such as gastric bypass are only generally considered when a patient has severe obesity and/or significant comorbidities such as sleep apnea.

> ### CLINICAL PEARL
>
> ▶ The third step in clinical problem solving is, in most cases, **tailoring the treatment** to the extent or stage of the disease.

FOLLOWING THE RESPONSE TO TREATMENT

The final step in the approach to disease is to follow the patient's response to the therapy. The "measure" of response should be recorded and monitored. Some responses are clinical, such as improvement (or lack of improvement) in a patient's abdominal pain, temperature, or pulmonary examination. Other responses can be followed by imaging tests such as a CT scan to determine the size of a retroperitoneal mass in a patient receiving chemotherapy, or with a tumor marker such as the level of prostate-specific antigen in a male receiving chemotherapy for prostatic cancer. For a closed-head injury, the GCS is used. The student must be prepared to know what to do if the measured marker does not respond according to what is expected. Is the next step to treat again, to reassess the diagnosis, to pursue a metastatic workup, or to follow up with another more specific test?

CLINICAL PEARL

▶ **The fourth step in clinical problem solving is to monitor treatment response or efficacy,** which can be measured in different ways. It may be symptomatic (the patient feels better) or based on a physical examination (fever), a laboratory test (prostate-specific antigen level), or an imaging test (size of a retroperitoneal lymph node on a CT scan).

Part 3. Approach to Reading

The clinical problem-oriented approach to reading is different from the classic "systematic" research of a disease. A patient's presentation rarely provides a clear diagnosis; hence, the student must become skilled in applying textbook information to the clinical setting. Furthermore, one retains more information when one reads with a purpose. In other words, the student should read with the goal of answering specific questions. There are several fundamental questions that facilitate **clinical thinking:**

1. What is the most likely diagnosis?

2. How can you confirm the diagnosis?

3. What should be your next step?

4. What is the most likely mechanism for this disease process?

5. What are the risk factors for this disease process?

6. What are the complications associated with this disease process?

7. What is the best therapy?

CLINICAL PEARL

▶ Reading with the purpose of answering the seven fundamental clinical questions improves retention of information and facilitates the application of book knowledge to clinical knowledge.

WHAT IS THE MOST LIKELY DIAGNOSIS?

The method of establishing the diagnosis has been covered in the previous section. One way of attacking this problem is to develop standard approaches to common clinical problems. It is helpful to understand the most common causes of various presentations, such as "The most common cause of serosanguineous nipple discharge is an intraductal papilloma."

The clinical scenario might be "A 38-year-old woman is noted to have a 2-month history of spontaneous blood-tinged right nipple discharge. What is the most likely diagnosis?"

With no other information to go on, the student notes that this woman has a unilateral blood-tinged nipple discharge. Using the "most common cause" information, the student makes an educated guess that the patient has an **intraductal papilloma.** If instead the patient is found to have a discharge from more than one duct and a right-sided breast mass is palpated, it is noted: "The bloody discharge is expressed from multiple ducts. A 1.5-cm mass is palpated in the lower outer quadrant of the right breast."

Then the student uses the clinical pearl: "The most common cause of serosanguineous breast discharge in the presence of a breast mass is breast cancer."

CLINICAL PEARL

▶ The most common cause of serosanguineous unilateral breast discharge is intraductal papilloma, but **the main concern is breast cancer.** Thus, the first step in evaluating the patient's condition is careful palpation to determine the number of ducts involved, an examination to detect breast masses, and mammography. If more than one duct is involved or a breast mass is palpated, the most likely cause is breast cancer.

HOW CAN YOU CONFIRM THE DIAGNOSIS?

In the preceding scenario, it is suspected that the woman with the bloody nipple discharge has an intraductal papilloma, or possibly cancer. Ductal surgical exploration with biopsy would be a confirmatory procedure. Similarly, an individual may present with acute dyspnea following a radical prostatectomy for prostate cancer. The suspected process is pulmonary embolism, and a confirmatory test would be a ventilation/perfusion scan or possibly a spiral CT examination. The student should strive to know the limitations of various diagnostic tests, especially when they are used early in a diagnostic process.

WHAT SHOULD BE YOUR NEXT STEP?

This question is difficult because the next step has many possibilities; the answer may be to obtain more diagnostic information, stage the illness, or introduce therapy. It is often a more challenging question than "What is the most likely diagnosis?" because there may be insufficient information to make a diagnosis and the next step may be to obtain more data. Another possibility is that there is enough information for a probable diagnosis and that the next step is staging the disease. Finally, the most appropriate answer may be to begin treatment. Hence, based on the clinical data, a judgment needs to be rendered regarding how far along one is in the following sequence.

> 1. Make a diagnosis → 2. Stage the disease →
> 3. Treat based on stage → 4. Follow the response

Frequently, students are taught to "regurgitate" information that they have read about a particular disease but are not skilled at identifying the next step. This talent is learned optimally at the bedside in a supportive environment with the freedom to take educated guesses and receive constructive feedback. A sample scenario might describe a student's thought process as follows:

Make a diagnosis: "Based on the information I have, I believe that Mr Smith has a small bowel obstruction from adhesive disease *because* he presents with nausea, vomiting, and abdominal distension and has dilated loops of bowel on radiography."

Stage the disease: "I do not believe that this is severe disease because he does not have fever, evidence of sepsis, intractable pain, leukocytosis, or peritoneal signs."

Treat based on stage: "Therefore, my next step is to treat with nothing per mouth, nasogastric tube drainage, and observation."

Follow the response: "I want to follow the treatment by assessing his pain (asking him to rate the pain on a scale of 1-10 every day), recording his temperature, performing an abdominal examination, obtaining a serum bicarbonate level (to detect metabolic acidemia) and a leukocyte count, and reassessing his condition in 24 hours."

In a similar patient, when the clinical presentation is unclear, perhaps the best next step is a diagnostic one such as performing an oral contrast radiologic study to assess for bowel obstruction.

CLINICAL PEARL

> ▶ The vague question "What is your next step?" is often the most difficult one because the answer may be diagnostic, staging, or therapeutic.

WHAT IS THE LIKELY MECHANISM FOR THIS DISEASE PROCESS?

This question goes further than making the diagnosis and requires the student to understand the underlying mechanism of the process. For example, a clinical scenario may describe a 68-year-old man who notes urinary hesitancy and retention and has a large, hard, nontender mass in his left supraclavicular region. This patient has bladder neck obstruction due to benign prostatic hypertrophy or prostatic cancer. However, the indurated mass in the left neck area is suggestive of cancer. The mechanism is metastasis in the area of the thoracic duct, which drains lymph fluid into the left subclavian vein. The student is advised to learn the mechanisms of each disease process and not merely to memorize a constellation of symptoms. Furthermore, in general surgery it is crucial for students to understand the anatomy, function, and how a surgical procedure will correct the problem.

WHAT ARE THE RISK FACTORS FOR THIS DISEASE PROCESS?

Understanding the risk factors helps the practitioner establish a diagnosis and determine how to interpret test results. For example, understanding the risk factor analysis may help in the treatment of a 55-year-old woman with anemia. If the patient has risk factors for endometrial cancer (such as diabetes, hypertension, anovulation) and complains of postmenopausal bleeding, she likely has endometrial carcinoma and should undergo endometrial biopsy. Otherwise, occult colonic bleeding is a common etiology. If she takes nonsteroidal anti-inflammatory drugs or aspirin, peptic ulcer disease is the most likely cause.

CLINICAL PEARL

▶ A knowledge of the risk factors can be a useful guide in testing and in developing the differential diagnosis.

WHAT ARE THE COMPLICATIONS OF THIS DISEASE PROCESS?

Clinicians must be cognizant of the complications of a disease so that they can understand how to follow and monitor the patient. Sometimes, the student has to make a diagnosis from clinical clues and then apply his or her knowledge of the consequences of the pathologic process. For example, a 26-year-old man complains of a 7-year history of intermittent diarrhea, lower abdominal pain, bloody stools, and tenesmus and is first diagnosed with probable ulcerative colitis. The long-term complications of this process include colon cancer. Understanding the types of consequences also helps the clinician to become aware of the dangers to the patient. Surveillance with colonoscopy is important in attempting to identify a colon malignancy.

WHAT IS THE BEST THERAPY?

To answer this question, the clinician not only needs to reach the correct diagnosis and assess the severity of the condition but also must weigh the situation to determine the appropriate intervention. For the student, knowing exact dosages is not as important as understanding the best medication, route of delivery, mechanism of action, and possible complications. It is important for the student to be able to verbalize the diagnosis and the rationale for the therapy.

CLINICAL PEARL

▶ Therapy should be logical based on the severity of the disease and the specific diagnosis. An exception to this rule is in an emergent situation such as shock, when the blood pressure must be treated even as the etiology is being investigated.

SUMMARY

1. There is no replacement for a meticulous history and physical examination.

2. There are four steps in the clinical approach to the patient: making the diagnosis, assessing the severity of the disease, treating based on severity, and following the patient's response.

3. There are seven questions that help bridge the gap between the textbook and the clinical arena.

REFERENCES

Doherty GM. Preoperative care. In: Doherty GM, ed. *Current Surgical Diagnosis and Treatment.* 14th ed. New York, NY: McGraw-Hill Publishers; 2015. 34-45.

Englebert JE. Approach to the surgical patient. In: Doherty GM, ed. *Current Surgical Diagnosis and Treatment.* 14th ed. New York, NY: McGraw-Hill Publishers; 2015. 1-5.

SECTION II

Cases

A 76-year-old man is undergoing evaluation for treatment of an 8-cm abdominal aortic aneurysm (AAA). His past medical history is significant for unstable angina that was treated by coronary artery angioplasty and stent placement 8 months ago. Since that time, he has been doing well without angina. His other medical problems include hypertension and gout. His home medications include metoprolol, allopurinol, aspirin, and clopidogrel. Recently, he has been active and walks approximately 1 mile daily. He had a 40-pack-year smoking history but quit 8 months ago, and he consumes alcohol socially. The patient denies any nocturnal dyspnea or respiratory symptoms. On physical examination, he appears well nourished. His blood pressure is 138/82 mm Hg, and his heart rate is 66 beats/minute. There is no jugular venous distension or carotid bruits. The lungs are clear bilaterally, and the heart sounds are normal. A nontender, pulsatile mass is present in the upper abdomen. No cyanosis or edema is noted in his extremities. Laboratory evaluations reveal a normal complete blood count and normal electrolyte values. The serum urea nitrogen and creatinine levels are 40 and 1.5 mg/dL, respectively. The urinalysis reveals trace proteinuria. The electrocardiogram (ECG) reveals a normal sinus rhythm and left ventricular hypertrophy. The CT angiography confirms the presence of an infrarenal AAA that is anatomically unfavorable for endovascular aneurysm repair (EVAR).

▶ What are the risks associated with surgical treatment of this patient's problem?
▶ What can be done to assess and optimize the patient's condition?

ANSWERS TO CASE 1:

Preoperative Risk Assessment and Optimization of High-Risk and Geriatric Patients

Summary: A 76-year-old man with a large AAA, hypertension, coronary artery disease, gout, and mild chronic renal insufficiency is undergoing evaluation for open AAA repair because his disease does not appear amendable to EVAR. Given his medical comorbidities, this patient can benefit from risk assessment, risk stratification, and optimization prior to his operation.

- **Surgical risks:** The risks associated with open AAA repair include the usual procedural risks in addition to significant risk of pulmonary, renal, and cardiac complications.

- **Optimizing the patient's status:** A thorough cardiac risk assessment should be made to define the current cardiac status, and to identify and quantify any end-organ dysfunction caused by hypertension and cardiac disease. Strategies to optimize the patient's condition include pharmacological therapy, coronary revascularization, and perioperative hemodynamic monitoring. Information gained from the cardiac risk assessment should help guide the plans for patient optimization.

ANALYSIS

Objectives

1. Learn the general approach to preoperative cardiac risk assessment.

2. Learn the principles of optimization of the medical conditions of the surgical patients.

3. Learn the principles of preoperative assessment of geriatric patients.

Considerations

The main goals of preoperative patient evaluation are to prevent perioperative complications and to avoid unnecessary testing that may cause care delays, unnecessary expenditures, and patient harm. For this patient with several cardiac risk factors, his preoperative assessment provides an excellent opportunity to have a discussion regarding maintenance of a healthy lifestyle and an opportunity to review and adjust his current medications. Elective open-AAA repairs are considered potentially highly morbid operations that are associated with a perioperative mortality rate of 3.7% based on the American College of Surgeons National Surgical Quality Improvement Program (NSQIP) data base report of U.S. surgical outcomes (2005–2011), with. Cardiac and renal complications are the most common causes of death; therefore, preoperative preparation of the patient is extremely important to help minimize adverse outcomes.

This patient has a history of coronary artery disease that has been previously treated with coronary angioplasty and stent placement. He also has a history of hypertension and subtle signs of chronic renal insufficiency, as demonstrated by a serum creatinine of 1.5 mg/dL and the presence of proteinuria. As we prepare him for his operation, it is critical that we carefully assess and optimize his cardiac and renal status. A favorable factor revealed in his history is that his angina has resolved since his coronary angioplasty and stent placement. Furthermore, it appears that his percutaneous coronary intervention has been successful, which has enabled him to walk a mile each day. It has been shown that the risks of perioperative cardiac deaths and/or myocardial infarctions are extremely low in patients who have undergone surgical coronary revascularization within 5 years or have undergone coronary angioplasty or stent placement from 6 months to 5 years prior, **providing that the patients' clinical conditions have normalized following the revascularization procedures.** Our patient is now active and asymptomatic, thus suggesting that extensive preoperative cardiac testing may not be necessary or beneficial.

This patient's preoperative evaluation should begin with a history and physical examination in addition to direct communications with his cardiologist and primary care physician. From these providers, we can gather information regarding past tests that have taken place and information regarding the status of his current CAD, hypertension, and renal insufficiency management. If not previously obtained, a 24-hour urine collection to help determine creatinine clearance might be useful to gauge the severity of his renal dysfunction. The serum creatinine level in an older adult without significant muscle mass can be deceptively low and may not clearly reflect his renal clearance functions. This information can be valuable to help direct dosing of medications in the perioperative period. The control of systolic hypertension is important to reduce perioperative cardiac complications, and blood pressure control should be accomplished prior to any elective operations.

A simple cardiac risk assessment model that is most frequently applied for the perioperative patients is the **revised cardiac risk index (RCRI).** The RCRI takes into consideration six factors: (1) history of ischemic heart disease; (2) history of congestive heart failure; (3) history of TIA or strokes; (4) history of diabetes mellitus requiring insulin; (5) serum creatinine >2 mg/dL; and (6) major surgery (such as supra-inguinal vascular surgery, intraabdominal, or thoracic surgery). This patient has an RCRI of 2 (history of CAD and major surgery), which puts him into a moderate-risk group with projected cardiac-related morbidity/mortality rate of 6.6%. Pharmacological interventions to reduce perioperative cardiac-related morbidity and mortality can be useful to further reduce his cardiac risk factors (Table 1–1). In the past, perioperative beta-blockade had been a standard prevention strategy for patients with significant cardiovascular risk factors. However, there have been **recent research findings that have suggested that perioperative beta-blockade is not beneficial, and in some cases, beta-blocker treatment has been found to be harmful.** Based on the recent findings, the current recommendations are that if the patient is already on a beta-blocker, then it should be continued in the perioperative period, but a beta-blocker should not be initiated in the perioperative period as a cardiac-risk reduction strategy. Statin administration has been demonstrated to

Table 1–1 • REVISED CARDIAC RISK INDEX		
Points	Class	Perioperative Cardiac Complication Rate (%)
0	I	0.4
1	II	0.9
2	III	6.6
≥3	IV	11

have cardiac-protective effects for patients undergoing cardiac surgery. In patients undergoing non-cardiac surgery, there is strong evidence to suggest that statin administration is associated with the reduction in cardiac complications; however, this practice is not yet clearly supported by high-quality clinical studies. The addition of statin therapy to his current risk-reduction regimen can be considered and discussed with his primary care physicians and cardiologist.

Our patient has a history of having undergone coronary stent placement 8 months ago. It is important to keep in mind that individuals with coronary stents in place are at risk for stent thrombosis in the perioperative period. At a minimum, patients with bare-metal stents require 1 month of dual antiplatelet therapy (ASA + clopidogrel). Patients with drug-eluting stents in place should receive a minimum of 3 months of dual antiplatelet therapy. Patients with paclitaxel stents should receive a minimum of 6 months of dual antiplatelet therapy. As a rule, one year of dual antiplatelet therapy should be strongly considered for any individual following coronary stent placement. Thus, it would important for him to continue his current antiplatelet regimen. Studies have shown that premature discontinuation of antiplatelet therapy can be associated with in-stent thrombosis rates of 25% to 30%; therefore, it is a common practice to extend the antiplatelet therapy beyond the minimal recommended time periods.

In summary, for this patient with a history of CAD and significant cardiac risk factors but who is asymptomatic following coronary revascularization 8 months ago, extensive cardiac testing is not necessary or beneficial. His hypertension management should be optimized and his renal dysfunction should be quantified with measurement of creatinine clearance. Continuation of his dual-antiplatelet therapy is important since he had coronary stent placement 8 months ago. A potentially beneficial pharmacologic protective strategy to consider is a statin, which has proven benefits in the perioperative period.

APPROACH TO:

Preoperative Assessment and Optimization of High-Risk Patients and Geriatric Patients

DEFINITIONS

AMERICAN SOCIETY OF ANESTHESIOLOGISTS (ASA) STATUS CLASSIFICATION SYSTEM: This is a standard physiological status classification system used by the anesthesiologist during their preoperative assessment. ASA (1) healthy person; ASA (2) mild systemic disease; ASA (3) severe systemic disease; ASA (4) severe systemic disease that is a constant threat to life; ASA (5) moribund individual who is not expected to survive without the operation; ASA (6) a declared brain-dead person undergoing organ procurement. An "E" is added to the end of the ASA class if the operation is an emergency procedure that cannot be delayed.

GERIATRIC PATIENT: Geriatric patient is a term often arbitrarily applied to a patient with age ≥65 years.

FRAILTY: This is a concept used to describe some geriatric patients. Frailty is used to describe an individual with diminished physiologic reserve across multiple organ systems, usually due to multiple cumulative comorbid conditions.

METABOLIC DEMAND (MET): A measure of aerobic demands of specific activities. The perioperative and long-term risks are increased for individuals who are unable to meet a four MET demand during their daily living (eg, activities of daily living such as dressing and cooking require 1-4 MET; climbing a flight of stairs, walking at 6 mph, and scrubbing the floor require 4-10 MET).

RESTING LEFT VENTRICULAR FUNCTION: Generally assessed by echocardiography. A left ventricular ejection fraction (LVEF) reflects the left heart's ability to pump blood to the body, and an LVEF less than 35% is associated with increased risk of perioperative cardiac complications; however, an LVEF greater than 35% does not reliably rule out perioperative complications. The difficult problem in preoperative cardiac evaluation is that testing does not help identify patients who have significant diastolic dysfunction.

VENTRICULAR DIASTOLIC DYSFUNCTION: Diastolic dysfunction is a term that describes a heart that does not adapt well to an increase in preload or an increase in intravascular volume. It is believed that a large percentage of perioperative cardiac events are related to diastolic dysfunction.

PROVOCATIVE CARDIAC TESTING: There are a variety of cardiac stress tests available to help identify patients who might have clinically silent CAD. These include standard exercise tolerance tests, and pharmacologic stress tests (persantinethalium scan and dobutamine stress echocardiography). These examinations are highly sensitive in identifying patients with CAD; however, their positive predictive values for perioperative cardiac complications are very low, as the majority of patients with CAD do not have complications. The negative predictive value of the stress test is excellent, since most patients without abnormalities do not develop cardiac complications. Because of the low predictive values of these tests, the role of perioperative testing has significantly reduced over the past decade.

CLINICAL APPROACH

When preparing a patient with significant medical comorbidities or risk factors for elective surgery, the patient's other medical conditions must be clearly identified, defined, and addressed to minimize adverse events. An assessment of comorbidities has been found to be especially important for patients undergoing vascular surgery procedures. Advanced vascular occlusive disease is very frequently associated with long-standing diabetes, atherosclerosis, and hypertension, and these conditions frequently contribute to multiple end-organ damage and a reduction in the patient's physiologic reserve. The assessment of cardiac risk consists of the eight steps listed in Table 1–2. Several major, intermediate, and minor clinical predictors have been identified to facilitate cardiac-risk assessment (Table 1–3). Some of the most valuable predictors can be easily gathered from the patient's history, current symptoms, and level of activity. It is important to keep in mind that cardiac-related

Table 1–2 • CONSIDERATIONS IN PREOPERATIVE CARDIAC RISK ASSESSMENT	
Step 1	What is the urgency of the surgical procedure? (If emergent, short-term medical optimization and perioperative monitoring may be indicated.)
Step 2	Has the patient undergone coronary revascularization during the past 5 y, and if so, have the symptoms resolved? (If yes, low risk.)
Step 3	Has the patient undergone an adequate cardiac evaluation during the past 2 y? (If yes and the results are favorable, repeated studies are unnecessary.)
Step 4	Does the patient have an unstable coronary syndrome or a major clinical predictor of risk? (If yes, the elective procedure should be postponed until these issues can be addressed.)
Step 5	Does the patient have an intermediate predictor of risk? (If yes, consideration of functional capacity and procedural risk are important in identifying patients who may benefit from further noninvasive testing.)
Step 6	(a) Intermediate-risk patients with moderate or excellent functional capacity generally undergo intermediate-risk procedures with low cardiac morbidity. (b) Further noninvasive testing may benefit patients with poor to moderate functional capacity undergoing high-risk procedures.
Step 7	Patients with neither major nor intermediate clinical predictors and with moderate to excellent functional capacity (≥4 MET) can generally tolerate noncardiac surgery; additional noninvasive testing is performed on an individual basis.
Step 8	(a) The results of noninvasive testing often identify the need for preoperative coronary intervention or cardiac surgery. (b) In general, cardiac intervention is undertaken if the morbidity associated with these interventions is less than that of the planned surgery. (c) If the morbidity of cardiac preoperative intervention exceeds that of the planned surgical procedures, coronary intervention is indicated only if it also significantly improves the patient's long-term prognosis.

Table 1–3 • CLINICAL PREDICTORS OF CARDIAC RISK		
Major Clinical Predictors	**Intermediate Clinical Predictors**	**Minor Clinical Predictors**
Unstable coronary syndrome	Mild angina pectoris	Advanced age
Decompensated CHF	Prior myocardial infarction	Abnormal electrocardiogram
Significant arrhythmias	Compensated CHF or prior CHF	Rhythm other than sinus
Severe valvular disease	Diabetes mellitus	Low functional capacity
		History of stroke
		Uncontrolled systemic hypertension

Abbreviation: CHF, congestive heart failure.

symptoms can remain silent due to limitations in activities in some patients. Furthermore, **CAD symptoms may be atypical in diabetic patients and women.** One of the important factors to not overlook is the type of operation planned and the anticipated physiologic stress that the operation produces. For example, body surface area operations such as breast biopsies, groin hernia repairs, and thyroidectomies are generally associated with minimal fluid shifts, blood loss, and hemodynamic fluctuations. On the other hand, vascular operations in the supra-inguinal region and lengthy open abdominal operations have the potential of causing large fluctuations in hemodynamic statuses and volume shifts. A 12-lead ECG can be valuable when assessing cardiac risks, especially if they can be compared to previously obtained ECGs. Echocardiography is noninvasive and may provide some information regarding the systolic functions of the heart; however, it is important to remember that a major limitation of echocardiography is that it does not provide information regarding function. **Ventricular diastolic dysfunction can be an important cause of perioperative cardiac morbidity, especially when significant fluctuations in intravascular volume and pressures are anticipated (eg, aortic surgery with cross-clamping).** In general, patients with moderate cardiac risk factors who are undergoing moderate- to high-risk operations may benefit from additional cardiac assessment, whereas, high-risk patients undergoing low risk operations generally would do well without additional testing.

One of the most important take-home messages in preoperative assessment is that the preoperative assessment should not lead to coronary revascularization just to get the patient through the operation. Several years ago, a VA medical center randomized controlled trial compared cardiac testing with prophylactic coronary revascularization to testing followed by pharmacologic management of the patients' conditions in patients undergoing vascular surgery. The results showed that prophylactic coronary revascularization did not lead to reductions in perioperative cardiac-related morbidities and mortality. In fact, patients who underwent preoperative coronary revascularization had significant delays in care.

Pharmacological Interventions

Perioperative beta-blockade had been the standard of care for high-risk patients; however, the results from the POISE Trial published in 2008 has led to significant change in this practice. This study demonstrated **increase in stroke-related deaths and complications in patients randomized to perioperative beta-block treatment.** The use of perioperative statins is potentially beneficial for high-risk patients, but this practice has not been examined by high-quality randomized controlled clinical trials.

PREOPERATIVE ASSESSMENT OF GERIATRIC PATIENTS

Statistically, nearly 50% of Americans will have an operation after the age of 65 years. Some will be life-saving emergency or elective operations, while the majority of the operations will be elective procedures to improve individuals' quality of life. The preoperative assessment of geriatric patients needs to include assessments that have already been described for patients with cardiovascular disease and/or cardiac risk factors. In addition, these patients need assessments of some geriatric-specific syndromes such as frailty, mobility-disability, malnutrition, mood/depression, and cognitive deficits. Some investigators have described **frailty** as the presence of three or more of the following items: (1) unintentional weight loss of ≥10 lbs in the past year; (2) self-reported exhaustion; (3) weakness in grip strength; (4) slow walking speed; and (5) low physical activity. The modified frailty index is another way that frailty has been quantified in national databases such as the National Surgical Quality Improvement Program (NSQIP). The modified index has a total of 11 items and scores represent the degrees of frailty (see Table 1–4).

Using the modified frailty scores (mFI), NSQIP data have been analyzed for patients age 60 and older, and the findings suggest that **ASA class, age, mFI, and wound class were the strongest predictors of perioperative mortality.** The ability to identify these risk factors is important in making decisions regarding whether or not to proceed with elective nonlife-saving operations.

Nutritional status, cognitive function, and mood disorders/depression are also important factors to assess/identify preoperatively in geriatric patients. Malnutrition has been estimated to occur in approximately 23% of the elderly population, and the presence of malnutrition can have significant impact on perioperative morbidity and mortality. In the elective surgery setting, preoperative nutritional

Table 1–4 • ELEVEN-ITEM MODIFIED FRAILTY INDEX*
History of diabetes mellitus
History of congestive heart failure
History of hypertension requiring medication
History of either transient ischemic attack or stroke
Functionally not independent (within prior 30 days)
History of myocardial infarction
History of either peripheral vascular disease or rest pain
History of cerebral vascular accident with neurologic deficit
History of COPD or pneumonia
History of percutaneous coronary intervention or CABG, or angina
History of impaired sensorium

*Scores range from 0 to 11 and describe absence, presence, and the degree of frailty.

support can be considered for the malnourished individuals. The preoperative functional statuses of geriatric patients are important to consider, since preoperative functional status can be helpful in identifying patients who may require long-term recovery and physical therapy in in-patient settings. Dementia and/or depression are common problems in the geriatric patient population, and both of these problems can contribute significantly to post-operative complications. Identifying these deficits in the preoperative setting will also help facilitate postoperative care for these individuals. In general, elderly individuals with dementia/cognitive defects will often demonstrate additional impairments in cognition following general anesthesia, and there is evidence to suggest that neuraxial anesthesia (epidural or spinal) is associated with less cognitive dysfunction than general anesthesia.

COMPREHENSION QUESTIONS

1.1 Which of the following patients can be classified as an American Society of Anesthesiologists (ASA)-class 5 patient?

A. 55-year-old with hypertension and type 2 diabetes that are well-controlled with medications and diet

B. 43-year-old man with history of hypertension and diabetes who is admitted to the hospital for DKA and found to have hypotension, tachycardia, and diffuse peritonitis from perforated gastric ulcer

C. 22-year-old man with type I diabetes that is well-managed by an insulin pump, who is an active individual with good performance status

D. 19-year-old tri-athlete with isolated open, comminuted left humerus fracture following a bicycle crash

E. 53-year-old man with history of CAD and two prior myocardial infarctions complicated by congestive heart failure

1.2 A 66-year-old man with a history of asymptomatic reducible left inguinal hernia is undergoing evaluation for elective hernia repair. He has a history of hypertension and elevated total cholesterol level with an unfavorable LDL-HDL ratio (low- to high-density lipoprotein ratio). He denies any history of chest pain or shortness of breath with exertion. His blood pressure in the office is 150/90 mm Hg. Which of the following is the best treatment plan?

A. Refer patient for an exercise stress test

B. Place patient on a beta-blocker one week before surgery and then schedule patient for surgery under local anesthesia

C. Discuss with patient about blood pressure control and long-term cardiac-risk reduction benefits and coordinate with his primary care physician to optimize his status

D. Place patient on a beta-blocker and statin one week before his operation then proceed with surgery under local anesthesia

E. Refer the patient to a cardiologist for cardiac catheterization and percutaneous revascularization

1.3 Which of the following statements regarding perioperative cardiac risk assessment and risk modification is most accurate?

  A. A major benefit of preoperative assessment is to identify patients with silent cardiac disease so that percutaneous or operative interventions can be implemented

  B. Beta-blocker initiation prior to surgery should be implemented in all patients with RCRI ≥ 2

  C. Coronary angiography is an evaluation tool that should be applied liberally to provide interventions prior to elective surgery in high-risk patients

  D. Preoperative cardiac risk assessment leads to unnecessary testing and interventions and is not beneficial

  E. Preoperative risk assessment is intended to lead to risk modification strategies in the perioperative setting and beyond

1.4 A 53-year-old man is being considered for surgical repair of a very symptomatic inguinal hernia. He has intermittent chest pain, and because of a chronic ankle injury, he is not able to complete an exercise treadmill test. Dobutamine echocardiography is ordered for further assessment. Which of the following statements is most accurate regarding dobutamine echocardiography?

  A. It is highly specific in identifying individuals who will develop perioperative cardiac complications

  B. It is highly sensitive in identifying patients who will develop perioperative cardiac complications

  C. When the findings are abnormal, it reliably predicts the occurrence of cardiac complications

  D. It is not useful unless the individual can complete a standard exercise treadmill protocol

  E. It is never indicated as a preoperative assessment tool

1.5 A 55-year-old man with unstable angina presents with acute abdominal pain, and he is found to have diffuse peritonitis, tachycardia, and chest pain. His ECG is consistent with a NSTEMI. Serum troponin levels are elevated. An upright CXR reveals pneumoperitoneum. Based on your history and physical findings, a perforated peptic ulcer is suspected. Which of the following is the most appropriate treatment for this patient?

A. Review his history, perform physical examination, order routine laboratory studies, initiate pharmacological interventions for his cardiac condition, and proceed with surgery for his perforated ulcer disease

B. Review his history, perform physical examination, order laboratory testing, and perform a dobutamine echocardiography prior to surgery

C. Review history, perform physical examination, attempt nonoperative management of his perforated ulcer disease because his cardiac condition precludes him from surgical intervention

D. Review history, perform physical examination, obtain a CT of chest to rule out pulmonary embolism, if negative then proceed with surgery

E. His current medical condition precludes him from any surgical interventions. Proceed with maximal supportive care

1.6 What is the American Society of Anesthesiologist (ASA) classification for the patient described in 1.5?

A. ASA Class 3E

B. ASA Class 4E

C. ASA Class 5E

D. ASA Class 5

E. ASA Class 6

1.7 Which of the following is NOT an item to be included in determining the Modified Frailty Index (mFI)?

A. History of impaired sensorium due to dementia

B. History of COPD

C. History of unintentional weight loss

D. History of congestive heart failure (CHF)

E. History of prior coronary artery bypass grafting

ANSWERS

1.1 **B.** ASA class 5 describes a moribund patient who is not expected to survive without the operation, and the description fits a 43-year-old man with history of DM and hypertension presenting with DKA and diffuse peritonitis from perforated peptic ulcer disease. Choice A describes an ASA class 2 patient. Choice C describes a class 2-3 patient. Choice D describes a class 1 patient, and choice E describes a class 3 patient.

1.2 **C.** This patient is seeking elective surgical repair of an inguinal hernia. His evaluation suggests that his hypertension may not be optimally controlled and that he has a high-risk lipid profile. A discussion with patient regarding the control of these risk factors and coordinating risk-reduction strategies with the primary care physician is the best choice listed.

1.3 **E.** The preoperative risk assessment is an opportunity to introduce risk-reduction strategies for the patient in the perioperative period and beyond.

1.4 **B.** The dobutamine echocardiography is a pharmacologic stress test performed to identify individuals with demand-induced cardiac ischemia. The study can be applied in patients who are not able to exercise. This study is highly sensitive in identifying demand-induced cardiac ischemia; unfortunately, abnormal studies have very low predictive value for perioperative ischemic events (low specificity).

1.5 **A.** This 55-year-old man presents with generalized peritonitis secondary to perforated peptic ulcer disease; at the same time, he has findings consistent with a NSTEMI. It is conceivable that his NSTEMI is the result of increased stress related to his perforated ulcer and continued nonoperative treatment of his ulcer disease will likely lead to worsening cardiac condition; therefore, the initiation of pharmacologic treatment for his NSTEMI and surgery are the best treatments.

1.6 **C.** The patient with generalized peritonitis from perforated ulcer who is also having NSTEMI requiring an emergency operation is classified as an ASA 5E.

1.7 **C.** History of dementia, history of COPD, history of CHF, and history of CABG are 4 of the 11 factors used in calculating the mFI. Unintentional weight loss is not included as one of the eleven factors.

CLINICAL PEARLS

▶ Most body surface operations (eg, hernia repair, breast surgery) can be safely performed with minimal physiologic stress to patients.

▶ Perioperative beta-blockade is a strategy that is no longer applied as a cardiac-risk-reduction strategy in the perioperative period, because of the increase in risk of cerebral ischemic events.

▶ Perioperative cardiac risk is low when patients have undergone successful surgical coronary revascularization within 5 years or percutaneous coronary interventions between 6 months to 5 years prior.

▶ The benefits of a thorough history and physical examination and adjustment of medications cannot be overlooked in the preoperative setting.

▶ Additional assessments for frailty, nutritional status, cognitive function, and reduced mobility are important in the preoperative assessment of geriatric patients.

▶ Cognitive function appears to be adversely affected when geriatric patients undergo general anesthesia as opposed to neuraxial anesthesia (spinal or epidural).

▶ 50% of Americans over the age of 65 years will have an operation; therefore, perioperative management of geriatric patients is very relevant and important.

REFERENCES

De Waal BA, Buise MP, Zundert AAJ. Perioperative statin therapy in patients at high risk for cardiovascular morbidity undergoing surgery: a review. *Br J Anaesthesia*. 2015;114:44-52.

Eagle KA, Vaishnava P, Froehlich JB. Peripeartive cardiovascular care for patients undergoing noncardiac surgical intervention. *JAMA Internal Med*. 2015;175:835-839.

Ghadimi K, Thompson A. Update on perioperative care of the cardiac patient for noncardiac surgery. *Curr Opin Anesthesiol*. 2015;28:342-348.

Kim S, Brooks AK, Groban L. Preoperative assessment of the older surgical patient: honing on geriatric syndromes. *Clin Intervent Aging*. 2015;10:13-27.

Kim SW, Han HS, Jung HW, et al. Multidimensional frailty score for the prediction of postoperative mortality risk. *JAMA Surg*. 2014;149:633-640.

CASE 2

During a rotation on the anesthesiology service, a third-year medical student is asked to perform preoperative evaluations and provide patient instructions regarding two patients who are scheduled to undergo elective gastrointestinal (GI) surgical procedures (laparoscopic colectomies) in 1 week's time.

The first patient is a 76-year-old man with a 4-cm sessile polyp in the sigmoid colon with a biopsy demonstrating adenocarcinoma. He has a history of atrial fibrillation and a left hemispheric stroke related to this process. In addition, he has a history of hypertension and diabetes. Because of the thromboembolic history, he is currently on rivaroxaban (direct factor Xa inhibitor) for this condition.

The second patient is a 48-year-old man with a partially obstructing sigmoid colon cancer and a history of acute coronary syndrome (ACS) for the past 10 days that required emergency cardiac catheterization, coronary angioplasty, and placement of drug-eluting stents in the left anterior descending coronary artery and the circumflex artery. Following coronary stent placements, his cardiac symptoms resolved, and the patient is currently on dual antiplatelet therapy with aspirin (ASA) and clopidogrel.

▶ How would you manage the antithrombotic and antiplatelet agents in these two patients in the perioperative period?
▶ What are the risks associated with the cessation of antithrombotic and antiplatelet therapies?
▶ What are the risks of continuing antithrombotic and/or antiplatelet therapy in the perioperative period?

ANSWERS TO CASE 2:

Perioperative Management of Antithrombotic and Antiplatelet Therapies

Summary: A 76-year-old man with atrial fibrillation and embolic stroke history is on an anti–factor Xa inhibitor (rivaroxaban) and a 48-year-old man with recent ACS requiring cardiac catheterization and drug-eluting coronary stent placement (two vessels) are being evaluated for colon surgery for colon cancers. You are asked to coordinate the management of the antithrombotic and antiplatelet therapies in these two patients during the perioperative period.

- **Management of antithrombotic or antiplatelet therapy during the perioperative period:** Management requires careful consideration of the bleeding risks of continuing these treatments versus the thromboembolic risks related to cessation of therapy.

- **Withholding antithrombotic therapy** in a patient with atrial fibrillation and thromboembolic history raises the risk of thromboembolic events. **Withholding antiplatelet therapy** in a patient with a recent placement of coronary stent increases the risk of stent thrombosis.

- **Continuation of therapy** can be associated with increased bleeding complications in both patients; however, the risks/benefits of continuing therapy versus bridging therapy versus stopping therapy need to be carefully considered.

ANALYSIS

Objectives

1. Become familiar with the management of vitamin-K antagonist, non–vitamin-K antagonists, and antiplatelet agents in patients scheduled to or have recently undergone operative treatments.

2. Become familiar with the need for antiplatelet therapy in patients with prior percutaneous coronary interventions.

Considerations

The management of anticoagulant and antiplatelet therapies in the perioperative period requires careful consideration of the risks/benefits of continuing therapy versus stopping therapy. If the decision is to continue anticoagulant therapy in the perioperative period, the next step is to decide whether transitioning or bridging the anticoagulation therapy during the perioperative period is necessary.

When considering the anticoagulant management of the 76-year-old man with atrial fibrillation, hypertension (HTN), diabetes mellitus (DM), and prior stroke, who is on a factor Xa inhibitor for stroke prophylaxis, one must take into account that his proposed operation is a laparoscopic colectomy, which is categorized as an operative procedure with an increased risk for bleeding at the anastomotic site. **Rivaroxaban's half-life is related to the patient's creatinine clearance;** therefore, it would be helpful to quantify the patient's creatinine clearance prior to surgery. The half-life of rivaroxaban in patients with creatinine clearance of greater than 50 mL/min is 5 to 9 hours, whereas the half-life in individuals with creatinine clearance of 30 to 49 mL/min is 9 to 13 hours. In patients with normal renal function who are undergoing procedures at high risk for bleeding, the last dose of rivaroxaban should occur 48 to 72 hours prior to surgery. If the patient's creatinine clearance is 30 to 49 mL/ min, the recommended last dose of rivaroxaban is 72 hours prior to surgery. For the patient to have abdominal surgery, consideration of whether an epidural catheter will be placed for perioperative pain management is important; for patients receiving epidural catheter placement, rivaroxaban needs to be stopped 24 hours prior to catheter insertion and the subsequent dose needs to be delayed until 22 to 26 hours after catheter insertion. There should be a 6-hour interval between epidural catheter removal and the reinitiation of rivaroxaban. The decision to initiate bridging anticoagulation therapy in the patient will ultimately be determined on the basis of his CHAD2 score. If his score puts him into the high-risk group, bridging therapy with an unfractionated heparin drip should be strongly considered during the perioperative period.

For the man with atrial fibrillation and prior stroke who is scheduled to undergo an operation that is considered a high risk for bleeding, most practitioners would not place the patient on bridging unfractionated heparin drip or subcutaneous therapeutic low-molecular heparin. The ultimate plan for this patient is to have his rivaroxaban stopped either at 48 to 72 hours preoperatively or at 72 hours preoperatively (based on his creatinine clearance), and the medication restarted at 48 to 72 hours after the operation.

For the next patient with partially obstructing colon cancer, the antiplatelet therapy management can be considered for the drug-eluting stents (two vessels) placed in his coronary arteries for the treatment of ACS 10 days previously. A recently published review of a large administrative database reported that 11% of the patients require surgery within 2 years of coronary stent placement and 4% of the patients require surgery within 1 year of stent placement. Stent thrombosis is a devastating complication in patients with coronary stents in place, and the mortality associated with this event is greater than 50%. To prevent stent thrombosis, patients are generally placed on antiplatelet therapy. The **general recommendation is to defer elective surgical procedures for at least 6 weeks after bare-metal stent placement and to defer surgery for 6 to 12 months after the placement of drug-eluting stents.** For this individual, we need to reassess to see if his operation can be delayed while chemotherapy is administered. However, if delaying his operation for 6 months is not an option, we will need to continue his dual anti-platelet therapy and proceed with his operation.

APPROACH TO:
Anticoagulant and Antiplatelet Management in the Perioperative Patient

DEFINITIONS

BRIDGING THERAPY: For anticoagulant therapy, bridging generally involves the termination of the standard oral anticoagulantion followed by the initiation of another shorter acting anticoagulation agent such as a heparin drip or low-molecular-weight heparin. Bridging therapy is indicated when the patient's risk of venous or arterial thromboembolic complication is considered high without treatment (eg, mechanical mitral valve prosthesis).

CHAD2 SCORE: This is a six-point clinical scoring system applied to estimate the risk of stroke associated with atrial fibrillation. The items for consideration in this scoring system include *congestive heart failure* (CHF) (1 point), *hypertension* with systolic BP greater than 160 mm Hg (1 point), *age* more than 75 years (1 point), *diabetes* (1 point), and *prior cerebrovascular accident* (CVA) (2 points). **High-risk group**: scores of 5 to 6; **moderate-risk group**: scores of 3 to 4; and **low-risk group**: scores of 0 to 2.

WARFARIN (VITAMIN-K ANTAGONIST): Perioperative management generally involves stopping warfarin 5 days before surgery and resuming warfarin dosing 12 to 14 hours after the operation. A patient with a mechanical valves, at high risk for venous thromboembolism, or atrial fibrillation with high stroke risk, and those undergoing low-bleeding-risk surgical procedures should receive bridging therapy with an unfractionated heparin drip or subcutaneous therapeutic doses of low-molecular-weight heparin. However, if the planned surgery has a high risk for the bleeding, the risk of bleeding may outweigh the benefits of the bridging therapy.

THROMBOEMBOLIC RISKS ASSOCIATED WITH MECHANICAL HEART VALVES: *High risk* includes any mitral prosthesis, any caged-ball or tilting disc aortic valve prosthesis, and recent stroke or TIA (within 6 months) with a prosthetic valve in place. *Moderate risk* includes a bileaflet aortic prosthetic valve and one or more risk factor (atrial fibrillation, prior stroke or transient ischemia attack [TIA], CHF, age > 75). *Low risk* includes aortic valve prosthesis without atrial fibrillation, no risk factors, and no history of stroke.

VENOUS THROMBOEMBOLIC (VTE) RISKS STRATIFICATION: *High risk* includes VTE within 3 months or a history of severe thrombophilia with protein C, protein S, antithrombin deficiencies, or antiphospholipid antibodies. *Moderate risk* includes VTE during the past 3 to 12 months, non-severe thrombophilia such as heterozygous factor V Leiden or prothrombin gene mutation, and active cancer within 6 months. *Low risk* includes VTE that occurred before the last 12 months and no other risk factors.

APPROVED CLINICAL APPLICATIONS FOR NEW ORAL ANTICOAGU-LANTS (NOACs): The NOACs have been approved for the prevention of strokes and embolic complications associated with atrial fibrillation, the treatment of deep vein thrombosis (DVT) and pulmonary embolism, secondary prevention of DVT, and DVT prevention following knee or hip replacements.

DABIGATRAN (PRADAXA): This is an oral direct thrombin inhibitor with a plasma half-life of 12 to 17 hours. This drug is contraindicated in patients with severe renal dysfunction. Prolonged activated partial thromboplastin time and prolonged thrombin time (TT) suggest that the drug effects are present. **If necessary, hemodialysis can be performed to speed up the reversal of the drug effects.**

RIVAROXABAN (XARELTO): This is an oral direct factor Xa inhibitor with a plasma half-life of 5 to 9 hours in healthy individuals and 11 to 13 hours in elderly individuals. This drug is contraindicated in patients with severe renal dysfunction. This drug is metabolized and cleared by the liver, and levels may increase in liver failure patients. This drug interacts with antifungal agents, protease inhibitors, and rifampin. The anticoagulant effects of rivaroxaban can be determined based on the prothrombin time (PT). If the PT is elevated and the reversal of anticoagulation effects is desired, this can be accomplished with the administration of activated prothrombin complex concentrate (aPCC) or prothrombin complex concentrate (PCC).

APIXABAN (ELIQUIS): This is an oral direct factor Xa inhibitor with a plasma half-life of 8 to 15 hours. The anticoagulant effects of apixaban can be measured by plasma anti-Xa levels (if available). The four-factor PCC or aPCC can be used to reduce bleeding in patients who develop excessive bleeding related to this medication.

CLINICAL APPROACH

Patients may receive anticoagulation or antiplatelet agents for therapeutic reasons or as preventive strategies. Some examples of therapeutic strategies include anticoagulation for patients with prosthetic mitral valves, caged-ball–type aortic prosthetic valves, or patients with history of recent PE or DVT. Prophylactic measures may include anticoagulation for patients with atrial fibrillation and high CHAD2 scores. Antiplatelet agents are indicated to prevent coronary stent thrombosis, reduce stroke risk in patients with cerebral vascular disease, or as a strategy to reduce cardiovascular events.

For any patient who is receiving anticoagulant therapy, our preoperative evaluation begins by identifying the indication for anticoagulant therapy and then to **stratify the individual's thromboembolic risk either as high risk, moderate risk, or low risk.** The next step is to determine the bleeding risk associated with the proposed procedure. In general, patients on anticoagulant therapy who are considered high risk for thromboemboli will usually need to have some form of bridging anticoagulation administered during the perioperative period. For moderate-risk patients, the decision to bridge the anticoagulation therapy is not entirely clear. For most low-risk patients, anticoagulation therapy can likely be stopped in the perioperative period without bridging therapy.

Antiplatelet Agents

The common antiplatelet agents that irreversibly inhibit platelet functions include ASA, clopidogrel, ticlopidine, and prasugrel; with each day the medication is stopped, there is a 10% to 14% restoration of platelet activity. In other words, the restoration of 100% platelet function requires the medication to be stopped for 7 to 10 days. There are several reversible antiplatelet agents whose effects are determined by the medication's half-life. **These reversible antiplatelet agents include dipyridamole, cilostazol, and the nonsteroidal anti-inflammatory drugs.** The optimal timing required to stop antiplatelet agents to minimize bleeding risks is unclear. For patients with high risk for cardiovascular or cerebral vascular events, it is recommended that antiplatelet therapies be continued during the perioperative period. For patients who are at moderate risk for cardiovascular events or are receiving antiplatelet agents for secondary prevention of cardiovascular diseases, the recommendation is to stop the antiplatelet therapy 7 to 10 days prior to surgery.

> **CASE CORRELATION**
>
> - See also Case 1 (Preoperative Risk Assessment and Optimization).

COMPREHENSION QUESTIONS

2.1 A 63-year-old man with chronic renal failure (creatinine clearance < 20 mL/min), who is on hemodialysis, develops atrial fibrillation with a CHAD2 score of 6, presents for possible long-term anticoagulation evaluation. Which of the following is the most appropriate strategy for managing this patient?

    A. No anticoagulant because the risk outweighs the benefits

    B. Rivaroxaban

    C. Dabigatran

    D. Warfarin

    E. Apixaban

2.2 A 63-year-old man with a recent bout of ACS was successfully managed with coronary angioplasty and placement of three bare-metal stents in his coronary arteries. He is interested in knowing how long he needs to continue his ASA and clopidogrel therapy. Which of the following is the most appropriate answer for this patient?

    A. These medications can be stopped once the coronary artery disease is treated

    B. The antiplatelet therapy should be continued for life

    C. A minimum of 3 years

    D. A minimum of 6 months

    E. A minimum of 6 weeks

2.3 A 78-year-old woman with atrial fibrillation is placed on dabigatran by her physician because she has a CHAD2 score of 6. While receiving this medication, she develops severe upper GI bleeding secondary to a gastric ulcer. Over a 6-hour period of time, she has received 6 units of packed red blood cells (PRBCs) and has continued to bleed. Which of the following is the best approach to reverse the effects of dabigatran?

A. Protamine infusion

B. Platelet transfusion

C. Hemodialysis

D. Stop the medication and wait for the drug effects to wear off

E. Fresh frozen plasma transfusion

2.4 A patient with atrial fibrillation is receiving rivaroxaban and develops epistaxis. How would you determine if this bleeding is caused by rivaroxaban?

A. Measure a bleeding time

B. Measure the partial thromboplastin time

C. Measure the prothrombin time

D. Measure the thrombin time

E. Measure the bleeding time

2.5 Which of the following is a favorable characteristic associated with the new oral anticoagulant treatment?

A. These medications can be prescribed for patients with chronic renal failure (creatinine clearance < 25)

B. These medications have fewer interactions with other medications

C. These medications only require monthly monitoring of effects

D. These medications are rarely associated with bleeding complications

E. These medications do not require reversal prior to emergency high-risk surgical procedures

2.6 For which one of the following patients is new oral anticoagulant (NOAC) indicated?

A. A 73-year-old man with mild renal insufficiency (creatinine clearance of 38 mL/min), atrial fibrillation, and CHAD2 score of 6

B. A 46-year-old man with atrial fibrillation and a CHAD2 score of 1

C. A 73-year-old man with atrial fibrillation following mitral valve replacement with a CHAD2 score of 6

D. A 73-year-old man with atrial fibrillation following mitral valve replacement and a normal creatinine clearance

E. A 66-year-old man with CHF following mitral valve repair and coronary artery bypass. He has atrial fibrillation and normal renal function

ANSWERS

2.1 **D.** For this 63-year-old man with chronic renal failure and creatinine clearance of less than 20 mL/min, atrial fibrillation, and CHAD2 score of 6, anticoagulation is indicated since he is at risk for thromboembolic complications. With a creatinine clearance of less than 20 mL/min, he should not receive rivaroxaban or dabigatran (contraindicated in patients with CrCl < 30) or apixaban (contraindicated in patients with CrCl < 25); based on these reasons, warfarin is the best anticoagulant for this patient.

2.2 **E.** It is recommended that the patient continue the dual antiplatelet therapy with ASA and clopidogrel for a minimum of 6 weeks following placement of bare-metal stents. Most practitioners would recommend a longer period of antiplatelet therapy because the outcomes associated with stent thrombosis are very devastating.

2.3 **C.** The anticoagulant effects of dabigatran can be reversed with hemodialysis. Reversal is indicated if the risk of bleeding is considered to outweigh the benefits of anticoagulation.

2.4 **C.** The PT is the most sensitive coagulation assay to detect the effects of rivaroxaban. A normal PT level suggests that the level of rivaroxaban activities is not excessive. Therefore, if a normal PT is found, we can determine that rivaroxaban overdose is not the contributing factor for the epistaxis.

2.5 **B.** The new oral anticoagulants have fewer drug-drug interactions than warfarin; however, drug-drug interactions between the NOACs and some of the antifungal medications are important to note. NOACs can contribute to bleeding complications and no drug level monitoring is usually required. There are tests that can be performed to determine if the effects of the NOACs are excessive. Reversal is indicated for surgery with high bleeding risks.

2.6 **A.** A patient with atrial fibrillation, CHAD2 score of 6, and creatinine clearance of 38 mL/min is the only patient listed here who does not have a contraindication to receive NAOC. The patient with CHAD2 score of 1 has low risk of thromboembolic complications and does not need anticoagulation. NAOCs are not recommended for the treatment of atrial fibrillation in patients with prosthetic valves.

CLINICAL PEARLS

▶ NAOCs are contraindicated in pregnant and/or breast-feeding patients.

▶ Rivaroxaban and dabigatran are contraindicated in individuals with CrCl < 30 mL/min; apixaban is contraindicated in individuals with CrCl < 25 mL/min.

▶ Dual antiplatelet therapy with ASA and clopidogrel is recommended for a minimum of 6 months following the placement of bare-metal coronary stents, and treatment is recommended for 6 to 12 months after the placement of drug-eluting stents.

▶ Bridging strategies are usually applied when oral anticoagulants are transitioned to intravenous anticoagulants in the perioperative period, such as transitioning from warfarin to heparin drip in patients with prosthetic mitral valves.

▶ Hemodialysis can be performed for the reversal of dabigatran effects.

REFERENCES

Darvish-Kazem S, Gandhi M, Marcucci M, Douketis JD. Perioperative management of antiplatelet therapy in patients with a coronary stent who need noncardiac surgery. *Chest.* 2013;144:1848-1856.

Franchi F, Rollini F, Angiolillo DJ. Perspectives on the management of antiplatelet therapy in patients with coronary artery disease requiring noncardiac surgery. *Curr Opin Cardiol.* 2014;29:553-563.

Lai A, Davidson N, Galloway SW, Thachil J. Perioperative management of patients on new oral anticoagulants. *Brit J Surg.* 2014;101:742-749.

Tran H, Young JL, McRae S, et al. New oral anticoagulants: a practical guide on prescription, laboratory testing, and peri-procedural/bleeding management. *Internal Med J.* 2014;44:525-536.

A 44-year-old woman is admitted to the ICU after having undergone a 3-hour abdominal operation for the debridement of infected necrotizing pancreatitis (infected pancreas necrosis). The operation resulted in 800 mL of blood loss, and she received 3000 mL of crystalloid, 2 units of packed RBC, and 2 units of fresh frozen plasma during the operation. Prior to the surgery, she was receiving imipenem, itraconazole, and micafungin for Gram-negative bacteremia and fungemia. The patient's skin appears warm and pink. She is intubated and mechanically ventilated. Her vital signs are pulse rate of 110 beats/minute, blood pressure of 94/60 mm Hg, and temperature of 39.1°C (102.4°F). Her breath sounds are present bilaterally and her abdomen is soft and distended. A chest radiograph reveals bibasilar atelectasis. A 12-lead ECG reveals sinus tachycardia. Complete blood count reveals WBC 24,000/mm³, hemoglobin 11 g/dL, and hematocrit 38%.

▶ What are the likely causes of this patient's low blood pressure?
▶ What should be the next steps in this patient's management?
▶ What are the best methods to provide ongoing assessment of this patient's condition?

ANSWERS TO CASE 3:
The Hypotensive Patient with Septic Shock

Summary: A 44-year-old woman has just undergone a 3-hour abdominal operation for debridement of infected pancreatic necrosis. The blood loss was 800 mL and the patient received 3000 mL of crystalloid, 2 units of PRBC, and 2 units of FFP during the operation. She is tachycardic and hypotensive postoperatively. She has been receiving antibiotic and antifungal therapy for bacteremia and fungemia.

- **Likely causes of low blood pressure:** Probably a combination of sepsis and blood loss.

- **Next steps in the management:** Initial efforts should be to restore intravascular volume with crystalloid fluids and blood products. The addition of a vaso-constrictive medication should be considered if volume replacement does not normalize her blood pressure and improve end-organ perfusion.

- **Best methods to provide ongoing assessment:** Place a central venous catheter for continuous CVP monitoring and an arterial catheter for ongoing blood pressure monitoring. Trans-thoracic echocardiography can be valuable to assess intravascular volume and evaluate cardiac functions. Serial measurements of serum lactate levels can be helpful to monitor progress during the resuscitation process.

ANALYSIS

Objectives

1. Recognize the signs and symptoms of shock and understand principles of early treatment.

2. Learn how to differentiate the causes of shock and manage patients with the various causes of shock.

3. Become familiar with the *Surviving Sepsis Campaign* treatment recommendations.

Considerations

This is a critically-ill patient with infected pancreatic necrosis, bacteremia, and fungemia who just underwent an operation directed at controlling the source of sepsis (debridement of the infected pancreas and peri-pancreatic tissue). Following the completion of the operation, she appears to be in septic shock with fever, tachycardia, and hypotension. Broad-spectrum antibiotic and antifungal agents are being administered as source control adjuncts. There are a number of monitoring parameters available to help provide the best supportive care to maintain optimal end-organ perfusion. The *Surviving Sepsis Campaign* has introduced a number of strategies regarding monitoring, resuscitation, and overall management of patients with sepsis and septic shock. These guidelines specify some parameters to follow such as central venous pressure (CVP), mean arterial pressure (MAP), and serum lactate. This campaign has also outlined strategies for introducing medications for support of septic shock patients (norepinephrine and vasopressin), and when adjuncts such as corticosteroids should be considered in the care of these patients.

APPROACH TO:

The Hypotensive Patient with Septic Shock

DEFINITIONS

SHOCK: A condition where the perfusion of end-organs is inadequate. Shock can be caused by insufficient intravascular volume such as during hemorrhagic shock or hypovolemic shock due to excess fluid loss or insufficient fluid intake. Shock can also be due to inappropriate distribution of circulatory volume, such as with neurogenic shock (loss of regulation in vascular tone) or with septic shock (vasodilation due to circulating endogenous vasodilators).

CENTRAL VENOUS CATHETER: An intravenous catheter of sufficient length to measure the pressures in the superior vena cava when placed through the internal jugular vein or subclavian vein.

ECHOCARDIOGRAPHY: Noninvasive imaging modality that can provide information about cardiac contractility, regional wall motion abnormalities, valvular abnormalities, and intravascular volume status. This imaging modality can be quite useful for the evaluation of critically ill, hemodynamically unstable patients.

SERUM LACTATE: When this end-product of anaerobic metabolism is elevated, it generally suggests a global deficit in oxygen delivery. Serum lactate can also become elevated as the result of inadequate clearance, such as with renal dysfunction.

PULMONARY ARTERY CATHETER: A centrally placed catheter that can measure left ventricular end-diastolic pressure and pulmonary artery pressures. These pressure measurements can help gauge the patients' left ventricular functions. Because of the invasive nature of this device and the limited information that it provides in comparison to CVP catheters, PA catheters are rarely used in the ICU settings now. The real advantage of a PA catheter over a CVP catheter is for the monitoring of patients with poor cardiac functions who are maintained on inotropic agents (such as acute heart failure patients).

CLINICAL APPROACH

Hypotension leading to shock can result from decreased intravascular volume, cardiac pump failure, and/or acute vasodilation without sufficient increase in intravascular volume. Persistent hypotension leads to deficits of perfusion to organ systems and predisposes to multiple organ dysfunction syndrome (MODS). A systematic approach to the hypotensive patient is important to minimize the duration and severity of organ hypoperfusion. **The cardiovascular system can be considered as an arrangement of pump, pipes, and fluid volume.** This simplistic idea translates to the three primary components of cardiovascular physiology: namely, cardiac output (pump), vascular tone (pipes), and intravascular volume (fluid). All components of the system need to be intact to maintain normal perfusion. Dysfunction in one or more of these components will often contribute to hypotension and shock. Evaluation of a patient with postoperative hypotension should include a review of the pertinent history including medications, a careful physical examination, the trend in vital signs and urine output. Table 3–1 lists the differential diagnoses of common causes of hypotension in the perioperative period, and Table 3–2 shows the hemodynamic characteristcs.

Diagnosis

The keys to assessment and management of hypotensive patients include **close monitoring of the vital signs, urine output, and clinical appearances.** It is important to note the changes in these parameters over time and after interventions. A Foley catheter for continuous urine output monitoring, serial arterial blood gas measurements for trends in base deficit and lactate levels, and arterial catheterization for continuous blood pressure measurements can be helpful. Similarly, serial hemoglobin measurements can be helpful to identify ongoing occult bleeding. (Caution: it is important to note that early hemoglobin values may not reflect active and acute blood loss, as the values may not change until hemodilution occurs after crystalloid administration.)

Central venous monitoring and echocardiography can provide valuable information about the causes of hypotension (differentiate between hypovolemic and cardiogenic causes) and help guide fluid resuscitation and pharmacologic therapy, especially when there is clinical uncertainty. The information gained from these diagnostic modalities must be considered within the proper clinical

Table 3–1 • CLASSIFICATION OF SHOCK	
Classification of Shock	**Etiologies**
Hypovolemic	Hemorrhage
	Dehydration
Distributive	Sepsis
	Neurogenic
	Anaphylaxis
	Medications
Cardiac: intrinsic	Acute coronary syndrome
	Cardiomyopathy
Cardiac: extrinsic	Cardiac tamponade
	Tension pneumothorax
	Massive pulmonary embolus
Mixed	Any combination of one or more of the above

context because CVP values and echocardiography findings should be used to confirm clinical suspicion and quantify the magnitude of abnormalities that are present.

Hypovolemia

Hypovolemic surgical patients who respond initially to crystalloid resuscitation but then experience subsequent drops in blood pressure may have ongoing bleeding that require operative intervention to control hemorrhage. It is very critical to remember that ongoing blood loss may be the cause for hypovolemia in surgical patients. Accordingly, the treatment is source control and not continued resuscitation. Also, in these settings, resuscitations are generally more effective with the administration of blood products rather than crystalloids. **Excess crystalloid administration to a bleeding patient can cause dilution of clotting factors and thrombocytopenia, which can cause further bleeding and create a vicious cycle of worsening hypotension, coagulopathy, and hypothermia.** For more details, refer to the chapter on hemorrhagic shock management (Case 8).

Distributive Shock

Hypovolemia can also be caused by changes in patients' a patient's vascular tone such as in the setting of neurogenic shock and inappropriate vasodilatory response from septic shock or anaphylaxis. In contrast to the bleeding patient, most patients with distributive shock exhibit gradual dips in blood pressure or minimal responses to fluid administration. This is due to microvascular leak syndrome or excess vasodilation. It is important to recognize these conditions, since **the appropriate treatments are administration of vasoconstrictive medications such as norepinephrine for septic shock or phenylephrine (apha-1 agonist) for neurogenic shock rather than continued fluid administration.**

Sepsis

Sepsis refers to the hyperdynamic and febrile responses to infections. **Severe sepsis** is defined as the occurrence of infection with septic host response and at least one end-organ dysfunction. **Septic shock is defined as sepsis with persistent hypotension despite fluid administration.** Early Goal-Directed Therapy is a treatment approach for sepsis that was introduced during the early 2000s; this approach is directed at early recognition of sepsis and early aggressive treatment to restore or minimize tissue hypoperfusion. It is important to recognize that severe sepsis can carry a mortality of 25% to 30% and septic shock can carry a mortality of 50%. **The two major treatment goals in septic shock are to identify and address the source of infection (source control), and to restore tissue perfusion as soon as possible to minimize remote organ hypoperfusion that can lead to organ dysfunction.** Ideally, these treatment priorities should be addressed simultaneously. Time to antibiotic initiation has been well documented to influence outcomes associated with sepsis; therefore, every effort should be made to select and administer the appropriate antimicrobial treatments as soon as sepsis is recognized.

The *Surviving Sepsis Campaign* is an international initiative to enhance the practice of sepsis management. The recommended end-points of resuscitation are target CVP of 8 to 12 mm Hg, a mean arterial pressure of >65 mm Hg, and urine output of >0.5 mL/kg/h. If fluids alone are insufficient to achieve the blood pressure goals, a norepinephrine (Levophed) drip is recommended to help achieve the target blood pressures once intravascular volume depletion has been corrected. If continued increases in norepinephrine infusion fail to achieve target blood pressures, a continuous infusion of vasopressin at a constant rate of 0.03 U/min can be initiated to help improve catecholamine receptor responsiveness. The use of physiologic doses of corticosteroids can be considered for individuals with septic shock who do not achieve sufficient responses to source control, fluid administration, and vasopressors.

Cardiogenic Shock: Intrinsic or Extrinsic (Mechanical)

Intrinsic conditions causing cardiogenic shock are due to primary cardiac dysfunction, and these include acute coronary syndrome, acute myocardial infarction, and heart failure. Conversely, a classic **extrinsic cause** of cardiogenic shock is tension pneumothorax where the mediastinal structures shift away from the side of the pneumothorax causing kinking of the vena cava and affecting cardiac filling. Another example of an extrinsic cause of cardiogenic shock is cardiac tamponade, in which pericardial pressure compromises venous return to the right heart and hypotension. The EKG, cardiac troponin levels, and echocardiography are helpful to evaluate hypotensive or hemodynamically unstable patients with history of cardiac disease or those with risk factors for having intrinsic cardiac disease. Chest auscultation, chest x-rays, and echocardiography are maneuvers and modalities that can be helpful to identify patients with extrinsic causes of cardiac dysfunction.

Mixed Causes of Shock

In some cases, hypotension and hemodynamic instability can be attributable to more than one cause. For example, an elderly man with a history of congestive heart failure with urinary tract sepsis can have hypotension due to the combined effects of cardiogenic and septic causes. For such an individual, echocardiography can be highly useful to determine cardiac function as well as intravascular volume status. The treatment of such a patient often requires prioritizing the more serious condition or sometimes requires simultaneous treatment of both conditions.

CASE CORRELATION

- See Case 4 (Postoperative Fever), Case 6 (Blunt Chest Trauma), Case 7 (Multiple Blunt Trauma), Case 8 (Hemorrhagic Shock [Trauma]), and Case 9 (Penetrating Abdominal Trauma).

Physiologic State	Cardiac Index	Systemic Vascular Resistance	Pulmonary Capillary Wedge Pressure	Prime Mover[a]
Table 3–2 • HEMODYNAMIC VARIABLES IN DIFFERENT SHOCK STATES				
Normal	2.4-3.0 L/min/m²	800-1200 dyne-s or dyne-s/cm⁵	8-12 mm Hg	Not applicable
Distributive (sepsis, neurogenic, anaphylaxis)	Elevated	Decreased (because of decreased vascular tone)	Low to normal	Decreased vascular tone
Cardiogenic (myocardial infarction, cardiomyopathy)	Decreased	Increased	Increased	Decreased cardiac contractility
Hypovolemic (hemorrhage, dehydration)	Decreased (because of decreased volume)	Increased (to attempt to maintain blood pressure)	Decreased	Decreased preload
Obstructive (tamponade, tension pneumothorax, pulmonary embolus)	Decreased	Increased	Normal to increased flow	Obstruction of blood flow

[a]The prime mover is the initial pathophysiologic change; this change then causes compensatory changes in other variables.

COMPREHENSION QUESTIONS

3.1 A 25-year-old man is noted to have a blood pressure of 60/62 mm Hg on the evening after laparotomy and small bowel resection for strangulated small bowel obstruction. His heart rate is 112 beats/minute, respiratory rate is 24 breath/minute, and temperature is 37.4°C (99.3°F); urine output is 20 mL over 2 hours and oxygen saturation by pulse oximeter is 95%. His preoperative serum hemoglobin value is 12.6 g/dL. Which of the following statements is most accurate regarding this patient?

A. A serum Hgb value of 12.4 g/dL obtained in the recovery room after surgery is good indication that his hypotension is not caused by blood loss

B. Intravenous furosemide (Lasix) should be administered to improve his urine output

C. This patient likely is affected by anxiety and a mild anxiolytic should be provided with close observation

D. The initial treatment should be a fluid bolus

E. CT imaging should be done to assess for possible bleeding or intra-abdominal infectious process

3.2 A 54-year-old woman is admitted to the ICU for management following an elective open AAA repair. The patient is noted to have low urine output, with only 20 mL collected over 3 hours. Her blood pressure is 90/55 mm Hg, heart rate is 110 beats/minute, and temperature is 35.5°C (96.1°F). Her serum cardiac troponin levels are elevated. Which of the following will most likely help establish the cause of her current condition?

   A. Return to the OR for re-exploration

   B. Renal ultrasound to evaluate for urinary obstruction

   C. Echocardiography and 12-lead ECG

   D. Blood culture and respiratory cultures

   E. Abdominal CT scan

3.3 A 52-year-old woman has undergone an open cholecystectomy 5 days previously. She has fever of 1-day duration and complains of shortness of breath and cough. Her pulse rate is 118 beats/minute, blood pressure is 110/70 mm Hg, temperature is 39.5°C (103.1°F), and respiratory rate is 46 breaths/minute. Her O_2 saturation by pulse oximetry is 89% on 60% FiO_2 O_2 by face mask. Auscultation of her lungs reveals rales and crackles in her left lung field. Her WBC count is 17,000 cells/mm³. Her chest radiography reveals infiltrates in the left low lobe. Which of the following statements is correct regarding her care?

   A. A higher FiO_2 should be avoided because it will cause oxygen toxicity

   B. Intravenous thrombolytic therapy should be given for her pulmonary embolism

   C. Antibiotics, mechanical ventilation, and transfer to the ICU are indicated

   D. A subhepatic abscess is the most likely cause

   E. Restriction of her fluid intake is indicated based on her pulmonary examination and CXR findings

3.4 Which of the following statements regarding fluid resuscitation is most true regarding volume repletion?

   A. 80% of crystalloid fluids given as a bolus will remain within the intravenous space

   B. Colloid resuscitation is preferable over crystalloid resuscitation in patients with septic shock

   C. PRBC should be transfused when the patient's Hgb value drops below 10 g/dL

   D. In patients with septic shock, blood product resuscitation is preferred over crystalloid

   E. The use of vasopressors such as norepinephrine is preferred over dobutamine for the initial resuscitation of septic shock patients

3.5 Which of the following choices best describes the difference between distributive shock and hemorrhagic shock?

A. Distributive shock requires treatment with vasoconstrictive agents only while hemorrhagic shock is treated with blood components and fluid repletion

B. The transfusion of blood products improves hemorrhagic shock but is not indicated in distributive shock

C. Both types of shock produce low urine output, but only hemorrhagic shock causes prerenal azotemia

D. CVP measurements allows for the differentiation between the two processes

E. Distributive shock is always associated with normal or low heart rates

3.6 Which of the following hypotensive patients may have increased cardiac output?

A. A 30-year-old man who is febrile and tachycardic from perforated appendicitis

B. A 61-year-old man with chest pain and new-onset left bundle branch block on 12-lead ECG

C. A 33-year-old man with gunshot wound to the abdomen with extensive amount of free fluid in the abdomen on ultrasound

D. A 38-year-old man who developed shortness of breath and hypotension after placement of a left subclavian vein catheter. His trachea is deviated to the right

E. A 18-year-old man with splenic laceration and pelvic fracture following a motorcycle crash

3.7 For which of the following hypotensive patients are a 12-lead ECG and chest radiograph unlikely to be helpful in identifying the cause?

A. 38-year-old man with facial swelling and urticuria after a bee sting

B. 42-year-old involved in a head-on motor vehicle crash with subcutaneous crepitus in the neck, multiple bilateral rib factures, and diminished breath sounds bilaterally

C. 78-year-old woman who underwent an emergency laparotomy for strangulated small bowel obstruction with several episodes of hypotension during the operation and ST-segment changes on her intraoperative ECG tracing

D. 42-year-old man with a single stab wound to the left lateral chest at the 4th intercostal space

E. 51-year-old man with a history of spontaneous pneumothorax in the past who collapsed at home with sudden onset of shortness of breath and chest pain. His breath sounds are diminished on the right

3.8 A 31-year-old man presents with a GSW to the abdomen. At presentation, his pulse rate was 130 and BP was 90/75. His abdomen was tender diffusely. The patient was taken to the operating room for an emergency exploratory laparotomy. During the operation, bleeding from a shattered right kidney was identified. He underwent a right nephrectomy. Following control of all bleeding, the patient was taken to the ICU. During the operation, he received 6 units of PRBC, 6 units of fresh frozen plasma, and 10 units of platelets. At the time of his arrival to the ICU, his blood pressure was 110/80 and pulse rate 96. The ICU admission laboratory studies revealed a hemoglobin value of 7.0 g/dL, and Hct of 29%. The serum lactate was 14 mmol/L (normal range: 0.6-2.1 mmol/L) during the operation and is 1.9 mmol/L at the time of arrival to ICU. Which of the following is the best treatment option at this time?

A. Immediate return to the operating room for ongoing bleeding

B. Observe the patient and repeat the serum lactate value in 4 hours

C. Transfuse the patient with four additional units of PRBC to achieve a Hgb value of >10 g/dL

D. Perform a CT scan to look for bleeding

E. Transfuse the patient with 4 units of PRBC and then return to OR for abdominal re-exploration

ANSWERS

3.1 **D.** This is a young man who is hypotensive following an operation for strangulated small bowel obstruction. His postoperative urine output is low (<0.5 mL/kg/h) and his pulse rate is elevated. Given the scenario of having strangulated small bowel obstruction that required a bowel resection, it is likely that he is hypovolemic secondary to the third-space fluid losses associated with his bowel obstruction and his recent laparotomy. Fluid bolus is the best choice at this point. Furosemide is not indicated unless there is clear evidence that his intravascular volume is normal or elevated. CT scan is not likely to provide useful information this soon following the operation.

3.2 **C.** This 54-year-old woman is hypotensive, tachycardic, with low urine output following open AAA repair. Her serum cardiac troponins are elevated. Based on the information provided, there is strong concern for possible myocardial injury and cardiogenic shock. An echocardiogram and 12-lead ECG are probably the most useful diagnostic studies for this patient at this time.

3.3 **C.** This patient has postoperative respiratory distress, cough, fever, leukocytosis, and physical examination findings suggestive of left sided pneumonia. The CXR findings of left lower lobe infiltrate confirm your clinical suspicion. The best treatments for her are mechanical ventilatory support, antibiotics, and transfer to the ICU for management and close monitoring of her sepsis.

3.4 **E.** The use of norepinephrine is indicated for the resuscitation of septic shock patients if the patients do not respond favorably based on physiologic parameters and laboratory parameters. Given the distributive nature of septic shock, an alpha agonist such as norepinephrine is the pharmacologic agent of choice. Dobutamine is an inotropic agent that produces increased cardiac contractility and some peripheral vasodilatation to decrease the afterload to the left heart. Dobutamine is an ideal pharmacologic support when there is intrinsic cardiac dysfunction leading to shock. Dobutamine use in the patient with septic shock will not likely improve tissue perfusion.

3.5 **B.** The transfusion of blood products will help address the hypovolemia associated with hemorrhagic shock; in addition, blood products will improve the oxygen carrying capacity in this setting. With distributive shock, the capacitance of the vascular system is increased, leading to a relatively hypovolemic state. Volume repletion with crystalloids or colloids will help improve the vital signs and tissue perfusion. CVP measurements will be low for both hemorrhagic shock and distributive shock. Some forms of distributive shock such as neurogenic shock will be associated with normal or low heart rate, but these findings are not present in all forms of distributive shock such as anaphylactic shock.

3.6 **A.** The 30-year-old man with sepsis from perforated appendicitis will have increased cardiac output because he has increased heart rate and normal intravascular volume. The patient described in choice "B" has cardiogenic shock and decreased contractility and reduced cardiac output. The patient described in "C" has hemorrhagic shock, and with decreased intravascular volume, the cardiac output is reduced. The patient described in "D" has tension pneumothorax that caused poor right heart filling and reduced cardiac output. The patient described in "E" has hemorrhagic shock due to decreased intravascular volume and with it decreased cardiac output.

3.7 **A.** Based on the history given, this patient has anaphylactic shock, which is a distributive shock. The chest x-ray and 12-lead ECG are not going to contribute to the diagnosis or treatment of this patient. The patient in "B" can have hypotension on the basis of tension pneumothorax and/or blunt cardiac injury, therefore both CXR and EKG may be contributory in directing his management. The patient described in "C" has cardiogenic shock secondary to acute coronary syndrome, and ECG and chest radiographs will likely help confirm the diagnosis. The patient described in "D" has either a tension pneumothorax, hemothorax, or cardiac tamponade and CXR and ECG can be helpful. The patient described in "E" likely has recurrent spontaneous pneumothorax with tension physiology, and CXR will be helpful.

3.8 **B.** Continued observation with close monitoring of vital signs and repeating the laboratory studies such as CBC and serum lactate in a few hours is the most appropriate course at this time. Based on the scenario, the patient had extensive blood loss and was likely in shock in the OR; however, following the control of bleeding, it appears that his vital signs and serum lactate levels have improved. Continued monitoring and repeating the serum lactate and CBC will help us trend the improvement or identify worsening values.

CLINICAL PEARLS

▶ The initial therapy for hypotension in most patients in whom sepsis is suspected should be fluid resuscitation and not vasopressors.

▶ Source control in patients with a surgical infection frequently requires appropriate procedures to control the infection (eg, drainage, debridement, bowel resection). For these types of patients, antibiotics alone will not be sufficient for source control.

▶ Clinical measures of perfusion status are adequate in most patients for determination of the adequacy of resuscitation.

▶ Monitoring devices and diagnostic modalities (CVP catheters and/or echocardiography) should be considered when the patient with septic shock fails to respond to initial fluid resuscitation.

▶ Do not be falsely reassured by a normal hemoglobin value in hypotensive surgical patients: they bleed whole blood so the hemoglobin and hematocrit values will not drop immediately.

▶ Patients younger than 30 years of age with a good cardiac reserve and patients on beta-blockers may not exhibit the expected tachycardia response to hemorrhage until late in the course of shock.

REFERENCES

Cioffi Jr WG, Connolly MD. The septic response. In: Cameron JL, Cameron AM, eds. *Current Surgical Therapy*. 11th ed. Philadelphia, PA: Elsevier Saunders; 2014:1262-1267.

Dellinger RP, Levy MM, Rhodes A, et al. Surviving sepsis campaign: international guidelines for management of severe sepsis and septic shock: 2012. *Crit Care Med*. 2013;41:580-637.

Kumar A, Roberts D, Wood KE, et al. Duration of hypotension before initiation of effective antimicrobial therapy is the critical determinant of survival in human septic shock. *Crit Care Med*. 2006;34:1589-1596.

A 58-year-old man underwent an emergency laparotomy with sigmoid colectomy and colostomy formation for a perforated diverticulitis 7 days previously. Since his operation, the patient has had intermittent fevers to 39.0°C (102.2°F). He has only tolerated minimal oral food intake since surgery secondary to abdominal bloating and distension. His indwelling urinary catheter was removed on postoperative day 2, and he denies any urinary symptoms. On examination, his temperature is 38.8°C (101.8°F), pulse rate is 102 beats/minute, and blood pressure is 130/80 mm Hg. His skin is warm and moist. The pulmonary examination reveals normal breath sounds in both lung fields, and his heart rate is regular without murmurs. His abdomen is distended and tender throughout, and the surgical skin incision is open without any evidence of infection. His current medications include maintenance intravenous fluids, morphine sulfate, and intravenous cefoxitin and metronidazole. A complete blood count reveals a white blood cell (WBC) count of 20,500/mm^3.

- ▶ What is the most likely diagnosis?
- ▶ What is the next step?
- ▶ Does this patient need another operation?

ANSWERS TO CASE 4:

Postoperative Fever (Intra-Abdominal Infection)

Summary: A 58-year-old has fever, abdominal distension, and delayed return of normal bowel functions following sigmoid resection and colostomy formation for complicated diverticulitis. His physical examination does not reveal respiratory, urinary, or superficial surgical site infection.

- **Most likely diagnosis:** Deep surgical space infection or intra-abdominal infection.

- **Next step:** A thorough fever workup including a complete physical examination for other potential sites of infections and a CT scan of the abdomen and pelvis.

- **Need for an operation:** Although his clinical course and current condition are concerning, he does not have a clear indication for re-exploration of the abdomen at this time. Operative intervention and percutaneous drainage are two important methods to achieve source control in a patient with deep surgical space infection, if confirmed.

ANALYSIS

Objectives

1. Recognize the sources of fever in postoperative patients and become familiar with diagnostic and treatment strategies for these patients.

2. Learn the principles of diagnosis and treatment of intra-abdominal infections in the postoperative patient.

3. Learn the pathogenesis of intra-abdominal infections.

Considerations

When a patient fails to improve and exhibits persistent fever following definitive surgical treatment for an intra-abdominal infectious process, we must first entertain the possibility that there are still untreated intra-abdominal infections. We must also consider other potential nosocomial infectious causes, as well as non-infectious causes for his fever. Given the picture of persistent ileus and fevers, the possibility of intra-abdominal (deep surgical space) infection should be at the top of our differential diagnosis. With his current picture, it is not unreasonable to initiate broad-spectrum antimicrobial therapy targeting GI tract microbial flora. A CT scan may be very useful. When identified, some intra-abdominal abscesses can be accessed and drained by percutaneous approaches (Figure 4–1). CT imaging may also identify inflammatory changes within the abdominal cavity but without abscesses (fluid collection); these, findings suggestive of persistent secondary peritonitis. Persistent secondary peritonitis can be the result of inappropriate or inadequate antimicrobial therapy, which can be addressed with additional antimicrobial therapy or modification of antimicrobial regimen.

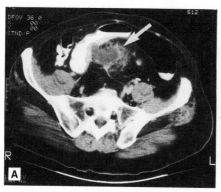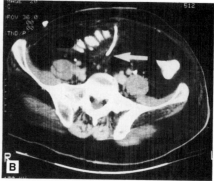

Figure 4–1. Diverticular abscess noted by arrow (**A**) and then evacuated by computer tomography–guided percutaneous drainage (**B**). *(Reproduced, with permission, from Schwarz SI, Shires GT, Spencer FC, et al, eds. Principles of Surgery. 7th ed. New York, NY: McGraw-Hill; 1999:1041.)*

APPROACH TO:

Fever and Intra-Abdominal Infection

DEFINITIONS

POSTOPERATIVE FEVER: There is no clear definition for fever; however, many clinicians arbitrarily define fever as oral temperature higher than 38.0 to 38.5°C (100.4-101.3° F).

SURGICAL SITE INFECTIONS: These are infections involving the skin and subcutaneous tissue and are further divided into *superficial* and *deep*.

SUPERFICIAL SURGICAL SITE INFECTION: These soft tissue infections involving the surgical site are above (superficial to) the fascia, comprising of a soft tissue infection involving the surgical site. They are treated primarily by wound exploration and drainage; systemic antibiotics may be added when there is extensive surrounding cellulitis (>2 cm from the incision margin) or if the patient is immunocompromised.

DEEP SURGICAL SITE INFECTION: These are infections involving the surgical site with involvement of the fascia and musculature. Deep surgical site infections may be a clinical manifestation of a deep surgical space infection. Patients with deep surgical site infections should have imaging such as CT to rule-out a deep surgical space infection.

DEEP SURGICAL SPACE INFECTION: In the case of patients with abdominal operations, the deep surgical space is the intra-abdominal space. This type of infection in the setting of postabdominal surgery can include *secondary peritonitis*, *tertiary peritonitis*, and *deep surgical space abscess*.

SECONDARY MICROBIAL PERITONITIS: Often the result of spillage of endogenous microbes into the peritoneal cavity following visceral perforation. The persistence of this infection can be the result of the microbial inoculum volume, the inhibitory and synergistic effects of a polymicrobial environment, and insufficient host response. Recurrence or persistence of this process can be due to insufficient antimicrobial therapy or insufficient control of contamination process (inadequate source control).

TERTIARY MICROBIAL PERITONITIS: This condition occurs in patients who fail to recover from intra-abdominal infections despite surgical and/or antimicrobial therapy. This is often caused by diminished host peritoneal response. Very often in these cases, low virulence or opportunistic pathogens such as *Staphylococcus epidermis*, *Enterococcus faecalis*, or *Candida* species are identified. The treatment for this condition is somewhat unclear because most cases are related to poor host immune responses. Generally, additional and/or prolonged antimicrobial therapy is prescribed.

INTRA-ABDOMINAL ABSCESS: A defined intraperitoneal collection of inflammatory fluid and microbes produced by a host compartmentalizing process in which fibrin deposition, omental containment, and ileus of the small bowel help to localize the infectious process. The response produces loculated, infected inflammatory fluid that cannot be eliminated by the host trans-lymphatic clearance process. When the abscesses are sizeable, surgical or percutaneous drainage are needed to resolve this process.

PREEMPTIVE ANTIBIOTIC THERAPY: This describes the administration of antimicrobial therapy when a large microbial inoculum is thought to have occurred, such as with disease processes associated with the spillage of GI tract contents. In these situations, the therapy should be initially broad and target Gram-positive and Gram-negative bacteria. The optimal therapeutic duration and end-points of treatment with this strategy remains controversial. In general, as the patients improve clinically and culture results become available, de-escalation of treatment is appropriate.

SEPSIS: Sepsis is defined as infection plus systemic manifestations of the host's response to the infection (ie, fever, tachycardia, hyperglycemia, and fluid sequestration). **Severe sepsis** is defined as sepsis plus sepsis-related organ dysfunction or hypoperfusion. **Septic shock** is defined as sepsis-induced hypotension that persists despite adequate fluid resuscitation. The **Surviving Sepsis Campaign** has introduced bundles of care for septic patients. These guidelines, based on basic science and clinical evidence, were initially introduced in 2001 and have been regularly updated, validated, and implemented internationally.

CLINICAL APPROACH

There are a variety of causes of fever in hospitalized surgical patients. These can include infections related to the original disease and the operative processes, such as secondary peritonitis, intra-abdominal abscess, and surgical site infection. In addition, hospital-acquired infections can also occur, including urinary tract infection, pneumonia, catheter-related bacteremia, and antibiotic-associated colitis. In some instances, patients can develop fever as the result of non-infectious causes such as systemic inflammatory response syndrome (SIRS), venous thromboembolic processes, endocrinopathies (adrenal insufficiency, thyrotoxicosis), drug reactions, and transfusion reactions. **The approach to a febrile postoperative patient who has undergone abdominal surgery is to presume that there is an intra-abdominal or surgical site related infectious complication until proven otherwise.**

Pathophysiology of Intra-Abdominal Infections

Perforation of the gastrointestinal (GI) tract results in microbial spillage into the peritoneal cavity. The severity of the peritoneal contamination is related to the intestinal location of the perforation, which determines the concentration and diversity of the endogenous microbes (ie, colon contents with 10^{11} to 10^{14} aerobic and anaerobic microbes per gram of contents versus stomach contents with 10^2 to 10^3 aerobic microbes per gram of contents). A number of adaptive host defense responses occur following the inoculation of bacteria into the peritoneal cavity. These include peritoneal macrophages and leukocyte (PMN) recruitment, development of ileus, and fibropurulent peritonitis to help localize the infection. Removal of the infection occurs with translymphatic clearance of the sequestered microbes and inflammatory cells to help resolve the process. Several factors can influence the effectiveness of the host response, and include the following: (1) the size of the microbial inoculum; (2) the timing of diagnosis and treatment; (3) the inhibitory, synergistic, or cumulative effects of microbes on the growth of other microbes; (4) effectiveness of the host peritoneal defense.

Treatment Goals

The goals in the management of secondary peritonitis are directed toward eliminating the source of the microbial spillage (eg, an appendectomy for perforated appendicitis or closure of a perforated duodenal ulcer) and early initiation of preemptive antibiotic therapy. With appropriate and timely therapy, secondary peritonitis resolves in most patients; however, approximately 15% to 30% of the treated individuals may develop complications such as recurrent secondary peritonitis, tertiary peritonitis, or intra-abdominal abscesses. Recurrent secondary peritonitis can be due to inappropriate antibiotics or insufficient antibiotic treatment duration. Patients suspected of having deep surgical space infections should undergo CT scan evaluation, and if identified and accessible, abscesses can be drained under CT guidance. The initial systemic antibiotics for patients with infections from GI sources should include coverage of the most likely pathogens. Table 4–1 contains some of the common antimicrobial agents or regimens that are used.

Table 4–1 • ANTIMICROBIAL THERAPY FOR INTRA-ABDOMINAL INFECTIONS

Dual-Agent Therapy:
- Second- or third-generation cephalosporin (cephtetan, cefoxitin, ceftriaxone, cefotaxime, cefepime) + metronidazole or clindamycin
- Fluoroquinolone (ciprofloxacin, levofloxacin, gatifloxacin) + metronidazole or clindamycin
- Aminoglycoside + metronidazole or clindamycin (This regimen should be applied with extreme caution for older patient or patients with compromised renal functions; close monitoring of levels is needed to avoid harm.)

Single-Agent Therapy:
- For treatment of mild or moderate infections such as perforated appendicitis in healthy individuals—Cefoxitin, cefotetan, ceftriaxone, ampicillin-sulbactam.
- For treatment of severe infections or infections in immunocompromised hosts—imipenem-cilastatin, meropenem, ertapenem, tigecycline, piperacillin-tazobactam, ticarcillin-clavulanate.

CASE CORRELATION

- See also Case 3 (Hypotensive Patient [Sepsis]).

COMPREHENSION QUESTIONS

4.1 A 66-year-old otherwise healthy woman undergoes exploratory laparotomy for peritonitis. A ruptured appendix with purulent drainage is noted in the lower abdomen. Which of the following statements is most accurate regarding this patient's condition?

A. The resulting infection is a difficult problem to resolve even with appropriate surgical treatment and antimicrobial therapy

B. The most common organisms involved in this infection are Candida and Pseudomonas

C. Treatment can be effectively accomplished with appropriate surgery and a first-generation cephalosporin

D. The patient should be sufficiently treated with operative removal of the appendix and copious irrigation of the peritoneal cavity

E. Persistent secondary peritonitis may result if inappropriate antibiotics are given or if the antibiotic treatment duration is too short

4.2 Which of the following is most accurate regarding patients who develop fever during the postoperative period?

    A. They should receive broad-spectrum antibiotics until the fevers resolve

    B. They require no specific treatments because fever is an expected host response to surgical stress

    C. The patients require immediate re-operation to address the source of fever

    D. Thorough searches for fever sources are required. Presumptive antibiotics can be given if patients exhibit physiologic signs of sepsis or if the patients are immunocompromised

    E. High doses of corticosteroids should be prescribed to blunt the physiologic responses to infection

4.3 A 39-year-old man who is on chronic corticosteroid treatment undergoes resection of the ileum with primary re-anastomosis for intestinal perforation related to his Crohn disease. Following surgery, he has persistent fever and abdominal pain despite the administration of ciprofloxacin and metronidazole. A CT scan reveals a loculated 6- × 5-cm heterogeneous fluid collection in the pelvis. Which of the following is the best treatment for this condition at this time?

    A. Broaden his antibiotic coverage with the addition of vancomycin and fluconazole

    B. Drain the fluid collection by percutaneous approach

    C. Administer intraperitoneal thrombolytic to dissolve this pelvic hematoma

    D. Drain the fluid collection by percutaneous approach and initiate broad-spectrum antibiotics treatment

    E. Perform re-operation of the abdomen to address this fluid collection

4.4 Which of the following statements is most accurate regarding secondary peritonitis?

    A. Treatment with appropriate antimicrobial regimen will successfully resolve this process

    B. Successful treatment cannot be accomplished with antimicrobial therapy alone

    C. Resection of the segment of the GI tract source producing the peritonitis will successfully address this process

    D. Antimicrobial therapy is not useful for secondary peritonitis, and treatment will only lead to the selection of resistant microbial species

    E. Fungal species are the most common pathogen isolated in secondary peritonitis

4.5 A 30-year-old man develops fever, abdominal distension, and leukocytosis 14 days following laparotomy and the repair of three small bowel perforations produced by a gunshot wound to the abdomen. A CT scan reveals a single large fluid collection in the left upper quadrant with extensive surrounding inflammatory changes. This collection is drained under CT guidance, and broad-spectrum antibiotics are started. Despite these treatments, the patient remains febrile and soon thereafter begins to have enteric contents draining from his drainage catheter. In addition, the patient develops drainage of purulent fluid from the inferior aspect of his midline surgical incision. Which of the following is the most appropriate treatment for this patient?

A. Add empiric treatment to cover for fungal infection

B. Repeat the CT scan

C. Perform a laparotomy to address the intestinal leakage and drain the fluid collection

D. Assess the patient for immunodeficiency, including skin anergy panel, lymphocyte count, and CD4 cell count measurement

E. Add antibiotics to cover for pseudomonas infection

4.6 A 29-year-old man underwent an exploratory laparotomy and lysis of adhesions for recurrent adhesive small bowel obstruction 14 days ago. His hospital course was unremarkable, and he was discharged from the hospital on postoperative day six. The patient was doing well but returned to the emergency department with abdominal pain and vomiting. A CT scan of the abdomen revealed that a loop of small bowel had herniated through a mid-abdominal fascia defect, and there is CT evidence of constriction of the herniated small bowel at the fascial defect with closed-loop obstruction of the herniated small bowel segment. Which of the following is the best treatment option for his current problem?

A. Non-operative management of small bowel obstruction for 7 days, and surgery if not improved

B. Attempt to reduce the hernia and obstruction by manipulation of the abdomen at the site of herniation

C. Provide intravenous sedation and muscle relaxants and attempt to manually reduce the hernia to relieve the obstruction manually

D. Take the patient to surgery to reduce the herniated intestine, and revise the fascial closure

E. Attempt nonoperative management for 14 days, while providing the patient with TPN and NG decompression. If the process does not resolve, then operate

4.7 A 48-year-old woman underwent laparotomy for sigmoid colon obstruction from a diverticular stricture. The patient developed a deep surgical site infection on postoperative day number 4. She remained in the hospital for close observation and wound care with frequent dressing changes. Six days later, the patient is noted to have a significant amount of purulent fluid draining into her wound through a 1-cm fascia defect in the lower aspect of her surgical incision. Which of the following is the best treatment for this patient?

A. CT scan, broad-spectrum antibiotics, and wound care
B. CT scan and surgery for abdominal re-exploration
C. Broad spectrum antibiotics and wound care
D. Extend the fascial defect to assess the contents within the abdominal cavity
E. Wound care and patient reassurance

ANSWERS

4.1 **E.** The patient described is a 66-year-old man with secondary peritonitis due to perforated appendicitis. He underwent appendectomy for source control. Properly selected antimicrobial therapy for sufficient duration of time is important to reduce the risk for tertiary peritonitis or intra-abdominal abscess formation. The appropriate antibiotics for this patient should be either a single agent or combination regimen covering Gram-negative and anaerobic activities. A first-generation cephalosporin is not the appropriate antibiotic for this patient.

4.2 **D.** Fever in the postoperative patient can be due to a variety of causes. Thorough search for a fever source is important in these patients. Not every patient with postoperative fever requires antimicrobial therapy; however, if the fever is also associated with signs of sepsis or if the patient is immunocompromised, preemptive antimicrobial treatment should be initiated while the search for fever source is ongoing.

4.3 **D.** The patient described here has Crohn disease and receives chronic corticosteroid treatment; he developed fever and a loculated intra-abdominal abscess following segmental small bowel resection. Drainage of the abscess by CT guidance is helpful to resolve the abscess, but given his fever and relative immunosuppressed condition (chronic steroid use), the addition of broad-spectrum antibiotics will be helpful to address the peritoneal inflammatory process and the systemic response to the infection.

4.4 **B.** By definition, secondary peritonitis is the result of another process that has produced the peritonitis. Within the abdominal cavity, a GI tract source of contamination is most common. Examples are appendicitis and perforated peptic ulcers. In both of these examples, control of the spillage by operative treatments (source control) is an essential component of the patient care. Antibiotic therapy without source control is insufficient; similarly, source control without antimicrobial therapy is also insufficient in the patient with secondary peritonitis.

4.5 **B.** The patient described here had definitive surgery to repair a gunshot wound to the small bowel. He develops a large postoperative abscess containing enteric contents in the left upper quadrant, and subsequent to that, he develops purulent drainage from his midline surgical site. At this time, there is strong concern for ongoing enteric leakage and a possible intra-abdominal abscess. A CT scan is need at this time to assess whether all intra-abdominal abscesses are being drained and to assess the need for CT-guided drainage or re-operation.

4.6 **D.** This patient underwent an abdominal operation for mechanical small bowel obstruction 14 days prior. His early postoperative course was uncomplicated, but he returns to the hospital with abdominal pain and vomiting. The CT scan suggests that the patient has developed an early fascial dehiscence with evisceration of the small bowel that has produced a mechanical small bowel obstruction. Based on the information provided, we do not know whether there is deep surgical space infection or deep surgical site infection that caused his fascial closure disruption. The CT scan demonstrates that incarceration of the small bowel at the fascial defect is causing mechanical small bowel obstruction. Manual reduction of early postoperative strangulating hernia is risky given the friability of the intestines. Nonoperative treatment is not appropriate when the cause of the small bowel obstruction is most likely early postoperative fascial closure failure due to technical complications. This patient should be returned to the operating room for wound exploration, inspection of the bowel and fascia, and reclosure of the wound.

4.7 **A.** The woman described here underwent sigmoid colectomy for diverticular stricture. She developed a deep surgical site infection on postoperative day 4, which was treated with opening of the skin wound and local wound care. Several days later she develops a small fascial defect with drainage of purulent fluid from this opening. To put it all together, she appears to have a deep surgical site infection that caused a secondary deep surgical space infection (through fascial erosion and extension of the subcutaneous infectious process); alternatively, she may have had a deep surgical space infection that manifested initially as a surgical site infection before spontaneously decompressing through a fascial opening. She will need a CT scan to fully assess the depth and extent of involvement of her infection and to assess for possible remaining undrained infection; in addition, broad-spectrum antibiotics and wound care are important for her care.

CLINICAL PEARLS

▶ Prolonged dysfunction of the GI tract following GI surgery frequently indicates the presence of intra-abdominal infectious complications, whereas the prompt return of GI function following surgery generally indicates the absence of generalized intra-abdominal infections.

▶ Atelectasis is the most common cause of fever in a patient during the first 24 hours following surgery.

▶ With the availability of many newer, effective antibiotics against Gram-negative organisms, aminoglycosides are rarely used as first-line therapy.

▶ The colon contains a high concentration of bacteria (10^{11}-10^{14} aerobes and anaerobes per gram of contents) versus small bowel containing 10^5 organisms per gram of contents, and stomach containing only 10^2-10^3 predominantly Gram positive aerobic bacteria per gram of contents.

▶ The spillage of colonic contents is associated with a much higher rate of septic complications than spillage from the stomach or small bowel.

▶ CT imaging is often helpful in identifying intra-abdominal infectious processes.

▶ Source control (treatment to address the spillage source) often goes hand-in-hand with antimicrobial therapy in the management of patients with secondary peritonitis.

▶ The preemptive antibiotic regimen is generally dictated by the pathogens that are presumed to be involved in the intra-abdominal infectious process. The prescribed regimen changes with anatomic source of the leakage and can vary based on the antibiotic susceptibility of the organisms at each specific treatment facility.

REFERENCES

Barie PS. Surgical infections and antibiotics use. In: Townsend CM Jr, Beauchamp RD, Evers BM, Mattox KL, eds. *Sabiston Textbook of Surgery: The Biological Basis of Modern Surgical Practice.* 19th ed. Philadelphia, PA: Elsevier Saunders; 2012: 240-280.

Fox AD, Livingston DH. The management of intra-abdominal infections. In: Cameron JL, Cameron AM, eds. *Current Surgical Therapy.* 11th ed. Philadelphia, PA: Elsevier Saunders; 2014: 1177-1181.

Rosenberger LH, Sawyer RG. Surgical site infections. In: Cameron JL, Cameron AM, eds. *Current Surgical Therapy.* 11th ed. Philadelphia, PA: Elsevier Saunders; 2014: 1172-1177.

Sartelli M. A focus on intra-abdominal infections. *World J Emerg Surg.* 2010;5:9-28.

A 38-year-old man fell 15 ft from a ladder while trying to rescue a cat from the roof. During the evaluation at the hospital, he was found to have fractures of his right femur, right radius and right ulna, and soft tissue contusions and abrasions on the right side of his body. The patient underwent open reduction and internal fixation of his femur fracture and external fixation of his forearm fractures without any apparent complications. On postinjury day 2, he began to complain of difficulty in breathing. On physical examination, his temperature is 38.4°C (101°F), pulse rate is 120 beats/minute, blood pressure is 148/86 mm Hg, respiratory rate is 34 breaths/minute, and Glasgow Coma Score is 15. The patient appears anxious and complains of having difficulty breathing and denies chest pain. Auscultation of the chest reveals diminished breath sounds bilaterally with scattered rhonchi. His cardiac examination is unremarkable. The abdomen is nondistended and nontender. Examination of the extremities reveals postinjury swelling. Laboratory studies reveal white blood cell (WBC) count of 16,000/mm^3, hemoglobin 10.8 g/dL, and platelet count of 185,000/mm^3. Arterial blood gas reveals pH 7.4, PaO_2 55 mm Hg, $PaCO_2$ 40 mm Hg, and HCO_3 24 mEq/L. A chest radiograph (CXR) reveals bilateral nonsegmental infiltrates and no effusion or pneumothorax.

► What are your next steps?
► What is the most likely diagnosis?
► What are the possible contributing factors?

ANSWERS TO CASE 5:
Postoperative Acute Respiratory Insufficiency

Summary: A previously healthy young man develops acute respiratory insufficiency after being injured in a fall and undergoing surgical repair of traumatic orthopedic injuries.

- **Next steps:** Administration of supplemental oxygen and transfer the patient to the intensive care unit for close observation and possible mechanical ventilation if the condition deteriorates or does not improve.

- **Most Likely Diagnosis:** Acute respiratory insufficiency secondary to acute lung injury (ALI).

- **Possible contributing factors:** ALI can occur following major injuries, and can be exacerbated by femur fractures and femur fixations. In addition, the possibility of missed injuries such as intra-abdominal hollow visceral injury needs to be considered. Direct blunt injuries to the lung parenchyma (pulmonary contusion) can also contribute to respiratory insufficiency.

Considerations

The timing of the patient's development of respiratory insufficiency is within the expected timeframe of pulmonary embolism (PE) and ALI. The patient's pulmonary examination reveals diminished breath sounds and scattered rhonchi, which are nonspecific findings that are compatible with ALI, atelectasis, and PE. His CXR findings reveal bilateral nonsegmental infiltrates, and the ABG reveals moderate hypoxemia. The CXR findings are not compatible with the PE, as patients with PE generally have relatively normal CXRs or may have segmental infiltrate associated with segmental pulmonary infarction. By strict definition, ALI diagnosis requires the respiratory insufficiency to be acute in onset (such as in this patient), associated with a $PaO_2/FiO_2 < 300$, nonsegmental infiltrates on CXR, and with a pulmonary capillary wedge pressure (PCWP) that is less than 18 mm Hg. Even though the initial presentation in this patient's case has several key features associated with ALI or ARDS, it is important to consider and rule out other possible causes, including aspiration pneumonitis, atypical pneumonia, atelectasis, and PE. In a setting of recent trauma, it is also important to consider the possibility of missed injuries within the abdomen as the cause of his current respiratory insufficiency. With these considerations in mind, our first priority for this patient is to address his respiratory insufficiency. Given the significant tachypnea and tachycardia that this patient is demonstrating, it is very reasonable to consider intubation and mechanical ventilation. The main reason for intubation is to help stabilize his respiratory status while we sort out the potential causes of his current problem.

> # APPROACH TO:
> ## Acute Respiratory Insufficiency

DEFINITIONS

ASPIRATION: Spillage of gastric contents into the bronchial tree causing direct injury to the airways, which can progress to a chemical burn or pneumonitis (especially if the pH is <3) and predisposes to bacterial pneumonia. When the aspirated gastric contents contain particulate matter, bronchoscopy may be helpful to help in clearing the airway. Roughly half of the patients with aspiration events will develop pneumonia; however, antibiotics treatment is not indicated unless the pneumonia develops.

PNEUMONIA: Pulmonary infection caused by impairment of the lung's defense mechanisms. Incisional pain frequently affects the patient's ability to clear airway mucus, leading to small airway obstruction and ineffective bacteria clearance. Most commonly, nosocomial organisms colonize the patients during the hospitalization.

ATELECTASIS: The collapse of alveolar units occurs in patients undergoing general anesthesia, which causes a reduction in functional residual capacity that is further reduced because of incisional pain. The subsegmental atelectasis may progress to obstruction and inflammation, leading to larger airway obstruction and segmental collapse. Most patients only have a low-grade fever and mild respiratory insufficiency.

CARDIOGENIC PULMONARY EDEMA: Myocardial dysfunction most frequently resulting from ischemia can produce left ventricular dysfunction, fluid overload, and pulmonary interstitial edema. The increase in the amount of interstitial water can cause compression of the bronchovascular structures and additional V/Q mismatches and worsening hypoxia.

PULMONARY EMBOLISM: A major source of morbidity and mortality in surgical patients. The prophylaxis, diagnosis, and treatment of PE are continuous concerns for the surgeon. Bed rest, cancer, and trauma increase the risk of deep vein thrombosis (DVT) and PE. PE can be clinically silent or symptomatic. In high-risk surgical patients, the risk of developing a clinically significant PE is 2% to 3%, and the risk of developing a fatal PE is close to 1%. The clinical hallmarks include acute-onset of hypoxia associated with anxiety leading to tachypnea and hypocarbia, which are often without significant CXR abnormalities.

PULMONARY CONTUSION: Blunt trauma to the chest is a common cause of pulmonary dysfunction resulting from direct parenchymal injury and impaired chest wall function. Injury to the chest wall and ribs can lead to impaired breathing mechanics that range from splinting secondary to pain to disrupted mechanics secondary to a flail chest. The morbidity from lung contusion is attributed to direct parenchymal injury and bronchoalveolar hemorrhage, causing ventilation/perfusion

(V/Q) mismatches and hypoxemia. This condition is worsened by chest wall injury pain, leading to atelectasis in the uninvolved lung.

ACUTE RESPIRATORY DISTRESS SYNDROME (ARDS): This is a severe form of ALI where the PaO_2/FiO_2 is less than 200. The patients generally have decreased oxygen exchange in addition to decreased pulmonary compliance. Pathologically, there is injury to the pulmonary endothelial cells with intense inflammatory responses. In general, the injury is inhomogeneous. Associated with the inflammatory changes are interstitial and alveolar edema, loss of type II pneumocytes, surfactant depletion, intra-alveolar hemorrhage, hyaline membrane deposition, and eventual fibrosis. These changes manifest clinically as severe hypoxia, decreased pulmonary compliance, and increase in dead space ventilation.

VENTILATOR BUNDLE: Consists of a combination of patient care strategies that have been demonstrated to reduce ventilation days, ICU length of stay, and mortality in mechanically ventilated patients. These interventions include: (1) elevation of head of bed; (2) stress ulcer prophylaxis; (3) DVT prophylaxis; (4) daily sedation interruption; (5) daily assessment of readiness for weaning and removal from ventilatory support.

VENTILATOR-INDUCED LUNG INJURY (VILI): Positive-pressure-ventilation-associated mechanical ventilators are capable of producing a variety of injuries to the lungs, and these injuries can occur secondary to over-inflation, overdistension, and repetitive opening and closing of the alveoli. High-oxygen delivery to the lungs can cause oxygen free radical formation and hyperoxic injuries. Ventilation strategies to reduce VILI include: (1) low tidal volume ventilation (5-7 mL/kg tidal volume); (2) reduction of FiO_2 to <60% within 48 to 72 hours; (3) application of positive end expiratory pressure (PEEP) to reduce atelectasis.

CLINICAL APPROACH

Patient Assessment

The initial priority in the management of a patient with acute respiratory distress is to assess and stabilize the ABCs. Prioritizing the ABCs is important, because acute respiratory distress can be a manifestation of a primary pulmonary, cardiac, or a systemic inflammatory/infectious process. The assessment of each patient should be directed at the patient's current status, as well as toward the anticipated condition of the patient. The inability to maintain PaO_2 of 60 mm Hg or an oxygen saturation of 91% with a supplemental nonrebreathing O_2 mask indicates significant alveolar-arterial (A-a) gradient, suggesting that mechanical ventilation should be instituted. An example of a patient with high likelihood of developing future respiratory failure is a patient with ALI who may not require immediate intubation and mechanical ventilatory support because he/she is able to maintain a high level of ventilatory efforts; however, if the condition is believed to be not amendable to immediate correction, the patient will not be able sustain his/her current level of respiratory effort and may benefit from ventilatory support to prevent the onset of respiratory failure at a later time.

In general, the ventilatory status of a patient is assessed based on respiratory rate, and respiratory efforts (use of accessory muscles), and subjective respiratory symptoms. **Hypoventilation** can be recognized by hypercapnia and respiratory acidosis on an arterial blood gas. **Hypoxemia** is detected often on the basis of patient's subjective respiratory complaint, low O_2 saturation by pulse oximetry, and a low PaO_2 on the blood gas. It is important to keep in mind the diagnosis of hypoxemia or hypoventilation should be based on the clinical assessment and a combination of factors, and not be based on a single laboratory parameter or a pulse oximetry reading.

Pathophysiology of Acute Lung Injury

Acute lung injury (ALI) encompasses a spectrum of lung disease from mild forms to severe lung injury or ARDS. The inciting event can be a direct or indirect pulmonary insult (Figure 5–1). The resultant cascade of events includes both cellular and humoral components that produce an inhomogeneous pattern of lung injury. The inflammatory response involves activated polymorphonucleocytes, which generate oxygen free radicals, cytokines, lipid mediators, and nitric oxide. The complement, kinin, coagulation, and fibrinolytic systems are also involved. Endothelial damage ensues with an increase in microvasculature permeability, leading to the accumulation of extravascular lung water, and resulting in diminished lung volume and decreased lung compliance. As the process progresses, lung compliance is further reduced due to sloughing of type I pneumocytes and a decrease in surfactant

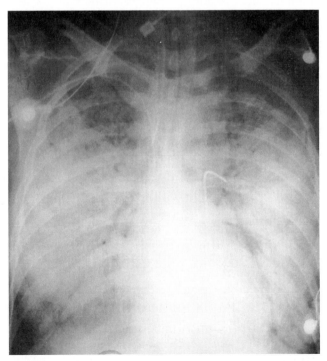

Figure 5–1. Chest radiography revealing the bilateral dense pulmonary infiltrates typical of acute respiratory disease syndrome. *(Reproduced, with permission, from Mattox KL, Feliciano DV, Moore EE, eds. Trauma. 4th ed. New York, NY: McGraw-Hill; 2000:526.)*

production by type II pneumocytes. Later in the process, there is an increase in interstitial edema, alveolar collapse, and lung consolidation. During the prodromal phase of ALI, a patient may simply complain of difficulty in catching their breath, leading to tachypnea. Hypoxia will generally follow as ALI progresses. Hyperventilation is often a key finding in ALI patients, and this is contributed by an increase in V/Q mismatches in the lungs causing increase in dead-space ventilation (leading to the need to increase respiratory effort to eliminate the usual amount of CO_2).

Noninvasive Respiratory Support

Some patients with acute postoperative respiratory insufficiency can be supported with supplemental oxygen therapy or noninvasive respiratory support such as the BIPAP mask. The use of the BIPAP mask provides the patient with some PEEP as well as higher levels of oxygenation than conventional masks. It should be applied with caution in individuals with conditions that are not readily correctable (such as atelectasis or fluid overload). The use of noninvasive ventilatory support is associated with an increase in aspiration events and should not be used in patients who are unable to cooperate or protect their airways effectively.

MECHANICAL VENTILATION MODES

Conventional Ventilation

Conventional ventilation or positive-pressure ventilation fills the lungs by supra-atmospheric pressure applied through an endotracheal tube in the airway. This creates a positive transpulmonary pressure that ensures inflation of the lungs. Exhalation is passive and occurs after the release of positive pressure in the ventilator circuit. The ventilator settings that are applied can be either volume controlled or pressure controlled.

High-Frequency Ventilation

High-frequency ventilation also uses an endotracheal tube to facilitate gas exchange; however, it delivers very small tidal volumes on the order of 1 mL/kg body weight at rates of 100 to 400 breaths/minute. This ventilatory mode has been shown to be beneficial for the support of infants with respiratory distress syndrome; however, the benefits of high-frequency ventilator support in adults are less clear.

Extracorporeal Life Support

Cardiopulmonary bypass of extracorporeal life support uses a heart-lung machine to take over the patient's respiratory and/or cardiac functions. If the cardiac function is adequate, a venovenous bypass circuit can be used to remove CO_2 and oxygenate the blood. As in the case of high-frequency ventilation, the greatest success has been achieved in neonates, and the application of these supportive modes in adults has not been well defined.

CASE CORRELATION

- See also Case 1 (Preoperative Risk Assessment and Optimization).

COMPREHENSION QUESTIONS

5.1 A 57-year-old woman develops acute respiratory distress 7 days following colectomy for adenocarcinoma of the colon. She had been doing well up until this time. The physical examination reveals diminished breath sounds at the lung bases. The CXR reveals atelectasis of the left lower lobe. Which of the following is the most appropriate treatment at this time?

A. Provide supplemental oxygen and chest physiotherapy

B. Provide supplemental oxygen, chest physiotherapy, and empiric antibiotics

C. Provide antibiotics and bronchoscopy to clear the airways

D. Provide supplemental oxygen therapy, obtain venous duplex scan of the lower extremities and CT angiography of the chest, consider empiric heparin therapy until the results of imaging studies are obtained

E. Encourage ambulation

5.2 Diagnostic bronchoscopy is most appropriate for which one of the following patients?

A. A 33-year-old man with right lower lobe hospital-acquired pneumonia

B. A 40-year-old man with AIDS who develops fever, acute respiratory distress, and bilateral pulmonary infiltrates

C. A 66-year-old man with dementia who develops a right upper lobe infiltrate following an episode of aspiration

D. A 30-year-old man with ARDS associated with fever and a loculated right pleural effusion

E. A 63-year-old man with tuberculosis, a right upper lobe cavitary lesion, and hemoptysis

5.3 A 34-year-old woman is hospitalized for septic shock caused by toxic shock syndrome. She is treated with intravenous nafcillins and noted to have hypoxemia. A CXR reveals diffuse infiltrates in bilateral lung fields. Which of the following would most likely differentiate ARDS from cardiogenic pulmonary edema?

A. Pulmonary artery catheter

B. Serum colloid osmotic pressure

C. Urinary electrolytes and partial excretion of sodium

D. V/Q scan

E. Bronchoscopy and bronchoalveolar lavage

5.4 A 46-year-old man suffered multiple rib fractures after sustaining a fall from a horse. He is otherwise healthy and has a one-pack per day smoking history for the past 24 years. Approximately 1 hour after arrival to the emergency center, his breathing appears to have become increasingly labored despite receiving several doses of morphine sulfate for pain. At this time, his respiratory rate is 36 breaths/minute, pulse rate is 120 beats/minute, blood pressure is 160/100 mm Hg, and his pulse oximeter indicates 92% on a 40% facemask. His breath sounds are diminished bilaterally but significantly less audible on the left. Which of the following is the most appropriate treatment at this time?

A. Administer a loop-diuretic

B. Perform endotracheal intubation and initiate mechanical ventilatory support

C. Replace his face mask with a BIPAP mask

D. Obtain an ABG and intubate the patient if his PaO_2 is less than 50 mm Hg or if his $PaCO_2$ is higher than 50 mm Hg

E. Obtain a CXR

5.5 A 34-year-old man slipped and fell in the bathroom at home and struck his anterior neck on the edge of some shelves. When he arrived in the emergency center, he had significant anterior neck pain, soft tissue crepitus, and stridor. The patient was successfully intubated after several difficult attempts. His initial CXR following intubation revealed a properly positioned endotracheal tube, diffuse bilateral nonsegmental infiltrates, and no evidence of pneumothorax or pleural effusion. Which of the following is the most appropriate treatment option at this time?

A. Bronchoscopy to identify the injury to the tracheal-bronchial tree

B. Supportive care including mechanical ventilation and fluid administration

C. Initiate broad spectrum antibiotics for aspiration pneumonia

D. Consult a pulmonologist

E. Extubation

5.6 A 26-year-old man with a gunshot wound to the abdomen underwent exploratory laparotomy and repair of several small bowel and colon injuries. Postoperatively, he is slow to have return of bowel functions and has persistent low urine output. On post-injury day number 9, he is noted to have fever, tachypnea, and tachycardia. During your evaluation of the patient, he complains of difficulty breathing and is noted to have diminished breath sounds bilaterally. His abdomen is distended with absence of bowel sounds. His WBC count is 18,000/mm³. Which of the following is the most appropriate management?

A. CT-angiography of the chest and empiric heparinization

B. Empiric broad-spectrum antibiotics and CT of the abdomen

C. Empiric broad-spectrum antibiotics and heparinization

D. Obtain blood cultures and continue to monitor the patient

E. Antibiotics therapy and re-exploration of the abdomen

ANSWERS

5.1 **D.** Provide supplemental oxygen, initiate a workup for PE, and consider empiric heparinization. This patient has increased risk factors for PE being post-op and with history of malignancy. What increases her probability of PE is that the patient was doing well and developed a sudden onset of respiratory distress.

5.2 **B.** Diagnostic bronchoscopy with bronchoalveolar lavage is indicated in the evaluation of an immunocompromised patient with acute respiratory distress with bilateral pulmonary infiltrates. This procedure is helpful to try to identify possible opportunistic respiratory infections.

5.3 **A.** Pulmonary artery pressures and pulmonary capillary wedge pressure measurements using a pulmonary artery catheter would help determine the patient's left ventricular end-diastolic pressure, and if the pulmonary artery wedge pressure is less than 18 mm Hg, the diagnosis of ARDS is more likely. If the pulmonary wedge pressure is elevated above 18 mm Hg, then cardiogenic pulmonary edema is the more likely diagnosis.

5.4 **E.** The patient's worsening respiratory distress and clinical deterioration can be attributed to several possible processes, including pneumothorax, pulmonary contusion, and atelectasis. An acute change in the patient's respiratory status requires a re-evaluation of the ABCs, which includes diminished bilateral breath sounds bilaterally with less audible breath sounds on the left. A chest x-ray would be very helpful at this point to determine if a pnemothorax is the cause of this problem. Intubation and mechanical ventilation is the right choice if the patient is in impending respiratory failure. ABG results are helpful for the revaluation of some patients with respiratory distress; however, the results in this patient would not help direct therapy. Diuretic therapy is not appropriate for a patient with respiratory distress and hyperdynamic status and no clear evidence of volume overload.

5.5 **B.** This patient's story and findings are highly suggestive of ALI secondary to forced inspiration against a closed or narrowed airway, resulting in "negative pressure pulmonary edema"; negative pressure pulmonary edema is an unusual variant of ALI and is often self-limiting with supportive care that includes mechanical ventilation and judicious fluid management.

5.6 **B.** This man develops fever, tachycardia, and tachypnea 9 days after exploratory laparotomy for GSW to the abdomen with multiple intestinal injuries. With slow return of bowel functions and distension of the abdomen, we should be concerned about the possibility of intra-abdominal sepsis, possibly related to an abscess or an anastamotic breakdown. CT scan plus antibiotics are probably the best option at this time, and exploration plus antibiotics are a second best option.

CLINICAL PEARLS

▶ Acute lung injury and ARDS are associated with increases in dead-space ventilation as there is significant ventilation and perfusion mismatches occurring in various parts of the lungs.

▶ The oxygen saturation should never be used as the sole parameter to determine when a patient should be intubated.

▶ The blood gas results should not be used as the sole criteria for intubation.

▶ Positive pressure ventilation can produce a variety of injuries that are known as VILI (ventilator-induced lung injury).

▶ Excess fluid administration is one of the leading contributors to respiratory distress in the surgical patient.

▶ Failure to terminate fluid resuscitation in patients with hemorrhagic shock and septic shock has been demonstrated to increase the pulmonary-related morbidity and mortality in ventilated patients.

REFERENCES

Malhotra A. Clinical therapeutics, low-tidal-volume ventilation in the acute respiratory distress syndrome. *N Engl J Med.* 2007;357:1113-1120.

Napolitano LM. Postoperative respiratory failure. In: Cameron JL, Cameron AM, eds. *Current Surgical Therapy.* 11th ed. Philadelphia, PA: Elsevier Saunders; 2014: 1219-1230.

The National Heart, Lung, and Blood Institute Acute respiratory Distress Syndrome (ARDS) Clinical Trial Network. Comparison of two fluid-management strategies in acute lung injury. *N Engl J Med.* 2006;354:2564-2575.

A 22-year-old man is brought to the emergency department by paramedics after being involved in a high-speed motor vehicle crash into a tree when his car veered off the highway. The patient apparently fell asleep at the wheel when this event occurred. He was restrained with three-point seatbelts, and the front and side airbags were deployed during the crash. In the emergency department, his blood pressure is 100/80, pulse rate is 114 beats/minute, respiratory rate is 28 breaths/minute, and Glasgow Coma Score (GCS) is 14. His oxygen saturation by pulse oximeter shows 92% saturation on 4 L/minute of O_2 by nasal cannula. The primary survey reveals intact airway, diminished breath sounds on the left, chest wall tenderness, and subcutaneous emphysema over the left anterior and lateral chest wall. The heart sounds are normal and there is no jugular venous distension. The secondary survey reveals no abdominal tenderness, a stable bony pelvis, and no extremity abnormalities. A chest radiograph revealed several rib fractures on the left, a large left-sided pulmonary contusion, a left pneumothorax, and a widening of the mediastinal structures.

▶ What are the most likely diagnoses?
▶ How would you confirm and address the injuries?
▶ What are the likely injuries produced by this motor vehicle accident mechanism?

ANSWERS TO CASE 6:
Chest Trauma (Blunt)

Summary: A 22-year-old man who was the restrained driver was involved in a high speed motor vehicle collision with a tree. He is tachycardic, borderline hypotensive, and tachypneic. Physical examination suggests findings that are compatible with left pneumothorax and rib fractures. The CXR shows a widened mediastinum.

- **Most likely diagnoses:** Blunt chest trauma with rib fractures, pneumothorax, possible pulmonary contusion, and possible blunt thoracic aortic injury.

- **Confirmation of injuries:** Chest radiography will help identify pneumothorax, hemothorax, rib fractures, and pulmonary contusion. CT angiography of the chest will help confirm and provide more details regarding all of the described injuries, in addition to assess for blunt thoracic aorta injury.

- **Injuries produced by his accident mechanism:** A restrained driver involved in a high-speed front end collision is at risk for blunt chest wall injuries, blunt cardiac injuries, pulmonary contusion, blunt abdominal injuries, traumatic brain injury, facial trauma, cervical and thoracic spine injuries, and lower extremity fractures.

ANALYSIS

Objectives

1. Learn the priorities in the treatment of patients with multiple blunt trauma.

2. Learn the diagnosis and treatment of pneumothorax, hemothorax, rib fractures, pulmonary contusion, and blunt thoracic aortic injuries following blunt trauma.

Considerations

The initial assessment of this patient should begin with the airway, breathing, and circulation (ABCs), followed by a secondary survey. Simultaneously, intravenous lines should be placed, blood specimens should be collected, vital signs should be monitored, and supplemental oxygen should be continued and titrated to achieve oxygen saturations >94% to 95%. Given his diminished left-sided breath sounds, chest wall tenderness, and chest wall crepitance, it is reasonable to perform a left tube thoracostomy (chest tube placement) for presumed left pneumothorax. In this patient's case, if a chest radiograph can be obtained quickly, the left tube thoracostomy can be delayed until a confirmatory CXR is obtained. However, a chest x-ray should never be the reason to delay care in a patient with findings compatible with having a pneumothorax. Frequent re-assessment of the patient's cardiopulmonary status is important to make sure that he maintains acceptable oxygenation and perfusion, and responds appropriately to the therapeutic interventions. If the patient's respiratory status worsens after chest tube placement, then intubation and mechanical ventilation should be considered to help restore respiratory stability. After the ABCs are adequately addressed, the patient should under go appropriate imaging to identify all potential injuries.

The evaluation and treatment of this patient is to assess, identify, and address all the injuries that could be produced by the traumatic energy transfer to the patient as the result of the automobile crash.

APPROACH TO:

Blunt Chest Trauma

DEFINITIONS

OCCULT PNEUMOTHORAX: This is a pneumothorax seen on CT scan but not visualized by CXR. This condition is identified in 2% to 10% of blunt trauma patients. A large observational study has reported that if a chest tube is not placed immediately, approximately 6% of the patients with this diagnosis go on to require chest tube placement during the observational period, and patients who require positive-pressure ventilation are more likely to require chest tube placement than those who are not on positive-pressure ventilation.

TENSION PNEUMOTHORAX: A pneumothorax that has increased in size to the point of causing a decrease in venous return to the heart and the potential for hypotension and cardiac arrest. Tension pneumothorax is a clinical diagnosis, but X-ray may reveal a shift of the mediastinal structures to the opposite side of the chest, and with shifting of the mediastinal structures.

PULMONARY CONTUSION: Lung parenchymal injury that occurs most commonly after high-energy blunt trauma to the chest. In most patients, the pulmonary contusions are associated with rib fractures or flail chest involving the overlying chest wall. Areas of the lung with pulmonary contusions are susceptible to capillary leakage and secondary inflammatory injuries, which can be made worse by pulmonary edema; therefore, excessive fluid administration should be avoided during the management of these patients.

FLAIL CHEST: Injury to the chest wall that causes a segment of the chest wall to become disrupted from the remaining chest wall. In all cases, this is associated with rib fractures that occur in more than one location, leading to that chest wall segment to move independently from the rest of the chest during respiration.

BLUNT DIAPHRAGMATIC INJURY: Rupture of the diaphragm can occur with high-energy blunt trauma to the chest and/or abdomen. This type of injury is more common on the left side. Rib fractures are commonly associated injuries.

COMPUTED TOMOGRAPHY ANGIOGRAPHY (CTA): CTA is a CT imaging technique obtained with the administration of intravenous contrast. This imaging sequence is designed to optimally assess arterial anatomy. The CTA is currently the

Table 6–1 • CAUSES OF INSTABILITY AFTER BLUNT CHEST TRAUMA	
Injury	Treatment
Tension pneumothorax	Tube thoracostomy Needle decompression
Hemothorax	Tube thoracostomy resuscitation Possible exploration, repair
Cardiac tamponade	Decompression (open, needle) Exploration repair
Blunt cardiac injury	Supportive care (inotropes); operative repair for cardiac rupture
Air emboli	Exploration, repair
Injury to great vessels	Exploration, repair or repair via endovascular approach

"gold standard" for the detection of blunt thoracic aortic injuries. The advantage of modern CTA techniques is that three-dimensional reconstructions can be rendered to visualize even minor abnormalities.

CLINICAL APPROACH

Blunt chest injuries are identified in 30% to 50% of patients with multiple blunt trauma, with motor vehicle crashes, fall from height, and automobile versus pedestrian crashes being some of the most common injury mechanisms. The approach to patients with multiple blunt traumas prioritizes the diagnosis and management of injuries in the sequence and time frame that are appropriate for the various injuries. A simple question to ask is: "What will kill the patient first?" and then address those issues first. **Tension pneumothorax, massive hemothorax, blunt cardiac injury, and thoracic aortic disruption are the leading causes of early death associated with blunt chest injuries.**

Rib fractures are common injuries that can be identified clinically based on focal tenderness by palpation, by plain radiography, or by CT imaging. Rib fracture diagnosis is important not only because these injuries can be a source of morbidity, in that the pain and discomfort associated with the fractures can lead to decreased respiratory efforts, splinting, and decrease mobility causing atelectasis, hypoxia, and pulmonary infections. Another important concern is the potential for injuries to structures beneath the ribs. For example, the presence of left lower rib fractures should raise our clinical suspicion for injuries to the spleen. Rib fracture diagnosis should raise our suspicion for associated conditions including pulmonary contusion, pneumothorax, and hemothorax. The presence of two or more rib fractures in patients over the age 45 has been reported to be associated with morbidity and even mortality. Therefore, older individuals with rib fractures should be recognized as patients who are at risk of developing complications, and admission to the hospital for pain control, monitoring, and chest physiotherapy is generally indicated. Pain control for patients with rib fractures is of critical importance, and this can be accomplished either with placement of epidural catheter or by patient controlled analgesia (PCA).

Sternal fracture in blunt trauma patients is not common. Patients with sternal fractures identified in the setting of multisystem injuries often have rib fractures, pneumothoraces, hemothoraces, and pulmonary contusion. Patients with isolated sternal fractures from blunt trauma do not have an increased risk of pulmonary injuries or cardiac injuries; therefore, many patients with isolated sternal fractures can be safely managed as outpatients.

Pneumothorax in the setting of blunt trauma is most commonly produced by disruption of the visceral pleura with the majority of injuries created by rib penetration or from direct impact causing disruption of the lung parenchyma. Patients with small and relatively asymptomatic pneumathorax can be treated with supplemental oxygen and monitored with repeat chest x-rays. It is important to monitor the patients with pneumothorax who are managed without chest tube placement, because simple pneumothorax will occasionally progress into tension pneumothorax. A symptomatic patient or a patient with a large pneumothorax should be treated with the placement of chest tube (tube thoracostomy) to help re-expand the lung and facilitate closure of the air leak. Following chest tube placement, the patient should be monitored for air leak and drainage volume. Most patients with chest tube placement will have resolution of the pneumothorax and can have chest tube removal about 48 hours after resolution of the pneumothorax. **If there is persistent large air leak and/or failure of lung re-expansion with the chest tube attached to suction, the possibility of a major tracheobronchial injury must be considered.** Recognition of this condition is important because patients with major tracheobronchial injuries may require operative treatments.

Hemothorax describes the accumulation of blood in the pleural cavity. Bleeding into the pleural space can range from minor self-limiting events to massive life-threatening processes. Hemothorax symptoms are related to the amount of blood accumulation. Blunt trauma-related hemothorax is diagnosed by chest x-ray, which demonstrates opacification of the involved hemithorax. Each pleural space can accommodate up to 3000 mL of fluid. Because the pleural spaces are potential sites for significant blood losses, all blunt trauma patients with the potential of having multiple injuries should have CXRs performed to look for potential bleeding in the pleural spaces. Patients who are hemodynamically unstable with large hemothoraces and no other sources of blood loss should undergo thoracotomy for control of bleeding. Similarly, most practitioners believe that **strong considerations for surgical treatment should also be given to patients with greater than 1500 mL of initial output with chest tube placement and patients with greater than 200 mL/h bloody output for 4 or more hours.**

Retained hemothorax is a problem that occurs in a small percentage of patients following chest tube placement for traumatic hemothorax. Some of the patients with retained hemothorax can go on to develop empyema and fibrothorax. Surgical evacuation is indicated for patients with large retained hemothoraces; whereas, most patients with less than 300 mL of retained hemothorax can be safely observed.

Blunt cardiac injury (BCI) is the cause of death in 45% to 76% of the victims who die following blunt trauma. Patients with BCI often have multiple injuries, including traumatic brain injury, thoracic aortic injuries, lung injuries, chest wall injuries, and vertebral injuries. The spectrum of BCI encountered in clinical practices can range from self-limiting sinus tachycardia, supraventricular tachycardia, and ventricular arrhythmias (rare), to the less common presentations of pump failure and cardiac rupture. The Eastern Association of Surgery for Trauma Guidelines published in 2012 recommended that an admission ECG be performed on all patients in whom blunt cardiac injuries are suspected (level 1 evidence), and that patients with new ECG abnormalities should undergo monitoring for cardiac rhythm or pump abnormalities for 24 hours (level 2 evidence). Most practitioners agree that if the initial ECG is normal and a serum troponin I is <0.4 ng/mL, the patient with suspected BCI can be safely discharged from the emergency center (level 2b evidence).

Traumatic rupture of the aorta (TRA) is the second leading cause of death from blunt trauma (traumatic brain injury is number 1). TRA should be suspected based on patients' injury mechanisms, with high-energy MVC and motorcycle crashes (MCC), auto-versus-pedestrian crashes, and fall from heights being the most common. The abnormalities observed on CXR in these patients include a left apical cap, mediastinal widening, obscured aortic knob, widening of the paravertebral stripe, downward deviation of the left mainstem bronchus, rightward deviation of the NG tube, and opacification of the aorto-pulmonary window. It is important to note that "normal CXR" has been reported in 7% to 13% of the patients with TRA. In the past, patients with suspected TRA underwent aortography for confirmation of injuries; however, CT-angiography (CTA) is now the preferred method of diagnosis of TRA. TRAs can range in severity from minimal intimal tears (<1 cm tear with minimal or no contrast extravasation), contained ruptures, to free-ruptures. Management choices for TRAs include conservative treatment,

Table 6–2 • ASSESSMENT OF CASE NO. 6's INJURIES, DIAGNOSIS, AND TREATMENT

Injury	Diagnosis	Treatment	Comment
Rib fractures	PE, chest radiograph rib series	Conservative, pain management; surgical plating if altered chest wall mechanics	Possible harbinger for other injuries, goal → pain control (epidural anesthesia) to prevent hypoventilation and associated pulmonary complications
Pneumothorax	PE, chest radiograph	Tube thoracostomy	Should achieve full re-expansion Failure to re-expand or persistent air leak → consider major tracheobronchial injury
Pulmonary contusion	Chest radiograph, CT scan	Supportive care with or without intubation	Ventilatory support on clinical grounds
Traumatic aortic rupture	CT angiography, TEE, aortography (much less commonly used)	Urgent repair by either open repair or endovascular repair	See Figure 6–1

Abbreviations: CT, computed tomography; PE, physical examination; TEE, transesophageal echocardiography.

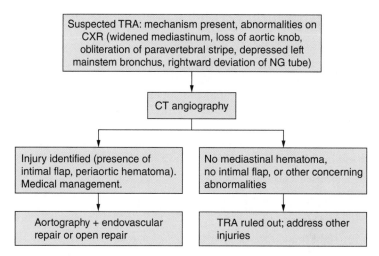

Figure 6–1. Diagnostic strategy for patients suspected of traumatic rupture of the aorta. NG, nasogastric. (Reproduced, with permission, from Mattox KL, Feliciano DV, Moore E. *Trauma*, 4th ed. New York: McGraw-Hill, 2000:562.)

thoracic endovascular aortic repairs (TEVARs), and open repairs. Treatment selection is mainly determined by the patient's clinical conditions, aortic injury type and severity, as well as patient co-morbidities and associated injuries. **All patients with TRAs should be initially managed with controlled hypotension to maintain a systolic BP of 100 mm Hg** until definitive repair or continued medical therapy is instituted. TEVARs are associated with lower rates of procedural-related complications; therefore in most centers, TEVARs have replaced open repairs as the preferred treatment approach.

CASE CORRELATION

- See also Case 8 (Hemorrhagic Shock [Trauma]) and Case 9 (Penetrating Abdominal Trauma).

COMPREHENSION QUESTIONS

6.1 An 18-year-old man is admitted to the intensive care unit for multiple blunt trauma approximately 12 hours ago. His injuries include bilateral femur fractures. He is noted to be confused and appears to have difficulties catching his breath. The pulse oximeter reads O_2 saturation of 93% with the administration of 100% oxygen by face mask. His lungs are clear bilaterally. His chest x-ray reveals clear lung fields bilaterally and a normal cardiac silhouette. Which of the following is the most likely cause of his clinical picture?

A. Pulmonary contusion

B. Occult pneumothorax

C. ICU psychosis

D. Fat embolism

E. Atelectasis

6.2 A 43-year-old man was involved in a motorcycle crash when the bike slipped on wet pavement and he hit a tree. In the emergency center, he is noted to have multiple rib fractures, a right tibia fracture, and left forearm fractures. During monitoring in the emergency center, he is found to have a brief period (3 minutes) of supraventricular tachycardia that resolved spontaneously. Which of the following is the most likely etiology for this rhythm abnormality?

A. Anxiety disorder

B. Fat embolism

C. Blunt cardiac injury

D. Caffeine-induced arrhythmias

E. Pain

6.3 Which of the following radiographic abnormalities seen on CXR is suggestive of traumatic rupture of the aorta (TRA)?

A. Pneumomediastinum

B. Sternal fracture

C. Enlarged cardiac silhouette

D. Widen mediastinum

E. Right-sided diaphragmatic rupture

6.4 A 36 year-old man is brought to the emergency department from the scene of a motor vehicle crash. He is found unconscious and is intubated in the field. Soon after intubation, he becomes hypotensive and is noted to have diminished right sided breath sounds leading to right needle thoracostomy that improved his blood pressure. In the emergency center, he is noted to have extensive subcutaneous emphysema in the neck and throughout the entire chest area. There is a moderate amount of blood in the endotracheal tube. A 40 French chest tube is placed on the right side. A subsequent CXR reveals a large right pneumothorax with proper chest tube positioning. The patient now has a large amount of air leakage associated with the right chest tube. His oxygen saturation on 100% FiO_2 is 89%. What is the best treatment at this time?

A. Perform bilateral thoracotomy and a laparotomy

B. Perform a bronchoscopy

C. Place an additional chest tube on the right

D. Place bilateral chest tubes

E. Perform a right thoracotomy

6.5 A 33-year-old woman is brought to the emergency center after a high-speed head-on collision with another car traveling in the opposite direction. She is noted to be hemodynamically stable with tenderness over the anterior chest. The CXR is normal. She undergoes CT scan evaluation of the brain, chest, abdomen and pelvis, where a 10% left pneumothorax is observed. After CT, she remains comfortable with respiratory rate of 24 and O_2 saturation of 97% on room air. What of the following is the best treatment for her condition?

A. Supplemental oxygen and continued observation

B. Left chest needle catheter placement

C. Left chest tube placement

D. Hyperbaric treatment

E. Thoracoscopic repair of lung injury

6.6 A 32-year-old man is brought to the emergency center from the scene of an automobile crash. He was unconscious at the scene and had witnessed bouts of emesis prompting orotracheal intubation in the field. At the time of his arrival to the emergency center, his pulse rate is 78, BP is 130/74, and GCS is 8T. His breath sounds are diminished on the left. His CXR in the emergency department revealed opacification of the left hemithorax with shifting of the mediastinum to the left. Which of the following is the best treatment for this condition?

A. Placement of 40 French chest tube on the left

B. Placement of 40 French chest tube on the right

C. Placement of bilateral chest tubes

D. Assess and adjust endotracheal tube position

E. Extubate the patient

6.7   A construction worker falls off a second story roof. He is brought to the emergency center. His blood pressure is 120/74, pulse is 100, respiratory rate is 22, and GCS is 14. His completed evaluation in the emergency center revealed a grade 2 splenic laceration with a small amount of fluid in the left upper quadrant. He also has six minimally-displaced rib fractures on the left, associated with flail chest and pulmonary contusion involving nearly 70% of the left lower lobe. The patient weighs approximately 70 kg. Which of the following is the most appropriate initial treatment for this patient?

A.   Supplemental O_2, lactated Ringers (LR) at 125 mL/h, morphine sulfate 4 mg intravenous push every 4 hours as needed

B.   Initial bolus of 1000 mL of lactated Ringers followed by 125 mL/h, morphine sulfate by patient controlled anesthesia pump (PCA), supplemental O_2

C.   Lactated ringers at 80 mL/h, morphine by PCA, supplemental O_2, oral ketoralac q6 h prn, supplemental O_2

D.   Operative fixation of the rib fractures, mechanical ventilation, LR at 80 mL/h, morphine by PCA, intravenous ketoralac

E.   Mechanical positive pressure ventilation, LR at 80 mL/h, morphine by PCA, and intravenous ketoralac

ANSWERS

6.1   **D.** 18-year-old man with multiple blunt trauma including femur fractures develops hypoxia and respiratory distress. His lungs are clear bilaterally and his CXR is relatively normal. There are several possible explanations for his current clinical condition. Fat embolism and acute pulmonary embolism are the two most likely causes of respiratory distress that are associated with normal breath sounds and relatively normal CXR. Occult pneumothorax can have a normal CXR but is unlikely to produce respiratory compromise to this extent. Pulmonary contusion is generally associated with CXR opacification. ICU psychosis can cause confusion and anxiety but does not cause hypoxemia. Similarly, atelectasis can cause hypoxemia but the condition is often associated with CXR findings.

6.2   **C.** This man has multiple injuries secondary to a motorcycle crash. He has developed a brief period of supraventricular tachycardia (SVT) that has spontaneously resolved. Given his recent major injury mechanism and multiple rib fractures, the period of supraventricular arrhythmia is likely due to blunt cardiac injury. Pain and anxiety disorder can cause sinus tachycardia but not SVT. Caffeine can cause some arrythmias but the SVT should not be attributed to that given the significant injuries that this patient has. Fat embolism is not often associated with any specific cardiac rhythm abnormalities.

6.3 **D.** Widened mediastinum along with left apical cap, obscured aortic knob, widening of the paravertebral stripe, downward deviation of the left mainstem bronchus, opacification of the aorto-pulmonary window, and rightward deviation of the NG tube are the CXR abnormalities associated with traumatic rupture of the aorta (TRA).

6.4 **E.** This man has extensive blunt chest injuries. Following intubation and the initiation of positive pressure ventilation, he develops tension pneumothorax on the right. With pleural decompression, the patient develops a large right-sided air leak and subcutaneous emphysema. He has persistence of right pneumothorax despite tube thoracostomy. At this time, he is becoming hypoxic from the air leakage and blood in the airway. His current findings and clinical course can be explained on the basis that he very likely has a major right sided bronchial injury, which should be treated by a right thoracotomy and repair of the airway injury. If the injury is more proximally located in the trachea, the incision can be extended by a median sternotomy to gain access to the trachea. Choice "A" is not chosen because he does not have an indication for a laparotomy.

6.5 **A.** This 33-year-old woman has an occult left pneumothorax following blunt chest trauma. Her pneumothorax is not seen by CXR and is only detected by CT scan. Observations from a large cohort of patients with occult pneumothoraces suggest that only 6% of the patients will develop worsening of the condition leading to chest tube placement. Patients on positive-pressure ventilation are at increased risk for this progression. The patient described here is comfortable, not in respiratory distress, and not on positive-pressure ventilation; therefore, close observation is appropriate.

6.6 **D.** This 32-year-old man is victim of a car crash who was intubated in the field because he was unconscious and vomiting. In the emergency center, his breath sounds are diminished on the left. The CXR obtained in the emergency center shows opacification of the left lung field with shifting of the mediastinum toward the left. These findings are compatible with either right mainstem bronchus intubation or a left bronchus obstructive process leading to collapse of the left lung and loss of left lung volume. It is reasonable to examine the CXR closely to see the position of the endotracheal tube, and if the tube appears to be too far in, we should adjust the position of the tube. Opacification of the hemithorax can also be caused by blood in that pleural space; however, if that were the case, there should not be a shift of the mediastinal structures toward the side of opacification.

6.7 **C.** This is a patient with splenic laceration, multiple rib fractures, flail chest, and a large pulmonary contusion. The management of this patient can be complicated, because he may need additional fluid/blood products for blood losses related to his splenic trauma, but at the same time his pulmonary contusion/flail chest would be better managed with relative fluid restriction and sufficient pain control. Because his blood pressure appears to be within normal range at this time, the choice selected offers a relatively low maintenance fluid rate, narcotic analgesia, and NSAID for pain control. The use of positive ventilatory support had been the corner stone of flail chest management in the 1970s to 1980s, but it is no longer applied routinely except when patients develop respiratory failure and need mechanical ventilatory support.

CLINICAL PEARLS

▶ Understanding amount of energy absorbed by the injured victim is helpful in the diagnosis and management of blunt trauma victims.

▶ The approach to chest trauma is to prioritize the diagnosis and treatment of injuries that will kill the patient first: tension pneumothorax, hemothorax, and pericardial tamponade.

▶ A widened mediastinum on chest radiograph in a patient with blunt chest trauma, including rapid deceleration injury should raise the suspicion for TRA.

▶ TRA can occur in patients with chest x-rays that do not demonstrate a widened mediastinum.

▶ The identification of two or more rib fractures in a patient with blunt trauma should prompt evaluation for other associated injuries, including pneumothorax, hemothorax, and pulmonary contusion.

▶ Patients with fractures of the left lower ribs are at risk for having blunt injury to the spleen.

▶ Blunt injury to the diaphragm should be considered in all patients with multiple rib fractures secondary to blunt trauma.

▶ CT angiography is the preferred method of diagnosis for TRA.

▶ Endovascular repair of TRA has emerged as the preferred method of repair for critically ill patients with this injury.

REFERENCES

Biffl WL. Thoracic trauma. In: Vincent JL, Abraham E, Moore FA, Kochanek PM, Fink MP, eds. *Textbook of Critical Care.* 6th ed. Philadelphia, PA: Elsevier Saunders; 2011: 1509-1517.

Coimbra R, Hoyt DB. Chest wall trauma, hemothorax, and pneumothorax. In: Cameron JL, Cameron AM, eds. *Current Surgical Therapy.* 11th ed. Philadelphia, PA: Elsevier Saunders; 2014: 1005-1009.

De Lesquen, H, Avaro J-P, Gust L, et al. Surgical management for the first 48 h following blunt chest trauma: state of the art (excluding vascular injuries). *Interactive Cardiovasc Thor Surg*. 2015;20: 399-408.

Estrera AL, Miller III CC, Guajardo-Salinas G, et al. Update on blunt thoracic aortic injury: fifteen-year single-institution experience. *J Thor Cardivasc Surg*. 2013;145:S154-S159.

Yousef R, Carr JA. Blunt cardiac trauma: a review of the current knowledge and management. *Ann Thorac Surg*. 2014;98:1134-1140.

A 23-year-old man was the restrained driver of an automobile involved in a high-speed head-on collision with an 18-wheeler that drifted across the highway divider. According to the paramedics, the front-seat passenger in the patient's vehicle was found dead at the scene. Extrication of the patient required approximately 30 minutes. His vital signs at the scene were pulse rate of 110 beats/minute, blood pressure of 90/60 mm Hg, respiratory rate of 14 breaths/minute, and Glasgow Coma Score (GCS) of 6. The paramedics performed endotracheal intubation, placed peripheral intravenous lines and initiated ventilation and fluid administration during transport to the hospital. His vital signs on arrival at the trauma center include a temperature of 36.2°C (97.2°F), pulse rate of 112 beats/minute, blood pressure of 88/70 mm Hg, assisted respiratory rate of 20 breaths/minute, and a GCS of 6T (M4, V1T, E1). A forehead hematoma and laceration is visible, and the patient also has multiple facial lacerations with bony deformity of the left cheek. The breath sounds are diminished on the left, and there is soft tissue crepitance in the left anterior chest wall. The abdomen is distended, with diminished bowel sounds. The bony pelvis is stable to palpation. Examination of the extremities reveal markedly swollen and deformed left thigh with a 10-cm laceration over the left knee. The peripheral pulses are present in all the extremities. No spontaneous movements of the lower extremities are noted.

▶ What should be the next steps in this patient's treatment?
▶ What are the most likely mechanisms causing this patient's current clinical picture?

ANSWERS TO CASE 7:

Blunt Trauma (Multiple)

Summary: A 23-year-old restrained driver has sustained multiple injuries follow-ing a high-speed front-end motor vehicle collision with a truck. He presents with tachycardia, hypotension, and a GCS of 6. The patient's initial assessment suggests the following injuries: traumatic brain injury, facial fractures, left pneumothorax, intra-abdominal injuries, and left femur fracture. The exact cause of the hypoten-sion is unclear at this time, but should be presumed to be hypovolemia until proven otherwise.

- **Next steps:** Placement of a left chest tube (tube thoracostomy) should be per-formed to address the suspected left pneumothorax, which should improve his ventilation and hypotension.

- **Likely responsible mechanisms:** The possible causes of the tachycardia, hypo-tension, and unresponsiveness in this patient include hemorrhagic shock, left tension pneumothorax, neurogenic shock, primary cardiac dysfunction, and severe traumatic brain injury (TBI).

ANALYSIS

Objectives

1. Learn the priorities and principles in the treatment of patients with multiple injuries, including blunt chest injuries, abdominal trauma, TBI, orthopedic injuries, and possible spinal cord injury.

2. Learn to recognize the causes of hemodynamic instability in a trauma patient and learn the methods of diagnosis for these problems.

Considerations

This young man is brought in with injuries sustained in a high-speed front-end collision MVC. He is hypotensive, tachycardic and has a GCS of 6. Clinically, his examination is suspicious for left pneumothorax, facial fractures, and a left femur fracture. Intubation, oxygenation, and ventilation are important for a patient with high likelihood of having severe TBI. With the findings of diminished left sided breath sounds and crepitance (subcutaneous emphysema) in the left chest wall, it is highly likely that the patient has a left pneumothorax and possibly a tension pneumothorax; therefore, immediate pleural decompression with chest tube place-ment is reasonable without first obtaining a CXR. Following chest tube placement, it is important to note if the patient's breathing and circulation statuses improve with the intervention. If the breath sounds improve and blood pressure remain low, the next step would be to perform a focused abdominal sonography for trauma (FAST) to determine if intra-abdominal hemorrhage is the cause of the hypoten-sion. If the FAST reveals intraperitoneal free fluid, this unstable patient should be immediately taken to the OR for exploration and control of bleeding with an abbreviated laparotomy so that a CT of the brain can be obtained immediately following the control of intra-abdominal bleeding. If the FAST does not reveal evidence of pericardial effusion or intra-abdominal free fluid, we should then presume that the source of low blood pressure is due to blood loss secondary to his lacerations, facial fractures, and long bone fractures. Transfusion with blood products to help support the blood pressure is a reasonable initial treatment in this patient with suspected TBI, as the combination of TBI and hypotension contribute to worsening of TBI. Once the patient's blood pressure is improved with blood products, our next priority would be to perform CT evaluation of the brain to further assess his traumatic brain injury. In many institutions, a pan-CT scan (brain, face, c-spine, chest, abdomen, and pelvis CT) would be performed to identify all the potential injuries and allow prioritization of management. In general, the priorities of injury management go from addressing injuries that affect oxygenation/ventilation, to blood loss, to bony injuries. A possibility of his hypotension is caused by neurogenic shock (from high spinal cord injury) must be considered as the patient has not been witnessed to move his lower extremities following his injuries. Although neurogenic shock is a possibility, the patient's current clinical picture is not exactly consistent with that diagnosis, due to his tachycardia.

APPROACH TO:
Multiple Blunt Trauma

DEFINITIONS:

FOCUSED ABDOMINAL SONOGRAPHY FOR TRAUMA (FAST): A quick ultrasound examination performed at the completion of the primary survey, designed to detect pericardial effusion and intra-abdominal free fluid. Four separate areas are evaluated, including the *pericardial space, right upper quadrant subhepatic space, left upper quadrant perisplenic space,* and *pelvis.* The FAST is especially helpful for evaluation of the hemodyamically unstable, multiple trauma patient.

DIAGNOSTIC PERITONEAL LAVAGE (DPL): The DPL is a bedside diagnostic procedure performed during the secondary survey in unstable patients to help identify intraperitoneal bleeding as the cause of the hypotension. Positive results can be based on aspiration of >10 mL of blood or enteric contents from the peritoneal cavity. If no blood is aspirated, a liter of warm saline is infused into the peritoneal cavity through a catheter and then retrieved for cell count analysis. A microscopic positive lavage is WBC count >500 cells/mm^3 or RBC count of >100,000 cells/mm^3. The DPL is highly sensitive in identifying intraperitoneal bleeding; unfortunately, this study lacks specificity. In hemodynamically stable, blunt trauma patient with positive DPLs, the laparotomies can be nontherapeutic in up to 30% of the patients. Because of increased utility of the FAST, DPLs are less commonly used today.

ABDOMINAL CT SCAN: A sensitive, specific diagnostic modality for solid organ injuries, retroperitoneal injuries, and peritoneal fluid in the blunt trauma setting.

Because of the time requirement for completion and the need for patient transportation to an uncontrolled environment, CT imaging is contraindicated for unstable trauma patients.

PAN-CT SCAN: In most institutions, the Pan-scan includes CT imaging of the brain, c-spine, chest, abdomen, and pelvis. The use of the pan-scan was originally introduced in Europe and has been proven in many European trauma centers to help identify and triage the multiple injured patients. Pan-scan application is increasing in North American trauma centers.

CLINICAL APPROACH

The initial treatment begins with **a primary survey consisting of airway (A), breathing (B), circulation (C), and D (disability) assessment** and optimization that are commonly referred to as the ABCs. The primary survey focuses on immediate life-threatening problems, which should be promptly identified and treated. Once the ABCs are addressed satisfactorily, a **secondary survey** is conducted via a head-to-toe examination and inventory of all injuries. Nasogastric tube and urinary catheters if needed are placed at the end of the secondary survey. In the multiple injured patient, an AP chest x-ray and an AP pelvis x-ray can be helpful to identify conditions that may need immediate attention. For patients who are stable and without injuries in the chest or abdomen that require immediate attention, the next step would be to obtain CT evaluations to rule-out TBI, spine injuries, intrathoracic and intra-abdominal injuries. Whenever a trauma patient experiences a significant change in clinical condition, a thorough evaluation that begins with re-evaluation of the ABCs should be done to identify the cause of the clinical deterioration. If a patient has ongoing bleeding, TBI, and orthopedic injuries, the bleeding source needs to be addressed first prior to addressing the TBI, and lastly the orthopedic injuries. Generally, the treatment of major orthopedic injuries not associated with significant bleeding can be delayed until an initial period of stabilization for 24 to 48 hours. Many hemodynamically stable patients with hemoperitoneum, liver, spleen, or kidney injuries can be successfully managed by nonoperative management with close monitoring.

CASE CORRELATION

- See also Case 6 (Blunt Chest Trauma), Case 7 (Multiple Blunt Trauma), and Case 8 (Hemorrhagic Shock [Trauma]).

COMPREHENSION QUESTIONS

7.1 Which of the following statements is accurate regarding the use of the Pan-CT scan?

   A. Pan-scans are routinely useful for all trauma patients including those with penetrating trauma

   B. Pan-scan allows rapid triage and identification of injuries in the unstable trauma patients

   C. Pan-scan consists of CT of the brain, c-spine, chest, abdomen, and pelvis

   D. Pan-scan is contraindicated in young adults due to the increased risk of radiation induced malignancies

   E. Pan-scan is helpful when FAST examination is not available

7.2 Which of the following factors is most likely to contribute to a worse outcome in a patient with a left subdural hematoma and a GCS of 9?

   A. Blood pressure of 70/50 mm Hg recorded for approximately 10 minutes prior to arrival to the hospital

   B. A right epidural hematoma

   C. Depressed skull fracture

   D. Pelvic fracture

   E. A 10% pneumothorax

7.3 A 32-year-old man is brought to the emergency center after having been stuck by a large branch that broke off a tree and hit the patient on the right side of his head and his right chest area. He is noted in the emergency department to have a large right parietal scalp hematoma, right cheek deformity, and right chest wall deformity associated with diminished right sided breath sounds. His pulse rate is 110 beats/minute, blood pressure is 120/70 mm Hg, respiratory rate is 30 breaths/minute, and GCS is 13. Which of the following is the most appropriate next step?

   A. Endotracheal intubation

   B. Right chest tube placement

   C. CT of the brain

   D. FAST

   E. Repair of the scalp laceration

7.4 A 40-year-old unrestrained man was the driver of a car that crashed into a tree when his car apparently veered of the road. He was brought to the emergency center, and after his initial resuscitation and evaluation, he is found to have multiple superficial scalp lacerations, a left subdural hematoma with no associated midline shift, and a GCS of 14. A 60% left pneumothorax was noted on CXR, and left tibia and fibula fractures with diminished left pedal pulses are noted. Which of the following is the most appropriate sequence of prioritization for this patient's injuries?

A. Brain injury, pneumothorax, lower extremity injuries, and facial lacerations

B. Pneumothorax, lower extremity injuries, facial lacerations, and brain injury

C. Pneumothorax, lower extremity injuries, brain injury, and facial lacerations

D. Brain injury, lower extremity injuries, pneumothorax, and facial lacerations

E. Pneumothorax, brain injury, lower extremity injuries, and facial lacerations

7.5 A 34-year-old man was an unrestrained passenger in a high-speed MVC and sustained fractured femur as well as blunt abdominal trauma. After stabilization of the patient, the trauma team ordered a CT scan of the abdomen. Which of the following statements is true regarding CT of the abdomen for blunt trauma evaluation?

A. It is costly and time consuming and should not be used when the FAST or DPL is available

B. Highly sensitive and specific for solid organ injury identification but lacks sensitivity for retroperitoneal injury identification

C. Highly sensitive and specific for solid organ identification but lacks sensitivity and specificity for hollow viscous injury identification

D. Highly sensitive and specific for solid-organ injuries and intraperitoneal blood identification, and useful for both stable and unstable patients

E. CT is not indicated when patients have no abnormalities on the abdominal examination

7.6 A 73-year-old man is seen after falling down a flight of stairs. He arrives on a backboard with C-collar in place. His initial pulse rate is 70 beats/minute, blood pressure is 160/80 mm Hg, respiratory rate is 10 breaths/minute, and GCS is 6. He has a large scalp hematoma, dilated and nonreactive left pupil, and a large bruise over his left flank. Which of the following is the most appropriate treatment?

A. O_2 by face mask, intravenous fluids, obtain a pan-CT scan, and request a neurosurgery consultation

B. Endotracheal intubation, intravenous fluids, obtain a CT of the brain and abdomen, and obtain a neurosurgical consultation

C. Endotracheal intubation, intravenous fluids, FAST examination, perform a bedside left decompressive craniotomy

D. Endotracheal intubation, request a neurosurgical consultation, transfer the patient to the operating room for a decompressive craniectomy

E. Endotracheal intubation, intravenous fluids, perform a FAST examination, CT of the brain, and neurosurgical consultation

ANSWERS

7.1 **C.** Pan-CT scan for trauma in most institutions consists of CT of brain, c-spine, chest, abdomen, and pelvis. The use of pan-scans has been shown to help rapid triage of multiple-injured blunt trauma patients. CT is not a safe place for unstable patients; therefore, the pan-scan is not advisable for the evaluation of hemodynamically unstable patients. The pan-scan is not intended to replace the FAST examination.

7.2 **A.** Persistent hypotension in a patient with TBI contributes to secondary brain injury and worse neurologic outcomes.

7.3 **B.** This is a patient with possible TBI (Mild based on GCS of 13), and blunt right-sided chest trauma with physical examination findings that are suspicious for right pneumothorax or hemothorax. Because his GCS suggests that his TBI is not the major issue at this point, endotracheal intubation is not indicated. Placement of a right chest tube should be the first intervention to try to improve his breathing.

7.4 **E.** This man was the driver involved in an MVC with multiple injuries, including a left subdural hematoma with no midline shift and a GCS of 14, a 60% left pneumothorax, left tibia/fibula fracture with possible compromised circulation to the left foot, and scalp lacerations. The prioritization of his injuries management goes from treatment of the pneumothorax with chest tube placement, to supportive care and monitoring of his TBI, to reduction of the fractured left lower extremity to improve the circulatory status to the left lower extremity, to repair of his superficial scalp lacerations.

7.5 **C.** CT scan of the abdomen is highly sensitive and specific for solid organ injuries identification as well as retroperitoneal injuries identification. CT lacks sensitivity or specificity for hollow viscous injury identification. CT is not recommended for the evaluation of hemodynamically unstable patients.

7.6 **E.** This is a 73-year-old man who fell down a flight of stairs and presents with signs and symptoms compatible with having severe TBI with GCS of 6 and some evidence of left hemispheric mass effect leading to left papillary dilatation. Intubation and ventilation is important for this patient to minimize secondary brain injury. A FAST is helpful to rule-out significant blood loss given the finding of left flank bruising. It is critical to obtain a CT of the brain and at the same time alert the neurosurgeon that the patient may need emergency decompressive craniectomy.

CLINICAL PEARLS

▶ Airway, breathing, and circulation should be reassessed whenever clinical deterioration develops in a trauma patient.

▶ Obtaining a detailed description of the traumatic event helps identify the injury mechanism and direct the evaluation process.

▶ TBI is rarely the cause of hemodynamic instability in a trauma patient; therefore, the evaluation should be directed toward identification of a bleeding source or mechanical source (such as tension pneumothorax).

▶ A low GCS in a patient with profound shock may result from inadequate brain perfusion, and the usual sequence of approach should not be altered.

▶ The CT scan is a valuable tool for the assessment of hemodynamically stable patients; however, obtaining a CT scan in a hemodynamically unstable patient can contribute to delays in addressing the cause of hypotension.

▶ Physical examination of the abdomen in a patient with multiple blunt trauma can be limited as the result of *distracting injuries* (such as rib fractures and long-bone fractures) or *altered sensorium* (due to TBI, alcohol intoxication, or other illicit substance influence).

REFERENCES

Peck G, Buchman TG. Initial assessment and resuscitation of the trauma patient. In: Cameron JL, Cameron AM, eds. *Current Surgical Therapy.* 11th ed. Philadelphia, PA: Elsevier Saunders; 2014: 981-984.

Weingart JD. The management of traumatic brain injury. In: Cameron JL, Cameron AM, eds. *Current Surgical Therapy.* 11th ed. Philadelphia, PA: Elsevier Saunders; 2014: 1001-1005.

A 20-year-old man was transported to the Emergency Department at a Level One Trauma Center after he sustained multiple gunshot wounds to the torso. He is conscious when he arrives to the Emergency Department and he has a BP of 80/60 with a heart rate of 100. He has multiple gunshot wounds to his chest and his thorax. He is able to communicate verbally but is clearly in distress. He has a Glasgow Coma Score of 15 and is awake and alert on physical exam. You perform your primary and secondary survey and you take a history. He has no medical problems, denies any medications, and he admits to consuming alcohol.

▶ What is your initial approach to the patient?
▶ How do you assess the degree of shock?
▶ How should you resuscitate this patient?

ANSWERS TO CASE 8:

Hemorrhagic Shock (Penetrating Trauma)

Summary: A 20-year-old patient presents in shock after sustaining multiple gunshot wounds to the torso. He is hypotensive and clinically in shock.

- **Initial approach:** Initial assessment and interventions to improve his hemodynamic status. The initial goal is not to normalize his vital signs but to identify the cause of shock and provide the appropriate interventions.

- **Degree of shock assessment:** This can be determined by vital signs and clinical appearance.

- **Resuscitation:** The goal of resuscitation is to keep him alive, while we determine the cause of his shock (eg, hemorrhage, cardiac tamponade, and tension pneumothorax are the major possible causes in this patient). The resuscitation in this situation has been described as hemostatic resuscitation.

ANALYSIS

Objectives

1. To understand the approach to the management of hemorrhagic shock.

2. To understand the use of blood products in patients who are injured.

3. To understand the assessment of the injured patient.

Considerations

The patient is a 20-year-old man who has sustained multiple gunshot wounds. The patient needs to be assessed quickly, resuscitated, and brought to the OR for definitive repair of his injuries as soon as possible. Each moment counts when a patient has sustained this type of injury. Every injured patients needs to be assesses based on the principles of Advanced Trauma Life Support (ATLS). Each patient needs an initial assessment that includes the primary and secondary survey based on ATLS principles. The primary survey is geared to assess a patient quickly for life threatening injuries and the secondary survey is a head to toe assessment of the patient's current status. In addition, the patient needs to have operative intravenous lines placed and foley catheter inserted as part of their initial assessment.

APPROACH TO

Hemorrhagic Shock, Penetrating Trauma

When a patient who presents with penetrating trauma and shock, every moment is vital, and interventions prioritized. The patient will be assessed according to the basic principles of ATLS.

The primary survey will consist of:

- Airway

- Breathing

- Circulation

- Disability

- Exposure

During the stage of resuscitation, the goal is to make sure the patient has all his lines in place for fluid resuscitation. A Foley is placed, and an NG tube if necessary. At that time there is a reassessment of the patient, as a summary of the findings and labs is sent to assess the degree of shock that the patient exhibits (see Table 8–1). We then proceed to the Secondary Survey where there is a complete assessment of his head, neck, chest, abdomen, pelvis, extremities, neurology exam that includes a Glasgow Coma Scale and an assessment of gross movement of all four extremities. There is no need to do a detailed neurologic examination in this setting. At the end of the secondary survey, typically, the patient is reassessed for any other injuries to make sure nothing is missed. In between the primary and the secondary survey, there is the stage of resuscitation. That is where the patient is reassessed and tubes and lines are placed. It is important at that point all aspects of the current status of the patient are reviewed. After the secondary survey, a decision is made about the course of action for the patient. If the patient has sustained a gunshot wound, operative intervention may be needed. If a tangential injury is sustained with low suspicion for vital torso injury in a hemodynamically stable patient, the patient can go to the CT Scan to assess the trajectory of the bullet.

The degree of shock is assessed by a review of the patient's vital signs followed by the physical exam. Many young patients in shock will only show tachycardia, even with a significant loss of blood volume. The pulse pressure will also narrow as an early sign of shock. Over reliance on the one physical sign may result in a under appreciation of the magnitude of the hypovolemic shock. The average 70 kg male has approximately 5 L of blood volume. The standard percentage shown

Table 8–1 • HYPOVOLEMIC SHOCK AND HEMORRHAGE				
	Class I	Class II	Class III	Class IV
Blood Loss (mL)	Up to 750	750-1500	1500-2000	>2000
Blood Loss (% Blood Volume)	Up to 15%	15-30%	30-40%	>40%
Pulse Rate	<100	>100	>120	>140
Blood Pressure	Normal	Normal	Decreased	Decreased
Pulse Pressure (mm Hg)	Normal or increased	Decreased	Decreased	Decreased
Respiratory Rate	14-20	20-30	30-40	>35
Urine Output (mL/h)	>30	20-30	5-15	Negligible
CNS/Mental Status	Slightly anxious	Mildly anxious	Anxious, confused	Confused, lethargy

above reflects the amount of blood loss the patient has the signs that go along with it. Table 8-1 is taken from ATLS and is a framework that allows trauma care providers to further assess the degree of shock sustained by the patient. Notice that the blood pressure can remain normal even if the patient has sustained a 30% to 40% of blood loss. Many times in the trauma room, there is too much focus on the patient's blood pressure and not as much on the other signs when the patient is initially injured. One measure to assess the degree of shock includes the physical exam. The presence of a hypoperfused patient that may be cool to the touch and diaphoretic can help trauma providers assess the degree of shock in the injured patient. Younger patients that are in excellent physical condition and children may just be tachycardic since they have a great reserve. They may not show the classic signs of shock until they enter decompensated shock and are near arrest. Laboratory tests are an adjunct to the signs and symptoms listed above and include the use of base deficit calculated from arterial or venous blood gas or lactate. Many trauma centers use both measures to assess the degree of shock.

The approach to resuscitation has changed over the years to include the early introduction of blood products into the resuscitation of the patient. The data from the military experience has influenced the civilian approach to trauma resuscitation, which can be referred to a hemostatic resuscitation of patients. Data from military surgeons revealed that if packed red blood cell:fresh frozen plasma:platelets in a ratio of 1:1:1, the patients had better outcomes from hemorrhagic shock. Many civilian trauma centers began to adopt Massive Transfusion Protocols to better prepare for blood product use in the patients over a decade ago and has led to improved survival. The partnership with the blood blank had allowed trauma centers and other providers to get access to blood products more rapidly consequently improving survival.

The ability of a civilian trauma centers to partner with the blood bank has saved lives. Several recent studies, including PROMMTT and PROPPR, have helped underscore the importance of early administration of blood products instead of crystalloid. The over use of crystalloid early on during resuscitations has lead gross fluid overload. Many experienced trauma surgeons, emergency physicians, and critical care physicians have refocused our attention on the early phase of resuscitation and the importance of early use of blood instead of isotonic resuscitation fluids. Damage control resuscitation or hemostatic resuscitation as it is now termed has been linked with improved survival of patients that have sustained trauma. These findings have caused a change in the administration of fluid and blood resuscitation to injured patients.

There is growing use of the Rotational thromboelastometry (ROTEM) and thromboelastography (TEGS) which assess the quality of the clot formation in the injured patient. These assays have become more useful in helping guide the resuscitation of patients. While these assays have been around for over two decades, they originally were used only by hematologists to help guide treatment of patients with bleeding diatheses. The use of these assays is becoming more standard in the initial evaluation of the injured patient at trauma centers. The information from these assays provide the surgeon, anesthesiologist, and emergency medicine physician to better guide the use of blood products since the test allows the physician to decide if the patient needs PRBCs, FFP, platelets, or cryoprecipitate.

> ## CASE CORRELATION
> - See Case 3 (Hypotensive Patient [Sepsis]), Case 6 (Blunt Chest Trauma), Case 7 (Multiple Blunt Trauma), and Case 9 (Penetrating Abdominal Trauma).

COMPREHENSION QUESTIONS

8.1 If a patient has a head injury and altered mental status with a history of treatment with Coumadin and an INR of 3.0, what treatment would reverse their coagulopathy most efficiently?

A. FFP

B. Vitamin K

C. Factor VII

D. Factor IX

8.2 If a patient presents with profound shock after a high-speed motor vehicle accident, what is the most important thing to do initially for the patient?

A. Intubate the patient

B. Obtain large bore IVs

C. Resuscitate the patient with crystalloid

D. Administer hemostatic resuscitation

8.3 What is the first line treatment for a patient in hemorrhagic shock after major trauma?

A. 2 L of crystalloid

B. 1 L hypertonic saline

C. FFP

D. Platelets

E. 2 units of PRBCs

8.4 If a patient is hypotensive from hemorrhagic shock and has a bleeding wound from their extremity, the first line of treatment should be:

A. Administer blood products

B. Apply direct pressure

C. Place a tourniquet above the wound

D. Perform emergency surgery in the emergency department

E. Initiate massive transfusion protocol

8.5 Hemostatic resuscitation means giving PRBCs/FFP/platelets in what ratio:

A. 1:2:1

B. 1:3:2

C. 1:1:1

D. 2:1:1

8.6 What are the indications for emergent exploration after penetrating trauma to the abdomen?

A. Evisceration

B. Intractable Shock

C. Peritonitis

D. All of the above

E. None of the above

8.7 If the patient is in shock with distended neck veins and midline trachea, what is the diagnosis for this patient?

A. Pericardial tamponade

B. Tension pneumothorax

C. Heart failure

D. Hemothorax

E. Tracheal injury

ANSWERS

8.1 **D.** The use of Factor IX has become an essential part of the management of patients who are on Coumadin treatment. If they receive the medication, their INR will typically normalize within one hour. That may be enough to arrest the hemorrhage in injured patients.

8.2 **A.** The initial priorities of the injured patient are always the same. Securing of the patient's airway is always the first priority in the initial management of the trauma patient.

8.3 **D.** Choices A, B, and C are three clear indications and are acceptable reasons to operate on the patient emergently when they are injured. The use of the CT scan has become routine, but if the patient has those findings, it is accepted practice to operate on the patient.

8.4 **B.** The first line of therapy is to apply direct pressure. That is followed by the placement of a tourniquet proximal to the injury on the extremity.

8.5 **C.** The patient should be given fluid resuscitation in the ration of 1:1:1 when they are injured. There may be a debate of how much to give, but determining the amount of blood product on the result of the ROTEM or the TEG which assesses the quality of clot formation is rapidly becoming the standard of care in injured patients.

8.6 **D.** Peritonitis, evisceration, and intractable shock are all indications for emergent exploration of the abdomen in a patient with penetrating abdominal trauma.

8.7 **A.** The answer here is pericardial tamponade. The pericardial sac acutely can only accommodate 100 to 150 mL of fluid. After that amount, there is equalization of pressures and neck veins become elevated and distended. A FAST study can detect the layer of fluid around the heart, so it is essential to perform the basics of ATLS and make sure the patient has an ultrasound study of the heart.

CLINICAL PEARLS

▶ The management of hemorrhagic shock in trauma patients is evolving. Over the past decade, the use of blood products early on has been associated with better outcomes.

▶ Nonoperative management has grown but there are still several conditions that mandate operative interventions after penetrating trauma including peritonitis, evisceration, and hemorrhagic shock.

▶ The use of factor IX prothrombin concentrates can reverse the coagulopathy associated with the use of Coumadin. This is essential for patients who are bleeding and have no margin for expansion of the process like in a closed head injury.

▶ The use of ROTEM or TEGs to assess the quality of the blood clot allows the physician who is administering blood products to decide which blood product needs to be given among PRBCs, FFP, platelets, or cryoprecipitate.

REFERENCES

Callcut R, Cotton B, Muskat P, et al. Defining when to initiate massive transfusion (MT): a validation study of individual massive transfusion triggers in PROMMTT patients. *J Trauma Acute Care Surg.* 2013 January;74(1):58-67.

Cotton B, Reddy N, Quiton, et al. Damage control resuscitation is associated with a reduction in resuscitation volumes and improvement in survival in 390 damage control laparotomy patients. *Ann Surg.* 2011 October;254(4):1-15.

Holcomb J. Optimal use of blood products in severely injured trauma patients. *Hem Am Soc Hematol Educ Program.* 2010;465-469.

Holcomb J, Tilley B, Barniuk S, et al. Transfusion of plasma, platelets, and red blood cells in a 1:1:1 vs a 1:1:2 ratio and mortality in patients with severe trauma: the PROPPR randomized clinical trial. *JAMA.* 2015;313(5):471-482.

Morrison J, Ross J, Dubose J, et al. Association of cryoprecipitate and transexamic acid with improved survival following wartime injury, findings form the MATTERs II Study. *JAMA Surg.* 2013;148(3):218-225.

A 22-year-old man presents to the hospital 1 hour after sustaining two stab wounds during an altercation. The patient admits to drinking alcohol prior to the incident. On examination, he appears intoxicated and grimaces during manipulation of the wounds. His temperature is 36.8°C, pulse rate is 86 beats/minute, blood pressure is 129/80 mm Hg, and respiratory rate is 22 breaths/minute. His physical examination reveals two stab wounds to the anterior truncal region. One wound is located at the anterior axillary line, 1 cm above the left costal margin; the second wound is located 4 cm left of the umbilicus. There is no active bleeding from either wound site. The breath sounds are present and equal bilaterally. The abdomen is tender only in the vicinity of the injuries. The patient claims that the knife used in the attack was approximately 5 in (12.7 cm) in length.

▶ What is your next step?
▶ What are the potential injuries?
▶ How do you decide if this patient needs an operation immediately?

ANSWERS TO CASE 9:
Penetrating Abdominal Trauma

Summary: A 22-year-old man presents to the emergency department with two stab wounds. He is intoxicated, hemodynamically stable, and does not exhibit evidence of peritonitis. His examination reveals one wound in the left thoracoabdominal region and a second wound in the mid-abdomen to the left of the umbilicus.

- **Next step:** Perform primary and secondary survey assessments with emphasis on the abdomen and thorax, and identify any other possible injuries. Obtain an upright chest radiograph to evaluate for possible pneumothorax, hemothorax, and pneumoperitoneum.

- **Potential injuries:** Heart, lung, diaphragm, intra-abdominal contents, and retroperitoneal structures.

- **Indications for immediate surgery:** Include hemodynamic abnormalities (eg, tachycardia and hypotension), large hemothorax, strong concerns for penetrating cardiac injury, evisceration, peritonitis, hematemesis, and impalement.

ANALYSIS

Objectives

1. Learn the various possible approaches in the selective treatment of patients with penetrating abdominal injuries.

2. Learn the benefits and limitations associated with the various diagnostic and treatment strategies.

3. Learn the evolving strategies in the initial management of hemodynamically unstable patients with abdominal injuries.

Considerations

This patient has sustained a left thoracoabdominal stab wound (SW) and an abdominal SW. The **primary survey** should focus on the patient's ABCs (airway, breathing, and circulation). With penetrating injuries below the clavicles, airway compromise is not usually a priority, and some practitioners have proposed that the correct sequence of evaluation for penetrating abdominal injury patients as "BCA" rather than "ABC", so that the more relevant issues are identified and treated first. Based on the information given, this patient appears to be stable from the respiratory and circulatory standpoints. Diagnostic studies such as upright chest x-ray (CXR) and the Focused Abdominal Sonography for Trauma (FAST) are generally obtained soon after completion of the primary survey. The CXR and FAST help us identify injuries that would require tube thoracostomy, and/or operative explorations of the thoracic cavities or abdominal cavity.

If the patient's condition remains stable and there are no immediate indications for thoracic or abdominal surgical interventions, several options are available to help us determine whether injuries to vital structures have occurred. One option is clinical observation with repeat physical examinations, repeat laboratory testing (complete blood count with differentials, serum amylase), and repeat CXR. Another option is a diagnostic peritoneal lavage (DPL) to identify blood (RBCs) and inflammatory changes (WBCs) within the peritoneal cavity. Alternatively, a computed tomography (CT) scan can be obtained to visualize the knife tracts and evaluate for potential structural injuries. One important consideration in the management of this patient is his recent alcohol consumption and intoxicated state, which can blunt his pain response and render the abdominal examination less reliable thus making clinical observation alone a less reliable option. Because of this concern, a CT scan should be obtained to visualize the trajectory and depth of penetration of the wounds. If the CT scan demonstrates that the knife tracts do not penetrate through the abdominal wall or chest wall, the patient does not require additional treatment or observation. However, CT scan is of limited reliability in defining knife tracts and extent of injuries within the abdomen, and most practitioners will proceed with either laparoscopy or laparotomy when the CT scan demonstrates peritoneal violation and secondary signs such as free fluid, free air, and inflammatory changes. The exceptions to this rule are that some stable patients with isolated penetrating liver injury and/or kidney injury can be monitored and treated with nonoperative management.

APPROACH TO:

Penetrating Abdominal Trauma

DEFINITIONS

SURFACE ANATOMY OF PENETRATING ABDOMINAL TRAUMA:

Anterior Abdomen—A body region bordered by the costal margins superiorly, anterior axillary lines laterally, and the inguinal ligaments inferiorly.

Flank—Superior borders are the costal margins, anterior borders are the anterior axillary lines, posterior borders are the posterior axillary lines, and inferior borders are the iliac crests.

Back—Superior border is a line drawn between the tips of the scapulas, lateral margins are the posterior axillary lines, and the inferior border is the posterior iliac crest.

Thoracoabdominal Region—The superior margin of this truncal region is bordered by a line drawn across the nipples anteriorly and connection circumferentially to a line drawn between the tips of the scapula in the back. The inferior border is the lower edge of the rib cage circumferentially. Penetrating wounds to this region have the potential of causing injuries to the diaphragms, thoracic, intra-abdominal, and retroperitoneal structures.

Cardiac Box—The cardiac box is the anterior truncal space defined superiorly by the clavicles, laterally by a line drawn from the clavicles to the anterior costal margins through both nipples, and inferiorly by a line drawn between the costal margins where the previously described lines intersect the costal margins. The majority of stab wounds to the heart originate with injuries to the "box"; therefore, it is vitally important to rule out a penetrating cardiac injury in patients with stab wound to this area. Stable patients with penetrating injuries to the "box" need to have early sonographic evaluation for pericardial effusions. This examination should be repeated in stable patients to make sure that there is no subsequent blood accumulation in this space.

FOCUSED ABDOMINAL SONOGRAPHY FOR TRAUMA (FAST): The FAST is useful for rapid assessment of hemodynamically unstable trauma patients because a FAST that demonstrates no free fluid can help rule-out intraperitoneal bleeding as the cause of instability. This ultrasound evaluation is performed following the primary survey. The FAST evaluates four separate areas: (1) the pericardial space for pericardial effusion and signs of cardiac tamponade; (2) subhepatic space at Morrison's pouch for free fluid; (3) perisplenic space for free fluid; (4) pelvic space for free fluid. The FAST is generally not sensitive enough to identify small amount of intraperitoneal fluid (<500 mL). FAST indications are not well defined in stable trauma patients.

CT SCAN FOR ABDOMINAL TRAUMA EVALUATION: CT scans are well accepted for the evaluation of stable patients with blunt trauma. The use of CTs for the evaluation of patients with penetrating trauma is slightly more controversial. Most groups administer some contrast material during the CT evaluations; however, there is no agreement among practitioners regarding the best type of CT to apply. Options include: CT of the abdomen/pelvis with intravenous contrast only (single-contrast), CT of the abdomen/pelvis with intravenous and oral contrast (double-contrast), and CT of the abdomen/pelvis with intravenous contrast, oral contrast, and rectal contrast (triple-contrast). Oral and rectal contrast administrations are associated with time delays and are not well-tolerated by some patients. The use of contrast allows improved visualization of various intra-abdominal structures and is helpful in identifying subtle abnormalities.

DIAGNOSTIC PERITONEAL LAVAGE (DPL): DPL is rarely performed today as the FAST has become the preferred modality for the evaluation of hypotensive trauma patients. The two components of DPL include initial aspiration of the peritoneal space and if there is not blood aspirated, the abdomen is then infused with 1000 mL of sterile saline followed by chemical analysis of this fluid after it is retrieved from the abdomen. Positive DPL criteria include: (1) 10 mL of aspirated blood or presence of bilious contents during aspiration; (2) >100,000 red blood cell count/mL and/or >500 white blood cell count/mL in the lavage fluid.

DAMAGE-CONTROL RESUSCITATION: The overriding principle of damage-control resuscitation is to support patients with hemorrhagic shock in ways to minimize additional bleeding and prevent the onset of coagulopathy. The initial goal is to recognize the patients with significant blood loss/bleeding so that the damage-control resuscitation strategy can be initiated. Permissive hypotension (maintaining a systolic blood pressure of 90 mm Hg) is a major component of the approach, except in patients with concomitant traumatic brain injury, who would benefit from higher blood pressure to minimize secondary brain injury. Along with permissive hypotension, the transfusion of packed RBC, fresh frozen plasma (FFP), and platelets in a 1:1:1 ratio is recommended.

TRANEXAMIC ACID (TXA): The early administration of this anti-fibrinolytic agent soon after major injuries (within 3 hours of injury) has been shown to produce lower transfusion requirement and improved survival in a randomized controlled clinical trial (CRASH-II Trial). Analysis of the CRASH-II trial also suggests that delayed administration after 3 hours was associated with worse outcomes.

MASSIVE TRANSFUSION: This is generally defined as greater than or equal to 10 units of PRBC transfusion over a 24-hour period. Patients that may require massive transfusion include systolic BP <110 mm Hg, HR >105, hematocrit <32%, and pH <7.25 in a trauma patient with high injury mechanism (high-speed motor vehicle crash, penetrating truncal injury, fall from height, and auto vs pedestrian crash).

DAMAGE-CONTROL LAPAROTOMY: Damage control operations are surgeries performed in a critically-ill, injured patient using the strategy of limiting the operation to life-saving procedures only, with planned return to the operating room for definitive repair when the patient's condition has improved. The damage-control approach was introduced following the recognition of the "lethal triad" of **hypothermia, acidosis,** and **coagulopathy** often associated with severe injuries and large volume blood losses. GI tract injuries can be controlled with simple closure or resection of the intestine without re-establishing GI tract continuity. Vascular damage control involves placement of intraluminal shunts in vital vessels, ligation of nonvital vessels, and placement of packing to control bleeding. Damage control operations are usually put into practice in conjunction with damage-control resuscitation.

CLINICAL APPROACH

Primary Survey and Resuscitation

Trauma patient treatment always begins with an evaluation and management of the ABCs, also known as the primary survey. This can be started with a brief conversation that includes a self-introduction, asking the patient to tell you what happened, or what the patient's name is. Listening to the patient's verbal response can help the examiner determine the adequacy of the airway, brain perfusion, the cooperativeness of the patient, and gross neurologic functions. Breathing is evaluated by listening to the patient's breath sounds and observing the individual's respiratory efforts. Absence of breath sounds on the same side of a penetrating injury is an indication for tube thoracostomy, especially if the patient has labored breathing or signs of cardiopulmonary compromise. In addition to vital signs measurement, the circulatory status can be assessed by palpation of the skin and observation of the capillary refill. Cool skin and diaphoresis along with delayed capillary refill (>2 seconds) are clinical signs of shock. The circulatory evaluation also includes examination of the jugular veins for distension and auscultation of the heart for muffled heart tones, which can indicate cardiac tamponade that requires immediate treatment.

Assessment of the patient's neurologic disabilities includes assessment of the patient's papillary response to light, and the motor and sensory functions. Near the completion of the primary survey, the patient's clothing should be completely removed for thorough examination of the entire body to identify any subtle signs of injuries. Following the primary survey, an upright CXR should be obtained to identify pneumothorax, hemothorax, major bony injuries, pneumoperitoneum, and retained foreign bodies (such as bullets or pellets). In patients with evidence of or history of thoracic penetrating injuries but no hemothorax or pneumothorax during the initial CXR, another CXR should be obtained after 4 to 6 hours to rule-out the possibility of delayed presentations of pneumothorax or hemothorax. For patients with gun shot wounds (GSWs) to the upper torso or abdomen, a FAST examination can be very useful in the early stages of the trauma evaluation. During the FAST examination, close attentions should be given to the pericardial view of the examination to identify for the possibility of pericardial effusion. The sensitivity of the FAST in detecting blood in the pericardial space is close to 100%; however, the sensitivity of FAST for identifying intra-abdominal injuries in stable trauma patients is only in the vicinity of 50%. Because of the low sensitivity, **initial negative FAST examinations do not reliably rule-out intra-abdominal injuries in stable patients with abdominal penetrating trauma.**

There have been significant paradigm shifts in the approach to the initial management of hypotensive trauma patients, with many of the strategies having been developed based on observations from the management of combat casualties during the military activities in Iraq and Afghanistan over the past several years. The basic principle guiding change is that the majority of hypotensive trauma patients have ongoing bleeding, so initial resuscitation should be directed toward minimizing bleeding rather than restoring normal vital signs. This approach is referred to as **hemostatic or damage-control resuscitation.** Hypotensive trauma patients without traumatic brain injury are purposely kept hypotensive with systolic blood pressures of 80 to 90 mm Hg until operative control of bleeding can be undertaken. The strategy minimizes crystalloid resuscitation to avoid dilutional coagulopathy and decreases in body temperature. In the operating room, resuscitation is accomplished with blood product components of **PRBC, FFP, and platelets in a 1:1:1 ratio.** A recent randomized controlled clinical trial comparing 1:1:1 to 2:1:1 transfusion strategies found that patients who received the lower ratio of PRBC to other blood products experienced earlier control of hemostasis and fewer deaths from exsanguination; however, no differences in 24-hour and 30-day mortality rates were observed between the two groups.

Secondary Survey

Following the primary survey, a careful secondary survey should be performed in all trauma patients to ascertain the extent of the patients' injuries. This is especially important when working with trauma patients with an unknown or unclear history of the injury events. The most important part of the secondary survey for patients with penetrating truncal injuries is the abdominal examination. Prominent physical findings such as **rigidity, guarding, or significant tenderness away from the skin wounds are signs of intraperitoneal inflammation and are indications for abdominal exploration.** It is important to note that the physical examination is not always reliable, as the result of distracting injuries and history of hallucinogen and/or alcohol consumption.

Treatment Options

Historically, patients with penetrating abdominal trauma have undergone mandatory surgical exploration. Unfortunately, that approach led to high rates of nontherapeutic operations with subsequent postoperative complications. From this experience, the practice of selective operative management has evolved, where exploration is limited to those patients with a high suspicion of having intra-abdominal injuries. In general, rates of intra-abdominal injuries are much higher among patients with GSWs to the abdomen compared to SWs with up to 90% of patients with GSW penetrating the peritoneal cavity requiring operative repairs. Selective management of patients with GSWs is acceptable in patients with normal hemodynamic status, absence of peritonitis, and GSW trajectories that are suspected to be tangential. Under these conditions, a CT scan of the abdomen and pelvis can be very useful to identify the bullet path.

Most patients who are hemodynamically normal and without evidence of peritonitis during the initial evaluation can be managed with clinical observation, with CT scan plus observation, with DPL plus observation, or with diagnostic laparoscopy. When considering these options, we seek the balance between timely treatments of potentially life-threatening injuries and minimizing the morbidity, mortality, and costs associated with nontherapeutic operations.

Observation of asymptomatic or minimally symptomatic patients with abdominal penetrating trauma for the development of positive clinical findings results in the lowest nontherapeutic laparotomy rates. Patients who are being observed require frequent evaluations for peritonitis, increasing tenderness, and systemic signs such as fever, tachycardia, tachypnea, or hypotension. Most reports have found the observation period for patients should be for a minimum of 24 hours. Ideally, patients being observed should be examined and evaluated by the same practitioner to minimize inter-observer variability. This observational approach is associated with the lowest nontherapeutic laparotomy rates, but can result in delayed treatment of patients or missed injuries.

Local exploration of stab wounds helps to identify patients with stab wounds that do not penetrate the abdominal wall and who are not at risk for having intra-abdominal injuries. The technique involves injecting the wound with local anesthesia and then extending the wound to visualize the subcutaneous tract and depth of the injury. If the tract penetrates the abdominal wall fascia, then it is presumed to be an injury that can potentially cause intra-peritoneal structural injuries. If the wound does not involve the fascia, the patient can have irrigation and repair of the wound followed by discharge. Patients with stab wounds that penetrate the fascia can be managed with laparotomy, laparoscopy, observation, or DPL.

Diagnostic peritoneal lavage (DPL) is a technique of sampling the intraperitoneal contents for blood, inflammation, or enteric contents. The DPL is performed with the placement of a catheter into the peritoneal cavity. With the catheter in place, an initial attempt is made to aspirate for free fluid or blood. If >10 mL of blood is aspirated or if enteric contents are aspirated, the result is considered positive and the patient then undergoes operative treatment. Patients with gross negative aspirations then undergo infusion of 1000 mL of sterile saline into the peritoneal cavity, followed by retrieval of the fluid for quantitative analysis for WBC and RBC. The criteria for microscopic positive DPL varies between institutions. The published thresholds range from RBC counts of 1000/mm^3 to 100,000/mm^3. The use of the lower RBC count criteria is associated with increase in diagnostic sensitivity to nearly 100%; however, the nontherapeutic laparotomy rates reported are as high as 30%. The use of lower RBC is associated with lower specificity but increased probability of nontherapeutic laparotomies. Over the past 10 years, the application of DPL has become greatly limited, as other diagnostic strategies such as FAST and CT scans have gained popularity and have become more accessible.

Computed tomography (CT) is being increasingly applied in the evaluation of patients with penetrating torso trauma. CT requires more time, and should only be used for the evaluation of stable trauma patients. CT scans performed without intravenous or enteric contrast material usually do not provide sufficient detail for the assessment of trauma patients; therefore, intravenous contrast is usually given during the CT scans. Some groups feel that the administration of oral contrast and rectal contrast can help improve visualization for the detection of hollow visceral injuries. The trade-off for additional contrast administration is time delay, patient discomfort, and aspiration risks. CT scans are highly sensitive in identifying injuries that do not violate the peritoneal space or the retroperitoneal space. It is however not reliable enough to rule-out bowel injuries in patients whose penetrating injuries have violated the peritoneal space. CT also lacks sensitivity in the detection of diaphragmatic injuries.

Diagnostic laparoscopy is an option for the evaluation of patients with penetrating abdominal trauma. It is very useful for the detection of peritoneal penetration, diaphragmatic injuries, and the evaluation of solid organ injuries. This approach can eliminate the need for open abdominal explorations but can be limited by the technical difficulty associated with evaluation and repair of the GI tract and other vital structures.

CASE CORRELATION

- See also Case 6 (Blunt Chest Trauma), Case 7 (Multiple Blunt Trauma), and Case 8 (Hemorrhagic Shock [Trauma]).

COMPREHENSION QUESTIONS

9.1 A 25-year-old man presents with a stab wound to the abdomen 2 cm above the umbilicus. He appears diaphoretic. His blood pressure is 95/70 and pulse rate is 115 beats/minute. His stab wound is not bleeding, and his abdomen is tender diffusely. Which of the following management options is most appropriate?

A. Abdominal CT scan

B. Diagnostic peritoneal lavage

C. Local wound exploration

D. Observation

E. Exploratory laparotomy

9.2 An 18-year-old man sustains a stab wound to the left upper quadrant of his abdomen. He complains of minimal pain. He is alert, hemodynamically normal, and his abdominal examination is essentially normal. Which of the following statements is TRUE?

A. An abdominal CT scan is sensitive in detecting injury to the diaphragm

B. The FAST examination reliably rules out intra-abdominal injury in this patient

C. If the local wound exploration reveals fascia penetration, it would be an absolute indication for abdominal exploration

D. Intra-abdominal injury is highly unlikely in this patient

E. The patient should be admitted for clinical observation for 24 hours

9.3 A 33-year-old woman presents with a stab wound located at the right anterior axillary line, 3 cm superior to the right costal margin. She is alert and has normal mentation. Her blood pressure is 198/60 mm Hg and pulse rate is 100 beats/minute. Which of the following is the most appropriate next step?

A. Listen to the patient's breath sounds

B. Obtain an upright CXR

C. Perform a FAST

D. Place a right chest tube

E. Perform a CT scan of the abdomen and thorax

9.4 A 36-year-old man was stabbed in the right lower quadrant of his abdomen one hour prior to presentation to the emergency center. He complains of pain at the wound site. His vital signs are normal. Local wound exploration reveals penetration of the anterior abdominal fascia, and a DPL performed reveals 7000 RBC/mm³ and 750 WBC/mm³. Which of the following is the most appropriate next step?

A. Repeat the DPL in 4 hours

B. Obtain an abdominal CT scan

C. Perform a diagnostic laparoscopy

D. Continue nonoperative management and observation

E. Perform a laparotomy

9.5 A 22-year-old man presents with a single stab wound to the epigastrium. The patient is diaphoretic and somnolent. His pulse rate is 120 beats/minute, blood pressure is 80/60 mm Hg, respiratory rate is 8, and GCS is 8. He has a single stab wound 6 cm below the xiphoid process. His CXR does not demonstrate evidence of hemothorax or pneumothorax. His FAST demonstrates free fluid in the pericardial space and free fluid in the subhepatic space. Which of the following is the best next step in management?

A. DPL

B. CT of the chest and abdomen

C. Exploratory laparotomy

D. Median sternotomy

E. Placement of bilateral chest tubes

9.6 Which of the following patients with a stab wound to the abdomen is the best candidate for laparoscopic treatment?

A. A 16-year-old boy with three separate stab wounds to the abdomen and peritonitis

B. A 44-year-old woman with a SW to the left lateral chest at the midaxillary line and 3 cm above the lower border of the rib cage. She is hemodynamically normal and has a normal abdominal examination. A CT scan reveals small amount of left pleural fluid and small amount of free fluid under the left hemidiaphragm

C. A 36-year-old man with a single SW to the left upper abdomen with CT scan demonstrating splenic laceration with active contrast extravasation

D. A 27-year-old man with prior history of SW to the abdomen 2 years ago, who underwent a laparotomy and small bowel resection. He now presents with a GSW to the abdomen just above the umbilicus and is tachycardic with pulse rate of 115 beats/minute

E. A 63-year-old man with a self-inflicted SW to the epigastium. He is hemodynamically normal and has a butcher knife impaled in his epigastrium. A cross table lateral x-ray indicates that the knife blade is approximately 8 in in length (~20.3 cm) and appears to be completely embedded in the abdomen

ANSWERS

9.1 **E.** This man has a single SW to the epigastric region and signs of shock that include diaphoresis, tachycardia, and marginally low blood pressure. In addition, he has diffuse abdominal tenderness that is suggestive of peritonitis. Exploratory laparotomy is the best treatment option for him.

9.2 **E.** Admission for clinical observation for 24 hours is a reasonable management option for this man and therefore is a TRUE statement. All the other choices listed are not true.

9.3 **A.** Even though it is sometimes tempting to proceed straight to diagnostic studies such as CXR, FAST, and CT scans, the primary survey should be competed first. Listening to her breath sounds is part of the primary survey. If the patient was hemodynamically unstable with this injury, placement of a right chest tube can be the correct choice; however, in this situation the patient is stable and does not need immediate pleural space decompression.

9.4 **E.** This patient with a SW to the abdomen has a wound that has penetrated the abdominal fascia based on local wound exploration. The DPL performed revealed 7000 RBC/mm^3 and 750 WBC/mm^3. The WBC count in the DPL can be elevated even without significant injuries, if the DPL is performed later than 6 to 7 hours after the injury. In this case, the patient sustained the SW 1 hour ago, therefore the elevated WBC count in the DPL fluid likely represents intestinal injury and the patient should undergo an exploratory laparotomy. Because of the nonspecific nature of WBC elevation in the DPL fluid, some groups have advocated adding amylase and alkaline phosphatase analysis to the fluid to improve sensitivity and specificity.

9.5 **C.** This patient has a single stab wound to the epigastric area, and based on the descriptions given, the stab wound is in the "cardiac box" where the majority of cardiac SW originate. The hemodynamic instability described in this patient can be due to either cardiac tamponade or blood loss. The patient's FAST examination has revealed the presence of pericardial fluid and fluid in the subhepatic space. With the information, the best approach is to proceed with a median sternotomy to explore the pericardial space, relieve the cardiac tamponade, and repair the cardiac injury. Following that procedure, we can proceed with exploration of the abdomen to address the intra-abdominal free fluid or bleeding that is seen by FAST. The cardiac injury should be addressed first in this unstable patient because it is a process that can produce fatality faster than intra-abdominal bleeding.

9.6 **B.** The patient with the SW to the left chest and radiographic suggestion of injury to the left hemidiaphragm is the best patient to undergo laparoscopy for evaluation of the left diaphragm. If a laceration of the left hemidiaphragm is seen, it can also be repaired by laparoscopic approach as well. The patients described in the other choices are either too unstable or may have injuries that are too complex to repair safely by the laparoscopic approach.

CLINICAL PEARLS

▶ Mandatory laparotomy for abdominal SW and GSW was considered the standard of care until the 1960s and late 1990s, respectively.

▶ Shock, peritonitis, impalement, and evisceration in the setting of penetrating abdominal trauma are generally considered indications for abdominal exploration.

▶ The false positive rate of DPL based on the WBC criteria increases in patients who undergo DPL in a delayed fashion (>6 hours from injury).

▶ The FAST is not sensitive in identifying injuries to retroperitoneal structures.

▶ When clinically normal patients with SW to the abdomen and anterior fascia violation identified by local wound exploration are taken to the operating room for exploratory laparotomy, the nontherapeutic laparotomy rate was 55%.

▶ A negative FAST in a patient with penetrating abdominal trauma does not rule-out intra-abdominal injuries.

▶ A 17% missed injury rate was reported by the Western Trauma Association Trial, when penetrating abdominal trauma patients were discharged based on a negative FAST.

▶ The "lethal triad" of trauma are acidosis, coagulopathy, and hypothermia.

▶ Damage-control operations and damage-control anesthesia are strategies developed to combat the "lethal triad" of acidosis, coagulopathy, and hypothermia.

REFERENCES

Biffl WL, Leppaniemi A. Management guidelines for penetrating abdominal trauma. *World J Surg.* DOI: 10.1007/s00268-014-2793-7.

Duke MD, Guidry C, Guice J, et al. Restrictive fluid resuscitation in combination with damage control resuscitation: time for adaptation. *J Trauma Acute Care Surg.* 2012;73:674-678.

Hicks CW, Haider A. Damage control operation. In: Cameron JL, Cameron AM, eds. *Current Surgical Therapy.* 11th ed. Philadelphia, PA: Elsevier Saunders; 2014: 1061-1067.

Holcomb JB, Tilley BC, Baraniuk S, et al. Transfusion of plasma, platelets, and red blood cells in a 1:1:1 vs a 1:1:2 ratio and mortality in patients with severe trauma. The PROPPR randomized clinical trial. *JAMA.* 2015;313:471-482.

A 63-year-old man is rescued from a house fire and brought to the emergency department. According to the paramedics at the scene, the victim was found unconscious in an upstairs bedroom of the house. His past medical history is unknown. His pulse rate is 115 beats/minute, blood pressure is 150/85 mm Hg, and respiratory rate is 30 breaths/minute. The pulse oximeter registers 91% oxygen saturation with oxygen by face mask. His face and the exposed portions of his body are covered with carbonaceous deposit. The patient has blistering open burn wounds involving the circumference of his left arm and left leg, in addition to his entire back and buttock areas. He does not respond verbally to questions and reacts to painful stimulation with occasional moans and withdrawal of extremities.

▶ What is the most appropriate next step?
▶ What are the immediate concerns and late complications associated with thermal injuries?

ANSWERS TO CASE 10:
Thermal Injury

Summary: A 63-year-old man presents with approximately a 40% total body surface area (TBSA) burn and inhalation injuries sustained in a house fie.

- **Next step:** Definitive airway management by intubation is critical in this patient with likely inhalation injuries, carbon monoxide (CO) poisoning, and major burns.

- **Immediate and late complications:** Airway compromise and tissue hypoperfusion are common early complications, while wound sepsis, functional loss, and psychological trauma are potential late complications associated with major burn trauma.

ANALYSIS

Objectives

1. Learn the initial assessment and treatment of patients with thermal injuries.

2. Learn the assessment and management of burn wounds.

3. Be familiar with the prognosis associated with thermal injuries.

Considerations

A 63-year-old man is found unconscious inside a burning house with an approximately 40% TBSA burn injury, and is brought to the emergency center. A burn patient found unconscious in a house fire has extremely high likelihood of having suffered smoke inhalation. Based on our initial assessment of his injury, the burn wound size is approximately 40% TBSA. Given the size of the wound, he will need to receive large volume of crystalloid fluids during the initial 48 hours of hospitalization. With the combination of smoke inhalation and fluid administration, his airway will become edematous and compromised. In addition, the combination of the patient's older age and large burn size are factors likely to contribute to pneumonia, acute lung injury and respiratory insufficiency. For all of these reasons, **intubation and the initiation of mechanical ventilation are the most critical interventions during his initial management.**

Once the airway is secured, we will need to start his fluid resuscitation with the infusion of Lactated Ringer solution. The initial infusion rate and volume can be estimated based on the formula of 2 to 4 mL/kg×% burn size. If the patient is not already at a facility with the capacity to provide specialized burn care, immediate arrangement should be made to transfer him to a specialized burn unit. The combination of this patient's age, burn wound size, and potential inhalation injuries are poor outcome prognosticators.

APPROACH TO:
Thermal Injury

DEFINITIONS

FIRST-DEGREE BURN WOUNDS: Superficial burns that involve only the epidermis. These wounds appear red and are not blistered.

PARTIAL-THICKNESS BURN WOUNDS: (Formerly known as second-degree burns) These are burns that extend beyond the epidermis and are classified as superficial or deep. **Superficial partial-thickness** wound appear as painful, pink wounds with blisters. With topical wound care such as silver sulfadiazine, superficial partial-thickness wounds often heal within 2 weeks without much impairment or scarring. **Deep partial-thickness** wounds are often dried, mottled, and variably painful. These wounds can also be healed with topical wound care; however, spontaneous healing is often associated with scarring and functional impairment; therefore, deep partial thickness wounds are often treated by excision and skin-grafting.

THIRD-DEGREE (FULL-THICKNESS) BURNS: Full-thickness burn of the skin involving the entire epidermis and dermis layers. These wounds are painless, appear white or black with a leather-like appearance. Spontaneous healing occurs only by contraction from the surrounding skin, leading to significant scarring and functional losses.

PARKLAND FORMULA: One of the most commonly applied strategies for initial burn resuscitation. This formula calculates the volume and rate of fluid administration for the first 24 hours for adults with major burns. (Affected TBSA%) × (4 mL of Lactated Ringer) × (weight of patient in kg). One-half of the calculated volume is given over the first 8 hours and the remainder given over the subsequent 16 hours. The rate and volume of administration are adjusted to keep urine output between 0.5 and 1.0 mL/kg/h.

MODIFIED BROOKE FORMULA: The main difference between this approach and the Parkland formula is the use of colloid solution during the second 24 hours. This formula can be applied for adults with burns and children weighing more than 10 kg, and the formula utilizes lactated Ringer 2 to 4 mL/kg×% TBSA during the first 24 hours, with one-half of the volume given in the first 8 hours and the remaining fluid in the subsequent 16 hours. During the second 24 hours, colloid fluid (5% albumin in lactated ringer) is given at 0.3 to 0.5 mL/kg×% TBSA titrated to maintain urine output of >0.5 mL/kg/h.

ELECTRICAL BURNS: The passage of electrical current through the body varies depending on the resistance of the tissue. Nerve, blood vessels, mucous membranes, and muscles have low resistance and are most susceptible to injuries from electrical currents. Skin, bones, fat, and tendons have higher resistance and tend to sustain less injury from electricity. Tissue injuries from electricity can include direct necrosis and ischemia due to vasoconstriction.

ESCHAROTOMY: Escharotomies are incisions made in the "leathery" and non-expansive full-thickness burn sites to help improve tissue perfusion if there is a circumferential burn wound in the extremities. Escharotomies can be made in the truncal regions for individuals with circumferential burn wounds to the torso causing compromised perfusion of abdominal organs and/or compromised expansion of the chest with ventilation.

FASCIOTOMY: Fasciotomies are incisions made in the fascia of extremities to help release pressures in swollen muscle compartments. Deep compartment swelling is most common following high-voltage electrical burns causing injuries to muscles and other deep structures.

SILVER SULFADIAZINE (SS): The most commonly applied topical agent for superficial burn wounds. The application of SS is generally soothing to the patients. SS lacks the ability to penetrate eschars and is not useful in infected burn wounds.

SULFAMYLON (MAFENIDE): A topical agent most useful for full-thickness, infected burns. This agent can penetrate eschars and is often used in the management of full-thickness burns. The drawbacks associated with sulfamylon are pain with application and metabolic acidosis relating to its carbonic anhydrase inhibition activities.

SILVER NITRATE: A topical burn wound agent. It has limited eschar penetrance and turns tissues a black color. Silver nitrate application can lead to leaching of sodium and chloride from the tissue, which can produce hyponatremia and hypochloremia, particularly if applied to large areas in children.

CLINICAL APPROACH

Burn injuries account for over 600,000 emergency department visits and approximately 50,000 hospital admissions in the United States each year. In the United States, more than 60% of the patients hospitalized for burn-related injuries are admitted to 125 specialized burn centers. Between 4% and 22% of burn patients require early admissions to the ICU. **Major burn wounds are generally defined as injuries with >20% TBSA involvement.** The skin is the largest organ of the body, and it is responsible for maintenance of fluid balance, temperature regulation, protein regulation, and serves as a barrier against bacteria and fungus. Patients with major burns require inpatient care; whereas, some patients with minor burn wounds can be managed in the outpatient setting with appropriate input and follow-up from practitioners who are knowledgeable about burn care.

Phases of Care for Major Burns

The hospital care of patients with major burn wounds can be viewed as three separate phases. The first phase encompasses day 1 to day 3, when complete evaluation of the patient and accurate fluid resuscitation are the primary goals. During the second phase, the main goals are initial wound excision and biologic wound coverage to prevent/minimize wound sepsis, systemic inflammation and sepsis. Ideally, second phase goals should be accomplished immediately following phase 1 treatments. The third phase priorities include definitive wound closure/coverage and treatment of injuries to complex anatomic regions such as the hands, face, and genitalia. Rehabilitation and some reconstructive processes are also undertaken during phase 3. It is important to bear in mind that the primary objectives in the care of hospitalized burn patients are to help patients return to work, school, community activities, and normal life.

Initial Assessment

The initial assessment of a burn patient is the same as for any other trauma patient (with attention to airway, breathing, and circulation—the ABCs). It is important to remember that many patients with burn injuries also suffer from injuries due to other mechanisms including blunt and penetrating trauma (examples include fires associated with explosions, fires following automobile crashes, and falls from height following electrical burns from power lines). Overall, concomitant injuries are encountered in roughly 10% of the burn victims.

Airway and Respiration

Airway assessment is the initial consideration. The upper airway can receive burn injuries from hot gases from a fire; whereas, pulmonary burns or burn injuries to the lungs rarely occur unless live steam or explosive gases are inhaled. The presence of facial burns, upper torso burns, and carbonaceous sputum should strongly increase our clinical suspicion regarding potential airway burns, and these findings should prompt an evaluation of the mouth and oral cavity for other signs of airway injuries. **If the oropharynx is dry, red, or blistered, then burn injury to the area is confirmed and the patient should undergo intubation for definitive airway management.** When indicated, endotracheal intubation should be performed before the progression of pharyngeal and/or laryngeal edema. Patients who are victims of house fires have the added risk of smoke inhalation, which can cause tracheobronchitis and bronchial edema as the result of exposure to the incomplete combustion of carbon particles and other toxic fumes.

Carbon monoxide (CO) poisoning is a cause of hypoxia in burn patients who sustain their injuries in enclosed-space fires. The inhalation of CO causes hypoxia, as CO has a 240-fold great affinity than oxygen (O_2) for binding to hemoglobin, thus shifting the oxyhemoglobin curve to the left. All victims rescued from the scene of closed-space fires should have their carboxyhemoglobin (COHgb) levels measured. A COHgb level of greater than 30% can produce permanent central nervous system (CNS) dysfunction, and a COHgb level greater than 60% can produce coma and death. It is important to be aware that a victim trapped in a smoky, house fire can develop COHgb level of 30% within 3 minutes. When inhalation injury is found in a patient with a burn that is greater than 20% TBSA, the patient has a 90% chance of requiring ventilator support. Oxygen therapy can help reduce the CO in blood. The half-life of CO in the blood in a patient receiving room air is 250 minutes; whereas, the half-life of CO in a patient receives 100% oxygen delivered through an endotracheal tube by a ventilator, is reduced to 40 to 60 minutes. The severity of CO associated injury can be underestimated because of the drop in level of COHgb associated with time elapse and oxygen therapy. To best determine the extent of the CO injury, we need to estimate the elapsed time between the injury and COHgb measurement, in addition to knowing the oxygen concentration that the patient received prior to arrival.

The work of breathing for patients with major burns involving the chest and/or abdomen can increase substantially once the patient receives fluid resuscitation with subsequent tissue edema formation. For patients with large torso burn wounds, early intubation and mechanical ventilation can be helpful prior to the onset of frank respiratory insufficiency. Another consideration is that patients with extensive or circumferential full-thickness burn wounds involving their chest may need escharotomy to allow for proper chest wall expansion during ventilation.

Resuscitation

Cutaneous burns produce accelerated fluid losses into interstitial tissue in the burned and unburned areas. Inflammatory mediators such as prostaglandins, thromboxane A2, and reactive oxygen radicals are released from injured tissues, which produce local edema, increased capillary permeability, decreased tissue perfusion, and end-organ dysfunction. Burn size exceeding 20% TBSA will produce systemic inflammatory responses and interstitial edema in tissues and organs away from the injured areas. With large burns, an initial decrease in cardiac output occurs and is later followed by hypermetabolic responses. Because of the tissue fluid losses and perfusion changes, burn resuscitation a key component in patient management. Organs, including the skin, can progress from a hypoperfusion state to permanent damage if resuscitation is not accomplished in a timely and appropriate manner.

Calculating the Burn Area

The "rule of nines" is a useful guide in estimating the extent of a person's burn (Table 10–1). This approach divides the body into anatomic regions that represent 9% or multiples of 9% of the TBSA. Another method of estimation is using the palm of the patient's hand (excluding the fingers) which represents approximately 1% of the adult patient's total body surface.

Burn Depth

When calculating the total percentage of burn involvement, the first-degree burns are not included. Different burn depths should be noted on a burn diagram form.

Table 10–1 • RULE OF NINES		
Location	Adult (%)	Infant (%)
Front of head with neck	4.5	9
Back of head with neck	4.5	9
Front of torso	18	18
Back of torso	18	18
Front of one arm	4.5	4.5
Back of one arm	4.5	4.5
Front of one leg (full length)	9	7
Back of one leg (full length)	9	7

Table 10–2 • BURN DEPTH				
	Location Affected	Characteristics	Course	Treatment
First-degree	Epidermis	Erythema and pain	Heals in 3-4 d without scarring. The dead epidermal cells desquamate (peel). Sunburns that blister are actually superficial dermal burns.	Lotions (like aloe) and nonsteroidal anti-inflammatory drugs
Second-degree or partial-thickness	Through epidermis and into dermis	Pink/red, weepy, swelling and blisters, very painful	Superficial dermal heal within 3 wk without scarring or functional impairment. Deep dermal heal in 3-8 wk but with severe scarring and loss of function.	Excise and graft deep dermal burns
Third-degree or full-thickness	All the way through dermis	White or dark, leathery, waxy, painless	Burns can heal only by epithelial migration from periphery and contraction. Unless they are tiny (cigarette burn size), they will need grafting.	Excise and graft

(Table 10–2). As burns marginate, the assessment of depth may change from those estimated during the initial assessment, and this is particularly true of scald burns that often do not appear to be as deeply involved during the initial assessments. Fourth-degree burns are wounds that extend through the skin, subcutaneous fat, and deeper soft tissue structures.

Calculating Resuscitation Fluid Requirements

Most adults with burns involving less than 15% TBSA can be resuscitated with oral fluids. For patients with larger wounds, isotonic solution such as lactated ringer (LR) solution is preferred over normal saline (NS) because NS given in large volumes causes hyperchloremic metabolic acidosis. Fluid resuscitation requirements are estimated based on burn wound size. The Parkland formula for adults and children over 10 kg in weight is calculated using 4 mL/kg×% TBSA burn, with half of the fluid given during the first 8 hours and remainder given over the subsequent 16 hours. The Modified Brooke Formula is calculated to given LR at 2 mL/kg×% TBSA burn, with half of the volume given during the first 8 hours and remainder given during the subsequent 16 hours. During the second 24 hours, 5% albumin in LR is given to help compensate for the increase in capillary permeability and protein leakage. The various formulas that have been developed help to guide initial fluid administration, and all patients need close monitoring for responses to the resuscitation. It is important to keep in mind that inhalation injury, deep burn, and delayed presentation are factors that cause greater fluid requirements than the volume calculated based on burn sizes alone. It is important to keep in mind that insufficient fluid administration as well as excess fluid administration ("fluid creep") can produce additional damages to the injured tissue; therefore, care should be taken to avoid under- or over-resuscitation in all patients.

Assessing the Adequacy of Resuscitation

Urine output measurement (UOP) is a generally useful method of assessing the adequacy of burn resuscitation. For most adults, UOP of 0.5 mL/kg/h is considered sufficient, for children an UOP of 0.5 to 1.0 mL/kg/h is desirable, and UOP of 1 to 2 mL/kg/h is strived for in the resuscitation of infants. Generally, UOPs are averaged over every 2 to 3 hours before changes in fluid resuscitation are made. Excess urine output should be avoided unless the patient is being intentionally treated for myoglobinuria. It is important to keep in mind that urine output can be falsely elevated when the patient has hyperglycemia associated with a large amount of glucose in the urine.

Compartment syndromes of the abdomen and extremities are unintended byproducts of volume resuscitation for burns. Bladder pressure monitoring is important in patients receiving large-volume fluid resuscitations. Bladder pressures >20 mm Hg plus at least one additional organ dysfunction are indications of abdominal compartment syndrome and are potential indications for abdominal decompression. Impaired capillary refill, increasing pain, and paresthesias in the extremities are signs of extremity hypoperfusion and suggest the need for decompressive procedures such as escharotomies and/or fasciotomies.

Temporary Wound Coverage

The skin is a vital structure in temperature regulation and in the defense against bacterial and fungal infections. Care must be taken to prevent hypothermia and burn wound infections in burn patients. Burn site infections can lead to systemic infections and sepsis. The use of steroids and other immunosuppressive agents should be limited when treating patients with burn wounds greater than 10% TBSA. Prophylactic intravenous antibiotics are not recommended because of their association with infections by resistant organisms. Several topical agents are used in the care of burn wounds, and these agents typically have local broad antimicrobial activities and are effective in preventing microbial colonization. Silver sulfadiazine (SS) is one of the most commonly applied topical agents; SS application is generally soothing to the patient and fairly well-tolerated. Wounds with eschars and infections are more effectively treated with sulfamylon based on its ability to penetrate the eschar. Temporary coverage of partial thickness burns and excised nongrafted wounds with biologic dressings are beneficial in preventing heat and fluid loss, reducing pain, and in promoting epithelialization. The coverage of burn wounds with biologic dressings becomes most relevant when dealing with patients who do not have sufficient amount of autologous donor skin for definitive coverage and in the management of patients with partial thickness burns undergoing spontaneous healing. Porcine or bovine xenografts, cadaver skin, and acellular dermal matrix are the major types of biologic dressings applied for temporary wound coverage. Study results show that burn wounds treated with biologic dressings epithelialized faster and with less hypertrophic scarring in comparison to wounds treated with topical antimicrobial agents alone. The major limitations associated with biologic dressings are the high costs and the transmission of infections (associated predominantly with human allografts).

DEFINITIVE WOUND COVERAGE

The optimal goal in the management of burn wounds is to excise the burn wounds as soon as the resuscitation phase is completed, and provide early coverage with autologous split-thickness skin graft to facilitate early wound coverage and to minimize the risk of wound sepsis. This goal is accomplishable when the wound size is smaller than the amount of viable skin available for harvesting, and when the patient is physiologically able to undergo the operative treatment. A single-stage approach is often not possible when the burn wound size exceeds the amount of viable skin available harvesting and wound coverage. Meshing of the skin graft is a technique that allows skin to spread out and cover a large surface area. When insufficient amount of skin is available for total wound coverage, biologic dressings as described above are some alternatives that can provide temporary coverage of wound; this would allow time for re-epithelialization of donors sites for future harvesting as needed.

BURN COMPLICATIONS

Systemic: Burns larger than 20% TBSA are associated with systemic hypermetabolic responses; this is an indication for transfer to a specialized burn center (see Table 10–3). These responses include activation of the complement and coagulation pathways leading to microvascular thromboses, capillary leak, and interstitial edema. The activation of the inflammatory cascade triggers a subsequent counter-regulatory anti-inflammatory response that produces immune-suppression and susceptibility to nosocomial infections and sepsis.

Neurologic: Transient delirium commonly occurs in patients with major burns. Mental status alterations require evaluations to identify causes such as anoxia and metabolic abnormalities.

Pulmonary: Pneumonias and respiratory failure requiring mechanical ventilation occurs commonly and causes are multifactorial.

Cardiovascular: Myocardial depression often occurs transiently following major burns, and this is caused by vasoactive and inflammatory mediators that are released by the injured tissue. In selective patients, inotropic agents may be indicated to help support end-organ perfusion during the first 24 to 48 hours following the injury. Venous thromoembolic events occur in 1% to 23% of the hospitalized burn patients, and the chemoprophylaxis should be administered to reduce the risk of this complication.

Gastrointestinal: Gastric and duodenal ulcers can develop secondary to decreased mucosal defenses resulting from the decrease in splanchnic blood flow. Early gastric feeding may be beneficial in the prevention of ulcer formations. As the result of regional hypoperfusion, patient with major burns are at risk for the development of acalculous cholecystitis, pancreatitis, and hepatic dysfunction.

Renal: Acute kidney injury is reported in up to 20% of patients with severe burns. Early on, this can occur as the result of inadequate resuscitation or myoglobinuria (more common with deep burns and high-voltage electrical injuries), and late onset acute kidney injury can be caused by sepsis, worsening of pre-existing renal dysfunction, and nephrotoxic agents (such as medications and intravenous contrast material).

Infection: Burn size and increased patient age are contributors of host immune suppression and increased susceptibility to infections after major burns. Infections can arise from the burns themselves or from treatment related interventions (such as urinary tract infections from indwelling urinary catheters, and bacteremia related to intravenous catheters).

Ophthalmic: Corneal abrasions or ulcerations may occur in burn patients as the result of the initial burn process. Patients with potential eye injuries, such as those produced by explosions, should undergo early eye examinations using fluoroscein to detect potential corneal abrasions. When identified, corneal abrasions should be treated with topical antibiotic lubrication. Early examinations should be performed prior to the onset of eyelid edema that makes examinations difficult.

Musculoskeletal and soft tissue: Burn scars can cause functional and cosmetic defects. Physical and occupational therapy, scar release, regrafting, and silicon prosthesis are some of the adjunctive treatments that can improve outcomes.

Psychological: Burns can be very traumatic as well as defacing. Patients often need counseling and supportive care to optimize their recovery.

Because of the specialized care required and the multidisciplinary aspects of burn treatment, the American Burn Association recommends that certain subsets of burn patients receive their care at specialized burn care centers.

OUTPATIENT MANAGEMENT OF BURNS

Some patients with minor burn injuries may be appropriately managed as outpatients. Candidates for outpatient treatments include some adults with partial-thickness burns measuring less than 10% TBSA, children and elderly patients with less than 5% TBSA burns, and adults with full-thickness burns measuring less than 2% TBSA. In order to qualify for outpatient management, the outpatient setting needs to be sufficient to address the patient's wound pain, with low-risk of wound contamination, and with sufficient resources for optimal wound healing

Table 10–3 • AMERICAN BURN ASSOCIATION RECOMMENDATIONS FOR TRANSFER TO BURN CENTERS
<10 y or >50 y with full-thickness burn >10% TBSA
Any age with TBSA burn >20%
Partial- or full-thickness burn involving face, eyes, ears, hands, genitalia, perineum, and over joints
Burn injury complicated by chemical, electrical, or other forms of significant trauma
Any patient requiring special social, emotional, and long-term rehabilitative support

Abbreviation: TBSA, total body surface area.

and functional recovery. In most cases, the important goals can be accomplished with home care, outpatient physical therapy, visiting home nursing, and frequent outpatient follow-ups.

CASE CORRELATION

- See also Case 3 (Hypotensive patient [Sepsis]) and Case 8 (Hemorrhagic Shock [Trauma]).

COMPREHENSION QUESTIONS

10.1 Which of the following is the best management option for a 30-year-old man with a deep partial-thickness burn over the anterior abdomen and chest measuring approximately 20% TBSA?

A. Burn wound excision and split-thickness skin graft application done in three separate stages over 10-day time period

B. Excision of entire burn wound with autologous split-thickness skin graft application

C. Excision of entire burn wound with immediate application of cadaveric skin for temporary coverage, followed by definitive coverage with autologous split-thickness skin grafting in 7 days

D. Application of silver sulfadiazine to the wound until epithelialization of wound is completed

E. Application of sulfamylon to wound until epithelialization of wound is completed

10.2 Which of the following patients is best managed in a specialized burn center?

A. A 40-year-old man with 10% TBSA partial thickness burn to anterior abdomen, who is also a member of the Jehovah's Witness Church

B. A 6-year-old boy with partial-thickness burn to the left anterior forearm

C. A 55-year-old unconscious man with deep-partial-thickness and full-thickness burns to the anterior chest and abdomen, and carbonaceous septum after being rescued from a house fire

D. A 3-year-old boy with partial-thickness scald burn to the left forearm after he pulled a pan of hot grease from the stove, and his mother is extremely tearful and guilt-riddeen

E. A 30-year-old man with partial-thickness burn to the anterior abdomen and anterior portions of both thighs

10.3 Which of the following is the most appropriate resuscitation strategy for a 30-year-old man weighing 70 kg with a 40% TBSA burn wound? Use the Parkland formula for this calculation.

A. D_5 0.45 NS at an initial rate of 700 mL/h for the initial 8 hours and then followed by an infusion rate of 350 mL/h for the subsequent 16 hours

B. Lactated Ringers solution at an initial rate of 350 mL/h for the first 8 hours followed by an infusion rate of 700 mL/h for the subsequent 16 hours

C. Lactated Ringers solution at an initial rate of 700 mL/h for the first 8 hours followed by infusion rate of 350 mL/h for the subsequent 16 hours

D. Lactated Ringers at 600 mL/h for the first 8 hours followed by infusion at 300 mL/h for the next 16 hours

E. Lactated Ringers at 700 mL/h for the first 8 hours followed by infusion of Lactated Ringers to titrate to urine output of 1 to 2 mL/kg/h for the subsequent 16 hours

10.4 Which of the following is the most appropriate next step for the patient described in question 10.3 if his urine output averaged over the initial 2 hours of resuscitation is 15 mL/h?

A. Change the resuscitation fluid to 5% salt-free albumin at the calculated rate

B. Adjust the rate of resuscitation fluid infusion to achieve a catch-up urine output rate of 1 to 2 mL/kg/h

C. Initiate dopamine drip at 0.5 µg/kg/min to optimize renal perfusion

D. Adjust the rate of infusion of Lactated Ringers to achieve an average urine output of 35 to 70 mL/h

E. Place a Swan-Ganz catheter to determine cardiac and hemodynamic parameters so that inotropic agents and or vasopressor agents can be initiated to optimize cardiac performance

10.5 Which of the following is a complication associated with sulfamylon application for a patient with a 30% TBSA full-thickness burn?

A. Bacterial colonization of the wound

B. Arterial blood gas findings: pH 7.32, PaO_2 92, $PaCO_2$ 48, HCO_3 30

C. Generalized seizure

D. Renal tubular acidosis

E. Arterial blood gas findings: pH 7.32, PaO_2 88, $PaCO_2$ 38, HCO_3 21

10.6 For which of the patients with burn injuries is outpatient management considered most reasonable?

A. A 2-year-old boy with scalding partial thickness burns involving both lower extremities in a "stocking-like" distribution

B. A 58-year-old man with scalding, partial-thickness burn over the posterior aspect of the deltoid sustained when a hot water pipe burst open in his house

C. A 26-year-old woman who sustained burns to both hands after she intentionally set the house curtains on fire

D. A workman who a sustained burn wound to the palmer surface of the right hand and a separate wound to the sole of the left foot when he accidently grabbed a high-voltage cable at the power plant

E. A 20-year-old college student who sustained 8% TBSA burns to the face and anterior neck while lighting an outdoor barbecue grill

10.7 Which of the following is the most appropriate treatment for a 19-year-old man who was found inside a burning house and without any evidence of burn injury? He appears lethargic and has a carboxyhemoglobin (COHgb) level 32%.

A. 100% oxygen by face mask

B. Exchange transfusion to reduce his COHgb level

C. Endotracheal intubation and mechanical ventilatory support with 100% FiO_2

D. Close observation with repeat examination of COHgb levels in 30 minutes, 1, and 3 hours

E. Initiate hemodialysis to reduce his COHgB level

ANSWERS

10.1 **B.** Total excision of the burn wounds and autologous split-thickness skin graft application is the treatment option that provides early complete coverage of the wound, which should provide this patient with the shortest treatment course and earliest recovery. The young age of the patient and the relatively small burn wound size (20%) makes this option feasible. Permanent coverage of the burn wound is generally done in separate stages when the size of the wound far exceeds the size of available autologous skin for coverage of the wound.

10.2 **C.** The 55-year-old unconscious man with deep partial and full-thickness burns to the chest and abdomen (~18% TBSA) sustained in a house fire should be managed at a specialized burn center because he likely has inhalation injury in addition to his burn wounds. The potential of having inhalation injuries worsens this patient's prognosis, therefore this patient deserves to be treated in a specialized burn center. The boy described in "D" is suspicious for being a victim of child abuse and needs to be reported to the child-protective services, but does not have clear indications for burn center admission.

10.3 **C.** The Parkland formula provides recommendation for resuscitation during the first 24 hours of treatment. The fluid calculation is based on (body weight in kg) × (%TBSA burn size) × 4 mL, with half of the calculated volume given in the first 8 hours and the remainder given over the subsequent 16 hours, which translates to 70 × 40 × 4 = 11 200 ml for first 24 hours, and with 5600 mL given during the first 8 hours at a rate of 700 mL/h and then the remaining 5600 mL is given over the subsequent 16 hours at a rate of 350 mL/h.

10.4 **D.** Low urine output of 15 mL/h during the first two hours of resuscitation suggests inadequate fluid administration. Even though the Parkland formula is used for initial fluid resuscitation, low urine output response in this young man with burns suggests inadequate fluid resuscitation, which is sometimes caused by under-estimation of burn size or delay in the initiation of fluid resuscitation. The fluid infusion rate should be increased to try to titrate to a urine output of 0.5 to 1.0 mL/kg/h, which translates to 35 to 70 mL/h urine output. Inotropic agents are not indicated unless the patient's intravascular volume depletion has been first addressed.

10.5 **E.** Sulfamylon administration can cause metabolic acidosis through carbonic anhydrase inhibition. The blood gas findings in "E" reflect metabolic acidosis, since the pH is low at 7.32, together with an nonelevated $paCO_2$, and low bicarbonate values.

10.6 **B.** The 58-year-old man with partial thickness scald burns over the posterior aspect of the deltoid does not have indications for inpatient care. The 2-year-old boy with stocking-like distribution of scalding burn over both lower extremities suggests that the injury pattern could be intentional and the result of child abuse; therefore, admission and social service consultation are indicated. The patient with burns to both hands after intentionally setting fire to the house needs specialized care to optimize functional recovery; in addition, she needs to undergo psychiatric evaluation for this behavior. The worker with electric burns to the hand and foot after contact with high-voltage wire needs observation to monitor for myoglobinuria and other clinical manifestations of high-voltage electric burns. The 20-year-old college student with flame burns to face and anterior neck would benefit from treatment in a burn center to optimize his functional recovery.

10.7 **C.** This unconscious man found inside a burning house has elevated carboxyhemoglobin level of 32%. This level of COHgb is likely the factor contributing to brain anoxia and his current lethargic state. CO has much greater affinity for binding with Hgb than O_2; however, bound CO can be displaced from Hgb more rapidly when patients are given high concentrations of O_2 to breathe. Intubation and mechanical ventilation support with 100% O_2 is a way to provide the patient with the highest O_2 concentration and will reduce the half-life of CO binding to Hgb from 250 minutes (on room air) to 40 to 60 minutes at a FiO_2 of 100%; therefore, intubation and mechanical ventilation is the best treatment choice to help reduce the anoxic effects of CO toxicity.

CLINICAL PEARLS

▶ A burn victims with a dry, red, or blistered oropharynx will likely require intubation.

▶ All burn victims from enclosed-space fires should have their COHgb values determined to assess for possible carbon monoxide poisoning.

▶ The rule of nines is a useful guide to estimate the size of burn wounds in burn victims. Body surface areas of various anatomic regions are divided roughly into multiples of 9%.

▶ The Parkland formula is a useful initial estimate of fluid resuscitation schedules for burn patients during the initial 24 hours (body weight in kg × %TBSA burn × 4 mL of Lactated Ringers, half of the calculate volume administered in the first 8 hours and the remainder given in the subsequent 16 hours).

▶ A full-thickness burn is typically leathery dry in appearance, and often nonpainful.

▶ The combination of smoke inhalation and burn injury increases the fluid requirement for the resuscitation and generally increases mortality.

▶ Compartment syndrome of the abdomen and extremities are complications associated with large volume fluid resuscitation for burns.

REFERENCES

Endorf FW, Ahrenholz D. Burn management. *Curr Opin Crit Care.* 2011;17:601-605.

Milner SM, Asuku ME. Burn wound management. In: Cameron JL, Cameron AM, eds. *Current Surgical Therapy.* 11th ed. Philadelphia, PA: Elsevier Saunders; 2014: 1128-1131.

Sheridan R. Practical management of the burn patient. In: Cameron JL, Cameron AM, eds. *Current Surgical Therapy.* 11th ed. Philadelphia, PA: Elsevier Saunders; 2014: 1131-1138.

Snell JA, Loh NEW, Mahambrey T, Shokrollahi K. Clinical review: the critical care management of the burn patient. *Crit Care.* 2013;17:241-250.

A 37-year-old (gravida 1, para 0) premenopausal, married woman presents with a painless left breast mass that she has noticed for the past 3 to 4 months. She is otherwise healthy and without any prior history of breast-related symptoms or family history of breast cancer. On physical examination, there is a 2-cm non-tender, indiscrete, hard mass in the upper outer quadrant of her left breast. There is no skin abnormality over the breast and no adenopathy in the axilla or supra-clavicular region. The remainder of her physical examination is otherwise normal. You perform a breast ultrasound examination that reveals a 1.8 × 2.5 cm solid, heterogeneous mass with irregular and indistinct borders.

▶ What are your next steps?
▶ What are the goals in this patient's management?

ANSWERS TO CASE 11:
Breast Cancer

Summary: A 37-year-old woman presents with a painless left breast mass. Physical examination reveals a palpable breast mass, no adenopathy, and no skin changes. The ultrasound appearance is highly suspicious for cancer (solid, heterogeneous mass with irregular and indistinct borders).

- **Next Steps:** You need to obtain tissue to confirm the diagnosis and characterize the tumor. After discussing the findings and your concerns with your patient, you can perform a core-needle biopsy under ultrasound guidance. Once cancer is verified by the pathologist, you will need to have in-depth discussions with the patient and her family regarding her diagnosis, prognosis, and treatment options. Her individual treatment plan will be best determined on the basis of her personal preference, the tumor characteristics (tumor size to breast size ratio, histologic grade, hormone receptors status, and biologic characteristics), and tumor stage (Tumor, Nodes, Metastases [TNM] stage). For most patients, treatments will include some combination of surgery, radiation therapy, chemotherapy, biologic therapy, and hormonal therapy. Before initiating treatment, baseline laboratory studies including liver function tests, bilateral mammography or bilateral breast magnetic resonance imaging (MRI), and chest x-ray should be obtained to identify or rule out other breast abnormalities and for tumor staging.

- **Treatment Goals:** The goals of treatment for this patient with suspected breast cancer are to establish a definitive diagnosis, obtain tissue to define tumor receptors and biologic characteristics, stage the disease, communicate with the patient regarding her surgical treatment options and preferences (breast conservation v. mastectomy with or without reconstruction), and help coordinate her multimodality treatments. In many practice settings, the patients' treatment recommendations are formulated at multidisciplinary Tumor Boards where practitioners from various specialties including surgery, medical oncology, radiation oncology, pathology, and radiology assemble to discuss individual patients' treatment strategies. The multimodality treatment of breast cancer is a process that often extends over months and sometime years; therefore, it is important to communicate the specific options early on with the patient and her family. Similarly, it is important to evaluate for emotional, social, and financial needs and barriers that could impact treatment compliance and outcomes. If indicated, it is important to make early referrals to social, medical, and community resources so that the patient and her family can receive emotional and social support to help them get through the long treatment course that would likely involve many visits to medical specialists over the course of months to years. **For this premenopausal woman, it is important to inquire regarding her desires for future fertility.** If she wishes to have children in the future, she and her spouse should be referred to a reproductive medicine specialist to discuss and explore options (such as oocyte retrieval) prior to starting any fertility altering treatments such as chemotherapy, biologic therapy, and antiestrogen therapy.

ANALYSIS

Objectives

1. Learn the diagnosis and staging of breast cancer.
2. Learn the locoregional and systemic treatment options for patients with breast cancers.
3. Learn the rationale for selecting various treatment options.

Consideration

When a woman presents with a dominant breast mass, the most important early goal is to "rule out" or confirm the diagnosis of breast cancer. If feasible, it is helpful to perform a core-needle biopsy during the initial visit, as this may provide information that will be pivotal for all subsequent discussions and therapeutic decisions. The diagnosis of breast cancer should be entertained whenever a woman or a man presents with an abnormality of the breast, such as a mass, skin change, nipple change, or axillary adenopathy.

A thorough evaluation of breast-related complaint needs to include *clinical evaluation* (history and physical examination), *imaging* (mammography, ultrasound, and/or breast MRI), and *pathology* (cytology or histology). **Together, the clinical, imaging, and pathology assessments are referred to as the "triple test." It it is critical to bear in mind that the triple test must be completed and found negative to sufficiently rule out breast cancer in any suspected individual.** For example, if the patient who presents with clinical and imaging findings that are highly suspicious for breast cancer and has a core-needle biopsy that revealed only benign breast tissue, a subsequent excisional biopsy of the mass would need to be performed because an inconsistency in the triple test can result from sampling error and would be insufficient to rule out breast cancer.

Once the biopsy confirms cancer, the patient should have staging work-up that includes bilateral mammography ± breast MRI, chest x-ray, chest and abdominal computed tomography (CT), or positron emission-CT (PET-CT). Based on her ultrasound measurements, the cancer is likely a T2 lesion (>2 cm and <5 cm). The treatment approach for a premenopausal woman with cancer of this size would certainly include some form of systemic therapy in addition to local regional treatment (ie, surgery and radiation therapy). **It is important that you convey to the patient that a partial mastectomy with radiation therapy offers her the same survival as a mastectomy.** In addition, a sentinel lymph node biopsy should be done to stage the axillary nodal status (N-stage), see Table 11–1.

Table 11–1 • BREAST CANCER AJCC STAGING				
Stage 0	Tis	N0	M0	Tx: Cannot assess
				T0: No evidence of primary tumor
Stage I	T1	N0	M0	Tis: In situ
				T1: ≤2 cm
Stage IIa	T0-T1	N1	M0	T1a: ≤0.5 cm
				T1b: >0.5 cm, 1 cm
	T2	N0	M0	T1c: >1 cm, ≤2 cm
				T2: >2 cm, <5 cm
Stage IIb	T2	N1	M0	T3: >5 cm
				T4: Extension to chest wall or skin
				T4a: Extension to chest wall
	T3	N0	M0	T4b: Edema or ulceration of the skin
Stage IIIa	T0-T2	N2	M0	T4c: Both chest wall extension and skin involvement
	T3	N1-N2	M0	T4d: Inflammatory carcinoma
				Nx: Cannot assess
Stage IIIb	T4	N0-N2	M0	N0: No regional nodal metastases
				N1: Mobile ipsilateral axillary nodal metastases
	T$_{any}$	N3	M0	N2: Fixed ipsilateral axillary nodal metastases
				N3: Ipsilateral internal mammary or supraclavicular nodal metastases
Stage IV	T$_{any}$	N$_{any}$	M1	Mx: Cannot be assessed
				M0: No distant metastases
				M1: Distant metastases

APPROACH TO:

Breast Carcinoma

DEFINITIONS

DOMINANT BREAST MASS: A three-dimensional breast mass that persists and remains relatively unchanged throughout the menstrual cycle.

FINE-NEEDLE ASPIRATION (FNA): A tissue sampling technique involving aspiration of the mass using a small-gauge needle. Cells aspirated are analyzed for cytology. This approach can identify malignant cells but cannot definitively differentiate in situ cancers from invasive cancers. FNA performed under ultrasound guidance is also valuable for cytologic assessment of axillary lymph nodes.

CORE-NEEDLE BIOPSY: A biopsy technique that is done via larger caliber needle with or without image guidance. Core biopsies can be done under mammographic guidance (stereotactic biopsy), MRI guidance, ultrasound guidance, or without image guidance (palpation alone). Image guidance is generally better to help verify actual sampling of the lesion in question and minimizes nondiagnostic results.

BREAST IMAGING REPORTING AND DATA SYSTEM (BIRADS): This is the standard reporting system originally developed for mammography results reporting and is based on the likelihood of a lesion being malignant. The BIRADS system is also used for the reporting of breast ultrasound and MRI results (see Table 11–2 for details).

BREAST DENSITY REPORTING AND IMPLICATIONS: Some radiology groups routinely comment on breast densities on mammogram reports; this is important because increased breast density increases cancer risks and diminishes the accuracy of mammography. Categories of 1 to 4 is often used, where 1 is <25% glandular tissue, 2 is 25% to 50% glandular tissue, 3 is 51% to75% glandular tissue, and 4 is >75% glandular tissue.

BREAST-CONSERVING TREATMENT (BCT): Surgical treatment that consists of partial mastectomy (also known as segmental mastectomy or lumpectomy) to conserve the breast. The patients undergoing BCT should receive whole breast irradiation following surgery or local radiation treatment with intraoperative radiation therapy.

INFLAMMATORY BREAST CANCER (IBC): An aggressive form of breast cancer that occurs more frequently in younger women of African-American descent. The clinical presentation of IBC is often rapid and dramatic with erythema and swelling of the breast occurring over a period of weeks to months. The skin of the involved breast is infiltrated with tumor cells; thus, it may display a thickening that is classically referred to as *peau d'orange* (orange peel-like). Regional lymph node involvement is common with IBCs. Most IBC patients are treated with neoadjuvant chemotherapy followed by surgery and radiation therapy. In general, IBC patients have worse prognosis, and patients' outcomes are significantly influenced by the lymph node statuses and responses to neoadjuvant therapy.

NEOADJUVANT SYSTEMIC THERAPY: Most commonly implemented in patients presenting with locally advanced disease. The systemic therapy (chemotherapy, biologic therapy, or hormonal therapy) is given prior to surgical treatment (locoregional Rx). The neoadjuvant approach has several proven benefits. (1) It improved success of breast-conserving treatment, especially for women presenting with cancers with unfavorable tumor size to breast size ratios. (2) Leaving the tumors in place provides clinicians with opportunities to modify systemic treatment regimens when favorable clinical responses are not produced by the initial treatments. (3) Neoadjuvant approach gives clinicians the opportunity to identify complete pathologic responses (cPR) in patients following systemic therapy, and patients who exhibit cPR have a much better prognosis in comparison to patients who do not achieve cPR.

MALE BREAST CANCERS (MBCs): These are much rarer than female breast cancers, accounting for only 1% of all breast cancers. Individuals with Klinefelter's syndrome (XXY) and *BRCA2* mutations have significantly increased risk of developing MBC, where an estimated 40% of MBCs are associated with *BRCA2* mutations. Treatments of MBC are mostly extrapolated from the treatment of female breast cancers. Stage for stage, MBCs carry similar prognosis as female cancers. Unfortunately, MBC patients generally present with more advanced disease stages than women; therefore, MBC patients as a group tend to have poorer survival than female breast cancer patients.

TRIPLE RECEPTOR NEGATIVE BREAST CANCERS (TNBCs): These are cancers that are estrogen, progesterone, and *HER2/neu* receptors negative. Although most TNBCs are classified as basal-like, not all basal-like breast cancers are TNBCs. TNBCs represent approximately 10% to 15% of all female breast cancers and are increasingly identified in premenopausal women of African-American descent. Although TNBCs are often chemosensitive, women with TNBCs frequently experience early (<3 years) visceral metastases and poorer survival in comparison to women with non-TNBCs. Women with *BRCA1* mutation-related breast cancers often have TNBCs or basal-like cancers.

GENE EXPRESSION ASSAYS FOR BREAST CANCER: Gene expression profile assays have been available since 2002. The two most commonly available commercial assays at the time of this writing are *Oncotype DX (21 gene profile)* and *MammaPrint (70 gene profile)*. Based on the gene array profile assessment of a patient's tumor, a recurrence risk score can be generated (report range of 0 to 100). The genetic profiles' recurrence risk determinations are useful to help decide whether a more aggressive systemic treatment is indicated, such as in deciding when systemic chemotherapy should be given to node (−) patients with ER(+) and Her2(−) tumors. See Table 11–3).

ANTIESTROGEN THERAPY: Antiestrogen therapy is effective in reducing cancer recurrences in patients whose cancers have high levels of estrogen and/or progesterone receptors expression. Antiestrogen therapy is most beneficial when given for ≥5 years. Tamoxifen is the main antiestrogen therapy for premenopausal women. Aromatase inhibitors (AIs) are more effective than tamoxifen; however, AIs are only effective for postmenopausal women and are the antiestrogen agents

Table 11–2 • BREAST IMAGING REPORTING AND DATA SYSTEM (BIRADS) CATEGORIES	
BIRADS 0	**Imaging is incomplete** (needs additional imaging or comparison to previous imaging)
BIRADS 1	**Negative** (resume routine screening mammography)
BIRADS 2	**Benign** (no signs of cancer but may contain benign changes; resume routine screening)
BIRADS 3	**Probably benign** (< 2% cancer probability); recommend shorter interval between imaging studies (eg, 6-month follow-up imaging)
BIRADS 4	**Suspicious abnormality** (biopsy should be considered). Some groups further subcategorize into 4A (low), 4B (intermediate), and 4C (high).
BIRADS 5	**Highly suggestive of cancer** (>95% cancer probability, therefore appropriate action should be taken).
BIRADS 6	**Known cancer**. Imaging of biopsy proven cancer

Table 11–3 • BREAST CANCER SUBTYPES BASED ON HORMONE RECEPTORS AND MOLECULAR CHARACTERISTICS

Subtype	Characteristics	Molecular Markers	Prognosis
Luminal A (50% of breast cancers)	Low histologic grade; High ER	ER(+); PR(+); HER2(−)	Best prognosis of all breast cancers
Luminal B (10% of all breast cancers)	High histologic grade; Low ER	ER(+); PR(±);HER2(±)	Intermediate Prognosis
HER2 (10% of all breast cancers)	High histologic grade	ER(−); PR(−); HER2(+)	Previously poor prognosis but with the anti-HER2 therapy prognosis has improved
Basal-like (30% of all breast cancers)	High proliferative index; TNBCs are included in this category	ER(−); PR(−); HER2 (−)	Poor prognosis due to high early recurrence rates following systemic therapy

of choice for postmenopausal women. Tamoxifen is associated with increase in the risk of uterine cancers; therefore, women on tamoxifen require monitoring. Joint pain and bony density losses are the major side effects of AI. **Bisphosphonate is often given together with AIs to minimize bone mineral losses and reduce osseous metastasis.** Tamoxifen can also be prescribed for men with breast cancers that express high levels of ER and/or PR receptors.

BIOLOGIC TREATMENTS TARGETING GROWTH FACTOR RECEPTORS: The *HER2* receptor is the most commonly targeted cell surface receptor in the epidermal growth factor family (EGF). Trastuzumab is a monoclonal antibody targeting the extracellular portion of *HER2* receptor. *Trastuzumab* + chemotherapy in the adjuvant setting for women with tumors that overexpress *HER2-neu* have been shown to produce significant survival advantage over adjuvant chemotherapy alone. In the neoadjuvant setting, trastuzumab has been shown to produce higher cPR rates in comparison to systemic chemotherapy alone. It is important to keep in mind that **trastuzumab causes cardiac toxicity**; therefore, to avoid treatment-related cardiac failure, cardiac-toxic chemotherapeutic agents such as doxorubicin (Adriamicin) should be avoided in patients with *HER2-neu* (+) tumors.

Antiangiogenic (anti-*VEGF*) monoclonal antibody treatments have been proven useful in the adjuvant treatment of lung, colon, and renal cell cancers; however, this treatment strategy has been disappointing in breast cancers treatment. In 2011, the Food and Drug Administration (FDA) withdrew the approval of anti-VEGF treatment for breast cancer patients because of high toxicity and lack of benefits.

BIOLOGIC TREATMENTS TARGETING DNA-REPAIR PATHWAYS: Poly(ADP-ribose) polymerases (PARPs) are a family of 17 DNA-repair enzymes. PARP inhibitors are monoclonal antibodies that target tumors with PARP mutations. **PARP inhibitors are particularly effective in the treatment of breast cancers with DNA-repair-gene mutations such as *BRCA1*, *BRCA2*, TNBCs, and basal-type cancers.**

DOSE-DENSE THERAPY: This strategy utilizes systemic treatment schedules with shortened intervals between treatment cycles (1-2 weeks v. 3-4 weeks). This approach is more effective but is associated with increased toxicity. Patient selection and growth factor support of bone marrow functions are important to minimize complications during dose-dense therapy.

CLINICAL APPROACH

The management steps for most patients with breast cancers consist of diagnosis, staging, locoregional therapy, and systemic therapy. The possibility of breast cancer is most often raised as the result of either some physical finding related to the breast or based on abnormalities identified by imaging, such as suspicious findings on screening mammogram. Whenever these abnormalities are encountered, tissue or cytology diagnosis should be strongly considered. FNA or core-needle biopsies are procedures that are done in the outpatient setting to help clinicians confirm or rule out cancer diagnoses. When small cancers or nonpalpable cancers are encountered, it is important to differentiate in situ (Tis) from invasive cancers (T_1 to T_4), because in situ cancers are managed differently and are curable with locoregional treatments alone.

Patients with clinically suspected stage I or II disease may not need additional whole body imaging to look for occult metastatic disease; whereas, patients with advanced local disease or suspected advanced diseases (stage III or IV) might benefit from additional imaging studies such as CT of the chest, abdomen, and pelvis to help identify synchronous occult metastases. Patients with bone-related symptoms should have bone scans to rule out osseous metastases. Patients with CNS-related symptoms should have CT or MRI of the brain to rule out or identify brain metastases. In some institutions, the systemic imaging survey is done using PET-CT, which may help identify and characterize overt and occult metastatic diseases.

Most patients with localized disease stages (stages I and IIa) will undergo locoregional treatment before systemic therapy; whereas, patients presenting with larger tumors or locally advanced disease (stages IIb and III) are often selected to undergo neoadjuvant systemic therapy prior to locoregional treatment. Neoadjuvant treatment has been demonstrated to improve the success of breast conservation treatments and is associated with improved cosmetic outcomes. However, no difference in survival outcomes has been demonstrated between patients receiving neoadjuvant and adjuvant therapies.

One area of controversy surrounding neoadjuvant therapy is in the timing of axillary staging. There is evidence to indicate that axillary staging is more accurate when SLNB is performed prior to neoadjuvant therapy. However, some practitioners believe that it is more important to know the axillary lymph node status after neoadjuvant therapy, as approximately 40% of patients have cPR in the axilla following neoadjuvant treatments, and cPR in the axilla following neoadjuvant therapy has great prognostic value. An approach that is popular currently is to utilize ultrasound evaluations of the axilla and perform FNA biopsy of suspicious lymph nodes prior to neoadjuvant therapy, and then perform axillary dissection or SLNB after the completion of neoadjuvant therapy.

The operative treatment of breast cancer has continued to evolve over the past three decades with a trend toward less aggressive surgical treatments. During the 1980s, randomized controlled trials showed that mastectomies did not offer any survival advantage over BCT consisting of partial mastectomy (lumpectomy), axillary dissection + radiation therapy. Clinical trials during the 1990s and 2000s demonstrated that routine axillary dissections (ALND) did not contribute to improved survival. These observations led to the elimination of routine ALND in patients with invasive breast cancers with negative SLNB.

In 2011, the ACOSOG Z0011 trial findings were published. This trial randomized breast conservation treatment (partial mastectomy + radiation) patients with primary tumors ≤5cm, clinically negative axilla, and with <3 (+) SLN to completion ALND versus no axillary treatment. The findings of the Z0011 trial showed that for patients with occult disease in the axilla found during SLNB, ALND did not produce additional survival or local disease control benefits over observation alone. The results of this trial have dramatically reduced the role of ALND in breast cancer patients.

Research discoveries and clinical trials over the past several decades have led to the development of more effective medical and biologic treatments. At the same time, medical advances have improved patients' abilities to tolerate aggressive systemic treatment regimens. Given these advances, **nearly all women with invasive breast cancers of >1 cm in size are now given some form of systemic therapy.** The current role of surgical treatment is to help stage the disease, control local and regional

---

CASE CORRELATION

- See also Case 12 (Breast Cancer Risk and Surveillance) and Case 13 (Nipple Discharge [Serosanguinous]).

---

disease while maintaining functional and cosmetic outcomes for the patients. Advances in tumor biology research and medical oncology have contributed to breast cancer prognosis improvements over the past two decades.

COMPREHENSION QUESTIONS

11.1 A 38-year-old woman has an asymmetric density in the left breast. FNA of the mass revealed malignant cells. Which of the following is the best next step?

A. Total mastectomy and SLNB

B. Partial mastectomy, SLNB, and radiation therapy

C. Core-needle biopsy

D. Partial mastectomy and radiation therapy

E. Neoadjuvant chemotherapy

11.2 A 54-year-old woman has a 1-cm breast mass that was demonstrated by core-needle biopsy as invasive ductal carcinoma. The patient undergoes partial mastectomy and axillary SLNB. The final pathology revealed invasive ductal carcinoma measuring 1.5 cm with one out of four SLNs being positive for metastatic disease. Which of the following is the most appropriate treatment plan for this patient?

A. Axillary lymph node dissection, whole-breast radiation, and adjuvant systemic chemotherapy

B. Whole breast, axillary, and chest wall radiation therapy, followed by systemic chemotherapy

C. Whole breast radiation and systemic chemotherapy

D. Mastectomy and axillary lymph node dissection

E. No additional treatment

11.3 A 43-year-old woman presents with painful enlargement of the left breast. The patient denies any antecedent events. On examination, her left breast is visibly larger than the right breast with skin thickening and redness. There is a 1-cm palpable lymph node in her left axilla. Which of the following is the most appropriate management?

A. Admit the patient to the hospital for intravenous antibiotics treatment

B. Give her a 7-day course of oral antibiotics and re-evaluate in 1 month

C. Give her a 7-day course of oral antibiotics, obtain bilateral mammography, and re-evaluate in 1 month

D. Perform ultrasound evaluation of the left breast and biopsy of any suspicious lesions

E. Obtain a PET scan to rule out cancer

11.4 A 60-year-old woman with a 3-cm left breast cancer underwent breast conservation therapy with complete excision of the tumor and SLNB. Her tumor is ER (+), PR (+), and *Her2* (−). The SLNB is negative and the metastatic work-up is negative. She has just completed a 6-week course of whole-breast radiation. Which of the following pieces of information is most helpful in deciding whether systemic chemotherapy should be given in addition to aromatase inhibitor treatment?

A. The results of her genetic expression profile assay

B. The PET-CT finding

C. The tumor size to breast size ratio

D. The patient's ethnicity

E. The location of the patient's tumor

11.5 A 46-year-old woman who underwent her first bilateral screening mammogram received a report that her mammography results were reported as BIRADS 0. In addition, the report commented that her breast density classification was 4 (>75% glandular tissue). Which of the following is the most appropriate next step?

A. Follow-up mammography in 6 months

B. Obtain bilateral breast ultrasound evaluation

C. Obtain bilateral breast MRI

D. Obtain image-guided core biopsies

E. Refer patient to a medical oncologist for breast cancer treatment

11.6 Which of the following is considered an appropriate treatment option for a 60-year-old woman who develops two liver metastases and a left lung metastasis 2 years following a modified radical mastectomy for invasive ductal carcinoma? The patient's tumor is ER (+), PR (+), and Her2 (−). She had completed a course of ACT (adriamycin/cyclophosphamide/taxotere) systemic chemotherapy just 1 year ago. She is currently on tamoxifen therapy.

A. Initiate trastuzumab treatment

B. Radiation therapy to the lung and liver

C. Resection of liver and lung metastases

D. Stop tamoxifen and begin aromatase inhibitor treatment

E. Initiate anti-VEGF treatment

ANSWERS

11.1 **C.** Even though the FNA has demonstrated malignant cells, this patient needs to have a core-needle biopsy or an excisional biopsy to determine if this tumor is an in situ or invasive cancer. Without knowing the difference, we would not have sufficient data to provide her with the most appropriate treatment.

11.2 **C.** Whole breast radiation and systemic therapy are the most appropriate treatments for this patient. She has T1 and N1 diseases. Based on the findings of the ACOZOG Z11 trial, axillary dissection will not offer any advantage over observation of the axilla alone. The systemic chemotherapy is indicated in this patient because she has stage IIA disease. Mastectomy is not necessary for this patient because there is no survival advantage in comparison to partial mastectomy with radiation therapy.

11.3 **D.** Ultrasound evaluation and image-guided biopsy are the most appropriate options. This patient's presentation is highly suggestive of inflammatory breast cancer. If imaging and biopsy prove that there is no cancer, then a trial of antibiotics therapy might be reasonable. A PET scan might be helpful after cancer diagnosis is verified but tissue diagnosis needs to be prioritized over the PET scan.

11.4 **A.** For this postmenopausal woman with ER (+), PR (+), Her2 (−), and node (−) breast cancer, information gain from a genetic expression profile assay may help identify patients with tumors that exhibit high-risk genetic profiles. Systemic chemotherapy in addition to aromatase inhibitor treatment may be more effective for patients with high-risk cancers. PET CT can be useful to determine the metabolic activities of cancers, and PET-CT results have been used in the selection of chemotherapy regimens in lymphoma patients. PET results are not used at this time to determine the course of initial breast cancer treatment.

11.5 **C.** This patient had mammography that was reported to be BIRADS 0, which indicated that the imaging was incomplete (inconclusive) and additional imaging studies should be obtained. Because the patient was noted to have dense breast tissue, additional imaging by breast MRI might be most helpful for further evaluation of her breasts that contain dense breast tissue. Breast MRI has higher sensitivity than mammography and ultrasound in the evaluation of women with dense breasts.

11.6 **D.** For this patient with ER/PR (+) breast cancer who develops liver and lung metastasis following systemic chemotherapy with ACT, there are a number of options remaining. Since the patient is postmenopausal, it is reasonable to discontinue tamoxifen and switch her over to aromatase inhibitor treatment. AI has been shown to be more effective than tamoxifen for patient with ER/PR (+) cancers. Radiation therapy and surgery are locoregional treatment strategies that are not likely to be of benefit in this patient with disease recurrence at distant sites. Trastuzumab is not effective in this patient with Her2 (−) cancer. Anti-VEGF treatment strategy has not been found effective in the treatment of breast cancer and is no longer approved by the FDA for breast cancer treatment.

CLINICAL PEARLS

▶ The initial workup for a dominant breast mass should involve tissue analysis and bilateral mammography to assess the lesion and look for other occult abnormalities.

▶ Negative triple-test confirmation is required before breast cancer can be definitively ruled out.

▶ Surgery and radiation therapy are locoregional treatment modalities, and chemotherapy, targeted biological therapy, and antiestrogen therapy are systemic treatment modalities.

▶ Patients with small invasive breast cancers (T1 or T2) and occult axillary lymph node metastasis involving two or fewer lymph nodes demonstrated by SLNB, who are undergoing partial mastectomy with whole breast radiation therapy do not need ALND to address the axillary lymph node involvement (ACOSOG Z11 trial).

▶ Patients with triple receptor negative tumors (ER (–), PR (–), and Her2 (–)) are at increased risk for developing visceral metastasis and have a poorer prognosis.

▶ Tamoxifen can be used for pre- or postmenopausal women and men with ER/PR (+) breast cancers.

▶ Aromatase inhibitors are more effective antiestrogen therapy than tamoxifen but are not effective for premenopausal women.

▶ Tamoxifen increases a woman's risk of developing uterine cancer.

▶ Increased breast tissue density is due to increased in glandular tissue, and this type of breast composition increases a woman's breast cancer risk and decreases our ability to identify the cancer using mammography.

▶ Breast MRI is more sensitive for the detection of breast cancers in women with dense breast tissue.

REFERENCES

Giuliano AE, Hunt KK, Ballman KV, et al. Axillary dissection vs no axillary dissection in women with invasive breast cancer and sentinel lymph node metastasis: a randomized clinical trial. *JAMA.* 2011;305:569-575.

Hunt KK, Green MC, Buchholz TA. Diseases of the breast. In: Townsend CM Jr, Beauchamp RD, Evers BM, Mattox KL, eds. *Sabiston Textbook of Surgery: The Biological Basis of Modern Surgical Practice.* 19th ed. Philadelphia, PA: Elsevier Saunders; 2012:824-869.

Krontiras H, Awonuga OO, Bland K. Molecular targets in breast cancer. In: Cameron JL, Cameron AM, eds. *Current Surgical Therapy.* 11th ed. Philadelphia, PA: Elsevier Saunders; 2014:579-583.

Lin JH, Giuliano AE. The management of the axilla in breast cancer. In: Cameron JL, Cameron AM, eds. *Current Surgical Therapy.* 11th ed. Philadelphia PA: Elsevier Saunders; 2014:595-599.

CASE 12

A 41-year-old woman underwent an initial screening mammography that revealed dense bilateral breast tissue. According to the evaluation by the radiologist, the evaluation was considered incomplete; therefore, additional imaging is recommended BIRADS-0). The patient's past medical history is unremarkable. She has never had previous breast masses, breast complaints, biopsies, or prior mammography. She is married and had onset of menarche at age 11 and her first child at age 27. Her family history is significant in that her mother died at the age of 45 from breast cancer. On examination, both breasts are firm but without specific abnormalities. No dominant masses or axillary adenopathy are appreciated.

▶ What is the most likely diagnosis?
▶ What concerns and complications associated with these changes?

ANSWERS TO CASE 12:

Breast Cancer Risks, Screening, and Surveillance

Summary: The patient is a 41-year-old woman with a high-risk profile for breast cancer based on history of maternal, premenopausal breast cancer, and the findings of bilateral dense breast tissue, which makes breast examinations and imaging less reliable.

- **Most likely diagnosis:** Dense breast tissue in a woman with breast cancer with a high-risk profile.

- **Concerns and complications:** The patient's family history suggests a high-risk profile. In addition, the presence of bilateral dense breast tissue affects the ability to detect abnormalities by physical examination and mammographic imaging. Furthermore, increased breast density is shown to correlate with increased risk in breast cancer occurrence.

ANALYSIS

Objectives

1. Learn the relationship between benign breast changes, borderline malignant changes, and malignant disease (Table 12–1).

2. Learn to assess (or estimate) a patient's lifetime risk of breast cancer.

3. Understand the management principles and options based on individual's cancer risk profile.

4. Appreciate the discrepancies between the American Cancer Society (ACS) Recommendations for mammographic screening and the United States Preventive Service Task Force screening mammography recommendations.

Table 12–1 • BENIGN BREAST LESIONS AND RELATIVE RISK OF BREAST CANCER
Benign breast histology not associated with an increased risk for breast cancer:
• Adenosis, apocrine metaplasia, cysts, ductal ectasia, fibroadenoma, fibrosis, mild hyperplasia, mastitis, squamous metaplasia
Risk increased 1.5- to 2.0-fold:
• Moderate or severe ductal hyperplasia, papillomatosis
Risk increased 5-fold:
• Atypical ductal hyperplasia
Risk increased 10-fold:
• Lobular carcinoma in situ
• Atypical ductal hyperplasia with family history of breast cancer

Considerations

For this 41-year-old woman whose mother died at the age of 45 from breast cancer, her initial screening mammographic study has to be extremely anxiety provoking. To make matters worse, her physical examination and mammography reveal bilateral dense breast tissue. These findings are associated with increased difficulties with the detection of cancers by physical and mammographic examinations. Furthermore, increased mammographic breast density is a well-established strong predictor of breast cancer risk. One of the most important discussions to have with the patient is regarding breast cancer risks and the rationale behind screening and surveillance strategies based on their risks. There are numerous breast cancer risk-stratification models that have been developed and are accessible through the Internet. (eg, the National Cancer Institute risk calculation http://www.cancer.gov/bcrisktool/). With the information given by this patient, we are able to calculate a lifetime risk of breast cancer of 19.8% and 5-year cancer risk of 1.3%. Her calculated lifetime risk is higher than the average population risk of 12%. This risk calculator does not take into account of breast density that is associated with additional breast cancer risks that would increase her lifetime risk above 20% (>20% lifetime risk is by definition "high risk" whereas, 15% lifetime risk is considered "moderate risk"). **Since 2007, the American Cancer Society has recommended the use of screening magnetic resonance imaging (MRI) as an adjunct for patients with lifetime cancer risks greater than 20% to 25%.** For this patient, screening breast MRI is further justified based on the difficulties associated with the interpretation of her mammographic study. If her initial MRI does not identify abnormalities, her future breast surveillance should include annual breast MRI based on a strong recommendation by the American Cancer Society.

Chemoprevention (Risk-Reduction) for High-Risk Women

The ultimate decision regarding screening, surveillance, treatment, and risk-reduction strategies is formulated based on the patient's risk factors and calculated lifetime risks. Tamoxifen and raloxifene are antiestrogen therapies that have been evaluated in chemoprevention trials for high-risk patients (defined as women with a 5-year cancer risk of >1.67%), and chemoprevention trials have demonstrated significant reduction in risk of breast cancer occurrences among high-risk women who received antiestrogen therapy for 5 years. The benefits of tamoxifen must be carefully weighed against the increased risk of uterine cancer (relative risk: 2.53) and risk of pulmonary embolism (relative risk: 3.10). The NSABP P-2 Star trial further compared tamoxifen to raloxifene in breast cancer chemoprevention and found no difference in cancer reduction rates between the two agents; however, raloxifene was found to be associated with significantly lower risk of venous thromboembolic events in comparison to tamoxifen. In addition, the raloxifene treated patients also had significantly lower risk of uterine cancers and uterine hyperplasia in comparison to patients receiving tamoxifen. Exemestane is another antiestrogen medication that is currently under investigation as a chemoprevention regimen. With a relatively short follow-up period, it appears that the uterine cancer risk associated with exemestane is similar to the risk associated with placebo treatment. Unfortunately, the long-term breast cancer reduction effectiveness of exemestane is not yet established. Based on our risk calculations, this patient's 5-year cancer risk of 1.3% does not fit her into the chemoprevention trial population (women with 5-year risk >1.67%); therefore, the relative risk benefit of chemoprevention for her is unclear.

APPROACH TO:
Screening, Surveillance, and Management of High-Risk Patients

DEFINITIONS

BREAST IMAGING REPORTING AND DATA SYSTEM: This is the quality assurance guide designed and published by the American College of Radiology to standardize breast imaging reporting and to facilitate outcome monitoring. The fifth edition of the Breast Imaging Reporting and Data System (BIRADS) atlas was published in 2012, and the classification system is applied to all reports on mammography, breast ultrasound, and breast MRI results. Images are categorized from 0 to 6, with specific recommendations attached to each of the categories.

Category 0: Assessment is incomplete. Additional imaging studies are needed.

Category 1: Negative. Routine annual screening mammography is recommended for women over the age of 40.

Category 2: Benign findings. Routine annual screening mammography is recommended for women over the age of 40.

Category 3: Probably benign findings. Initial shortening of imaging follow-up (usually in 6 months) is recommended. (Malignancy rate is <2%.)

Category 4: Suspicious abnormality. Biopsy should be considered; category 4 is often subdivided into 4A, 4B, and 4C, with malignancy rates ranging widely from 3% to 94% depending on the subcategorization.

   4A: Findings need intervention but with *low suspicion* for malignancy

   4B: Findings with *intermediate suspicion* for malignancy

   4C: Findings with *moderate concern but not classic* for malignancy

Category 5: Highly suggestive of malignancy and it requires biopsy or surgical excision (>95% malignancy).

Category 6: Known biopsy proven malignancy.

DOMINANT BREAST MASS: This term describes a breast mass that is palpable and persistent throughout the menstrual cycle. It can be discrete or ill-discrete in character. This term generally suggests that the mass is not related to fibrocystic changes that vary in characteristics during the menstrual cycle.

BREAST ULTRASONOGRAPHY: This imaging modality is often used to further assess masses or abnormalities detected by physical examinations or mammography. This modality can be used to characterize cystic and solid lesions. In general, cysts without solid components or septations are more likely benign, and solid lesions are more likely cancers when they are irregularly shaped, taller-than-wide, and hypoechoeic.

CONCORDANCE: This term indicates that all diagnostic modalities together support the potential diagnosis. When history, physical findings, diagnostic imaging results, and cytologic/histologic results are discordant, additional steps need to be taken to clarify the discordance. In general, additional imaging and/or tissue sampling would need to be obtained to help sort out the conflicting data.

***BRCA1* AND *BRCA2* MUTATIONS:** The *BRCA* genes are tumor suppressor genes responsible for DNA (deoxyribonucleic acid) repairs. Only 5% to 10% of patients with breast cancers have *BRCA* mutations, and *BRCA* mutations account for 20% to 25% of the hereditary breast cancers. *BRCA* mutations are rare and occur only in 0.25% to 0.5% of the general population. In the Ashkenazi Jewish population, *BRCA* mutations are reported in 8% to 10% of the population. *BRCA1* mutations are associated with early-onset breast cancers, ovarian cancers, and fallopian tube cancers. *BRCA2* mutations are associated with breast cancers in men and women, ovarian cancers, prostate cancers, melanomas, and pancreatic cancers. **It is estimated that 55% to 65% of women with a *BRCA1* mutation, and 45% of women with a *BRCA2* mutation will develop breast cancer by the age of 70.** It is estimated that 35% to 40% of women with *BRCA1* mutation and 11% to 17% of women with *BRCA2* will develop ovarian cancer by age 70. (See Table 12–2 for management of high risk patients).

INVASIVE LOBULAR CARCINOMA: This makes up only 10% to 15% of all breast cancers. These tumors tend to be less discrete-appearing in comparison to invasive ductal carcinoma. Clinically, the appearance can be described as asymmetric focal thickening rather than dominant breast masses. Mammographically, these

---

Table 12–2 • NATIONAL COMPREHENSIVE CANCER NETWORK HIGH-RISK SCREENING ALGORITHM (>25 Y OF AGE)

Prior thoracic chest radiation: Annual mammogram and physical examination every 6 mo beginning 10 y after the XRT.

GAIL[a] model risk >1.67% (>35 y of age): Annual mammogram and physical examination; consider risk-reduction strategies.

Family history or genetic predisposition (mutations of *BRCA1* or *BRCA2*): Annual mammogram and physical examination every 6 mo starting at age 25 or 5-10 y prior to the earliest familial case. Breast MRI starting at age 30 and consider risk-reduction strategies.

Lobular carcinoma in situ: Annual mammogram and physical examination every 6-12 mo; consider risk-reduction strategies.

[a]GAIL, mathematical model risk factors: age, menarche, age at first live birth, number of first-degree relatives with breast cancer, number of previous benign breast biopsies, atypical hyperplasia in previous biopsy, race. The percent estimation refers to the annual probability of cancer development.

lesions can also appear negative. Detection is based on physical examination, MRI, and ultrasonography.

ATYPICAL DUCTAL HYPERPLASIA (ADH): This diagnosis is histologically very similar to ductal carcinoma in situ (DCIS), and some believe that this histology pattern is along the progression to DCIS and invasive carcinoma. When ADH is encountered by core biopsy, an excisional biopsy of the area should be obtained because 25% to 35% of the patients will have DCIS identified at the excisional biopsy.

LOBULAR CARCINOMA IN SITU: This is a histologic abnormality involving cells in the breast lobule. The abnormality probably represents a spectrum of abnormalities that implies risk of subsequent lobular and ductal carcinoma development in the ipsilateral and contralateral breasts. In some patients, lobular carcinoma in situ (LCIS) is an actual precursor to invasive lobular carcinoma.

SCREENING MAMMOGRAPHY: An imaging modality applied for early detection of breast cancers. Mammography is associated with 10% to 15% false-positive and 10% false-negative rates; however, in younger women (ages 40-49), the false-negative rate can be as high as 25%. There have been ongoing debates regarding the cost-benefit of screening for 40 to 49-year-old women. **It is important to recognize that the recommendations for screening from the ACS and the US Preventive Services Task Force (USPSTF) are different and these discrepancies have cause significant confusion among medical practitioners and patients.** The ACS recommends annual screening mammography beginning at age 40, whereas the USPSTF 2009 guidelines recommend initiation of screening mammography at age 50 with repeat examinations every 2 years (Table 12–3).

GAIL MODEL: A mathematical model developed at the NCI to risk-stratify patient's breast cancer risk. This model is the most commonly used model and takes account of **patient age, age of menarche, age of first live birth, number of first-degree relatives with breast cancer, number of previous benign biopsies, atypical hyperplasia on previous biopsy,** and **patient race.** The model is used to tabulate 5-year and lifetime risks of breast cancer. Because this model was developed on the

Table 12–3 • AMERICAN CANCER SOCIETY (ACS) AND US PREVENTIVE SERVICES TASK FORCE (PSPSTF) BREAST CANCER SCREENING RECOMMENDATIONS		
	ACS Recommendations	2009 USPSTF Recommendations
Age of first mammogram	40 years old	50 years old
Mammogram frequency	Yearly	Every 2 years
Self breast examination (SBE)	Optional	Recommends against SBE
Clinical breast examination (CBE)	Annually	Insufficient evidence to assess additional benefits of CBE beyond screening mammography

basis of data accumulated from Caucasian women, it is less accurate for risk prediction in other races. The GAIL model was also developed before the discovery of *BRCA1* and *BRCA2* mutations; therefore, the model does not take into account the *BRCA* status of patients.

CHEMOPREVENTION: Tamoxifen (20 mg per day for 5 years) has been the Food and Drug Administration approved as a chemoprevention strategy for high-risk women. The benefits of tamoxifen have to be weighed against the increased risk of venous thromboembolic events and uterine cancer development.

STAR (STUDY OF TAMOXIFEN AND RALOXIFENE) TRIAL: After tamoxifen was shown to reduce breast cancer development in high-risk women in the NSABP P-1 trial, the STAR trial randomized 19,000 high-risk women to chemoprevention with tamoxifen or raloxifene. This study showed that women who received raloxifene had similar rates of breast cancer risk reduction and 29% fewer venous thromboembolic events in comparison to women who received tamoxifen. In addition, women who received raloxifene had a lower risk of uterine cancer development in comparison to women who received tamoxifen. This study suggests that raloxifene is a superior chemoprevention strategy in comparison to tamoxifen.

BREAST MRI: A useful technique to define the local extent of breast cancers. Breast MRI is more sensitive than mammography for identifying small breast cancers (sensitivity 90%-95%); however, abnormalities seen on MRI may or may not be cancerous (low specificity). The specificity of breast MRI increases as the cancer rate in the population increases. Since 2007, MRI has been recommended as an adjunct to screening mammography for patients with *BRCA* mutations, untested first-degree relatives of patients with *BRCA* mutations, patients with lifetime cancer risk greater than 20% to 25%, patients with prior chest wall radiation, and patients and first-degree relatives with the Li–Fraumeni syndrome (*p53* mutations).

SCREENING DUCTAL LAVAGE: This is a technique that is sometimes applied to the surveillance of high-risk patients. This involves aspiration of the nipple–areolar complex to induce nipple discharge. The effluent produced is analyzed by cytology. Screening duct lavage may help identify patients with early lesions who may benefit from more aggressive screening strategies, including ductography, ductoscopy, or MRI.

CLINICAL APPROACH

Epidemiology

Breast cancer is the most commonly diagnosed cancer in women in the United States and accounts for 29% of all newly diagnosed cancers in women. Breast cancer accounts for 15% of cancer mortality in women in the United States. According to the Surveillance Epidemiology and End Results data, breast cancer mortality has declined 2.3% each year between 1990 and 2003, and the percentage of women surviving at least 5 years after breast cancer diagnosis is 88% with 5-year survival reported at 98% for women diagnosed with localized disease (nonmetastatic disease). The improved survival has been attributed to advances in screening, diagnosis, and treatment.

Breast cancer rates differ by race and ethnicity. African-American women have a lower overall incidence of breast cancer in comparison to Caucasian women; however, African-American women have a high incidence of breast cancer before the age of 35 years in comparison to Caucasian women. For reasons that are not well understood, the breast cancer mortality in African-American women is higher at all ages in comparison to Caucasian women with the disease. Some of the disparities can be explained on the basis of access to care; however, genetic susceptibility and difference in tumor characteristics are likely contributing factors as well. Appreciation of breast cancer epidemiology and risk factors are important in the selection of screening, surveillance, and treatment strategies.

Familial Risk Factors

The risk of breast cancer increases **1.8-fold** in a woman whose **mother or sister** has had breast cancer diagnosed. This risk is further increased if the cancer was diagnosed in the **first-degree relative at a premenopausal age (3.0-fold risk)** or if **the cancer occurred in both breasts (4.0-5.4-fold if postmenopausal and 9.0-fold if premenopausal)**. In addition, some families carry a genetic predisposition for breast cancer with mutations in the *BRCA1* or *BRCA2* genes. It is estimated that only 5% to 10% of the breast cancers are associated with mutations in the *BRCA* genes. *BRCA1* or *BRCA2* mutations increase the breast cancer risks in carriers by 3- to 17-fold in comparison to noncarriers.

Approach to Patient Management

Options to address a patient's breast abnormalities vary depending on individual patient's risk factors and personal concerns regarding cancer risk versus breast cosmesis. Another very important factor contributing to the selection of diagnostic and follow-up strategies is the patient's ability and willingness to continue close surveillance. Low-risk, benign lesions can be observed or excised based on the patient's clinical presentation and/or preference. For a patient with high-risk lesions or a patient with high-risk history/profile, the options may include excision of the lesion, close surveillance with or without antiestrogen agents for chemoprevention. Selective patients with strong family history or known BRCA mutations may be treated with bilateral prophylactic mastectomies and/or bilateral oophorectomy. Prior to proceeding with prophylactic surgeries, the patients and their families need to receive extensive counseling regarding risks and all treatment and surveillance options. Regardless of the management strategy selected, all high-risk patients need to be followed with annual imaging studies (either mammography or MRI), clinical breast examinations, and receive instructions regarding monthly breast self-awareness (Table 12–4).

CASE CORRELATION

- See also Case 11 (Breast Cancer) and Case 13 (Nipple Discharge [Serosanguinous]).

Table 12–4 • NATIONAL COMPREHENSIVE CANCER NETWORK HIGH-RISK SCREENING ALGORITHM (AGE >25)
History of thoracic radiation therapy: Annual mammography and physical examination every 6 months beginning 10 years after radiation treatment.
GAIL model 5-year risk >1.67% (women from >35 years of age): Annual mammography and physical examination; consider risk reduction strategies (chemoprevention)
Family history or genetic predisposition (*BRCA1* or *BRCA2* mutations): Annual breast imaging and physical examinations every 6 months, starting at age 25 or 5 to 10 years prior to earliest familial case. Breast MRI starting at age 30 and consider risk-reduction strategies.
Lobular carcinoma in situ: Annual mammography and physical examinations every 6 to 12 months; consider risk-reduction strategies.

COMPREHENSION QUESTIONS

12.1 A 44-year-old woman underwent a stereotactic biopsy of a suspicious mammographic lesion in the left breast. The biopsy revealed LCIS. The patient's past medical history is significant for left femoral vein thrombosis that occurred after 18-hour air travel. Which of the following is the most appropriate management recommendation for this patient?

A. Left total mastectomy with mirror image biopsy of the right breast

B. Left partial mastectomy and whole-breast radiation therapy

C. Tamoxifen, clinical examinations, and mammography every 2 years

D. Raloxifene, clinical examinations, and mammography every 6 to 12 months

E. Tamoxifen, clinical examinations, and mammography every 6 to 12 months

12.2 Which of the following is associated with the greatest risk of developing breast cancer in a woman?

A. Age greater than 40

B. First-degree relative with breast cancer

C. Prior benign breast biopsy

D. Mutation of the *BRCA1* gene

E. History of LCIS on biopsy

12.3 A 37-year-old woman with multiple family members with breast cancer is noted to have *BRCA1* mutation during genetic testing. She is counseled about a 55% to 65% lifetime probability of breast cancer. She asked whether mastectomy would be advisable. Which of the following statements regarding prophylactic mastectomy is most accurate?

A. Prophylactic mastectomy is an acceptable treatment option

B. Prophylactic mastectomy is rarely indicated because chemoprevention, diagnostic, and surveillance strategies are sufficient to identify and treat cancers at a treatable stage

C. Unilateral mastectomy is preferable over bilateral mastectomies

D. Prophylactic mastectomy should only be done if the patient will be able to undergo immediate reconstruction procedure

E. Prophylactic mastectomy is only indicated for women who fail chemoprevention

12.4 Which of the following statement is most accurate regarding mammography?

A. The radiation exposure can lead to pulmonary malignancies, especially in smokers

B. Its primary purpose is to differentiate benign from malignant processes when a mass is detected by physical examination

C. Its main purpose is to identify and characterize nonpalpable abnormalities

D. It is more accurate in young women

E. Annual mammography is effective in identifying greater than 99% of all breast cancers in the "preclinical" stages

12.5 A 47-year-old woman, whose mother was diagnosed with breast cancer at the age of 61 years, underwent a stereotactic breast biopsy of the left breast and was found to have ADH. Which of the following is the most appropriate treatment option?

A. Tamoxifen chemoprevention

B. Raloxifene chemoprevention

C. Left breast biopsy with needle localization

D. Left modified radical mastectomy

E. Tamoxifen chemoprevention and surveillance mammogram every 6 months

12.6 A 33-year-old woman has a strong family history of breast cancer. Her mother has had breast cancer diagnosed at the age of 43 and her sister has had breast cancer diagnosed at the age of 41. She is concerned about her own risk of breast cancer development but does not wish to have prophylactic mastectomies. Which of the following options is considered most acceptable?

A. Prophylactic breast radiation and raloxifene

B. Initiate annual screening mammography and clinical breast examinations

C. Recommend counseling, genetic testing, initiate annual mammography, breast MRIs, clinical breast examinations, and raloxifene therapy

D. Recommend mammography, breast MRIs, and clinical examinations every 3 to 6 months

E. Recommend counseling and genetic testing; if no abnormalities are seen, begin surveillance mammography and clinical examinations at age 40

12.7 Which of the following statements is TRUE of BRCA1 and BRCA2 mutations?

A. The BRCA1 mutation is associated with increased risk of breast cancer in both men and women

B. The breast cancer and ovarian cancer risks are higher for women with BRCA1 mutations than those with BRCA2 mutations

C. The breast cancer risk is higher in BRCA2 mutation patients in comparison to BRCA1 patients

D. The BRCA mutations are linked to 45% of all breast cancers encountered in women

E. BRCA mutations are encountered exclusively in the Ashkenazi Jewish patient population

12.8 A 52-year-old woman underwent annual mammography, and the report indicated that there were findings in the left breast that were categorized as BIRADS category 3 abnormalities. Which of the following is the most appropriate action to take at this time?

A. Follow-up with repeat mammogram in 1 year

B. Obtain bilateral breast MRI

C. Perform a needle-localization biopsy of the abnormal area

D. Recommend chemoprevention with Raloxifene for 5 years

E. Repeat her mammogram in 6 months

ANSWERS

12.1 **D.** The findings of LCIS carry a 10-fold increase in risk of breast cancer compared to the general population, and this increase in risk is bilateral. For most cases, LCIS is generally considered a marker for subsequent cancer rather than an early stage of breast cancer. The subsequent cancers that develop in these patients can be ductal carcinoma or lobular carcinoma; patients with LCIS can benefit from chemoprevention with tamoxifen as shown by the NSABP-P1 trial results. The -P2 (STAR) trial results demonstrated that raloxifene was equally effective as tamoxifen in the prevention of cancer occurrence, but raloxifene had the added benefits of causing fewer venous thromboembolic complications and uterine malignancies. Chemoprevention with raloxifene, intensive clinical and radiographic surveillance are most appropriate for this patient. Mastectomy with mirror image biopsy of the contralateral breast had been a treatment approach in the past but is no longer indicated with our current knowledge regarding this diagnosis. The NCCN guidelines suggest that a more aggressive clinical evaluation and imaging surveillance approach is indicated in LCIS patients (Table 12–4).

12.2 **D.** Women with mutations of the *BRCA1* gene have approximately a 55% to 65% lifetime risk of developing breast cancer. Women with LCIS have a lifetime breast cancer risk of 35% to 40%. First-degree relative with breast cancer and increase in age are risk factors for breast cancer development, but the risks associated with these factors are substantially lower than those associated with *BRCA1* mutation or diagnosis of LCIS.

12-3 **A.** Prophylactic mastectomy is an acceptable treatment option for properly counseled and properly selected women with high-risk profiles. This should only be done after the patient has been extensively counseled regarding risks and benefits associated with all treatment options. Most often, prophylactic mastectomy is done bilaterally and often done with immediate reconstruction. In this patient with BRCA1 mutation, prophylactic mastectomies and prophylactic bilateral oophorectomy are reasonable treatment after appropriate counseling.

12-4 **C.** The main purpose of diagnostic mammography is to help detect breast cancers before they are detectable by physical examination. Patients should be informed that mammography is less effective in detecting lobular carcinoma that makes up approximately 15% of all breast cancers, and because of this limitation, mammography alone is insufficient in the detection of breast cancers in women; clinical breast examinations, self-examinations, breast MRI, and breast ultrasonography all contribute to the detection of breast cancers in selective settings.

12.5 **C.** This patient with a core needle biopsy demonstrating ADH needs to have a needle localization excisional biopsy of that area of the breast. ADH is often found adjacent to DCIS; in fact, when patients with core biopsy diagnosis of ADH undergo excisional biopsy, approximately 30% of the time, DCIS is found on the subsequent biopsy.

12.6 **C.** This patient has two first-degree relatives with history of premenopausal breast cancer, which raises the suspicion of familial breast cancer syndromes including BRCA mutations and P53 mutations. Genetic testing is a reasonable recommendation after the patient has received appropriate counseling regarding implications, consequences, and management options for the patient and her family members who may be affected. For high-risk individuals such as this woman, the screening and surveillance recommendations include clinical examinations and surveillance imaging with mammography and/or MRI beginning at age 25 or at age 5 to 10 years before the age of onset of earliest familial case. Chemoprevention with antiestrogen therapy has been demonstrated to be beneficial in high-risk patients, and raloxifene is a very appropriate option given the lower complications and side-effect profile of raloxifene in comparison to tamoxifen. This patient should be placed on a surveillance schedule that includes clinical examinations and imaging studies every 6 to 12 months.

12.7 **B.** The breast cancer and ovarian cancer risks are greater for BRCA1 affected patients than BRCA2 affected women. Approximately, 55% to 60% of women who are BRCA1 mutation carriers will develop breast cancer during their lifetime, and approximately 35% to 40% of the BRCA1 carrier women will develop ovarian cancer. Whereas, approximately 45% of the BRCA2 affected women will develop breast cancer and 11% to 17% of these women will develop ovarian cancers.

12.8 **E.** A BIRADS category **3** indicates that there is or are abnormal finding(s); however, the findings are probably benign. An initial short period (6 months) of follow-up and repeat imaging is recommended to confirm that these findings are benign.

CLINICAL PEARLS

▶ The primary role of mammography is the detection of nonpalpable breast abnormalities.

▶ Having one or more first-degree relative with breast cancer, especially if the affected relative is premenopausal and the disease is bilateral, represents significant risk factor for the development of breast cancer.

▶ Mammography in young women under 30 years of age tends to be less sensitive because of increased breast density and fibrocystic changes.

▶ Raloxifene is just as effective as tamoxifen in chemoprevention for high-risk patients, and it is associated with fewer complications and side-effects.

▶ Women with *BRCA1* mutations have a 55% to 60% lifetime risk of developing breast cancers and 35% to 40% risk of developing ovarian cancers.

▶ Women with *BRCA2* mutations have a 45% lifetime risk of developing breast cancers and 11% to 17% risk of developing ovarian cancers.

▶ Men with *BRCA2* mutations are at risk of developing breast cancers, prostate cancers, melanomas, and pancreatic cancers.

▶ *BRCA1*, *BRCA2*, and *P53* mutations are associated with familial breast cancer syndromes and follow an autosomal dominant inheritance pattern.

REFERENCES

Gadd MA. Screening for breast cancer. In: Cameron JL, Cameron AM, eds. *Current Surgical Therapy*. 11th ed. Philadelphia, PA: Elsevier Saunders; 2014:568-571.

Heywang-Kobrunner SH, Hacker A, Sedlacek S. Magnetic resonance imaging: the evolution of breast imaging. *Breast*. 2013;22:S77-S82.

Houssami N, Lord SJ, Ciatto S. Breast cancer screening: emerging role of new imaging techniques as adjuncts to mammography. *MJA*. 2009;190:493-498.

Nelson HD, Tyne K, Naik A, et al. Screening for breast cancer: systematic evidence review update for the U.S. Preventive Service Task Force. *Ann Intern Med*. 2009;151:727-742.

A 43-year-old woman presents with blood-tinged discharge from her right nipple. She indicates that this problem has been occurring intermittently over the past several weeks, and the discharge occurs spontaneously without any manipulations. Her past medical history is significant for hypothyroidism. She has no prior history of breast complaints. The patient is premenopausal and is not lactating. Her medications consist of oral contraceptives and levothyroxine. On physical examination, she has minimal fibrocystic changes in her both breasts. There is slight thickening in the right retroareolar region. A small amount of serosanguineous fluid can be expressed from a single duct opening in the right nipple. There is no evidence of nipple discharge or any dominant masses in the left breast.

▶ What should be your next step?
▶ What is the most likely diagnosis?

ANSWERS TO CASE 13:

Nipple Discharge

Summary: A 43-year-old premenopausal, nonlactating woman presents with unilateral nipple discharge that is serosanguineous.

- **Next step:** The evaluation should begin with bilateral mammography to evaluate for potential breast lesions and ultrasonography to evaluate the retroareolar thickening. A ductogram or biopsy should be considered.

- **Most likely diagnosis:** Intraductal papilloma.

ANALYSIS

Objectives

1. Become familiar with an approach to the evaluation of nipple discharges in women by categorizing the conditions as physiologic or pathologic.

2. Appreciate the relative cancer risks of patients presenting with nipple discharge.

Considerations

This is a premenopausal woman who presents with spontaneous serosanguineous discharge from a single duct in the right nipple. The patient has a history of hypothyroidism and no prior history of breast diseases. The discharge is coming spontaneously from only one nipple, and a single duct, further diagnostic evaluations are needed to determine the cause of this process. **Cytology of the discharge fluid is associated with very low diagnostic yield and therefore should not be pursued.** This patient's history of hypothyroidism is a "red herring." Hypothyroidism is a condition often associated with elevated prolactin levels and can predispose her to have galactorrhea or a form of physiologic "milky" nipple discharge; however, this is not relevant for this patient because her discharge is from only one nipple and is not milky. Diagnostic imaging such as breast ultrasonography and mammography can be very helpful for the initial evaluation, and if a suspicious mass is demonstrated biopsies can be obtained. If no suspicious lesions are seen on mammography and ultrasound, a ductography should be obtained to look for a filling defect within the duct from which the discharge is arising. Lesions identified by ductography can be excised utilizing localization techniques.

The majority of patients (~95%) with nipple discharge from isolated ducts have benign intraductal lesions; therefore, it might be desirable to provide this patient with some early reassurance that her condition is unlikely due to cancer, and she should be informed that the treatment goals are to confirm the benign nature of the process and control the nipple discharge.

APPROACH TO:

Nipple Discharge

DEFINITIONS

PHYSIOLOGIC NIPPLE DISCHARGE: There are a variety of causes leading to physiologic nipple discharge, and these include lactation, pregnancy, hypothyroidism, hormone therapy, medications, renal insufficiency, and excessive breast/nipple stimulation. Physiologic discharge is characterized as bilateral, involving multiple ducts, nonspontaneous, and appears clear or milky. Physiologic discharges do not occur spontaneously and occur only with nipple or breast manipulations. Patients with physiologic nipple discharges do not require specific diagnostic work-ups related to the breasts.

PATHOLOGIC NIPPLE DISCHARGE: Pathologic nipple discharge may present as serous, serosanguineous, purulent, or bloody. Pathologic discharge can be recognized as discharge from only one nipple and often from a single duct. The discharge occurs spontaneously. Intraductal papilloma (a benign ductal growth) contributes to 35% to 60% of all cases of pathologic nipple discharges, with the typical effluent being serosanguineous or bloody. Patients with breast cancers can present with pathological discharge; however, the overall rate of cancer in women with nipple discharge is below 5%. Papillary breast cancer is a rare form of breast cancer that arises from the central ducts, and these lesions can be visualized with breast ultrasonography (see Table 13-1 for causes).

INTRADUCTAL PAPILLOMA: A benign epithelial lesion most commonly arising from major ducts near the nipple, these lesions are mostly microscopic but can grow to 2 to 3 mm. Clinically, patients present with bloody nipple discharge from a single duct. Treatment consists of removal of the involved duct(s).

DUCT ECTASIA: These are duct dilatations that occur as the result of elastin loss in the duct walls. Ductal ectasia is a condition that is related to tobacco use, as the condition does not occur in nonsmokers. Ectasia may occur following chronic inflammation of the duct wall. Nipple discharges associated with duct ectasia are often purulent appearing. Treatment of the condition involves identification of the involved duct(s), followed by duct excision.

DUCTOGRAPHY: This is a radiographic study of the duct that is obtained with the injection of contrast material into the duct. Tumors along the duct walls will appear as filling defects or irregularities.

DUCTOSCOPY: This is often an office-based procedure involving the introduction of a small-diameter flexible endoscope into the suspicious duct(s) to visualize and obtain cytologic assessment of the duct and ductal contents. Some groups have utilized this diagnostic study to select patients for duct excisions.

Table 13-1 · DIFFERENTIAL DIAGNOSIS FOR NIPPLE DISCHARGE

Diagnosis	History	Tests[a]	Treatment
Pregnancy	Reproductive age and female. This diagnosis is the most common reason for nipple discharge. Milk can be secreted intermittently for as long as 2 y after breast-feeding, particularly with stimulation.	Pregnancy test.	Remember to consider this diagnosis in all women of reproductive age.
Infection and/or mastitis or abscess	Purulent discharge; nipple is erythematous and tender.	Gram stain and culture of discharge. Complete blood count (CBC).	Antibiotics and/or drainage.
Galactorrhea secondary to pituitary adenoma	Galactorrhea of all causes is usually characterized by bilateral milky white discharge.	Prolactin level to rule out pituitary adenoma (if pregnancy is excluded). If pregnancy test results are negative, magnetic resonance imaging. (Tumors usually seen only for levels ~ 100 ng/mL.[b])	Treatment as per pituitary adenomas.
Galactorrhea secondary to medications	Patient taking phenothiazines, metoclopramide, oral contraceptives, α-methyldiphenylalanine, reserpine, or tricyclic antidepressants.		Change medications if possible and exclude other causes.
Galactorrhea secondary to hypothyroid	May have symptoms of hypothyroidism, but may exclude with testing.	Thyroxine and thyroid-stimulating hormone levels.	If hypothyroid, treat with appropriate medications.
Fibrocystic changes	Nodularity of breasts, often varying with menstrual cycle. May have mastodynia. Discharge can be yellow, brown, or green.	Hemoccult test. Ultrasound is helpful in delineating cystic lesions and fibroglandular tissue. Mammogram may be appropriate.	If discharge is from fibrocystic changes, observe and reassure. Consider abstention from methyl-xanthines (caffeine) for mastodynia. If lesion is suspicious, perform a biopsy, but otherwise there is no increased risk of breast cancer for fibrocystic changes.

Intraductal papilloma	Usually unilateral serous or bloody discharge.	Consider ductogram. Ultrasound may be helpful during work-up.	Subareolar duct excision to confirm diagnosis. No increased risk of breast cancer.
Diffuse papillomatosis	Serous rather than bloody discharge, often involves multiple ducts more distant from the nipple, and can be bilateral. Discharge can recur if entire portion of ductal system is not removed.	Ductogram to identify duct system. Needle localization following ductogram may assist in excision. Ultrasound may be helpful during work-up.	Excision of involved ducts. This diagnosis is associated with an increased risk of breast cancer.
Carcinoma	Bloody or serous nipple discharge (or none), newly inverted nipple, abnormal skin changes, suspicious mass on examination or mammogram.	Prior to diagnosis, consider ductogram and ultrasound in work-up, or needle localization if not palpable.	Biopsy and then treatment as per breast cancer.

aBilateral mammograms should be obtained for the evaluation of all these diagnoses except for milky discharge related to pregnancy.
bMinor elevations in prolactin without a tumor can be caused by polycystic ovary or Cushing syndrome or can be idiopathic.

CLINICAL APPROACH

Nipple discharges are broadly categorized as **physiologic or pathologic.** Physiologic discharges are typically bilateral, clear or milky, involving multiple duct orifices, and occur nonspontaneously (eg, generally with stimulation or manipulation of the nipple or breast). Specific radiographic imaging studies of the breasts are generally not indicated for the work-up of physiologic discharges. Imaging studies can be obtained as a part of routine breast cancer screening if indicated. Most patients with physiologic discharges simply require treatments to address any potential causes, reassurance, and follow-up.

The approach to women with pathologic nipple discharges is initially directed at characterizing the discharged material (serosanguineous, purulent, or serous). **Pathological discharges most often occur unilaterally and involve single ducts.** Occasionally, discharge related to fibrocystic breast changes can be difficult to differentiate from old blood. The drainages related to fibrocystic changes are generally nonspontaneous. Appropriate breast imaging such as mammography and/or ultrasonography should be obtained as the initial assessment for all patients presenting with pathologic nipple discharges. Patients with abnormalities identified by imaging will need biopsies performed. Patients without abnormalities identified by breast imaging studies should undergo ductography to help identify potential isolated ductal lesions. If intraductal lesions are seen by ductography, excisional biopsies should be performed. Patients with pathologic nipple discharges with no abnormalities identified by mammography, ultrasound, and ductography may be closely followed and imaging studies repeated if symptoms continue.

Surgical treatment for intraductal masses identified during the work-up of pathologic nipple discharges can consist of partial duct excision or complete central duct excision. A more extensive procedure is associated with better control of the nipple discharge but can affect the patient's ability to breast feed in the future, and this possibility should be discussed with the patients prior to proceeding with total duct excisions.

CASE CORRELATION

- See also Case 11 (Breast Cancer Surveillance) and Case 12 (Breast Discharge).

COMPREHENSION QUESTIONS

13.1 A 35-year-old woman with two children and no previous medical problems presents with recent onset of increased fatigue and whitish discharge from both nipples with minor manipulation. Which of the following is the best next step?

A. Obtain a thyroid-releasing hormone level

B. Image the sella turcica

C. Measure a serum human chorionic gonadotropin level

D. Ultrasound the breasts

E. Initiate treatment with bromocriptine

13.2 A 38-year-old woman is noted to have nipple discharge. She is concerned about the association of nipple discharge with breast cancer. Which of the following conditions is associated with increased breast cancer risks?

A. Fibrocystic changes

B. Hypothyroidism

C. Intraductal papilloma

D. Diffuse atypical papillomatosis

E. Pregnancy

13.3 A 44-year-old woman with nipple discharge is seen by her physician. Blood tests and imaging studies are obtained. Which of the following findings in a work-up requires additional evaluations?

A. Ultrasonography demonstrating ductal ectasia

B. A ductogram demonstrating no filling defects or irregularities

C. An ultrasound demonstrating fibrocystic changes and a 3-mm simple cyst

D. A 3-mm lobular, smooth mass within the breast parenchyma

E. Serum prolactin of 100 ng/mL

13.4 A 65-year-old woman who takes a tricyclic antidepressant and metoclopramide has serosanguinous discharge from her right nipple. She has no palpable breast abnormalities, normal bilateral mammograms, and a right breast ultrasound that does not demonstrate any abnormalities. Her right breast ductogram reveals a cutoff at 3 cm from the nipple. Which of the following is the best treatment for this patient?

A. Observe and instruct her not to manipulate the nipple or breast

B. Change her medications

C. Check her prolactin level

D. Duct excisional biopsy

E. Mammographic-guided biopsy

13.5 Which of the following statements is TRUE regarding nipple discharge in women?

  A. It is a common presenting symptom for ductal carcinoma of the breast

  B. Nipple discharge, breast pain, and breast mass are the three most common complaints related to the breast

  C. Dopamine stimulates prolactin and causes nipple discharge

  D. Hyperthyroidism causes nipple discharge

  E. The concern for breast cancer is raised when the nipple discharge occurs from multiple ducts

13.6 For which of the following patients is a diagnostic duct excision indicated?

  A. A 23-year-old woman with right nipple discharge following manipulation. She has a family history of breast cancer. Her ultrasound and breast magnetic resonance imaging (MRI) are normal

  B. A 48-year-old woman with spontaneous right nipple discharge. Her mammogram and breast ultrasound studies are normal. The right breast ductoscopy revealed no evidence of duct abnormalities

  C. A 43-year-old woman with hypothyroidism and nipple discharge with stimulation only. Her serum prolactin level is elevated. Her family history is significant for breast cancer diagnosis in her 52-year-old elder sister

  D. A 38-year-old woman with left nipple discharge with normal mammogram and ultrasound demonstrating fibrocystic changes

  E. A 33-year-old woman with left nipple bloody discharge with a small filling defect seen on ductography

ANSWERS

13.1 **C.** This is a woman of child-bearing age who presents with some nonspecific symptoms including fatigue and apparent physiologic nipple discharge. These symptoms can be consistent with pregnancy; a pregnancy test is indicated as the initial evaluation. Other possibilities include hypothyroidism, but that can be evaluated once pregnancy is ruled out.

13.2 **D.** Papillomatosis is a benign condition associated with papillary proliferation of the ductal epithelium, which can fill up the ducts and cause distension of the ducts. Papillomatosis without atypia is not associated with the increase in cancer risk; however, papillomatosis with atypia carries a 4- to 5-fold increase in breast cancer risk. None of the other choices given here are associated with significant increase in breast cancer risks.

13.3 **E.** Prolactin level in the range of 100 ng/mL or greater is abnormally elevated and can be caused by a pituitary adenoma, and this finding should be followed up by an MRI of the brain. Other findings that are described do not require specific work-ups.

13.4 **D.** The finding of an abrupt cutoff on ductography in this 65-year-old woman with pathologic nipple discharge needs to be further evaluated by diagnostic duct excision.

13.5 **B.** Nipple discharge, breast pain, and breast mass are the three most common breast-related complaints leading to medical consultations. Nipple discharge is an unusual symptom related to breast cancers, and only 5% to 12% of women with nipple discharge are found to have breast cancers.

13.6 **E.** Diagnostic duct excision is indicated for the 33-year-old woman with bloody nipple discharge and a filling defect seen on ductography.

CLINICAL PEARLS

► The causes of nipple discharge can be grouped as pathologic or physiologic. This grouping helps in direct evaluation and treatment. Patients who require surgical evaluation have spontaneous, unilateral, and recurrent nipple discharges.

► Nipple discharge is a disturbing complaint for the patient; notably, only 4% to 6% of the women with nipple discharge that is not associated with a breast mass have breast cancer. The cancer risk is increased among postmenopausal women, when discharge is associated with abnormal findings on breast imaging, or when a mass is associated with nipple discharge.

► The most common cause of unilateral serosanguineous nipple discharge in the absence of a breast mass is an intraductal papilloma.

► Pathologic nipple discharge evaluation needs to include evaluation to rule out breast cancers.

► Antihypertensive medications, phenothiazines, antidepressants, and antipsychotic medications can all cause nipple discharges. (Medications that block the secretion of dopamine can cause galactorrhea.)

REFERENCES

Morgan HS. Primary care management of the female patient presenting with nipple discharge. *Nurse Pract.* 2015;40(3):1-6.

Nelson RS, Hoehn JL. Twenty-year outcome following central duct resection for bloody nipple discharge. *Ann Surg.* 2006;243:522-524.

Patel BK, Falcon S, Drukteinis J. Management of nipple discharge and the associated imaging findings. *Am J Med.* 2015;128:353-360.

A 39-year-old man presents for evaluation of burning epigastric pain and substernal pain that has occurred frequently over the past 6 months. He indicates that the symptoms generally occur after meals and especially when he is lying down. The patient has been prescribed a proton pump inhibitor (PPI) and has taken it regularly for the past 3 months with significant symptomatic improvement. He has no other major medical problems and denies any recent weight loss. He reports moderate consumption of tobacco and alcohol. On examination, he is moderately obese but without any cardiopulmonary or abdominal findings. The main reason for his visit at this time is to inquire how long he will need to continue his medication and whether there are other therapeutic options.

▶ What is the most likely diagnosis?
▶ What are mechanisms that can contribute to this problem?
▶ What are complications associated with this disease process?
▶ Is surgery a good treatment option for this patient?

ANSWERS TO CASE 14:

Gastroesophageal Reflux Disease

Summary: A 39-year-old man with a history of frequent substernal and epigastric burning pain that occurs mainly after meals and while lying supine. He has been taking a proton pump inhibitor for 3 months, which has relieved much of his symptoms.

- **Most likely diagnosis:** Gastroesophageal reflux disease (GERD).

- **Mechanisms potentially contributing to the problem:** Defective lower esophageal sphincter (LES) function, impaired esophageal clearance, excess gastric acidity, and abnormal esophageal response to acid exposure are all potential contributors to GERD.

- **Complications associated with GERD:** Peptic stricture of the esophagus, Barrett's esophagus, and extra esophageal (respiratory and upper airway) complications.

- **Surgery as an option for GERD treatment:** Operative and endoscopic treatment options are available and are quite effective for the treatment of GERD.

ANALYSIS

Objectives

1. Learn the pathophysiology of GERD.

2. Learn the diagnostic work-up and treatment for patients with GERD.

3. Be familiar with the controversies and uncertainties related to the treatment of GERD.

Considerations

This patient's clinical presentation is typical for GERD. His symptoms occur mainly after meals, and appear to be aggravated by being in the supine position; in addition, he reports that taking a PPI has produced significant symptomatic improvement. Given this information, you can make a presumptive diagnosis of GERD. During the interview, you should try to illicit history or complaints related to GERD complications, which may include airway symptoms related to aspiration and esophageal obstructive symptoms from peptic stricture formation.

A patient with GERD who responds favorably to pharmacologic therapy also will generally respond favorably to surgical treatments, thus making this patient a good candidate for antireflux treatment procedures. Surgical fundoplication is the traditional operative option. Endoscopic or endoluminal techniques are newer options in antireflux interventions that produce symptoms improvement in 70% of the patients; however, the durability of endoscopic treatments is not yet determined. The patient in this case has a choice regarding how he wishes to manage his GERD symptoms.

Surgical treatment and antisecretory medications are highly effective for the treatment of GERD, and there is no definitive evidence to suggest that surgery offers any advantages over medical treatment. This patient currently consumes tobacco and alcohol, which can exacerbate GERD symptoms; therefore, it is important to counsel him regarding the benefits of tobacco and alcohol cessation. Other lifestyle modifications that may also help reduce GERD symptoms include weight loss, elimination of caffeine and fatty foods, restriction of food and liquid consumption prior to bed time, and elevation of the head of bed at night. If this patient chooses to pursue surgical antireflux treatment, most surgeons would obtain **ambulatory pH monitoring** to measure the pattern and severity of acid reflux and esophageal manometry to confirm that the patient has LES dysfunction and that there is no esophageal dysmotility. A very commonly selected surgical option for GERD patients in the United States is a complete (360°) fundoplication procedure (Nissen fundoplication) performed by the laparoscopic approach. Most patients stay in the hospital for only 1 day following this type of surgery. While in the hospital, the patient will begin on liquid diet and will go home with instructions to remain on this diet for approximately 1 week while the distal esophageal swelling resolves. After that, patients may resume a regular diet.

APPROACH TO:

Gastroesophageal Reflux

DEFINITIONS

AMBULATORY pH MONITORING: This is the gold standard test for confirmation of GERD. This study is helpful to confirm GERD in patients who have typical symptoms but do not have esophagitis on endoscopy and patients who do not have good responses to medical treatment. In addition, pH monitoring may be helpful to make the diagnosis in patients presenting with atypical symptoms. Prior to the pH monitoring study, patients need to discontinue antisecretory medications for 1 week.

LOWER ESOPHAGEAL SPHINCTER: The primary role of the LES is to prevent the reflux of gastric contents into the esophagus. The LES is not a distinct anatomic structure but rather a physiologic entity. The LES is a high-pressure zone enforced by the distal esophageal musculature, sling fibers of the gastric cardia, extrinsic pressure on the distal esophagus contributed by its abdominal location, and presence of the diaphragmatic crura.

ESOPHAGEAL MANOMETRY: This examination consists of a thin flexible tube with a pressure sensor, which is passed through the nose into the esophnagus. This study provides information regarding esophageal motility and swallowing response (ie, coordination of esophageal peristalsis with LES relaxation). Manometry also quantifies LES length and pressure. Many surgeons feel that this is an essential study prior to antireflux surgery.

NONEROSIVE REFLUX DISEASE (NERD): Up to 50% of the GERD patients have no esophagitis seen during endoscopy. Patients with NERD generally do not respond as favorably to medical or surgical management. It is believed that some of the patients with NERD have hypersensitivity of the esophageal epithelium and relatively normal (nonpathologic) acid exposure patterns. Esophageal pH monitoring is important in this patient group to rule out or rule in GERD as the cause of symptoms.

HIATAL HERNIA: These are anatomic findings that occur in many individuals. GERD is often associated with hiatal hernias, but not all hiatal hernias will cause GERD. Type I hiatal hernia is a sliding hernia where the GE junction slides above the diaphragmatic opening. Type II hiatal hernia is a rolling hernia where the GE junction remains in its normal location and the intra-abdominal contents such as stomach and colon herniate above the diaphragm and can produce obstructive symptoms. Type III hernia is a combination of type I and II hernias. **Indication for hiatal hernia repair is based on symptoms related to the hernia and not simply based on the presence of hernia.**

SURGICAL ANTIREFLUX OPERATIONS: There are a variety of surgical procedures that involve the construction of an external distal esophageal sphincter mechanism using the gastric fundus (ie, a fundoplication). The fundoplication (or the wrap) can involve the entire esophageal circumference (360°) or to a lesser extent (90°-270°). Selection of a fundoplication is often based on the surgeon's choice and patient's factors such as esophageal dysmotility. The surgical fundoplication procedure can be performed through a variety of approaches including left thoracotomy, open transabdominal, or laparoscopic. Most often, the procedure is performed laparoscopically.

ENDOLUMINAL GERD TREATMENT: These are endoscopic techniques developed to enhance the LES function in patients with GERD. The available techniques include controlled delivery of radiofrequency energy to the distal esophagus to induce scarring and mucosal thickening, and endoscopic fundoplication with intraluminal stapling of the distal esophagus and gastric fundus. Short-term results are good with these approaches, while long-term outcomes are still being accumulated.

BARRETT'S ESOPHAGUS: This describes the pathologic replacement of the esophageal squamous epithelium with intestinal-like columnar epithelium. Barrett's esophagus changes are presumably due to chronic exposure of the esophagus to acidic and bile-containing contents. It is estimated that 5% to 15% of patients with GERD develop Barrett's changes. **Barrett's esophagus is reported to be associated with a 40-fold increase in the risk of adenocarcinoma** development in the esophagus in comparison to individuals without GERD and Barrett's changes. Barrett's esophagus can be associated with varying degrees of dysplastic changes that range from no dysplasia to high-grade dysplasia. The presence and severity of dysplasia correlate with cancer risks. The cancer progression risk from high-grade dysplasia to cancer is estimated between 0.9% and 14% per year.

CLINICAL APPROACH

The typical symptom associated with GERD is postprandial, epigastric, and substernal burning pain. Approximately 50% of the patients also report acidic taste in their mouths. Atypical GERD symptoms are produced by chronic microaspirations, which include reactive airway symptoms, morning hoarseness, coughing spells during sleep, recurrent pneumonias, and even pulmonary fibrosis. Patients who are being treated with antisecretory medications are less likely to report heartburn and are more likely to report atypical symptoms. Occasional GERD-like symptoms occur in 20% to 40% of adults. Only about 60% of patients with GERD-like symptoms have reflux, and symptoms from cardiopulmonary diseases, gallstone diseases, or peptic ulcer disease can produce symptoms that mimic those produced by GERD. When patients present with atypical or typical symptoms do not respond to pharmacologic treatment, it is important to confirm the diagnosis with physiologic testing (pH monitoring and manometry).

With low-dose PPI treatment, nearly all patients report improvement or resolution of GERD symptoms initially; however, on low-dose PPI treatment, it is expected that approximately half of the patients will develop breakthrough symptoms within 5 years. Patients who develop these symptoms will respond well to escalation of medical treatment to a high-dose PPI regimen. The expectation is that patients with chronic, severe GERD will require life-long PPI treatment to help control their symptoms.

Many medical practitioners who have recommended the Nissen fundoplication procedures for GERD treatment have hoped that the surgery would lead to the elimination of long-term medication use for GERD patients. Unfortunately, a drawback that has been observed is that for reasons that are not entirely clear, roughly half of the patients postoperatively developed abdominal complaints that ultimately requires placement back on antisecretory medications.

Pathophysiology

There are a number of physiologic mechanisms in place to prevent GERD in most individuals. These include adequate length and pressure of the LES, and normal esophageal neutralization and clearance mechanisms to address small amounts of refluxed gastric contents. GERD in most individuals is produced by some combination of excess acidity, decreased esophageal clearance, defective LES function, or hypersensitivity of the esophageal epithelium. In some cases, the LES dysfunction and GERD are associated with the presence of a hiatal hernia.

Work-up

Patients with mild GERD symptom or symptoms that respond to lifestyle modification and/or pharmacological treatment may be simply monitored without further work-ups. Patients with long-standing history of symptoms, atypical symptoms, or persistence of symptoms during pharmacologic treatments are candidates for 24-hour pH monitoring to document that symptoms are actually related to GERD. For some of the patients, other diagnostic studies listed in Table 14–1 may also be indicated.

Treatment

The initial treatment of GERD consists of lifestyle modifications (Table 14–2) and medications as needed. For patients with documented esophagitis and patients

Table 14–1 • DIAGNOSIS OF GASTROESOPHAGEAL REFLUX DISEASE	
Test	Purpose of Test
Endoscopy	Evaluates for erosive esophagitis or Barrett esophagus, or alternative pathology. Biopsy for suspected dysplasia or malignancy.
Barium esophagogram	Identifies the location of the GE junction in relation to the diaphragm. Identifies a hiatal hernia or shortened esophagus. Evaluates for gastric outlet obstruction (in which case fundoplication is contraindicated). Can demonstrate spontaneous reflux.
pH Monitoring for 24 h	Correlates symptoms with episodes of reflux. Quantitates reflux severity.
Pharyngeal pH monitoring	Correlates respiratory symptoms with abnormal pharyngeal acid exposure.
Manometry	Evaluates the competency of the lower esophageal sphincter. Evaluates the adequacy of peristalsis prior to planned antireflux surgery. Partial fundoplication may be indicated if aperistalsis is noted. Can diagnose motility disorders such as achalasia or diffuse esophageal spasm.
Nuclear scintigraphy	May confirm reflux if pH monitoring cannot be performed. Evaluates gastric emptying.

with frequent symptoms, the mainstay of treatment is consistent acid suppression or antisecretory therapy with a PPI. Escalation to high-dose PPI (twice-a-day dosing) is often needed when patients develop breakthrough symptoms on low-dose PPI. In some cases, when patients have nighttime reflux breakthrough, the

Table 14–2 • TREATMENT OF GASTROESOPHAGEAL REFLUX DISEASE	
Behavioral therapy	Avoidance of caffeine, alcohol, and high-fat metals Avoidance of meals within 2-3 h of bedtime Elevation of the head of the bed Weight loss in obese individuals Smoking cessation
Medical therapy	Antacids H_2 blockers Proton pump inhibitors Prokinetic agents
Surgical therapy	Laparoscopic or open antireflux procedure
Endoscopic therapy	Radiofrequency energy directed to the GE junction Endoscopic endoluminal gastroplication

addition of an H2-antagonist at night can be beneficial. Most patients with severe and frequent GERD symptoms will benefit from lifelong high-dose PPI treatment. Because PPI is effective in relieving GERD symptoms in >95% of the patients with the diagnosis, individuals who do not respond to high-dose PPI should undergo additional diagnostic studies to rule out other causes of symptoms. It is now recognized that many patients with NERD or refractory GERD have visceral hypersensitivity as the cause for their symptoms. For some of these patients, the addition of a tricyclic antidepressants, trazadone, or selective serotonin re-uptake inhibitors for esophageal pain modulation can help improve their symptoms.

Laparoscopic fundoplications have been applied for the treatment of GERD since the 1990s. The pH measurements obtained in patients following Nissen fundoplication operations suggest that operative treatment is an effective and durable method of reducing acid reflux. The ideal surgical candidate is a patient with GERD who responds to antisecretory therapy but is unwilling to continue life-long medical treatment. Many of the patients currently being referred for surgical management are individuals whose symptoms are not responding to medical treatments. Unfortunately, fundoplication procedures in these patients are also less effective, with only 60% to 70% of the patients having satisfactory results postoperatively. One of the most perplexing long-term observations following the Nissen fundoplication procedures is that despite adequate control of acid reflux in most postoperative patients, **50% of the patients develop recurrent abdominal symptoms that require placement back on PPI.** Since it is required to resume PPI in many postoperative patients, laparoscopic Nissen fundoplication does not appear to be an effective strategy in eliminating long-term pharmacologic therapy in patients with GERD. The therapeutic limitations associated with laparoscopic Nissen fundoplication have prompted recent researches and developments in endoscopic antireflux treatment options.

Barrett's esophagus development is the result of long-standing GERD and occurs in 10% to 15% of patients undergoing upper gastrointestinal (GI) endoscopy for reflux symptoms. The presence of Barrett's esophagus increases the risk of esophageal adenocarcinoma development by 30 to 125 times. The prevalence of Barrett's esophagus in the United States is approximately 5.5% with an annual cancer risk of 0.5% per year. Surveillance and treatment recommendations are variable and based on the presence and severity of dysplasia identified within the Barrett's changes. Patients with Barrett's esophagus need treatments to control acid reflux, and there is no convincing evidence to suggest that antireflux operations offer any additional advantages over PPI treatment.

CASE CORRELATION

- See also Case 15 (Esophageal Perforation), Case 16 (Esophageal Carcinoma), and Case 17 (Peptic Ulcer Disease).

COMPREHENSION QUESTIONS

14.1 A 66-year-old man with congestive heart failure and emphysema reports substernal burning and regurgitation after meals and at bedtime. He has had partial relief of his symptoms with ranitidine that he has purchased over the counter. Esophagoscopy has revealed distal esophagitis. Which of the following is the most appropriate next step?

A. Refer the patient for laparoscopic Nissen fundoplication

B. Schedule the patient for 24-hour pH monitoring and esophageal manometry studies to confirm that patient has GERD

C. Prescribe a PPI

D. Reassure that the symptoms will improve and that some breakthrough symptoms are expected

E. Recommend dietary changes

14.2 A 51-year-old woman with a history of hypertension and hyperlipidemia presents with 3-month history of daily substernal chest pain and vague abdominal discomfort. She has been prescribed a PPI by her primary care physician without relief of symptoms. Her upper GI endoscopy revealed a small hiatal hernia but no evidence of esophagitis. Which of the following is the best next step?

A. Barium esophagram to evaluate her hiatal hernia

B. Refer the patient for evaluation of atypical chest pain and to rule out cardiac origin of symptoms

C. Refer the patient to a psychiatrist for possible conversion reaction

D. Perform a computed tomography (CT) scan of the chest and abdomen

E. Refer the patient for esophageal manometry to rule out achalasia and diffuse esophageal spasm

14.3 A 50-year-old man with the diagnosis of GERD for 3 years has been managed with ranitidine with partial symptoms relief. He has some residual symptoms that prompted an upper GI endoscopy. At endoscopy with biopsy, Barrett's esophagus without dysplasia was identified. Which of the following is the best treatment recommendation for this patient at this time?

A. Stop the ranitidine and initiate low-dose PPI

B. Advise the patient to have an esophagectomy to prevent cancer progression

C. Keep patient on his H2-blocker and schedule him for follow-up endoscopy in 3 months

D. Recommend Nissen fundoplication because it is a more effective treatment against Barrett's progression

E. Add misoprostol (PGE1 analog) to help improve mucosal protection

14.4 Which of the following is NOT an indication for laparoscopic Nissen fundoplication in a 48-year-old woman with pH study proven GERD?

A. Lack of desire to continue PPI treatment

B. Incomplete relief of symptoms with PPI treatment

C. Nissen fundoplication is more effective than PPI in controlling the progression of Barrett's esophagus.

D. Inability to pay for long-term PPI therapy

E. Inability to tolerate PPI

14.5 The Nissen fundoplication is contraindicated in which of the following situations?

A. A 50-year-old woman with diabetic gastroparesis causing bloating and reflux symptoms

B. A 44-year-old man with pH study proven GERD and Barrett's esophagus without dysplasia

C. A 38-year-old man with GERD and a prior Nissen fundoplication with significant symptoms relief, postoperatively. He now has recurrent symptoms and is found to have herniation of the repair into the mediastinum.

D. A 60-year-old man with GERD symptoms and pH study and EGD confirmation of disease who has incomplete response to PPI treatment

E. A 50-year-old man with GERD that is well managed with PPI who wishes to discontinue medication treatment

14.6 For which of the following patients is esophageal manometry study most likely to help in determining the treatment?

A. A 40-year-old man with GERD-like symptoms with initial good response to low-dose PPI treatment but now has developed occasional breakthrough symptoms

B. A 47-year-old man with GERD-like symptoms and dysphagia to solids and liquids

C. A 70-year-old man with 4-month history of progressively worsening dysphagia, inability to tolerate solid food, and 15 pound (6.8 kg) weight loss

D. A 53-year-old man with atypical chest pain with no evidence of cardiac ischemia demonstrated by a stress test

E. A 48-year-old man with a history of peptic ulcer disease and *Helicobacter pylori* infection who has incomplete healing of his duodenal ulcer after a course of *H. pylori* treatment

ANSWERS

14.1 **C.** This is a 66-year-old man with significant cardiopulmonary comorbidities and typical GERD-like symptoms that are partially relieved with an H2-blocker. Given this history of partial response, switching to a PPI is the best option at this time. Choice A is not a good answer because Nissen fundoplication may be risky for a patient with significant cardiopulmonary comorbidities; in addition, operative treatment may not be needed as he has not yet received the best medical treatment. Esophageal physiology studies are appropriate to determine if GERD is the cause of his symptoms if he fails to respond to PPI treatment. Dietary recommendation should be provided for all patients but is not the best answer at this time. Reassurance is not an appropriate answer because the patient's symptoms are not yet adequately addressed.

14.2 **B.** This is a 51-year-old woman with cardiac risk factors and symptoms suggestive of GERD. The patient has been taking a PPI without symptoms relief. Given her history of cardiac comorbidity (hypertension and hyperlipidemia), evaluations for her atypical chest pain are indicated. She would likely benefit from cardiac stress test and other cardiac evaluations to rule out coronary artery disease. This patient has a hiatal hernia which occurs commonly and may not have any relevance to her GERD symptoms; therefore, specific work-up of this is not indicated at this time. CT of the abdomen and pelvis can be helpful to identify mass lesions or other structural abnormalities responsible for her symptoms, but without additional symptoms such as obstructive symptoms or constitutional symptoms, this imaging study is not indicated at this time. Esophageal pH monitoring is a test that could likely help us determine if the cause of her symptoms is GERD-related, but tests to rule out cardiac disease should be done first. Patients with achalasia can present with GERD-like symptoms; however, cardiac causes need to be ruled out first.

14.3 **A.** This 50-year-old man has a history of GERD and Barrett's esophagus without evidence of dysplasia. Patients with Barrett's esophagus should have treatment to optimally address their GERD; therefore, he should switched to a PPI which is a better pharmacologic choice than H2 antagonist treatment. Esophagectomy is an option for the management of patients with Barrett's esophagus containing severe dysplasia. Nissen fundoplication has not been proven to control Barrett's esophagus progression better than PPI treatment. Misoprostol is helpful for gastric mucosal protection, especially in patients taking nonsteroidal anti-inflammatory drugs, but this agent plays no role in preventing Barrett's progression.

14.4 **C.** Antisecretory treatment and Nissen fundoplications are effective in reducing progression of Barrett's in GERD patients; however, antireflux surgery is not proven to be more effective than PPI treatment. Unwillingness to continue with PPI treatment, incomplete response to PPI treatment, and inability to tolerate or pay for PPI treatments are all reasonable indications to consider antireflux surgery options.

14.5 **A.** Nissen fundoplication is contraindicated in a patient with gastroparesis, bloating, and GERD. Since the reflux of gastric contents in this situation is likely secondary to overdistension of the stomach produced by poor gastric motility, a fundoplication might reduce reflux symptoms but will cause worsening of bloating and distension. A displaced fundoplication causing symptoms is an indication for re-operation. A fundoplication procedure is an appropriate treatment option for a patient with Barrett's changes without dysplasia or a patient with GERD and incomplete relief with medical treatment. Although not all patients with GERD are able to discontinue antisecretory therapy following fundoplication procedures, the procedure is not contraindicated for a patient who wishes to discontinue pharmacologic treatment.

14.6 **B.** A 47-year-old man with dysphagia to solids and liquids and GERD-like symptoms could have achalasia. Patients with achalasia often have undigested and fermented food remaining in their esophagus secondary to esophageal dysmotility and poor esophageal emptying. Fermented food with bacterial overgrowth in the esophagus can cause esophagitis and GERD-like symptoms. The patient with breakthrough of GERD-like symptoms following initial response to low-dose PPI treatment does not raise a suspicion for alternative causes of the symptoms; therefore, manometric study would not likely contribute to the care. The patient with incomplete healing of his duodenal ulcer after a course of *H. pylori* treatment needs biopsy to see if the infection has been eradicated.

CLINICAL PEARLS

▶ A 24-hour pH monitoring study is the most objective indicator of GERD.

▶ A patient's response to PPI is one of the best clinical indicators of GERD.

▶ Adenocarcinoma of the esophagus is a complication of long-standing GERD.

▶ Gastroparesis or delayed gastric emptying can cause GERD-like symptoms, but these symptoms are usually accompanied by bloating and abdominal distension.

▶ The long-term efficacy of PPI and antireflux operations in reducing esophageal cancer develop in GERD patients appears to be equivalent.

▶ Achalasia can produce GERD-like symptoms because undigested and fermented food in the esophagus can produce esophagitis.

▶ Endoscopic or operative antireflux procedures are indicated in patients with documented GERD whose symptoms are incompletely controlled with PPI, or in patients who do not wish to continue or are unable to tolerate long-term PPI treatment.

REFERENCES

Elmadhun N, Kent M. Endoscopic treatment of Barrett's esophagus. In: Cameron JL, Cameron AM, eds. *Current Surgical Therapy*. 11th ed. Philadelphia, PA: Elsevier Saunders; 2014:23-27.

Jobe BA, Hunter JG, Peters JH. Esophagus and diaphragmatic hernia. In: Brunacardi FC, Andersen DK, Billiar TR, et al., eds. *Schwartz's Principles of Surgery*. 9th ed. New York, NY: McGraw-Hill; 2010:803-887.

Telem DA, Rattner DW. Gastroesophageal reflux diseases. In: Cameron JL, Cameron AM, eds. *Current Surgical Therapy*. 11th ed. Philadelphia, PA: Elsevier Saunders; 2014:9-14.

Teran MD, Brock MV. The management of Barrett's esophagus. In: Cameron JL, Cameron AM, eds. *Current Surgical Therapy*. 11th ed. Philadelphia, PA: Elsevier Saunders; 2014:19-23.

Wang YK, Hsu WH, Wang SW, et al. Current pharmacological management of gastroesophageal reflux disease. *Gastroenterol Res Pract*. 2013;2013:983653.

Wendling MR, Melvin WS. Endoluminal approaches to gastroesophageal reflux disease. In: Cameron JL, Cameron AM, eds. *Current Surgical Therapy*. 11th ed. Philadelphia, PA: Elsevier Saunders; 2014:14-18.

A 23-year-old man comes to the emergency department with severe chest pain and upper abdominal pain that began approximately 6 hours ago. The patient says that he had attended a party where he consumed food and a large amount of alcohol that made him ill. He vomited several times before going to sleep. Within a short time after going to bed, he was awakened with severe pain in the upper abdomen and midportion of his anterior chest. His past medical history is otherwise unremarkable. On physical examination, the patient appears extremely uncomfortable and anxious. His temperature is 38.8°C (101.8°F), pulse rate is 125 beats/minute, blood pressure is 106/80 mm Hg, respiratory rate is 32 breaths/minute. His head and neck examination is unremarkable. His cardiopulmonary examination is significant for tachycardia and diminished breath sounds at the left inferior lung fields. His laboratory studies revealed a white blood cell count of 20,000/mm^3. His hemoglobin, hematocrit, and electrolytes are within normal limits. The serum amylase and lipase, bilirubin, aspartate transaminase (AST), alanine transaminase, and alkaline phosphatase values are all within normal limits. A 12-lead electrocardiogram shows sinus tachycardia. The chest radiograph reveals left pleural effusion and pneumomediastinum.

► What is the most likely diagnosis?
► What is your next step?
► What are your options for treatment?
► How do you decide which is the most appropriate treatment option?

ANSWERS TO CASE 15:
Esophageal Perforation

Summary: A 23-year-old man presents with spontaneous perforation of the thoracic esophagus following retching and vomiting (Boerhaave syndrome). The patient has pneumomediastinum, left pleural effusion, and exhibits a septic picture as the result of leakage of esophageal luminal contents that is causing mediastinitis.

- **Most likely diagnosis:** Spontaneous esophageal rupture (Boerhaave syndrome).

- **Next step:** Resuscitation and source control are the immediate priorities. He should be given supplemental oxygen, intravenous fluid, and broad-spectrum antibiotics. Simultaneously, arrangements should be made to have the patient undergo water-soluble contrast esophagram to identify the exact location of the perforation.

- **Treatment options:** Treatment options include antibiotics, nothing by mouth (NPO), operative drainage, percutaneous drainage, operative or endoscopic esophageal repair, esophageal diversion, esophageal covered stent placement, and esophageal resection.

- **Selection of appropriate treatment option:** Treatment selection is based on location, severity, and cause of perforation. Additional factors influencing treatment selection include patient's clinical condition, and existence of underlying esophageal pathology. Resource and expertise availability are also important in treatment selection.

ANALYSIS

Objectives

1. Recognize the clinical settings, early signs and symptoms, and complications of esophageal perforations.

2. Learn the diagnostic and therapeutic strategies for patients with suspected esophageal perforations.

Considerations

This is a young man with a history of forceful retching followed by the onset of chest pain, abdominal pain, and fever. His chest radiograph reveals pneumomediastinum which is likely due to air leakage from the esophagus into the mediastinum. In addition, his left pleural effusion suggests that esophageal contents likely have leaked into the left pleural space. Early recognition and treatment of this potentially deadly condition is essential. Delays in recognition and treatment do occur because most physicians do not have extensive experiences dealing with such unusual clinical condition. Given his history and the location of his pain, the site of perforation is most likely in the distal esophagus. The treatment priorities are to initiate fluid resuscitation as needed along with broad-spectrum antibiotics targeting upper gastrointestinal (GI) tract microbes. To locate and characterize his perforation, we can obtain an esophagram using water-soluble contrast or a computed tomography (CT) scan with administration of oral water-soluble contrast. Depending on the perforation site, treatment options include drainage of the periesophageal space, stent coverage, or operative repair of the perforation.

APPROACH TO:
Suspected Esophageal Perforation

DEFINITIONS

ESOPHAGEAL PERFORATION: This is a transmural disruption of the esophagus associated with contamination of the surrounding spaces by oral and/or gastric secretions. All patients with esophageal perforations should be managed initially with NPO and broad-spectrum antibiotics.

LOCATION OF PERFORATION: Perforation sites are broadly categorized as **cervical, thoracic,** or **abdominal.** Most cervical perforation can be managed with NPO and antibiotics, and drainage if there is significant luminal content extravasation. Thoracic perforation is the most common location with a variety of treatment options. Abdominal esophageal perforation treatments are similar to those for intrathoracic perforations.

BOEHAAVE SYNDROME: Spontaneous esophageal perforation is often secondary to forceful retching, coughing, or vomiting. The site of perforation is often in the distal esophagus near the gastroesophageal (GE) junction. Frequently, the perforation extends to the proximal stomach.

PNEUMOMEDIASTINUM: Air within the mediastinum. The presence of air in the mediastinum should raise immediate suspicion for esophageal perforation either in the chest or neck. This condition is often associated with the tracking of air into the neck, therefore a physical finding that is sometimes present is soft tissue crepitus in the neck. Pneumomediastinum is most commonly diagnosed by chest radiography or chest CT scan.

ESOPHAGEAL PERFORATION SEVERITY SCORE: This scoring system was introduced by Abbas et al. from the University of Pittsburg. The scores range from 0 to 18. From their original report, patients with scores <2 had 23% risk of complications and 2% risk of mortality; patients with scores of 3 to 5 had 32% risk of complications and 3% risk of mortality; patients with scores >5 had 81% risk of complications and 28% risk of mortality; mortality for patients with scores >9 was 100% (see Table 15–1).

CLINICAL APPROACH

Esophageal perforation is a rare but potentially life-threatening condition. Morbidity and mortality associated with the condition are influenced by the site of

Table 15–1 • ESOPHAGEAL PERFORATION SCORE	
Variables	Score
1. Age >75 y 2. HR >100 bpm 3. WBC >10,000/mm³ 4. Pleural effusion of CXR or CT	1 point each
1. Temperature >38.5°C 2. Noncontained leak on CT or esophagram 3. Respiratory rate >30 breaths/minute or requiring mechanical ventilation 4. Time to diagnosis >24 hours	2 points each
1. Cancer 2. Hypotension	3 points each
Total possible score	18

perforation, the underlying pathology, treatment delays, and methods of treatment. Historically, most nontraumatic perforations were spontaneous occurrences associated with coughing, retching, vomiting, or foreign body ingestions. In the modern era, the majority of perforations are associated with instrumentation of the esophagus, including GI endoscopy, transesophageal echocardiography, pneumatic dilatation, esophageal or gastric tube placement, and operative procedures near the esophagus such as spine surgery. Patient outcomes are influenced by several factors: (1) the cause and location, (2) the underlying esophageal pathology, (3) time interval to diagnosis and treatment, and (4) patient comorbid conditions. Most patients with esophageal perforations describe pain associated with the occurrence. Patients with cervical esophageal perforation may describe neck and chest pain, whereas patients with thoracic or abdominal esophageal perforation generally describe chest and/or abdominal pain. Cervical perforations can produce spreading infections in the deep spaces of the neck and the anterior and posterior mediastinum. Thoracic and abdominal esophageal perforations can produce contaminations and infections in the posterior mediastinum, pleural cavities, and abdomen.

Early recognition of the condition, immediate support of airway, breathing, and circulation, along with antibiotics administration are critical for good treatment outcomes. Diagnosis is often confirmed with contrast esophagram or CT esophagram. In some instances, CT-guided drainage can be performed and may help limit the extent of leakage and contamination. Treatment options for patients range from NPO + antibiotics, NPO + antibiotics + drainage, NPO + antibiotics + endoscopic repair or endoscopic stent placement, NPO + antibiotics + surgical debridement, repair, and drainage. Because of the rarity of the condition, treatment recommendations and strategies have not been developed based on high-level clinical evidence.

Cervical esophageal leaks are rarely life-threatening as long as they are recognized and addressed in a timely fashion, and in most cases, only supportive care, antibiotics + drainage is required. Only a small percentage of the patients with perforations in the neck require drainage or repairs. Ideally, thoracic and abdominal esophageal perforations should be directly repaired if the patients' condition can

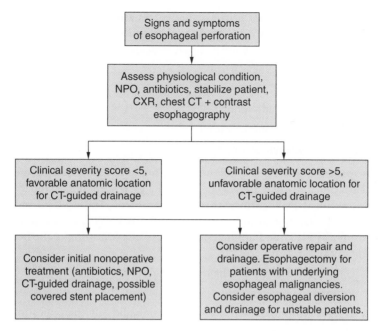

Figure 15–1. Algorithm for evaluation and management of suspected esophageal perforation.

tolerate the operations. Perforations that are associated with underlying esophageal pathology (such as esophageal cancer and achalasia) generally carry a worse prognosis and are more likely to require stent placement, resection, or repairs and myotomies. In selective cases, patients with small thoracic esophageal perforations with contained leakage and no underlying esophageal pathology can be managed with NPO + antibiotics and observation alone (See Figure 15-1).

COMPREHENSION QUESTIONS

15.1 A 63-year-old man with abdominal pain and chest pain is diagnosed with esophageal perforation. Which of the following is the most common cause of this condition?

A. Congenital defects

B. Trauma

C. Spontaneous rupture

D. Iatrogenic

E. Caustic ingestion

15.2 A 53-year-old man with achalasia undergoes esophageal dilatation. Shortly following the procedure, he develops chest pain and tachycardia. Which of the following diagnostic studies is best to assess his condition?

A. Barium esophagram

B. Esophagoscopy

C. Upright chest radiograph

D. Water-soluble contrast esophagram

E. CT scan without contrast

15.3 The patient described in Question 15.2 is found to have a thoracic esophageal perforation approximately 8 cm above the gastroesophageal junction with noncontained leakage into the posterior mediastinum. The radiologist indicated that the location is amendable to percutaneous drainage. In addition to NPO and antibiotics, which of the following is the best treatment option for this patient?

A. CT-guided drainage of the mediastinal space

B. Endoscopic covered stent placement

C. Operative drainage, esophageal myotomy, and full fundoplication

D. Operative drainage, esophageal myotomy

E. Operative drainage, esophageal myotomy, partial fundoplication

15.4 After drinking several beers and eating a left-over, stale pizza, a 21-year-old college senior presents to the emergency room with a 16-hour history of chest pain that began after a bout of vomiting. His temperature is 39.0°C, pulse rate is 120 beats/minute, and blood pressure is 96/60 mm Hg after fluid resuscitation. A CT esophagram reveals a distal esophageal perforation with extensive contrast extravasation. Which of the following is the best treatment?

A. Esophageal diversion

B. Endoscopic repair

C. NPO and observation

D. Surgical repair

E. NPO and feeding gastrostomy tube placement

15.5 Which of the following factors is NOT a prognostic factor for patients with esophageal perforation?

A. Patient age

B. Noncontained leakage

C. Size of perforation

D. White blood cell count

E. Time interval between perforation and treatment

15.6 Which of the following statements regarding esophageal perforation is TRUE?

   A. Treatment protocol is well defined and based on high-quality clinical evidence

   B. Nonoperative management is best

   C. Operative repair is best when perforation is diagnosed within 24 hours

   D. Percutaneous drainage is best when it is performed within 24 hours

   E. Diagnosis cannot be made without endoscopic confirmation

ANSWERS

15.1 **D.** Esophageal instrumentation leading to iatrogenic injury is the most common cause of nontrauma-related esophageal perforations. Traumatic esophageal injuries are most commonly the result of penetrating trauma.

15.2 **D.** Esophagram with water-soluble contrast is the best diagnostic study to help confirm esophageal perforation. This study also helps us to determine if the leakage is large and whether it is contained. Esophagoscopy can identify a perforation and provide information regarding its size and location. Unfortunately, the procedure is invasive; with the air introduction into the esophageal lumen during the procedure, perforation can be worsened. CT scan with intravenous contrast only has limited diagnostic value for esophageal perforation.

15.3 **E.** Operative drainage with distal esophageal myotomy and a partial fundoplication is the best treatment choice for the man with esophageal perforation that occurred during esophageal dilatation. Because achalasia is associated with poor esophageal emptying, simply repairing the perforation without performing a myotomy would not be sufficient because with persistent distal obstruction, the repair has a higher chance of failure. A myotomy alone with repair would produce significant gastroesophageal reflux and compromise the patient's quality of life. Therefore, the best option is to repair the perforation, perform the myotomy, and create a partial fundoplication. Because patients with achalasia have esophageal dysmotility, a full circumferential wrap can result in postoperative dysphagia.

15.4 **D.** Surgical repair is the preferred treatment for patients with thoracic esophageal perforations. Esophageal diversion and drainage is generally applied when patients present late (>24 hours) and/or if the clinical condition is poor, or when the patient is a poor surgical candidate. For this 21-year old patient, an operative repair should be well tolerated and would provide him with the best long-term outcome.

15.5 **C.** The size of the esophageal perforation has not been found to be a prognostic indicator for esophageal perforation. Older age, noncontained leakage, white blood cell count, and time interval between perforation and treatment are established prognostic indicators for patients with esophageal perforations.

15.6 **C.** Operative treatment is best performed within 24 hours of perforation. With the increase in elapsed time between perforation and repair, the patient's overall condition generally deteriorates and with increased contamination of the mediastinum, the tissue at the edges of the perforation may become more inflamed and edematous. With deterioration in clinical condition, patients are less likely to tolerate an aggressive surgical procedure. With delays and increased inflammatory changes in the esophagus and the surrounding areas, there is increased likelihood of repair failure. Nonoperative treatment is generally applied when the perforation occurs in the cervical esophagus or if the leakage is well contained and not causing sepsis. Diagnostic endoscopy is generally not performed to diagnose esophageal perforation because it can make the condition worse. Endoscopy is performed in selective patients for treatment, and endoscopic treatments available include endoscopic closure of perforation and stent placement to seclude the site of perforation.

CLINICAL PEARLS

▶ Spontaneous esophageal perforation should be suspected in a patient presenting with chest pain after vomiting.

▶ Indicative findings of esophageal perforation include subcutaneous crepitus over the neck and Hamman's sign on chest auscultation. Chest radiograph demonstrating pneumomediastinum and/or left pleural effusion are common.

▶ A high index of suspicion is needed because delays in treatment compromise patient outcomes.

▶ Patient's age and physiologic conditions at presentation are important prognostic factors.

▶ Most spontaneous esophageal ruptures occur in the distal third of the esophagus.

▶ Most iatrogenic perforations are associated with endoscopy.

▶ Patients with esophageal perforations and underlying esophageal pathology (eg, cancer and achalasia) generally require more complex treatments that include treatments of the underlying pathology.

REFERENCES

Abbas G, Schuchert MJ, Pettiford BL, et al. Contemporaneous management of esophageal perforation. *Surgery.* 2009;146:749-756.

Biancari F, D'Andrea V, Paone R, et al. Current treatment and outcome of esophageal perforations in adults: systematic review and meta-analysis of 75 studies. *World J Surg.* 2013;37:1051-1059.

Ferguson CM. Esophageal perforation. In: Cameron JL, Cameron AM, eds. *Current Surgical Therapy.* 11th ed. Philadelphia, PA: Elsevier Saunders; 2014:64-68.

Kuppusamy MK, Hubka M, Felisky CD, et al. Evolving management strategies in esophageal perforation: surgeon using nonoperative techniques to improve outcomes. *J Am Coll Surg.* 2011;213:164-172.

A 54-year-old man complains of chest pain and difficulty with swallowing and weight loss. The patient states that over the past 4 to 5 weeks, he has noticed a worsening ability to tolerate solid foods. During this time, he has had pain and discomfort with swallowing, along with a sensation of "the food being stuck in his chest." Because of these symptoms, he has switched over to a liquid diet essentially consisting of soups, juices, and tea that he has tolerated relatively well. The patient has noticed a 20-lb (9.1-kg) weight loss. His past medical history is significant for hypertension and self-diagnosed and self-treated "indigestion." His medications include metoprolol and a proton pump inhibitor (PPI) that he has obtained over the counter. The patient appears thin with significant temporal wasting. His vital signs are normal, there is no evidence of adenopathy, and the remainder of the physical examination is unremarkable. His white blood cell count is normal, hemoglobin is 12 g/dL, and the hematocrit is 40%. His serum electrolytes, liver enzymes, and glucose are within normal limits.

▶ What is the most likely mechanism causing this process?
▶ What is the most appropriate next diagnostic step?
▶ What are the risk factors associated with this process?

ANSWERS TO CASE 16:
Esophageal Carcinoma

Summary: A previously healthy 54-year-old man presents with dysphagia and weight loss.

- **Most likely mechanism:** Mechanical obstruction from a neoplastic process.

- **Most appropriate next step in diagnosis:** Esophagoscopy with biopsy.

- **Risk factors associated with the process:** Known risk factors associated with squamous cell carcinoma include caustic burns, alcohol consumption, tobacco smoking, and nitrite- and nitrate-containing food. Gastroesophageal reflux disease (GERD) is a known risk factor for gastroesophageal junction (GEJ) adenocarcinoma (odds ratio of 7.7). Other suspected risk factors of this disease include Western diets and acid-suppression medications.

ANALYSIS

Objectives

1. Learn the approach to local and systemic staging of esophageal and gastroesophageal (GE) junction carcinomas.

2. Learn to apply staging information and clinical assessment to help determine the optimal treatment course for patients with esophageal carcinomas.

Considerations

This patient describes dysphagia to solid foods that has developed over a fairly short period of time (several weeks). The timing of symptoms progression along with a history of self-medication with a PPI suggests that he may have had a history of GERD and perhaps now has developed adenocarcinoma of the distal esophagus. If the patient were to describe a more protracted course of symptoms progression (months to years), other differential diagnoses such as benign strictures, congenital malformations, and achalasia could be more likely. However, given the time course of his symptoms evolution, the most likely diagnosis is an obstructive malignant neoplasm.

Critical issues for his management are to determine the nature and location of his obstruction. This can be accomplished in a number of ways, but an esophagogastroduodenoscopy is probably the most direct and expeditious approach, allowing us to localize, visualize, and biopsy the lesion. If the biopsy should demonstrate the presence of esophageal cancer, the next step is to proceed with local and systemic staging of the disease process. A computed tomography (CT) scan of the chest and abdomen is helpful for both local and distant disease assessment and staging. For local staging, the endoscopic ultrasound is very helpful to characterize the local extent of the tumor. A positron emission tomography (PET) CT scan is often helpful to assess for local and distant diseases.

It is important to bear in mind that many patients with foregut malignancies, such as esophagus and stomach cancers, often present with very similar symptoms (dysphagia and inability to eat), and imaging and/or endoscopy are the modalities that allows us to differentiate these problems. Precise location of the tumor is essential for the planning of treatment. There have been several large international clinical trials published examining multimodality treatment strategies for these patients. Details regarding disease location, histology, and staging are critical to determine the best treatment plan for this patient.

Nutritional assessment and optimization are critical prior to the initiation of therapy and during therapy. If the nutritional assessment demonstrates that he is significantly malnourished, intense nutritional support plans need to be implemented during his initial evaluation and staging work-up. Pretreatment nutritional support may simply involve nutritional supplementation by mouth. However, if the patient is unable to tolerate sufficient oral feedings, placement of a durable enteral nutritional access such as a feeding gastrostomy or feeding jejunostomy should be considered.

APPROACH TO:
Esophageal and Gastroesophageal Junction Cancers

DEFINITIONS

ENDOSCOPIC ULTRASONOGRAPHY (EUS): This is currently the preferred imaging modality for assessment of the local extent of esophageal and GE-junction tumors (T stage) and for the assessment of regional lymph nodes (N stage). In patients with lymphadenopathy, EUS-guided fine-needle aspirations the regional lymph nodes can be performed for cytologic diagnosis.

NEOADJUVANT THERAPY: This describes preoperative treatment. One of the current approaches is a combined chemoradiation therapy regimen before operative resection for patients with invasive but resectable esophageal cancers.

SIEWERT CLASSIFICATION OF GE JUNCTION ADENOCARCINOMAS (Types I-III): Type I tumors are centered in the esophagus, at more than 1 cm above the GEJ (surgical treatment typically is an esophagectomy). Type II tumors are "at the GE junction", within 1 cm above the GEJ and up to 2 cm distal to GEJ, and surgical resection consists of esophagectomy with resection of the proximal stomach. Type III tumors are located in the cardia of the stomach, >2 cm distal to the GEJ and treatment consists of total gastrectomy.

EARLY ESOPHAGEAL CANCER AND ESOPHAGEAL DYSPLASIA ENDOSCOPIC TREATMENT OPTIONS: Intramucosal/noninvasive cancers and high-grade dysplasia associated with Barrett's esophagus can be treated with either endoscopic mucosal resection techniques or with radiofrequency ablation techniques. Prior to mucosal resections, the cancer depth and extent need to be accurately assessed with endoscopy and endoscopic ultrasound.

CLINICAL APPROACH

The incidence of esophageal cancer has increased six-fold over the past 25 years, where this tumor is the sixth most common malignancy encountered in the United States. Although squamous cell carcinoma continues to account for the majority of cancers encountered in developing countries, adenocarcinoma is the predominant cancer encountered in North America (about 70%).

Curative Therapy

Historically, the prognosis for patients with esophageal cancers has been dismal, with 5-year survival rates reported at 25% to 30%; however, over the past decade, multimodality approaches have significantly improved patient prognosis to the point that some groups are now reporting 5-year survival rates around 50% for patients with resectable disease. Cancer stage remains as the most important predictor of survival following treatments (see Tables 16-1 and 16-2 for staging systems).

Table 16–1 • 2010 AJCC TNM DEFINITIONS FOR ESOPHAGEAL CANCERS				
Primary Tumor (T)		**Regional Lymph Nodes (N)**		**Distant Metastasis (M)**
T0	No evidence of primary tumor	**N0**	No regional lymph node involvement	**M0**- No distant metastasis
Tis	High-grade dysplasia			
T1	Tumor invades lamina propria, muscularis mucosa, or submucosa	**N1**	Metastasis to 1-2 regional lymph nodes	**M1**- Distant metastasis present
T1a	Tumor invades lamina propria, muscularis mucosa			
T1b	Tumor invades submucosa			
T2	Tumor invades muscularis propria	**N2**	Metastasis to 3-6 regional lymph nodes	
T3	Tumor invades adventitia	**N3**	Metastasis to >7 regional lymph nodes	
T4	Tumor invades adjacent structures			
T4a	Resectable tumor invading pleura, pericardium, or diaphragm			
T4b	Unresectable tumor invading other adjacent structures, such as aorta, vertebral body, and trachea			

Table 16–2 • 2010 AJCC ESOPHAGEAL CANCER STAGING		
Stage	Squamous Cell Carcinoma	Adenocarcinoma
0	Tis, N0, M0, G1, any location	Tis, N0, M0, grade 1,
IA	T1, N0, M0, G1, any location	T1, N0, M0, grades 1-2
IB	T1, N0, M0, any location, grades 2-3 or T2-T3, N0, M0, lower, grade 1	T1, N0, M0, grade 3 or T2, N0, M0, grades 1-2
IIA	T2-3, N0, M0, grade 1, upper or middle or T2-3, N0, M0, grades 2-3, lower	T2, N0, M0, grade 3
IIB	T2-3, N0, M0, grades 2-3, upper and middle or T1-2, N1, M0, any grade, any location	T3, N0, M0, any grade or T1-2, N1, M0, any grade
IIIA	T1-2, N2, M0, any grade, any location or T3, N1, M0, any grade, any location or T4a, N0, M0, any grade, any location	T1-2, N2, M0, any grade or T3, N1, M0, any grade or T4a, N0, M0, any grade
IIIB	T3, N2, M0, any grade, any location	T3, N2, M0, any grade
IIIC	T4a, N1-2, M0, any grade, any location or T4b, any N, M0, any grade, any location or any T, N3, M0, any grade, any location	T4a, N1-2, M0, any grade or Tab, any N, M0, any grade or any T, N3, M0, any grade
IV	Any t, any N, M1 disease	Any T, any N, M1, any grade

Grade 1: low grade; grade 2: moderate grade; grade 3: high grade.

Evidence-Based Treatments

Two high-profile, randomized controlled clinical trials over the past 10 years have significantly influenced the management of esophageal cancer patients. Both trials have been influential in establishing the importance of neoadjuvant therapy in the care of patients with esophageal cancers. The "MAGIC" trial, published in the New England Journal of Medicine in 2006, investigated patients with adenocarcinoma of the GE junction and stomach. Patients were randomized to a sandwich-treatment approach with preoperative chemotherapy (epirubicin, cisplatin, 5-FU) followed by surgical resection and then postoperative chemotherapy versus surgery alone. The findings demonstrated that **patients randomized to the sandwich therapy arm had higher rates of complete resections and significant improvements in overall and disease-free survivals.**

The next influential trial was the "CROSS" trial that was published in the New England Journal of Medicine in 2012. This trial randomized patients with squamous cell carcinoma of the esophagus or adenocarcinoma of the esophagus to surgery alone versus preoperative chemoradiation therapy (carboplatin + external beam radiation) followed by surgery. Based on the intention to treat, patients who received neoadjuvant treatments had a mean 5-year survival of ~50% versus ~35%

Table 16–3 • ESOPHAGEAL CANCER SURGICAL OPTIONS		
Procedure	Surgical Resection	Applications
Transhiatal Esophagectomy	Abdominal incision, tabularizing of the stomach; transhiatal dissection; left neck incision; anastomosis of gastric conduit to cervical esophagus	Best for distal esophageal cancers; hazardous for tumors in the midesophagus; less physiologic insult from the respiratory standpoint
Ivor–Lewis Esophagectomy	Abdominal incision, tubularization of stomach; right thoracotomy and resection of esophagus to proximal esophagus; anastomosis of esophagus to gastric conduit in right chest	Operation is best for midesophageal lesions; associated with more pain and greater degree of respiratory impact postoperatively
Three-Field Esophagectomy	Abdominal incision, tubularization of stomach; right thoracotomy to dissect and resect the entire thoracic esophagus; cervical incision to create cervical esophagus to gastric conduit anastomosis in neck	Theoretically provides the best oncologic resection in the chest; because of the three field approach, this operative approach also is associated with the greatest physiologic insult for the patients
Distal Esophagectomy with Left Thoracotomy and Laparotomy	Thoracoabdominal incision extending from abdomen into left chest. Stomach is tabularized; distal esophagus resected through left chest and anastomosis is created between thoracic esophagus and gastric conduit in the left chest	This operative approach causes pain and respiratory compromise; also limits the extent of the esophageal resection
Minimal Invasive Esophagectomy	Laparoscopy to tabularize the stomach; transhiatal laparoscopic dissection of the esophagus; right thoracoscopic dissection of the thoracic esophagus; cervical dissection and anastomosis of esophagus to gastric conduit in the neck.	Well tolerated by most patients. The procedure is more cumbersome

with surgery alone, and subgroup analysis showed that patients with squamous cell carcinoma had approximately 55% to 60% 5-year survival (see Table 16–3 for surgical options).

Targeted therapy has also been evaluated for the treatment of patients with gastric and GE-junction adenocarcinoma (trastuzumab for gastric cancer trial). This study suggested that in patients with tumors that overexpressed human epidermal growth factor receptor 2 (*HER2*), the combination of chemotherapy + trastuzumab provided additional survival benefits.

Palliative Care

Palliation for patients with esophageal cancer is directed at preserving the quality of life for patient in whom cure would not be possible. Because the most common complaint that affects patients' quality of life is dysphagia, the primary goal of palliative care is rapid relief to dysphagia with minimal hospitalization and with the

Table 16–4 • PALLIATIVE MODALITIES FOR ESOPHAGEAL CARCINOMA

Palliative Modality	Effectiveness, Advantages, and Disadvantages
Endoscopic stent placement	**Advantages:** Rapid relief of dysphagia; treatment of choice for tracheoesophageal fistula; short procedural time; outpatient procedure **Disadvantages:** Recurrence due to stent migration, tumor overgrowth, food impaction; transient pain following placement; gastroesophageal reflux; and increased risk of late hemorrhage
Photodynamic therapy and Nd:YAG laser	Endoluminal destruction of obstructing lesions **Advantages:** Works well with exophytic lesions; generally low complication rates **Disadvantages:** Often available only in specialized centers; special expertise required; repeat treatment every 4-8 weeks is needed
Single-dose brachytherapy	Intraluminal radiotherapy **Advantages:** Long-term dysphagia improvement is better than stent placement; long-term quality-of-life score was better when compared with stent placement; lower rate of hemorrhage than stent placement **Disadvantage:** Dysphagia relief is delayed in comparison to stent placement
Palliative chemotherapy Epirubicin, cisplatin, and 5-FU (ECF) is the chemotherapy combination that has been established as the optimal palliative chemotherapy regimen at this time	**Advantages:** Treatment improves median survival; responders may have improved quality of life due to relief of obstruction **Disadvantages:** Response to obstruction is variable; therefore, additional treatment for obstruction may be needed; relief from obstruction may be delayed

preservation of swallowing function. Secondarily, palliative care may be directed at the prevention of bleeding, perforation, and tracheoseophageal fistula (TEF) formation. Palliative modalities include endoscopic therapies (stent placement, laser, and photocoagulation), radiation therapy (external beam or intraluminal), chemotherapy, and feeding tube placement. Factors that determine the selection of palliative therapy for any given patient include the availability of technology, local expertise, patient condition, tumor location and characteristics, and the expected length of survival (see Table 16–4 for details).

CASE CORRELATION

- See also Case 14 (Gastroesophageal Reflux Disease), Case 15 (Esophageal Perforation), and Case 17 (Peptic Ulcer Disease).

COMPREHENSION QUESTIONS

16.1 A 53-year-old man is found to have invasive squamous cell carcinoma of the distal esophagus. Imaging studies including PET-CT scan and EUS suggest that the disease is resectable. Which of the following is the best treatment approach for this patient?

A. Endoscopic mucosal resection

B. Induction chemotherapy with epirubicin, cisplatin, and fluorouracil (5-FU) followed by esophagectomy and postoperative chemotherapy

C. Induction chemoradiation therapy with carboplatin and external beam radiation therapy followed by surgical resection

D. Radiation therapy and trastuzumab

E. Esophagectomy

16.2 Which of the following is a risk factor for adenocarcinoma of the esophagus?

A. Smoking

B. Alcohol consumption

C. Gastroesophageal reflux

D. Nitrite- and nitrate-containing foods

E. Hypertension

16.3 Which of the following is an advantage of transhiatal esophagectomy over the Ivor–Lewis esophagectomy?

A. The Ivor–Lewis approach is associated with less pulmonary complications but leakages are better tolerated with the transhiatal approach.

B. The transhiatal approach is less stressful from the physiologic standpoint.

C. The transhiatal approach is a better approach to tumors in the midesophagus.

D. The transhiatal approach avoids an abdominal operation.

E. The transhiatal approach follows the principles of oncologic surgery better.

16.4 Which of the following statements regarding squamous cell carcinoma of the esophagus is accurate?

A. Squamous cell carcinoma of the esophagus incidence has dramatically increased

B. Gastroesophageal reflux disease is a major risk factor

C. This tumor is most amendable to surgical resection when it is located in the cervical esophagus

D. The 5-year survival exceeds 80% when completely resected

E. This tumor is highly responsive to radiation therapy

16.5   Which of the following is a major limitation to endoscopic stent placement for the palliation of esophageal cancer?

A.   Recurrent esophageal obstruction

B.   Patients often have a several-week delay before symptom improvement occurs.

C.   Endoscopic stent placement eliminates the possibility of surgery at a later time.

D.   The presence of TEF is a contraindication.

E.   Endoscopic stent placement is helpful in limiting gastroesophageal reflux.

16.6   A 45-year-old man is diagnosed with an exophytic adenocarcinoma of the distal esophagus that penetrates to but does not penetrate through the muscularis propria and biopsy reveals low-grade histology. A PET CT demonstrates localized disease in the distal esophagus without distant metastasis. Which of the following is the most appropriate treatment?

A.   Placement of endoscopic stent to relieve the obstruction and initiate definitive chemoradiation therapy

B.   Initiation of chemoradiation followed by esophagectomy

C.   Treat with radiation therapy and trastuzumab

D.   Nutritional therapy for 8 weeks followed by esophagectomy

E.   Endoscopic mucosal resection

ANSWERS

16.1   **C.** Induction therapy with carboplatin and radiation therapy followed by esophagectomy is the choice listed here that offers the patient the best opportunity for long-term survival. This regimen is the one introduced by the CROSS trial. In that study, the 5-year survival reported for patients with squamous cell cancers was between 55% and 60%. The regimen described in option "B" was used in the MAGIC trial that included only patients with adenocarcinoma of the stomach and GE junction. Anti-*Her2* strategies have been found to benefit patients with gastric adenocarcinoma and GE-junction adenocarcinomas.

16.2   **C.** Gastroesophageal reflux is a known risk factor for adenocarcinoma of the esophagus and confers a relative risk of 7.7-fold. Smoking, alcohol consumption, and nitrite and nitrate containing foods are risk factors associated with squamous cell carcinoma of the esophagus.

16.3   **B.** The transhiatal esophagectomy when compared to the Ivor–Lewis esophagectomy (abdomen + right chest) is associated with less physiologic insult and lower respiratory complication rates. However, the operation is theoretically less oncologic because clear radial margins are not sought. Because the anastomosis is in the neck, leakages are not usually lethal complications following transhiatal esophagectomies.

16.4 **E.** Squamous cell carcinoma of the esophagus is highly radiation responsive. The incidence of squamous cell carcinoma of the esophagus has not increased over the past 10 years; the increase in esophageal cancer has been associated with the increase in adenocarcinoma of the esophagus.

16.5 **A.** Recurrent obstruction may develop as the result of tumor progression and stent migration. Following stent placements, esophageal obstructions usually improve fairly quickly. TEF is not a contraindication to stent placement, in fact covered stent placement is a palliative treatment for TEF. Worsening GE reflux is common after stent placement.

16.6 **B.** This patient has a stage IB adenocarcinoma of the esophagus, with this depth of penetration, regional LN metastasis and distant micrometastatic disease are highly likely; therefore, the treatment needs to be systemic in addition to esophagectomy. The treatment described in option "B" is the one introduced by the CROSS trial and offers this patient the best long-term survival.

CLINICAL PEARLS

▶ The incidence of adenocarcinoma of the esophagus and GE junction is rapidly increasing in westernized, developed countries.

▶ Treatment outcome of esophageal cancers is improved with multimodality treatment.

▶ Esophagectomy is primarily performed in patients with potentially curable esophageal cancers.

▶ Induction chemoradiation therapy followed by esophagectomy is currently the best approach for patients with invasive and resectable esophageal cancers.

▶ The best treatment for esophageal cancer has evolved over the past 10 years thanks to well-conducted randomized controlled clinical trials.

REFERENCES

Lada MJ, Peters JH. The management of esophageal carcinoma. In: Cameron JL, Cameron AM, eds. *Current Surgical Therapy.* 11th ed. Philadelphia, PA: Elsevier Saunders; 2014:47-54.

Rizk NP. Neoadjuvant and adjuvant therapy of esophageal cancer. In: Cameron JL, Cameron AM, eds. *Current Surgical Therapy.* 11th ed. Philadelphia, PA: Elsevier Saunders; 2014:54-58.

Van Hagen P, Hulshof MCCM, van Lanschot JJB, et al. Preoperative chemoradiotherapy for esophageal or junctional cancer. *N Engl J Med.* 2012;366:2074-2084.

A 45-year-old man presents with a 2-month history of epigastric abdominal pain. He describes the pain as burning and says that it occurs at night or early in the morning. The patient has found that eating food generally improved these symptoms. He admits to having had similar symptoms intermittently over the past few years, and over-the-counter H_2 antagonists have usually resolved his symptoms. Unfortunately, over the past few weeks, self-medication has not resolved his pain. He denies any weight loss, vomiting, or melena. He has no family history of significant medical problems. His physical examination reveals normal head, neck, and cardiopulmonary findings. The abdomen is nondistended, minimally tender in the epigastrium, and without masses. A digital rectal examination reveals Hemoccult-negative stool. Laboratory studies reveal normal values for white blood cell (WBC) count, hemoglobin, hematocrit values, platelet count, electrolyte values, serum amylase, and liver function tests.

▶ What is your next step?
▶ What is the most likely diagnosis?
▶ What are the treatment options?

ANSWERS TO CASE 17:
Peptic Ulcer Disease

Summary: A 45-year-old man has signs and symptoms consistent with peptic ulcer disease (PUD). The patient has self-medicated with H_2 antagonists in the past with success, but the symptoms are currently unrelieved with medications.

- **Next step:** Perform diagnostic esophagogastroduodenoscopy (EGD).

- **Most likely diagnosis:** Peptic ulcer disease.

- **Treatment options:** Testing for *Helicobacter pylori* should be performed, and if the result is positive, treatment to eradicate *H. pylori* should be administered. If the *H. pylori* status is negative then conventional pharmacological treatment should be attempted.

ANALYSIS

Objectives

1. Be familiar with the five types of gastric ulcers and relationship between ulcer type, pathogenesis, and treatment.

2. Be able to discuss the relationship between *H. pylori* and PUD.

3. Become familiar with the mechanisms of action and the efficacy of PUD therapy.

4. Become familiar with the indications for surgery in the treatment of patients with PUD.

Considerations

This is a 45-year-old man with recurrent "burning" epigastric pain that improves with food ingestion. His history suggests a diagnosis of PUD that is somewhat refractory to medical management. Even though his story is highly suggestive of PUD, our differential diagnoses should include other potential causes such as gastritis, pancreatitis, biliary colic, and gastric malignancy. In this case, an upper abdominal endoscopy can be very helpful to evaluate for evidence of ulcers, other mucosal lesions, and neoplasms. In addition, endoscopic biopsy of the stomach can be obtained to test for *H. pylori*. If endoscopy does not identify a potential source of his symptoms, then gallbladder ultrasonography and computed sonography (CT) scan of the abdomen are indicated to evaluate for potential liver, pancreas, or biliary pathology. If the work-up indeed confirms that the patient is suffering from PUD, it is important to inquire if the patient has been compliant with medical therapy, and to determine if he has previously been tested and/or treated for *H. pylori* infections. The failure of optimal medical management for patients with PUD does not occur very often. Whenever medical ineffectiveness is encountered, it is important to consider potential causes of refractory PUD, which include excess gastrin production (hypergastrinemia) from gastrinoma(s) and/or the ingestion of noxious agents such as nonsteroidal anti-inflammatory drugs (NSAIDs).

> # APPROACH TO:
> ## Ulcer Disease

CLINICAL APPROACH

Ulcer Treatment Trends

With advances in pharmacologic inhibition of gastric acid secretions and the treatment of *H. pylori*, surgeries for ulcer complications such as intractability and gastric outlet obstruction have been dramatically reduced. However, surgery has remained important in the treatment of patients with other PUD complications such as bleeding and perforation. The fact is that mortality from PUD bleeding and PUD perforation has not been significantly reduced with medical advances. Bleeding ulcers requiring hospitalization still carry mortality rates of 10% to 30%, and perforated ulcers are still associated with mortality rates of 5% to 35% with higher mortality rates reported in older patients. The availability of newer and more effective ulcer medications have enabled surgeons performing operations for ulcer complications to select less aggressive forms of operations with fewer post-operative side effects for the patients needing surgical interventions. For example, many surgeons feel that simple closure of perforated ulcers without the addition of vagotomy procedures are highly acceptable for most individuals presenting with perforated ulcers. Similarly, highly selective vagotomy or vagotomy with drainage rather than vagotomy and antrectomy is increasingly used in patients with bleeding ulcers.

PATHOPHYSIOLOGY OF PEPTIC ULCERS—BENIGN GASTRIC ULCER

The number of hospitalizations and operations for patients with benign gastric ulcers may have increased slightly over the past decade because of the greater use and abuse of NSAIDs, particularly among women. As shown in Table 17–1, there are five types of gastric ulcers. Type I gastric ulcers are the most common and accounts for 60% to 70% of gastric ulcers. This type of ulcer is located on the lesser curve and are at or just proximal to the incisura angularis. The pathogenesis of a type I ulcer is believed to be related to mucosal vulnerability in the epithelial tissue between the body of the stomach and the antrum. Even though hypersecretion of acid is not the main cause of this ulcer, acid does play a permissive role in ulcer development and progression. Recent evidence suggests that *H. pylori* plays a role in the formation of type I ulcers. Type II gastric ulcers account for 20% of gastric ulcers, and these ulcers are located in the same location as type I ulcers but these ulcers coexist with ulcers in the duodenum. Type II ulcer development is related to acid hypersecretion. Type III gastric ulcers are pre-pyloric ulcers located usually within 2 cm from the pylorus. Development of type III ulcers is believed to be

Table 17–1 • GASTRIC ULCER TYPES			
Type	Location	Acid Secretion	Surgical Treatment
I	Gastric body-antrum junction, usually lesser curve	Low	Distal gastrectomy or vagotomy with drainage
II	Gastric body and associated with duodenal ulcer	High	Vagotomy with drainage or highly selective vagotomy
III	Prepyloric region	High	Vagotomy and drainage
IV	High on the lesser curve	Low	Subtotal gastrectomy or ulcer excision and vagotomy with drainage
V	Anywhere in the stomach	Associated with NSAIDs exposure. No relationship to excess acid	Surgery rarely indicated

related to hyper acidity and pyloric dysfunction. Type IV gastric ulcers are on the lesser curve of the stomach and within 2 cm from the gastroesophageal junction. These ulcers are rare and not usually associated with increase acid production but are believed to be due to mucosal vulnerability in older individuals. Type V gastric ulcers are ulcers related to NSAID exposure and can occur anywhere in the stomach (Table 17–1).

DUODENAL ULCERS

Hospitalization and operations for duodenal ulcer disease have dramatically decreased over the past three decades. However, the number of urgent operations for this disease has increased. Currently, patients with duodenal ulcer complications tend to be older and more often already hospitalized for other medical conditions. Duodenal ulcer disease has multiple etiologies. The most common contributing mechanisms to PUD are acid and pepsin secretion in conjunction with *H. pylori* infections or the ingestion of NSAIDs. Gastric acid secretions are usually increased in patients with duodenal ulcers. There is strong evidence that *H. pylori* infestation in the stomach contributes to resistance and recurrences following standard antisecretory therapy. Therefore, it is important to clarify in all PUD patients whether there is *H. pylori* involvement. For duodenal ulcer patients with *H. pylori* infections, eradication of *H. pylori* with antisecretory treatment will produce sustainable ulcer healing in 98% of the treated patients.

MEDICAL TREATMENT OF UNCOMPLICATED PEPTIC ULCER DISEASE

Following a review of the patient's history, physical examination, and routine laboratory studies, endoscopy is generally performed (Figure 17–1). Testing for *H. pylori* should be performed because *H. pylori* infections are common in most patients with gastric ulcers (60%-90%) and in more than 90% of the patients with duodenal ulcers. Most *H. pylori* negative patients tend to be NSAID users. Nearly all the currently available tests for the detection of *H. pylori* have good

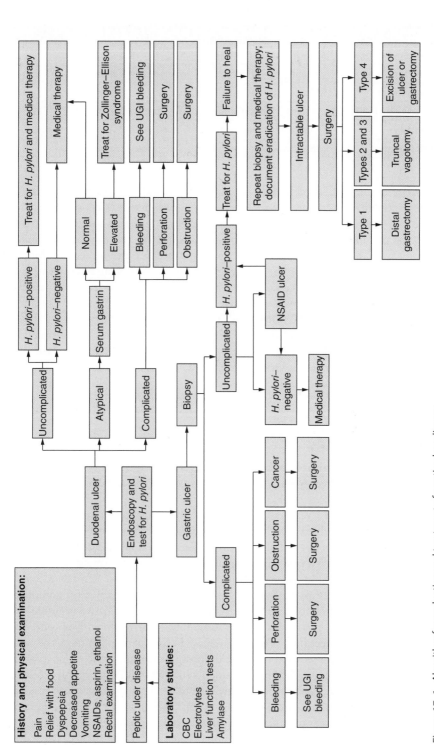

Figure 17–1. Algorithm for evaluation and treatment of peptic ulcer disease.

Table 17–2 • MEDICAL THERAPY FOR PEPTIC ULCER DISEASE	
Agent	**Mechanism of Action**
Antacids	Neutralize gastric acidity and decrease activity of pepsin
H$_2$ antagonist	Blocks H$_2$ parietal cell H$_2$ receptor
Proton pump inhibitors	Inhibits H$^+$-K$^+$-adenosine-triphosphatase pump
Sucralfate	Complexes with pepsin and bile salts and binds to proteins in mucosa
Prostaglandins	Inhibit acid secretion, increase endogenous mucosal defense

sensitivity and specificity. The less invasive tests include an immunoglobulin G serology test that does not correlate necessarily with active infections. Another of the noninvasive tests is the urea breath test, which is highly specific in detecting active infections. The useful invasive studies include the rapid urease assay performed on biopsy specimens and histologic studies performed on biopsy samples. Patients with PUD and *H. pylori* infections should undergo treatment for *H. pylori* eradication. **The failure to eradicate *H. pylori* will lead to an annual relapse rate of 58%, as opposed to relapse rate of 2% with eradication.** Common treatment regimens are **OAC, OMC,** and **OAM** (**O**, omeprazole or other PPI; **A**, amoxicillin; **C**, clarithromycin; and **M**, metronidazole) for a treatment duration of 1 to 2 weeks. In general, triple therapy regimen is more successful than dual therapy or monotherapy; For patients with PUD who are *H. pylori* negative, treatment with PPI or H$_2$ blocker should be initiated, and if the patients are taking NSAID, co-therapy with misoprostol (a prostaglandin analogue) is helpful to improve ulcer healing (see Table 17–2).

SURGICAL THERAPY

For patients with gastric or duodenal ulcers, surgical therapies are directed at treating complications related to the disease. Ulcer disease is generally considered intractable if the process persists for 3 months despite appropriate medical therapy, if the ulcer recurs within 1 year after initial healing despite appropriate maintenance therapy, or if the ulcer disease is characterized as having cycles of prolonged activity with only brief periods of remission. **Gastric ulcers should be biopsied early during the course of treatment to rule out malignancies.** Operative treatment for patients with gastric ulcers should include ulcer excision at a minimal. Several operative options are available for patients undergoing surgical therapy for ulcer complications, and the magnitude of operations ranges from highly selective vagotomy to truncal vagotomy with gastric drainage to vagotomy + antrectomy to subtotal gastrectomy to total gastrectomy. With the increase in operative magnitude, the risks of ulcer recurrences are reduced but risks of "postgastrectomy" and/or "postvagotomy" syndromes increase. With the introduction of PPIs which are highly effective antisecretory agents, most surgeons are inclined to perform less aggressive surgical options in most situations. Most ulcer operations can now be performed laparoscopically, which provides patients with additional recovery benefits.

Surgical treatment of type I gastric ulcers can be accomplished with distal gastrectomy to include the area of the ulcer and reconstruction with a gastroduodenostomy (Bilroth I) or a gastrojejunostomy (Bilroth II). For patients who are not able to tolerate a lengthy operation, an alternative procedure is ulcer excision with vagotomy and pyloroplasty. For patients with type II gastric ulcers, the operation of choice is an acid-reducing procedure, which can be highly selective vagotomy, truncal vagotomy, and pyloroplasty. Operative treatment for patients with type III gastric ulcers should include either highly selective vagotomy or truncal vagotomy and the addition of pyloroplasty to correct the pyloric dysfunction. For type IV ulcers, operative treatment can be a subtotal gastrectomy to include the ulcer area or in patients who are unable to tolerate the operation, the procedure can be ulcer excision plus vagotomy and drainage.

Most patients who present with perforated duodenal ulcers and without extensive prior history of ulcers and/or ulcer treatments can have omental patch closure of the ulcers and medical management + *H. pylori* eradication rather than formal acid-reducing operations.

> ## CASE CORRELATION
>
> - See also Case 14 (Gastroesophageal Reflux Disease), Case 15 (Esophageal Perforation), and Case 16 (Esophageal Carcinoma).

COMPREHENSION QUESTIONS

17.1 Which of the following patients is best managed by surgical treatment?

A. A 44-year-old man with a 1-cm duodenal ulcer that is causing epigastric pain for 3 weeks. His *H. pylori* serology is positive

B. A 68-year-old woman who has been consuming NSAIDs for osteoarthritis develops melena. She has remained hemodynamically stable and on **esophagogastroduodenoscopy** (EGD) is found to have superficial mucosa erosions throughout the stomach

C. A 40-year-old man with epigastric pain and coffee-ground emesis. His EGD reveals a small ulcer in the gastric antrum and a second ulcer in the duodenal bulb. His *H. pylori* serology is positive

D. A 90-year-old man with decompensated congestive heart failure and active upper gastrointestinal (GI) bleeding from a duodenal ulcer that is visualized by EGD

E. A 57-year-old man with a history of gastric ulcer that was biopsied 4 months ago and found to be benign. He has received treatment for *H. pylori* and has been maintained on PPI and continues to have pain. Repeat EGD reveals persistent gastric ulcer involving the lesser curve of the stomach near the incisura angularis

17.2 A 35-year-old man is diagnosed with duodenal ulcer. He asks about the indications for surgical therapy. For which of the following situations is surgical treatment indicated?

A. Development of diabetes mellitus

B. Persistent *H. pylori* infection

C. Chronic gastric outlet obstruction

D. Need for taking NSAIDs

E. Occult gastrointestinal bleeding

17.3 Which of the following is correct regarding medical therapy of PUD?

A. PPI and H_2 antagonists have approximately equal efficacy in controlling ulcer symptoms

B. Prostaglandin compounds such as misoprostol promote resolution of gastric ulcers by inhibiting the proton pump, thereby decreasing acid production

C. NSAID-induced ulcers are sometimes associated with *H. pylori* and require antibiotics treatment

D. H_1 receptors are associated with gastric acid secretion

E. Patients with NSAID-induced ulcers generally do not respond to medical therapy

17.4 A 33-year-old stock broker has midabdominal pain throughout the day, which is relieved somewhat by meals and antacid intake. A gallbladder ultrasound is negative. He undergoes an upper GI endoscopy which reveals a duodenal ulcer. Which of the following best describes characteristics of duodenal ulcer disease?

A. It is rarely associated with hypersecretion of acid

B. It is a disease of multiple etiologies

C. Complete eradication of *H. pylori* is difficult and associated with frequent recurrences

D. *H. pylori* infections usually occur in the gastric cardia

E. Duodenal ulcer predisposes the patient to subsequent malignancy

17.5 A 41-year-old woman has progressive epigastric pain which has improved somewhat with PPI. She underwent upper endoscopy and a gastric ulcer is diagnosed. Which of the following best describes a characteristic of gastric ulcers?

A. Type I gastric ulcers are usually not associated with excess acid secretion

B. Type I gastric ulcers are usually located in the prepyloric region of the stomach

C. Type II gastric ulcers are usually associated with gastroesophageal reflux

D. Type V gastric ulcers are associated with chronic steroid usage

E. Type III gastric ulcers are not associated with excess acid production

17.6 Which of the following is a true statement regarding the surgical treatment of PUD?

A. Most surgery for PUD is done to treat patients after failure of pharmacologic therapy

B. Ulcer surgeries remain highly effective for the control of acid secretion

C. With improved pharmacologic therapy, surgery has been eliminated in the treatment of PUD

D. Surgery for PUD results in better quality of life than medical therapy

E. Surgical therapy is almost exclusively performed for the treatment of gastric outlet obstruction due to PUD

17.7 A 54-year-old man presents with a type I gastric ulcer. He was given 2 weeks of antibiotics therapy for *H. pylori* eradication and 4 weeks of PPI therapy. Three months later, he presents with progressive weight loss and gastric outlet obstruction. Which of the following is a true statement regarding this sequence of events?

A. His *H. pylori* infection likely recurred

B. Biopsy of his ulcer at his initial evaluation might have prevented the gastric outlet obstruction

C. Two weeks of *H. pylori* treatment was insufficient for eradication of *H. pylori*

D. Highly selective vagotomy should have been performed at the time of his ulcer diagnosis

E. Gastric outlet obstruction from refractory ulcer disease is the most common cause of gastric outlet obstruction

17.8 Which of the following is a true statement regarding operations for peptic ulcer disease?

A. Truncal vagotomy and antrectomy are associated with lower rate of ulcer recurrence and better postoperative functional outcomes than truncal vagotomy and pyloroplasty

B. Ulcer recurrence is the most important concern when selecting an ulcer operation for a patient with refractory PUD

C. Complications following vagotomy are extremely rare and do not influence the decision in operative treatment selection

D. Patients who develop recurrence following vagotomy and antrectomy should undergo gastric acid analysis and serology testing for gastrin levels

E. A patient who develops recurrent PUD after vagotomy and pyloroplasty should undergo total gastrectomy

ANSWERS

17.1 **E.** A gastric ulcer that is refractory to medical therapy after 4 months should be considered for surgical therapy. The operation to be performed can be excision of the ulcer and vagotomy with drainage procedure or a partial gastrectomy that includes the ulcer and the distal stomach. *H. pylori* eradication with ulcer medication should be the treatment for the patients described in choices A and C. The treatment for the patient with NSAID-associated gastric erosion is medical therapy with PPI and misoprostol.

17.2 **C.** Chronic gastric outlet obstruction associated with PUD is an indication for surgical treatment which can be either vagotomy with drainage or vagotomy with antrectomy. Patients with PUD taking NSAIDs can be managed with *H. pylori* treatment and PPI. Occult GI bleeding does not necessarily require surgical treatment.

17.3 **C.** Patients with NSAIDs-induced ulcers are not uncommonly associated with *H. pylori*. If infection is documented, treatment will include antibiotics to eradicate *H. pylori* and antisecretory medication (PPI). PPI is much more effective than H_2 antagonist in reducing gastric acid production.

17.4 **B.** Duodenal ulcer pathogenesis can be multifactorial. The end result is generally hyperacidic gastroduodenal environment that can be aggravated by *H. pylori* infections and perhaps low blood flow conditions (eg, shock-related ulcers and stress-related ulcers).

17.5 **A.** The patient described has a type I gastric ulcer and this ulcer is not usually contributed to by hyperacidity. Type II ulcers are classic gastric ulcer and duodenal ulcer and are related to hyperacidity. Type III ulcer is a prepyloric ulcer related to hyperacidity and pyloric emptying dysfunction. Type IV is a proximal gastroesophageal ulcer. Type V ulcer is an NSAID-induced mucosal ulcer that can occur in any location in the stomach.

17.6 **B.** Ulcer surgeries are highly effective at reducing acid production from the stomach. The drawbacks of surgical treatment are motility disorders affecting gastric emptying and reduction in gastric capacity. Surgical treatment is most commonly performed today to address bleeding that is refractory to medical interventions and to address perforated ulcer disease.

17.7 **B.** The patient with an apparent gastric ulcer undergoes medical therapy and 3 months later, develops gastric outlet obstruction. A plausible explanation for this sequence of events is that the gastric ulcer thought to be benign in nature is actually a gastric malignancy that has progressed over the ensuing 3 months to cause gastric outlet obstruction.

17.8   **D.** Patients who develop recurrent ulcers following vagotomy and antrectomy suggest unusual causes of their ulcer diseases such as excess gastrin production related to gastrinomas (Zollinger–Ellison syndrome). An ulcer recurrence following vagotomy and pyloroplasty can be salvaged with the addition of an antrectomy rather than a total gastrectomy.

CLINICAL PEARLS

▶ Appreciation of the type of gastric ulcer that a patient has helps identify the underlying pathogenesis and the selection of the most appropriate treatment strategy.

▶ Prevention of ulcer recurrence requires *H. pylori* eradication rather than treatment alone in the selected cases.

▶ In general, gastric ulcers should be biopsied to rule out malignancy.

▶ Type V gastric ulcers are related to NSAIDs or aspirin use, and these ulcers rarely need surgical therapy.

▶ The indications for surgery for PUD are obstruction, hemorrhage, perforation, and intractable symptoms.

▶ Acid-reduction therapy such as PPI and surgery can be beneficial for patients with ulcers that are not related to hyperacidity (eg, type I gastric ulcer), and the reason is that acid aggravates the healing of these ulcers.

REFERENCES

Beaulieu RJ, Eckhauser FE. The management of duodenal ulcers. Periampullary carcinoma. In: Cameron JL, Cameron AM, eds. *Current Surgical Therapy.* 11th ed. Philadelphia, PA: Elsevier Saunders; 2014:76-80.

Lanas A, Carrera-Lasfuentes P, Arguedas Y, et al. Risk of upper and lower gastrointestinal bleeding in patients taking nonsteroidal anti-inflammatory drugs, antiplatelet agents, or anticoagulants. *Clin Gastroenterol Hepatol.* 2015;13:906-912.

Testerman TL, Morris J. Beyond the stomach: an updated view of *Helicobacter pylori* pathogenesis, diagnosis, and treatment. *World J Gastroenterol.* 2014;28;20:12781-12808.

A 37-year-old man presents with 1-day history of abdominal pain, nausea, and vomiting. The patient reports that the pain was colicky in nature at the onset but has become dull and persistent over the past few hours. He indicates that the symptoms developed shortly after dinner the previous evening. Thinking that he had some bad food, the patient went to bed hoping that it would resolve. He woke up four times during the night and vomited copious amount of bilious material. The patient was well up to the time when symptoms began, and since the onset of symptoms, he has not passed flatus or stool. He has no current medical problems, except that 2 years ago, he had a laparotomy for perforated appendicitis. On physical examination, his temperature is 38.5°C (100.5°F), pulse rate is 105 beats/minute, blood pressure is 130/84 mm Hg, and respiratory rate is 28 breaths/minute. His abdomen is distended, mildly tender throughout, and without peritonitis. His white blood cell (WBC) count is 16,000/mm^2 with 88% neutrophils. His serum chemistry studies are within the normal ranges. His abdominal radiograph is shown in Figure 18–1. An abdominal computed tomography (CT) scan was performed with a representative image shown in Figure 18–2.

▶ What is your next step in the management?
▶ What are the complications associated with this disease process?
▶ What is the probable therapy?

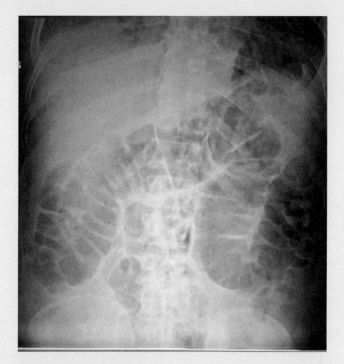

Figure 18–1. Supine abdominal radiograph.

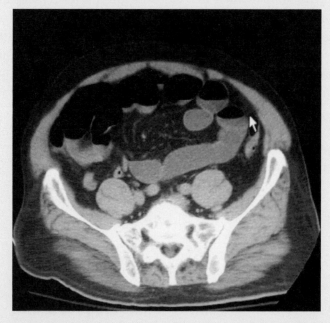

Figure 18–2. Axial CT image of small bowel obstruction. Note the fluid-filled, dilated small bowel loops and decompressed small bowel seen in the right lower quadrant. The arrow points to decompressed descending colon.

ANSWERS TO CASE 18:
Small Bowel Obstruction

Summary: A 37-year-old man presents with colicky abdominal pain and vomiting but the pain pattern has become persistent over the past few hours. His abdominal radiograph demonstrates a dilated stomach and dilated small bowel. All of the findings together are compatible with the diagnosis of mechanical small bowel obstruction.

- **Next step in management:** Place a nasogastric (NG) tube to help decompress his stomach and relieve his vomiting, initiate fluid resuscitation, place a Foley catheter to help monitor urine output and determine his response to fluid resuscitation.

- **Complications associate with this disease process:** Mechanical small bowel obstruction may cause bowel strangulation, bowel necrosis, bowel perforation, and sepsis. Vomiting may cause aspiration pneumonitis. When unrecognized and untreated, intravascular fluid loss (from third-space fluid loss and vomiting) can cause prerenal azotemia and acute kidney injury.

- **Probable therapy:** Exploratory laparotomy or exploratory laparoscopy, because his clinical presentation raises the concern for high-grade obstruction and the potential for bowel necrosis.

ANALYSIS

Objectives

1. Learn the clinical and radiographic signs associated with mechanical small bowel obstruction (SBO), and learn to recognize patient presentations that should raise our clinical suspicion for complicated SBO.

2. Learn the management strategy for mechanical small bowel obstruction.

Considerations

An otherwise healthy 37-year-old man presents with the sudden onset of colicky pain, vomiting, abdominal distension, and obstipation, which are typical signs and symptoms compatible with intestinal obstruction. The bowel obstruction in this case is likely SBO, as obstruction of the small bowel is much more common than obstruction of the large bowel. For an otherwise healthy man with a prior history of a laparotomy for perforated appendicitis, a large cohort study has reported the prevalence of SBO to be 1.0% for those with prior open appendectomy and 0.4% for those with prior laparoscopic appendectomy. The etiology causing SBO in this patient is most likely postoperative intra-abdominal adhesions. The other potential causes of SBO include incarcerated hernias, Crohn disease, and tumors. Therefore, we need to carefully direct our history and physical examination to determine whether one of these other less common causes can be the reason for his current condition. This patient's abdominal radiograph demonstrates dilated small bowel and a paucity of air in the colon, which are again consistent with SBO. The change in this patient's pain pattern is concerning, as **persistent pain associated with SBO raises the concern for bowel ischemia or severe bowel distension.** Severe distension of the intestine is problematic because as the bowel gets more distended, venous congestion increases in the bowel wall, which in turn contributes to the vicious cycle of increased venous congestion, bowel edema, worsening obstruction, and eventually bowel ischemia. Other concerning features of this patient's presentation include fever, tachycardia, leukocytosis, and radiographic signs of high-grade small bowel obstruction.

Mechanical bowel obstruction causes "third-space" fluid losses, since there is shift of fluid from the intravascular space into the bowel lumen, the bowel wall, as well as fluid loss into the peritoneal cavity. The tachycardia and leukocytosis in this patient with SBO can be due to dehydration from fluid losses or can indicate a septic response to bowel strangulation. His initial response to fluid resuscitation will tell us whether bowel ischemia or dehydration is the problem. If his vital signs and clinical appearance improve significantly within the first 1 to 2 hours, then his initial presenting symptoms are more likely related to fluid loss rather than bowel ischemia/necrosis. Because delayed operative intervention for patients with complicated SBO is associated with significant patient morbidity and mortality, most surgeons faced with this patient's clinical presentation would proceed with immediate resuscitation followed by operative intervention if the patient does not respond clinically.

This patient had a CT scan performed as a part of his diagnostic work-up. The abdominal CT scan can provide valuable information regarding whether a tumor or Crohn disease may be the reason for the SBO. In addition, there are CT features that are useful to assess the perfusion status of the bowel wall, and/or determine the severity and location of the obstruction. CT scans are useful when a patient presents with partial SBO and without clinical signs that would prompt an early operative intervention. In these patients, the CT helps determine the severity of SBO and provide reassurance for surgeons to proceed with an initial nonoperative strategy. An advantage of CT in a preoperative patient is that the study can help identify the number and locations of the obstructions so that a laparoscopic approach can be undertaken. One of the drawbacks of CT scan in a patient with SBO is that if the patient is severely dehydrated during the CT examination, contrast-induced acute kidney injury can occur. Therefore, prior to obtaining a CT scan, it is important to make sure that the patient's intravascular volume depletion is corrected with fluid resuscitation. Another disadvantage of CT scannig is that the examination can lead to delays in patient treatment, especially if the patient already has indications for surgical treatment. Therefore, it is always important to weigh the risks/benefits of CT scan before obtaining it.

APPROACH TO:
Small Bowel Obstruction

DEFINITIONS

EARLY POSTOPERATIVE SMALL BOWEL OBSTRUCTION: This is defined as SBO that occurs within 30 days of an abdominal operation. Early postoperative SBO is almost uniformly treatable by a nonoperative approach, as the adhesions causing this process is often less organized and are less likely to lead to bowel strangulation. Most early postoperative SBO will resolve with NG decompression and supportive care.

COMPLICATED SMALL BOWEL OBSTRUCTION: This is not a standard term but can be applied to a patient with SBO that is complicated by intestinal ischemia or intestinal strangulation. When clinicians are faced with a patient with SBO, it helps them to recognize whether there are no concerning features for bowel ischemia and/or strangulation (uncomplicated SBO) or if there are concerning clinical features, such as pain out of proportion to clinical examination, fever, tachycardia, hypotension, peritonitis, leukocytosis, and elevated serum lactate. To provide timely and appropriate treatment for patients with SBO, it is critical for clinicians to recognize signs, symptoms, laboratory findings, and radiologic findings associated with complicated SBO.

CLOSED-LOOP OBSTRUCTION: This develops when an intestinal blockage occurs at the proximal and distal ends of a bowel segment. Examples include small bowel incarceration in a tight hernia defect, intestinal volvulus, and a tight adhesive band obstructing the intestine in two areas. Closed-loop obstructions are unlikely to resolve without surgical treatment.

ILEUS: Distension of the small intestine and/or colon due to nonobstructive causes. Common causes include localized and systemic inflammatory/infectious processes, metabolic derangements, recent abdominal surgery/trauma, and medications. Common examples include ileus associated with acute pancreatitis, ileus associated with an appendicitis abscess, and postoperative ileus.

INTERNAL HERNIA: This is a congenital or acquired defect within the peritoneal cavity through which the intestine can become trapped and blocked. When this finding is associated with SBO, surgical repair is generally needed.

GALLSTONE ILEUS: This describes an intestinal blockage from a large gallstone in the bowel. The usual passage of the gallstone in this situation is through an opening between the gallbladder and the adjacent duodenum (cholecysto-duodenal fistula). The obstructive point is most commonly in the distal ileum where the luminal diameter is smaller. Air in the biliary tree or in the gallbladder in a patient with SBO should raise the suspicion for this diagnosis.

ABDOMINAL CT FOR SBO: This study is usually obtained with intravenous contrast and enteric contrast administration. Intestinal distension and intestinal wall perfusion can be assessed with this study. The study can help identify intestinal necrosis and high-risk features indicating high-grade obstruction, and intestinal volvulus. CT scans are helpful to localize the point of obstruction and provide a "road map" for a more focused operative approach such as a laparoscopic approach.

GASTROGRAFIN CHALLENGE: This is a diagnostic and therapeutic maneuver involving Gastrografin (datrizoatemeglumine/diatrizoate sodium) infusion into the bowel (by NG tube). Gastrografin is a water-soluble contrast material, and because of its hyperosmolar properties, Gastrografin the intestinal lumen causes fluid to shift into the bowel lumen. This fluid shift decreases the edema within the intestinal wall and may promote resolution of the obstruction. Randomized control studies have reported that Gastrografin challenge led to earlier resolution of partial SBO in adults with adhesions related SBO. In addition, this approach has been reported to be safe in patients with SBO and a history of intraperitoneal or pelvic malignancies.

CLINICAL APPROACH

History

Mechanical SBO is a common clinical problem. For adult patients, the most common causes of SBO are postoperative adhesions, hernias, malignancies, inflammatory bowel disease (Crohn disease), and gallstone ileus. In neonates, infants, and young children, hernias, malrotation, meconium ileus, Meckel diverticulum, intussusception, and intestinal atresia are the common causes of intestinal obstruction. Important factors to inquire during the initial assessment include history of prior abdominal surgery, history of prior GI or GU malignancies, history of inflammatory bowel disease, history of prior SBO, and history of hernias. Clinically, when a patient presents with abdominal distension, vomiting, and obstipation/constipation, the diagnosis can be either intestinal obstruction or ileus. Often, **a history of cramp-like pain will help differentiate mechanical obstructions from ileus.** With mechanical bowel obstruction, the intestinal peristalsis often remains intact despite intestinal narrowing or blockage. Therefore, patients with SBO will generally describe cramp-like pain, while patients with ileus generally will complain of constipation and distension without cramps. The goals in patients' evaluation are to diagnose the bowel obstruction, determine if the obstruction is partial or complete, and identify patients who might require timely surgical interventions (see Figure 18–3).

Physical Examination

Abdominal distention is a finding that occurs commonly with SBO. However, when the obstruction is located in the proximal small bowel (jejunum), patients may not have significant abdominal distention; instead, these patients may present with frequent vomiting. Most patients with SBO will initially present with low-grade fever and mild tachycardia secondary to dehydration and low-grade inflammatory changes. However **when fever and tachycardia do not improve with initial fluid resuscitation and NG decompression, the possibility of complicated SBO should be entertained.** The presence of localized abdominal tenderness is indicative of a high-grade

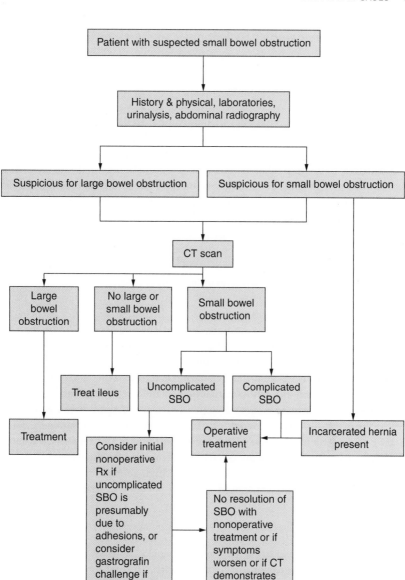

Figure 18-3. Algorithm for small bowel obstruction management.

obstructive process with focal bowel ischemia or impending ischemia. Patients presenting with these findings should be considered for early surgical treatment. Auscultation of the abdomen in a patient with SBO will often reveal high-pitched bowel sounds with occasional fluid-rushing sounds. However, as bowel ischemia and/or necrosis develop in the setting of complicated obstructions, auscultation of the abdomen may reveal absence of bowel sounds.

Laboratory and Radiographic Evaluations

Laboratory studies for patients with suspected SBO should include complete blood count with a differential count, serum electrolytes and amylase, urinalysis, and arterial blood gas (especially for patients who are toxic appearing and patients exhibiting respiratory distress). With dehydration and the host physiologic responses to the bowel obstruction, even patients with uncomplicated SBO may initially present with mild leukocytosis (WBC of 10,000-14,000 cells/mm³) and/or a left shift in the cell count differential. Following appropriate hydration, most patients' WBC will normalize, and the persistence of leukocytosis should raise the suspicion of complications and prompt consideration for early surgical intervention. An elevation in the serum amylase can occur in the setting of complicated SBO but may also suggest pancreatitis as the cause of the abdominal pain and distension. The serum lactate level is often relied on as an indicator of bowel ischemia. Unfortunately, elevation in this laboratory value is often observed only after bowel ischemia/necrosis has already occurred, and **serum lactate value has not been found as a sensitive indicator to help identify patients with impending bowel ischemia.**

Abdominal radiographs are frequently obtained during the work-up of patients with suspected SBO. These films often reveal dilated small bowel with or without colonic air. However, these findings are not specific for SBO and may occur with intestinal ileus. Abdominal radiographs can be useful to help determine if the obstructive process is partial or completed. One of the drawbacks of relying on abdominal radiography in the initial evaluation is that patients with advanced SBO can have predominantly fluid-filled small bowel, and the absence of air-fluid levels in the bowel can contribute to miss-diagnosis. A common application of abdominal radiographs is to follow the progress of patients with SBO undergoing initial nonoperative management. **Because of the limited specificity and sensitivity associated with abdominal radiographs, many groups are advocating for the use of CT scans for the initial evaluations.** Abdominal CT scan has high sensitivity and specificity for the diagnosis of SBO but is associated with risk of **contrast-associated acute kidney injury** in patients with hypovolemia.

Nonoperative Treatment

The nonoperative treatment of patients generally includes NPO, NG-decompression, and intravenous fluid resuscitation. Patients with SBO who are initially selected for this nonoperative treatment typically have partial SBO related to postoperative adhesions. Patients presenting with concerning findings such as fever, hypotension, and localized tenderness should not be managed with a nonoperative approach. The Gastrografin challenge is an option for patients deemed appropriate for nonoperative treatment. This challenge can promote earlier resolution of obstruction in some patients. It is critical to closely monitor patients undergoing nonoperative treatment. For, such as frequent re-evaluation of temperature, pulse rate, urine output, NG output, abdominal physical examination, and WBC. Failure to improve with nonoperative treatment within 24 to 48 hours should prompt additional radiographic evaluation such as a Gastrografin challenge or surgical treatment.

Surgical Treatment

Prior to surgery, patients should receive broad-spectrum antibiotics with coverage for enteric flora. For patients with SBO due to postoperative adhesions, the anticipated procedure is lysis of adhesions, which can be approached either by laparoscopy or open laparotomy. The laparoscopic approach is ideal for patients with few adhesions and in whom the obstructive sites have been localized by CT imaging. When successfully implemented, the laparoscopic approach is associated with faster patient recovery and less postoperative pain. However, laparoscopy can be extremely challenging when dense adhesions or extensive bowel distension are encountered.

Patients with SBO due to incarcerated hernias, obstructing tumors, and small bowel intussusception should undergo early surgical management following initial fluid resuscitation. Patients with SBO secondary to exacerbation of Crohn disease should be treated with escalation of pharmacological treatments as initial treatment strategy. It is important to coordinate the care of patients with inflammatory bowel disease and intestinal obstructions with the patients' gastroenterologists so that these patients do not undergo unnecessary operations.

Outcomes

The mortality associated with SBO has improved over the past 50 years with improved medical imaging, supportive care, and perioperative care. Despite this overall improvement in patient outcomes, patients with complicated SBO continue to experience higher morbidity and mortality than patients with uncomplicated SBO. As medical providers, it is imperative for us to recognize the signs, symptoms, laboratory findings, and radiographic signs associated with the existence or the likely progression to complicated SBO. Once these patients are recognized, early resuscitation and early surgical intervention are vital to minimize the harm associated with SBO.

> ## CASE CORRELATION
> - See also Case 21 (Short Bowel Syndrome), Case 24 (Abdominal Pain [Right Lower Quadrant]), and Case 28 (Diverticulitis).

COMPREHENSION QUESTIONS

18.1 A 66-year-old woman without prior history of abdominal surgery presents with intermittent abdominal distension and pain for approximately 1 week's duration and persistent vomiting for the past 1 day. Her physical examination does not reveal any abdominal or groin hernias. She is afebrile and has normal vital signs. Her WBC count is 5200/mm^2, and abdominal x-ray reveals dilated small bowel and no air within the colon and rectum. Which of the following is the most appropriate next step?

A. Place an NG tube and attempt nonoperative treatment for 48 hours

B. Perform a Gastrografin challenge

C. Obtain a serum carcinoembryonic antigen level (CEA)

D. Proceed with immediate laparotomy

E. Perform a CT scan of the abdomen

18.2 Which of the following patients with small bowel obstruction is most likely to have resolution of the obstruction without an operative intervention?

A. A 1-year-old child with SBO due to midgut volvulus

B. A 73-year-old woman with SBO due to gallstone ileus

C. A 27-year-old man with complete SBO for 3 days due to an incarcerated right inguinal hernia

D. A 33-year-old man with SBO 11 day following an exploratory laparotomy and repair of the transverse colon after a stab wound to the abdomen

E. A 55-year-old man with carcinoid tumor involving the ileum and SBO

18.3 A 72-year-old man with a history of hypertension and an exploratory laparotomy for splenic injury following an automobile crash at the age of 20 years presents with signs and symptoms compatible with SBO. He is afebrile. His abdomen is distended and tender below the umbilicus. His WBC count is 19,000/mm^2. His serum electrolytes reveal sodium of 140 mEq/L, potassium of 4.2 mEq/L, chloride of 105 mEq/L, and bicarb of 14 mEq/L. Which of the following is the best treatment option?

A. Place an NG tube and a urinary catheter and initiate nonoperative treatment

B. Perform a colonoscopy to relieve his sigmoid volvulus

C. Treat the patient for *Clostridium difficile* infection

D. Surgical therapy

E. Broad-spectrum antibiotics to target enteric organisms

18.4 A 33-year-old woman with a history of three prior c-sections presents with partial small bowel obstruction diagnosed by plain radiography of the abdomen. She is initially treated by nonoperative management. On the second day of NPO, intravenous fluids, and NG suction, her abdomen is less distended; however, her NG output volume remains relatively high at 600 mL/24 hours. Which of the following is the most appropriate option at this time?

A. Place a central venous catheter to initiate total parenteral nutrition and continue nonoperative treatment for another 10 days

B. Remove the NG tube and initiate oral diet

C. Prescribe an enema to stimulate bowel movement

D. Obtain a CT scan

E. Perform a laparotomy

18.5 A 27-year-old man underwent a laparoscopic appendectomy for perforated appendicitis. He is doing well and discharged from the hospital on postoperative day 3. Eight days after hospital discharge, the man returns to the the emergency department with nausea and vomiting. His temperature is normal. His abdomen is distended and mildly tender at the incision sites. A CT scan demonstrated findings compatible with partial small bowel obstruction. Which of the following is the best treatment for this patient?

A. Exploratory laparotomy

B. Gastrografin challenge

C. Diagnostic laparoscopy

D. Barium enema to rule out colonic obstruction

E. Initiate broad-spectrum antibiotics treatment

18.6 A 40-year-old man with acute appendicitis is concerned about undergoing appendectomy because he has a history of SBO that has required four separate inpatient hospital stays. Which of the following information is true regarding postoperative SBO?

A. The incidence of SBO is lower following nonoperative treatment of acute appendicitis

B. Open appendectomy is associated with a lower incidence of postoperative SBO

C. Laparoscopic appendectomy is associated with a lower incidence of postoperative SBO

D. Small bowel obstruction occurrence goes down after the age of 30 years

E. Small bowel obstruction occurrence is unlikely after an appendectomy

ANSWERS

18.1 **E.** For this 66-year-old woman without a prior history of abdominal operations presenting with these signs and symptoms, and abdominal radiography indicating high-grade SBO, there are a couple of options that may be reasonable. One option is to obtain a CT scan to help delineate what is causing this process (eg small bowel neoplasm, obstructing cecal caner, or internal hernia). A second option is to proceed with immediate operation and determine what the problem is in the operating room. Because this patient does not have concerning evidence for complicated obstruction, there is no urgency in proceeding with immediate operation. Therefore, the best choice is to perform a CT scan to help delineate what is causing her obstructive symptoms.

18.2 **D.** The 33-year-old-man with early postoperative (postoperative day 11) SBO is most likely to have resolution of the bowel obstruction without operative treatment. The 1-year-old patient with a midgut volvulus needs early operative treatment because there is a high rate of ischemic necrosis associated with this process. The patient with complete SBO and incarcerated inguinal hernia should be treated with operative treatment rather than an attempt at reduction of the inguinal hernia, because the obstructive symptoms have been on-going for 3 days, and there is an increased risk of bowel ischemia when hernia incarceration and SBO have been going on for more than just a few hours. For the other remaining patients, operative treatment is preferred because the obstructions are all associated with conditions that are not likely to resolve spontaneously.

18.3 **D.** This 72-year-old man with history of prior abdominal operation presents with signs and symptoms consistent with SBO. Because there are several clinical signs (abdominal focal tenderness) and laboratory indicators (leukocytosis and low bicarb value) suggestive of complicated obstruction, the best treatment option is to proceed with early abdominal exploration.

18.4 **D.** A CT scan can help provide additional information regarding the location and extent of the obstructive process in this patient with partial resolution of her obstruction with nonoperative management. The high NG output suggests that the obstructive process has not completely resolved; therefore, feeding the patient at this time may actually worsen her condition. Another strategy not listed here is a Gastrografin challenge that might help promote earlier resolution of her obstruction.

18.5 **B.** This 27-year-old man has early postoperative SBO (SBO occurring within 30 days of an abdominal operation). Most cases of early SBO can be successfully managed without operative intervention. A Gastrografin challenge is the best option provided here.

18.6 C. The incidence of postoperative SBO following laparoscopic appendectomy is lower than the rate of postoperative SBO following open appendectomy. The rate of SBO following medical treatment of acute appendicitis is relatively unknown. The patient's age is not a known factor that influences postoperative SBO occurrence.

CLINICAL PEARLS

▶ Persistent pain, fever, tachycardia, localized abdominal tenderness, elevated serum amylase, and reduced serum bicarbonate level are findings suggestive of complicated SBO.

▶ Patients with closed-loop obstruction require early operative intervention.

▶ CT scan is helpful to differentiate SBO from ileus, because it can identify a point of caliber change in the small bowel ("transition point").

▶ CT feature suggestive of complicated SBO includes intraperitoneal free fluid, decreased bowel wall perfusion, and presence of a swirl sign.

▶ Air in the gallbladder or biliary tree (pneumobilia) in a patient with SBO is highly suggestive of gallstone ileus.

▶ As many as 10-15% of patients with gallstone ileus may have a second stone in the gastrointestinal tract; therefore, the entire small bowel should be examined during the operation for gallstone ileus.

▶ A cecal carcinoma may cause obstruction at the ileal–cecal valve, thus mimic a small bowel obstruction.

▶ A patient with SBO from an incarcerated hernia associated with overlying edema and/or inflammatory changes has a high likelihood of ischemic or necrotic bowel at the site of strangulation, and these patients should undergo surgery rather than attempts at hernia reduction.

REFERENCES

Biondo S, Pares D, Mora L, et al. Randomized clinical study of gastrografin administration in patients with adhesive small bowel obstruction. *Br J Surg.* 2003;90:542-546.

Khasawneh MA, Ugarte ML, Srvantstian B, et al. Role of gastrografin challenge in early postoperative small bowel obstruction. *J Gastrointest Surg.* 2014;18:363-368.

Kodadek LM, Makary MA. Small bowel obstruction. In: Cameron JL, Cameron AM, eds. *Current Surgical Therapy.* 11th ed. Philadelphia, PA: Elsevier Saunders; 2014:109-113.

McKenzie S, Evers BM. Small intestine. In: Townsend CM Jr, Beauchamp RD, Evers BM, Mattox KL, eds. *Sabiston Textbook of Surgery: The Biological Basis of Modern Surgical Practice.* 19th ed. Philadelphia, PA: Elsevier Saunders; 2012:1227-1278.

A 46-year-old man presents to the emergency department with tarry stools and a feeling of light-headedness. He indicates that over the past 24 hours, he has had several bowel movements containing tarry-colored stools, and that during the past day, he has been feeling light-headed whenever he stood up to walk around. His past medical and surgical history is unremarkable except for back pain over the past 3 weeks after slipping on a wet floor at work. His back pain has improved with the use of 12 to 14 tablets of ibuprofen daily over the past 2 weeks. He denies significant alcohol use and does not use tobacco products. On examination, the patient is nonicteric, his temperature is 37.0°C (98.6°F), heart rate is 106 beats/minute, blood pressure is 108/80 mm Hg, and respiratory rate is 22 breaths/minute. His abdomen is not distended, but is mildly tender in the epigastrium. The rectal examination reveals melanotic stool and no rectal masses.

▶ What is your next step?
▶ What is the best initial treatment?
▶ What is the role of surgery?

ANSWERS TO CASE 19:
Nonvariceal Upper Gastrointestinal (GI) Tract Hemorrhage

Summary: A 46-year-old man presents with signs and symptoms of acute GI tract hemorrhage. The patient has no history or evidence of liver disease or portal hypertension, and he has recent history of nonsteroidal anti-inflammatory drug (NSAID) ingestion; therefore, the source of the bleeding is likely nonvariceal in origin.

- **Next step:** The first step in the treatment of patients with upper GI hemorrhage is to address the effects of blood loss. The etiology, rate of bleeding, and physiologic status of the patient are helpful in stratifying the risk of further bleeding, as well as complications and mortality from the bleeding.

- **Best initial treatment:** Prompt attention to the patient's airway, breathing, and circulation is mandatory with all patients with acute upper GI bleeding. This patient needs close monitoring and resuscitation as well as early upper GI endoscopy (within the initial 24 hours), which is helpful to identify the source of bleeding, determine whether the bleeding is active, and determine the risk for recurrent bleeding. In addition, endoscopic therapy can be applied.

- **Role of surgery:** The role of surgery for patients with acute nonvariceal upper GI hemorrhage is mainly to control bleeding when endoscopic treatments and/or arterial embolizations fail. A less common surgical indication is to perform antiulcer operations in a patient whose GI bleeding is related to peptic ulcer disease that does not respond to medical therapies such as *Helicobacter pylori* eradication and antisecretory medications.

ANALYSIS

Objectives

1. Be able to outline initial management strategies for patients presenting with acute nonvariceal upper GI bleeding.

2. Learn the likely causes of acute nonvariceal GI bleeding.

3. Learn the prognosticators associated with adverse outcomes in patients with acute nonvariceal upper GI bleeding.

Considerations

This is a 46-year-old man who presents with melena and symptomatic anemia from his acute GI bleeding. Most healthy adults can compensate physiologically and maintain relatively normal vital signs even in the face of significant active hemorrhage; therefore, the absence of hypotension should not lead us to believe that his condition is clinically stable. In fact, the mild tachycardia and normal blood pressure in this patient are compatible with class II hemorrhagic shock associated with approximately 750 to 1500 mL of blood loss. **Once the patient's clinical problem is recognized, the appropriate priorities in this patient's management are (1) address the anemia and intravascular volume, (2) diagnosis, and (3) treatment, in that order.** His initial management should include placement of reliable large-bore intravenous catheters while blood samples are simultaneously sent for complete blood count, liver functions test, coagulation studies, and type and cross-matching. In a patient with acute GI bleeding, the use of nasogastric tube (NG tube) is somewhat controversial, but in selective cases, an NG tube can help reduce the patient's aspiration risks and help confirm or rule out an upper GI tract bleeding source. If the NG aspirate is bilious and without blood or "coffee grounds" materials, the probability of on-going upper GI bleeding is remarkably low. If this individual should develop agitation or lethargy secondary to hemorrhagic shock, he may benefit from early oral–tracheal intubation to help maintain his airway and to minimize aspiration of gastric contents.

A critical step in the initial management of patients with acute upper GI bleeding is to **determine whether the bleeding is nonvariceal in origin or due to portal hypertension and bleeding from gastric and/or esophageal varices.** This patient's history and physical findings strongly suggest that nonvariceal bleeding is the cause, because he does not exhibit any stigmata of cirrhosis such as ascites and jaundice, and he has no known history of cirrhosis. The fact that he is currently taking an NSAID for treatment of back pain further raises our suspicion that his bleeding may be related to gastric/duodenal erosive processes associated with NSAID ingestion (see Table 19–1). Patients with suspected variceal bleeding should receive octreotide and broad-spectrum antibiotics, empirically. For this patient with presumed nonvariceal bleeding, we need to initiate **high-dose proton-pump inhibitor (PPI), consisting of 80 mg omeprazole intravenous bolus followed by 8 mg/h intravenous drip for 72 hours.** Based on the patient's initial presentation, he would likely benefit from early (within 24 hours) upper GI endoscopy and possibly endoscopic intervention.

Table 19–1 • PREDICTORS OF UPPER GI BLEEDING TYPE		
Variables	Variceal Bleeding	Nonvariceal Bleeding
Diagnosis of cirrhosis	Yes	
History of variceal bleeding	Yes	
Ascites	Yes	
Thrombocytopenia	Yes	
High INR	Yes	
High bilirubin	Yes	
NSAIDs use		Yes
Anticoagulant use		Yes

NSAID, nonsteroidal anti-inflammatory drug.

APPROACH TO:

Suspected Nonvariceal Upper GI Bleeding

DEFINITIONS

MALLORY–WEISS TEAR: A proximal gastric mucosal tear following vigorous coughing, retching, or vomiting. The bleeding is generally self-limiting, mild, and amendable to supportive care and endoscopic management.

DIEULAFOY'S EROSION: This is a rarely encountered lesion. GI bleeding associated with this process occurs when erosion causes bleeding from aberrant submucosal artery located in the stomach. This type of bleeding is frequently significant and requires prompt diagnosis by endoscopy and endoscopic or operative control of bleeding.

ARTERIOVENOUS MALFORMATION: A small mucosal lesion located along the GI tract. Bleeding usually occurs abruptly, but the rate of bleeding is usually slow and the process often self-limiting.

ISOLATED GASTRIC VARICES: Isolated gastric varices most commonly develop as the result of splenic vein thrombosis, which then produce "left-sided" or sinistral portal hypertension. With thrombosis of the splenic vein, blood return from the spleen can only return from the spleen through the short gastric veins, thus causing increase in pressure and size of the short gastric veins. **This condition is correctable by splenectomy.**

ESOPHAGITIS: Mucosal erosion that frequently results from gastroesophageal reflux, infections, or medications. Patients generally present with occult bleeding, and treatment consists of correction or avoidance of the underlying conditions.

HEMORRHAGIC SHOCK SEVERITY: Severity of hemorrhagic shock is classified by ATLS as classes I–IV.

- *Class I:* Well-compensated shock with generally normal vital signs and up to 15% or 750 mL blood loss in an average sized adult.

- *Class II:* Slight tachycardia, normal systolic blood pressure with elevated diastolic blood pressure, associated with up to 30% or 750 to 1500 mL blood loss in an average adult.

- *Class III:* Tachycardia to 120 associated with hypotension. Patient is generally anxious appearing and diaphoretic. The patient can have up to 40% blood volume loss or up to 2000 mL in an average size adult.

- *Class IV:* Tachycardia to 140 associated with severe hypotension. Patient is generally unresponsive with decreased mentation. The associated blood loss is greater than 40% of circulating volume or over 2000 mL.

NSAID-ASSOCIATED UPPER GI BLEEDING RISKS: Study results suggest that there is a significantly increased risk for upper GI bleeding associated with

Table 19–2 • RELATIVE RISK OF UPPER GI BLEEDING ASSOCIATED WITH NONSTEROIDAL ANTI-INFLAMMATORY DRUGS (NSAIDs)	
NSAID	**Relative Risk of Bleeding**
Ibuprofen	2.7
Meloxicam (Mobic)	4.0
Diclofenac (Voltaren)	4.0
Naproxen (Naprosyn)	5.2
Indomethacin (Indocin)	5.3
Ketoprofen	5.7
Piroxicam (Feldene)	9.3
Ketorolac	14

NSAID use, and the risk of bleeding is increased when the patient is using NSAIDs (odds ratio: 4.8) or using NSAIDs with concurrent *H. pylori* infection (OR: 6.1). The relative risks of upper GI bleeding associated with different NSAIDs are variable and these are listed in Table 19–2.

CLINICAL APPROACH

Upper GI bleeding describes bleeding from an anatomic location that is proximal to the ligament of Treitz. Overall, **upper GI bleeding is far more common than lower GI bleeding and accounts for 80% of all GI bleeding cases.** The majority of patients with acute upper GI bleeding should be admitted to a unit in the hospital where they can be closely monitored and receive transfusions and resuscitation as needed. At most institutions, the intensive care unit or the step-down unit are the most appropriate places for admissions. In most practice settings, 70% to 90% of the patients presenting with acute upper GI hemorrhage have nonvariceal bleeding causes. Each year, approximately 400,000 admissions to hospitals in the United States are for nonvariceal upper GI bleeding. The prevalence of nonvariceal upper GI bleeding is twice as high in men as it is in women, and the prevalence for both sexes increase with age. **The in-hospital mortality from acute upper GI bleedings is approximately 10% to 15%, where most deaths are attributable to exacerbation of existing medical illnesses secondary to blood loss and shock. Rebleeding in hospitalized patients with nonvariceal upper GI bleeding is approximately 15%, and rebleeding is a major contributor to adverse patient outcomes.**

The treatment of patients with suspected upper GI bleeding begins with an initial assessment to determine if the bleeding is occult or acute. Acute upper GI bleeding should be suspected when the patient presents with hematemesis, coffee-ground emesis, melena, or bloody stools; in contrast, the patient with occult blood loss presents with normal vital signs, no overt evident of GI blood loss, and iron-deficiency anemia. A critical part of the initial management is to determine the intravascular volume status and estimate the extent of the patient's blood loss. It is important early in the management process to stratify the patient's need for early endoscopy, and estimate his/her risks for morbidity, rebleeding, and death. Risk stratification is important to help determine resource and expertise needs for each patient. The **Glasgow Blatchford score (GBS)** is a commonly used scoring system that takes into account patient's pulse rate, systolic blood pressure, hemoglobin, blood urea nitrogen level, and medical comorbidities. The GBS ranges from 0 to 23, and the score has been found to correlate with the patient's need for early endoscopic interventions. The **Rockall score** is a scoring system that combines clinical parameters and endoscopic findings, and the calculated scores have been shown to help predict individual patient's rebleeding and mortality risks.

NG tube placement is indicated for patients presenting with hematemesis, as NG suction can help reduce aspiration events in these patients. Gastric lavage through the NG tube had been a common practice in the management of upper GI bleeding patients but is now rarely performed because of the increased aspiration risk associated with this maneuver. **There has been a recent major change in the transfusion strategy for patients with acute upper GI hemorrhage, which now utilizes a restrictive transfusion approach.** The evidence supporting the newer approach is based on results of a randomized controlled trial reported by Villanueva et al. in the *New England Journal of Medicine* in 2013. This multicenter trial randomized variceal and nonvariceal upper GI bleeding patients to blood transfusions when the patients' hemoglobin fell below either 9 g/dL (liberal transfusion group) or below 7 g/dL (restrictive transfusion group). The results demonstrated that patients in the restrictive transfusion arm received fewer transfusions, had less bleeding, suffered fewer adverse events, and had improved survival in comparison to patients in the liberal transfusion group.

Evidence-based consensus guidelines recommend upper GI endoscopy within 24 hours of presentation, and recent limited data suggest that endoscopy within 12 hours of presentation may be beneficial for patients who present with acute severe hemorrhage. Upper GI endoscopy is valuable for diagnosis, treatment, and risk stratification and prognostication (Table 19–3). Patients who are found with high-risk stigmata (eg, active bleeding, visible vessel, or adherent clot) during endoscopy benefit from endoscopic hemostasic techniques. The applications of endoscopic hemostatis have contributed to significant reductions in patient morbidity, mortality, and their need for surgical interventions. Endoscopic hemostasis techniques include epinephrine injections, thermal application techniques, and clip applications. Epinephrine injections have been reported to be effective in stopping

Table 19–3 • NONVARICEAL BLEEDING CAUSES	
Bleeding Cause	**Frequency Among Bleeding Patients**
Gastroduodenal peptic ulcer disease	20%-50%
Gastritis/duodenitis	8%-15%
Esophagitis	5%-15%
Mallory–Weiss tear	8%-15%
Arteriovenous malformation	5%
Other conditions (eg, Dieulafoy's lesions and malignancies)	<5%

Table 19–4 • PREVALENCE AND RISK OF REBLEEDING OF PEPTIC ULCERS BASED ON ENDOSCOPIC APPEARANCES

Endoscopic Appearance	Prevalence	Rebleeding without Endoscopic Treatment	Rebleeding after Successful Endoscopic Treatment
Active arterial bleeding	10%-15%	90%	15%-30%
Visible vessel	20%-25%	50%	15%-30%
Adherent clot	10%	33%	5%
Oozing but without visible vessel or arterial bleeding	10%-15%	10%	<5%
Flat spot	10%	7%	<5%
Clean ulcer base	30%-40%	3%	<5%

bleeding but without additional thermal or clip applications, rebleeding can often occur. Once bleeding is controlled endoscopically, pharmacologic treatments are continued and patients can be discharged from the intensive care unit if no further bleeding occurs and/or if low-risk endoscopic stigmata are reported. There is no evidence to support routine second look endoscopy; however, second-look and repeat endoscopic hemostasis is indicated for selective high-risk patients with high-risk lesions (see Table 19-4 for risk factors for rebleeding).

Angiography and Transarterial Embolization (TAE)

In some practice settings, TAE has emerged as an alternative to surgery for patients in whom endoscopic treatments have failed to control bleeding. TAE utilizes angiography to access the bleeding vessels and then control the bleeding either with the infusion of vasoconstrictive medication (vasopressin) or with mechanical occlusion by embolization. The ideal candidates for TAE are individuals whose bleeding sources have already been located by endoscopy so that they can proceed directly to TAE without undergoing a diagnostic angiogram to identify the vessel involved. TAE is an excellent option at institutions that have the resources and personnel available to provide consistent around the clock care for these patients. Unfortunately, there have not been any randomized controlled studies performed comparing surgery and TAE for patients who fail endoscopic treatment.

Surgery for Nonvariceal Upper GI Bleeding

The indication for surgical control of nonvariceal bleeding is to achieve hemostasis when endoscopic therapies fail. There is evidence to suggest that for a patient with peptic ulcer disease, when recurrent bleeding develops following an initially successful endoscopic treatment, a second endoscopic intervention produces better patient outcomes than surgical intervention. Surgery is infrequently performed in the modern era because endoscopic and angiographic treatments are highly effective for the control of acute bleeding. When necessary, most surgeons operate for the control of bleeding, rather than to address the underlying ulcer disease. With the availability of proton-pump inhibitors and medical regimen for *H. pylori* eradication, operations to specifically treat ulcer diseases are infrequently required in patients in these emergency settings. In general, surgical control of bleeding involves the creation of a gastrotomy or duodenotomy to access the bleeding area directly, followed by placement of sutures to control the bleeding areas.

Outcome

The bleeding in nonvariceal upper GI bleeding patients is self-limiting approximately 80% of the time. Recurrent or continuing bleeding is reported in approximately 20% of the patients. The in-patient mortality in this patient population is 10% to 15% and has remained relatively unchanged over time. Factors associated with increased mortality include rebleeding, increased patient age, major comorbid conditions, and patients who develop bleeding while hospitalized for another medical condition.

> ## CASE CORRELATION
>
> - See also Case 20 (Upper GI Bleeding [Variceal]).

COMPREHENSION QUESTIONS

19.1 A 55-year-old man underwent upper GI endoscopy. He was told by his gastroenterologist that the lesion identified is a common cause of anemia but rarely a cause of acute blood loss. Which of the following is the most likely diagnosis?

A. Gastric ulcer

B. Duodenal ulcer

C. Dieulafoy's lesion

D. Gastric cancer

E. Gastric varices

19.2 A 32-year-old otherwise healthy man arrives to the emergency center with a history of vomiting "large amounts of bright red blood" and his blood pressure is 100/88 mm Hg. Which of the following is the most appropriate first step in the management of this patient?

A. Perform a history and physical examination

B. Determine his hemoglobin and hematocrit levels

C. Place IV and administer intravenous fluids

D. Insert a nasogastric tube

E. Perform urgent endoscopy

19.3 A 63-year-old man arrives to the emergency center with acute upper GI bleeding. An NG tube was placed and revealed a large amount of blood in the stomach. Which of the following statements is true regarding this man's condition?

A. Statistically, there is a 20% chance the bleeding will not stop or will recur after stopping

B. The mortality for patients like him is much longer today than it was 10 years ago

C. Mesenteric ischemia is a likely cause for his condition

D. Hypertension is a risk factor for this condition

E. Emergency surgery is the best approach for this man's condition

19.4 A 63-year-old man develops acute upper GI bleeding while in the hospital recovering from his total knee replacement. The upper endoscopy revealed a duodenal ulcer with a visible vessel. The endoscopist injected the area with epinephrine and applied endoscopic clips. The patient is placed on high-dose PPI therapy; 12 hours after the procedure, the patient develops rebleeding but remains hemodynamically stable. Which of the following is the best treatment at this time?

A. Angiography and embolization

B. Surgery to control bleeding

C. Repeat endoscopy

D. Transfuse the patient to a hemoglobin value of 10 g/dL

E. Bilateral truncal vagotomy with antrectomy

19.5 Which of the following is NOT a parameter used in calculating the Glasgow-Blatchford score that is used to identify patients who might benefit from early endoscopy?

A. Age

B. Pulse rate

C. Blood pressure

D. Blood urea nitrogen

E. Hematocrit

19.6 Which of the following is considered standard care for patients with severe acute nonvariceal upper GI bleeding?

A. NG lavage with saline

B. Octreotide

C. Transfusion triggering a hemoglobin value of <9 g/dL

D. Endoscopy within 24 hours

E. Second-look endoscopy

ANSWERS

19.1 **D.** Gastric cancer is a common cause of occult upper GI bleeding but an unusual cause of overt upper GI bleeding. All the other choices listed are commonly associated with acute and overt bleeding.

19.2 **C.** Place IV and administer fluids. This patient is presenting with acute upper GI bleeding and possible hemorrhagic shock. Placement of a secured IV and initiation of fluids are important priorities. The history and physical examination are important but are secondary in this patient with questionable hemodynamic status. NG tube placement and endoscopy are important but are secondary. The patient's initial hemoglobin and hematocrit are not helpful to guide initial treatment in this man who is acutely bleeding.

19.3 **A.** Statistically, 20% of upper GI bleeding patients will continue to bleed or develop recurrent bleeding, while 80% of the patients will stop bleeding. The mortality of upper GI bleeding patients remains high at 10% to 15%, and this figure has not changed over the past 20 years. It is likely that GI bleeding patients encountered in modern times are older and sicker; therefore, despite medical advances, the mortality remains high.

19.4 **C.** Repeat endoscopy. There is randomized controlled clinical evidence to show that patients who rebleed after initially successful endoscopic interventions do better when they undergo repeat endoscopic treatments rather than emergency surgery to control their bleeding. There is no clear evidence that compares outcomes with repeat endoscopy versus angiographic embolization. Transfusion to a hemoglobin value of 10 is not indicated. Surgical treatments to address ulcer disease when patients develop rebleeding are likely to produce higher perioperative complications than repeat endoscopic treatment; therefore, surgery is not the first-line treatment in this situation.

19.5 **A.** Age is not used for GBS calculation. The parameters applied in the calculations of GBS include pulse rate, systolic blood pressure, blood urea nitrogen, hemoglobin, chronic medical conditions (eg, liver disease, heart failure, melena, and syncope).

19.6 **D.** Endoscopy within 24 hours of presentation is considered standard care for a patient presenting with severe upper GI bleeding. Endoscopy within 6 to 12 hours after presentation has also been investigated and found not to produce advantages over endoscopy at 24 hours. Transfusion trigger or threshold of hemoglobin value of 7 g/dL has been found to produce less bleeding and better outcomes in comparison to a trigger of 9 g/dL. Routine second-look endoscopy has not been found to produce better outcomes than re-endoscopy only when indicated.

CLINICAL PEARLS

▶ Risk assessment to stratify patients into high- and low-risk categories is helpful to help determine the level of care, optimal timing for endoscopy, and need for admission.

▶ Gastric lavage through the NG tube is not necessary for diagnosis, prognosis, visualization, or therapy. This practice is associated with pulmonary aspiration risks.

▶ Patients with significant acute upper GI bleeding associated with hemodynamic abnormalities should undergo upper GI endoscopy within 24 hours after presentation.

▶ Epinephrine injections should not be used alone for the control of bleeding during endoscopy. This treatment should be combined with a second treatment modality such as coagulation therapy or clip placement.

▶ Repeat endoscopy is indicated for patients with recurrent bleeding after endoscopic therapy and in patients with high-risk stigmata (such as spurting vessel and visible vessel).

▶ Surgery or embolization should be considered if a patient rebleeds after two endoscopic treatment attempts.

▶ Intravenous infusion of erythromycin (250 mg 30 minutes before endoscopy) may improve gastric motility and visualization during endoscopy.

▶ Discharge from the emergency department without in-patient endoscopy can be considered for patients with systolic blood pressure ≥110 mm Hg, pulse rate <100 beats/minute, hemoglobin ≥13 g/dL (men) or ≥ 12 g/dL (woman), blood urea nitrogen <18.2 mg/dL, and the absence of melena, syncope, heart failure, and liver disease. **Overall, requirement for intervention is less than 1%.**

REFERENCES

Khamaysi I, Gralnek IM. Acute upper gastrointestinal bleeding (UGIB)–initial evaluation and management. *Best Pract Res ClinGastroenterol*. 2013;27:633-638.

Laine L, Jenson DM. Management of patients with ulcer bleeding. *Am J Gastroenterol*. 2012;107: 345-360.

Lu Y, Loffroy R, Lau JYW, Barkun A. Multidisciplinary management strategies for acute non-variceal upper gastrointestinal bleeding. *Br J Surg*. 2014;101:e34-e50.

Villanueva C, Colomo A, Bosch A, et al. Transfusion strategies for acute upper gastrointestinal bleeding. *N Engl J Med*. 2013;368:11-21.

A 46-year-old man with a known history of alcoholic cirrhosis is found unconscious at home on the bathroom floor. He is transported to the emergency center by ambulance. The physical examination reveals a pulse of 102 beats/minute, blood pressure of 92/60 mm Hg, and respiratory rate of 23 breaths/minute. He does not appear to have suffered any external signs of trauma. According to a friend, the patient had contacted her by phone and informed her that he began vomiting blood an hour prior and needed help. On physical examination, the patient appears lethargic with blood around his mouth and clothing. His skin is mildly jaundiced; his cardiopulmonary examination is unremarkable; his abdomen is nontender and nondistended. The patient's friend indicates that the patient has been hospitalized in the past for alcohol-related problems and has known history of cirrhosis.

▶ What is the most likely diagnosis?
▶ What are the most appropriate next steps in management?
▶ How do you determine the prognosis for this patient?

ANSWERS TO CASE 20:

Acute Upper Gastrointestinal (GI) Hemorrhage: Variceal Bleeding

Summary: A 46-year-old man with known history of alcoholic cirrhosis presents with acute and overt upper GI bleeding.

- **Diagnosis:** Acute upper GI bleeding that is likely due to gastroesophageal varices.

- **Next steps in management:** Secure the airway by performing endotracheal intubation because patient's current level of response and consciousness puts him at risk for aspiration. The patient will also need to have placement of secured intravenous access and should be transferred to an intensive care unit for monitoring and early upper endoscopy.

- **Prognosis of acute variceal bleeding:** This is determined by the significance of the bleeding and hemodynamic compromise that the bleeding produces. In addition, the status of the patient's liver also determines the prognosis.

ANALYSIS

Objectives

1. Learn the initial management and resuscitation for patients presenting with acute variceal hemorrhage.

2. Learn the options for the definitive management of patients with gastroesophageal variceal hemorrhage.

Considerations

This is a 46-year-old man with a known history of alcoholic cirrhosis who presents with altered mental status and acute upper gastrointestinal hemorrhage. The patient has dried blood around his mouth and lethargy at presentation; thus, the initial concern should be directed at the patient's airway. Most practitioners would proceed with early orotracheal intubation in this situation to prevent aspiration events. Once the airway is secured, our next priority is the assessment of hemodynamic status and initiation of resuscitation. Early on during the evaluation process, it is also helpful to obtain laboratory studies (complete blood count, chemistry panel including liver function tests and coagulation studies) to determine the severity of the patient's liver dysfunction.

The resuscitation of patients with hemorrhagic shock does not necessarily require that we restore normal vital signs and normal hemoglobin values, as recent studies suggest that restoration of normal vital signs may contribute to increased bleeding, and the **resuscitation of GI hemorrhage patients to a hemoglobin target of 7 g/dL has been shown to be associated with better outcomes than resuscitation** to a target hemoglobin of 9 g/dL. Another recent trend that has evolved from trauma resuscitation practice suggests that crystalloid products should be administered sparingly during the initial resuscitation, as excessive crystalloid administration can produce coagulopathy, hypothermia, and worsening bleeding. If available, we should administer blood products such as packed red blood cells, fresh frozen plasma, and platelets at a ratio of 1:1:1. When considering the causes of upper GI hemorrhage in the general population, 70% of the patients have nonvariceal bleeding sources and 30% of the patients have variceal bleeding sources. **However, in cirrhotic patients, 90% of the time bleeding is related to variceal sources.** The initiation of pharmacologic therapy is helpful to reduce portal pressure and decrease variceal bleeding, and the choices of pharmacologic therapy include octreotide (bolus + infusion), somatostatin (infusion), terlipressin (not available in the United States given in boluses), or vasopressin (infusion). Prior to endoscopic verification of variceal bleeding sources, it is reasonable to begin high-dose proton-pump inhibitor (PPI) treatment (omeprazole 80 mg intravenous bolus followed by 8 mg/h drip for 72 hours) which would be helpful if the bleeding source was nonvariceal in origin. Because of the high rates of infectious complications encountered in patients with variceal hemorrhage, the most recent clinical guidelines recommend **broad-spectrum antibiotics prophylaxis in all patients with suspected variceal hemorrhage.** Based on these recommendations, we need to initiate a third-generation cephalosporin intravenously or oral quinolones.

If the patient is stabilized with our initial efforts, the next step would be to obtain an upper GI endoscopy to help identify and address the bleeding varix with variceal banding. The recommendation is to proceed with the initial endoscopy within 24 hours of hospital admission. If the patient continues to bleed and remains unstable prior to endoscopy becoming available, our options include placement of a Sengstaken–Blakemore tube or another type of balloon tamponade device to temporarily control the bleeding. The balloon devices are helpful for temporary control but can only remain in place for approximately 24 hours; patients have high rebleeding rates following tube removal. At most institutions, balloon tamponade is only used to temporize the bleeding before the implementation of definitive care such as transjugular intrahepatic portal-systemic shunt (TIPS), endoscopic therapy, or self-expanding intraesophageal stent placement (see Table 20–1).

Table 20–1 • CHILD-TURCOTTE-PUGH SCORE			
Variable	1 Point	2 Points	3 Points
Bilirubin level	<2 mg/dL	2-3 mg/dL	>3mg/dL
Albumin level	>3.5 g/dL	2.8-3.5 g/dL	<2.8 g/dL
INR	<1.7	1.7-2.2	2.2
Encephalopathy	None	Controlled	Uncontrolled
Ascites	None	Controlled	Uncontrolled

Class A: 5 to 6 points
Class B: 7to 9 points
Class C: 10 to 15 points

APPROACH TO:
Upper Gastrointestinal Bleeding: Variceal Bleeding

DEFINITION

PRIMARY PROPHYLAXIS OF VARICEAL HEMORRHAGE: This describes strategies for prevention of variceal hemorrhage in a cirrhotic patient with known gastroesophageal varices that have not previously bled. Pharmacologic prevention with noncardioselective beta-blocker (propranolol 40 mg bid initially and titrate the medication to reach a target heart rate of 50 to 55 beats/minute) has been shown to prevent variceal bleeding. Alternatively, prophylactic variceal banding has also been demonstrated to help prevent variceal bleeding.

CARVEDILOL: This is a noncardio-selective beta-blocker that is often used for primary prophylaxis for variceal hemorrhage. In addition to its beta-blockage activities, this agent is a vasodilator because of its alpha-1 receptor blocking properties. Hemodynamic studies suggest that this agent reduces portal pressure more effectively than propranolol.

SURVEILLANCE ENDSOCOPY: There is good evidence to support initial upper endoscopy for all patients at the time of their initial diagnoses of cirrhosis; for patients with no varices seen during the initial endoscopy, surveillance endoscopy is recommended every 2 to 3 years. Patients with grade-I varices identified are recommended to have annual surveillance endoscopy. If the endoscopy reveals grade-II or grade-III varices or varices with red signs, the recommendation is to initiate primary prophylactic therapy with either propranolol or endoscopic banding if the patient is unable to tolerate the medication.

RED WALE SIGN: This refers to an endoscopic finding consisting of linear, red streaks that are noted on an esophageal varix; this finding is suggestive of a recent or impending bleeding. The finding represents a thinned out portion of the varix wall.

TRANSJUGULAR INTRAHEPATIC PORTOSYSTEMIC SHUNT: This is an endovascular approach that creates a portosystemic shunt within the liver parenchyma. This approach is attractive because it does not require open surgery, and does not result in increased technical difficulties for patients who may undergo liver transplantation. The drawback of the procedure is that it can produce or worsen encephalopathy in some patients. Because the shunt is placed within the liver parenchyma, an additional limitation is restenosis and occlusion of the shunt can occur.

CLINICAL APPROACH

Acute GI bleeding is a common cause of hospital admissions, with bleeding in roughly 80% of the patients coming from the upper GI tract (proximal to the ligament of Treitz). When all upper GI bleeding cases are considered, variceal bleeding sources are the cause of bleeding in less than 30% of these patients. Cirrhosis is a common problem worldwide. During the course of disease, approximately 90% of patients with cirrhosis will develop esophageal varices, and variceal hemorrhage is associated with mortality rates of 7% to 15%. The known risk factors associated with variceal bleeding include variceal diameter (>5-mm), presence of a red wale sign, and impaired liver functions.

The presentation of variceal bleeding is often dramatic, with hematemesis as the most common presenting symptom. When suspected, the patient should have immediate stabilization of the airway and placed under close monitoring. Clinical and laboratory evaluations to determine the patient's liver reserve should be undertaken (see Table 20–2). Hemodynamically unstable patients should receive fluids, blood products, and vasoactive agents for blood pressure support. The transfusion target for patients with variceal hemorrhage should be with a restrictive strategy to target a hemoglobin level of 7 g/dL, because higher levels of hemoglobin have been demonstrated to increase portal pressures and worsen the rate of bleeding. Medical therapy has been demonstrated to help reduce bleeding, and the choices of pharmacologic therapies include somatostatin, octreotide, terlipressin, and vasopressin. Both **octreotide and somatostatin have better safety profiles** than terlipressin and vasopressin. High-dose PPI has not been demonstrated to provide any benefits to patients with variceal hemorrhage, and this should not be utilized except in cases where a nonvariceal bleeding source is suspected. (See Figure 20-1 for algorithm).

In 80% to 90% of the times, variceal bleeding episodes can be successfully controlled with endoscopic treatments. Endoscopic band ligation technique was first introduced in 1988, and it is currently the preferred endoscopic treatment for patients with bleeding varices. **Endoscopic band ligation is preferred treatment over endoscopic sclerotherapy** because bleeding in most cases can be controlled with a single banding session as opposed to multiple treatment sessions that are needed for the control of bleeding with sclerotherapy.

When available, TIPS is also very effective in controlling variceal bleeding even in patients with bleeding that is refractory to endoscopic treatments. The drawback

Table 20–2 • CLASSIFICATION OF LIVER LESIONS
Benign
Cyst
Hemangioma
Focal nodular hyperplasia
Adenoma
Biliary hamartoma
Abscess
Malignant
Hepatocellular carcinoma
Cholangiocarcinoma (bile duct cancer)
Gallbladder cancer
Metastatic colorectal cancer
Metastatic neuroendocrine cancer (carcinoid)
Other metastatic cancers

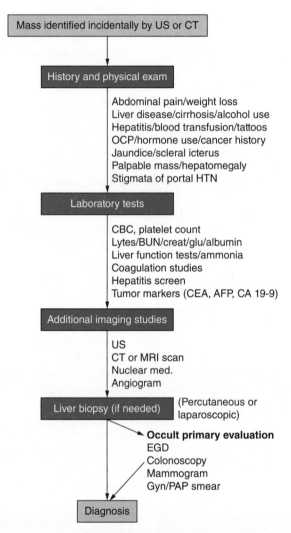

Figure 20–1. Algorithm for diagnostic work-up of an incidental liver lesion. The evaluation includes history and physical examination, blood work, imaging studies, and liver biopsy (if needed). AFP, α-fetoprotein; BUN, blood urea nitrogen; CA 19-9, cancer antigen 19-9; CBC, complete blood count; CEA, carcinoembryonic antigen; creat, creatinine; CT, computed tomography; EGD, esophagogas-troduodenoscopy; glu, glucose; Gyn, gynecologic; HTN, hypertension; MRI, magnetic resonance imaging; OCP, oral contraceptive pill; PAP, papanicolaou; US, ultrasound. *Source:* Reproduced, with permission, from Brunicardi FC, Andersen DK, Billiar TR, et al. *Schwartz's Principles of Surgery.* 10th ed. New York, NY: McGraw-Hill Education, 2010, 1112, Figure 31-17.

is that TIPS shunts blood away from the portal venous system. With the diversion of blood flow away from the portal system, new or worsening encephalopathy can occur in 30% to 45% of the patients following TIPS. Previously, bare-metal stents were deployed during TIPS procedures and placements were associated with a restenosis rates of up to 45%. However, more recent procedures are being performed with the placement of Polytetrafluroethylene (PTFE)-covered stents, which is reported with reduced dysfunction rate of roughly 15%.

Urgent or emergent surgery for patients with variceal bleeding is rarely performed presently, especially in centers with ready access to TIPS and therapeutic endoscopy. In some centers, after patients recover from an episode of variceal bleeding, an elective selective portal-systemic shunting procedure is performed as a secondary prevention strategy.

CASE CORRELATION

- See also Case 19 (Upper GI Bleeding [Nonvariceal]) and Case 23 (Lower GI Bleeding).

COMPREHENSION QUESTIONS

20.1 Which of the following describes an advantage of endoscopic banding over TIPS?

    A. Banding is associated with lower rates of postprocedural encephalopathy

    B. Banding is more effective in the treatment of hepatic vein thrombosis

    C. Banding procedures can be repeated as needed

    D. Banding procedures causes less perihepatic scarring in patients who have liver transplant

    E. Banding is associated with lower rate of infectious complications

20.2 A 43-year-old man with cirrhosis presents with variceal bleeding that is now controlled endoscopically. His bilirubin is 3.3 mg/dL, serum albumin is 2.9 g/dL, and INR is 1.9, and he has encephalopathy and ascites that are controlled with medical therapy. What are his Child-Turcotte-Pugh Score and class?

    A. Score of 11 and class B

    B. Score of 8 and class B

    C. Score of 11 and class C

    D. Score of 15 and class C

    E. Score of 7 and class B

20.3 Which of the following pharmacologic interventions has not been shown to benefit patients with acute variceal hemorrhage?

    A. High-dose proton pump inhibitor

    B. Somatostatin

    C. Octreotide

    D. Broad-spectrum antibiotic prophylaxis

    E. Terlipressin

20.4 For which of the following patients has primary prophylaxis with beta-blockers been demonstrated to prevent variceal hemorrhage?

A. Child B cirrhotic with 4-mm varices without red wale sign identified in the gastroesophageal junction

B. Child C cirrhotic with grade-3 varices without red wale sign identified in the GE junction

C. Child C cirrhotic with grade-1 varices and bleeding related to gastritis

D. Child C cirrhotic with grade-3 varices that was banded as a primary prophylactic procedure

E. Child C cirrhotic with several 3-mm gastroesophageal varices without red wale signs

20.5 Which of the following statements is true regarding TIPS?

A. The procedure performed with PTFE-covered stents is associated with lower rates of shunt dysfunction than those performed with bare-metal stents

B. The procedure is associated with new or worsening encephalopathy in 10% of the patients

C. The procedure can benefit patients with portal vein thrombosis

D. The procedure is contraindicated in patients who are candidates for liver transplantation

E. When successfully performed, the procedure is associated with improvement in encephalopathy

20.6 Which of the following statements regarding surveillance endoscopy in cirrhotic patients is true?

A. Surveillance endoscopy is recommended in all patients within the first 5 years after diagnosis of cirrhosis

B. If the initial surveillance endoscopy reveals no evidence of varices, the procedure needs to be performed annually thereafter

C. If grade-I varices are identified during the initial endoscopy, the procedure should be repeated in 6 months

D. If grade-II varices are identified, then the procedure should be repeated in 3 months

E. Patients with red wale sign identified during surveillance endoscopy should undergo pharmacologic prophylaxis with noncardio-selective beta-blocker

20.7 Which of the following statements is true regarding carvedilol?

    A. This agent is inferior to primary prophylaxis against variceal hemorrhage in comparison to propranolol

    B. This is a cardioselective beta-blocker

    C. The combination of its beta-blockade actions and alpha-1 blockade actions makes it more effective in reducing portal venous pressure than propranolol

    D. Carvedilol is contraindicated in patients with hepatitis-C-induced cirrhosis

    E. Carvedilol is contraindicated in patients after variceal banding

ANSWERS

20.1 **A.** The most important advantage of banding over TIPS is that banding does not produce or worsen hepatic encephalopathy, whereas TIPS is reported to cause new or worsening encephalopathy in 30% to 45% of the patients. Both TIPS and banding can be repeated as needed. Both procedures are designed to not cause excessive scarring around the liver that might create technical difficulties in patients who are liver transplantation candidates. Infectious complication risks do not appear to be influenced by banding or TIPS.

20.2 **C.** This patient has bilirubin 3.3, 3 points; albumin 2.9, 2 points; INR 1.9, 2 points; encephalopathy controlled, 2 points; and ascites controlled, 2 points. With a total of 11 points, it places this patient as a class C cirrhotic.

20.3 **A.** High-dose PPI has not been shown to benefit patients with acute variceal bleeding. All the other choices listed have been demonstrated to improve outcomes in a patient with acute variceal hemorrhage.

20.4 **B.** Primary prevention with beta-blocking agents has been shown to prevent variceal bleeding in patients with grade II or III varices or varices with red wale signs.

20.5 **A.** PTFE covered stents placed during TIPS are associated with lower rates of shunt dysfunction than procedures involving the placement of bare metal stents (15% vs 45% shunt dysfunction rates).

20.6 **E.** Patients with red wale signs seen during surveillance endoscopy are recommended to undergo primary prophylaxis with noncardioselective beta-blocker therapy or endoscopic banding. Initial surveillance endoscopy is recommended at the time of cirrhosis diagnosis. If no varices are seen during initial endoscopy, repeat endoscopy is recommended every 2 to 3 years. If grade-1 varices are seen, repeat endoscopy at 1 year is recommended. Patients with grade-II or -III varices identified during surveillance endoscopy are recommended to undergo primary prevention with beta-blocker therapy or endoscopic banding.

20.7 **C.** Carvedilol has been observed to be more effective than propranolol as a primary prevention against variceal bleeding. Carvedilol is a noncardioselective beta-blocker with alpha-1 blocking activities, and these properties are effective in reducing portal pressures.

CLINICAL PEARLS

▶ Upper GI endoscopy within 24 hours of admission is recommended for all patients presenting with suspected variceal upper GI hemorrhage.

▶ Varices will develop in approximately 90% of patients with cirrhosis.

▶ Variceal hemorrhage is the source in bleeding in approximately 30% of the patients presenting with upper GI bleeding; however, in a patient with a known history of cirrhosis, variceal hemorrhage accounts for acute upper GI bleeding approximately 90% of the time.

▶ The Child-Turcotte-Pugh score helps determine the prognosis of patients who present with acute variceal bleeding.

▶ TIPS can cause new or worsening encephalopathy in 30% to 45% of the patients.

▶ Infections are one of the major causes of morbidity and mortality associated with acute variceal hemorrhage; therefore, prophylactic broad-spectrum antibiotics administration has been shown to improve patient outcomes.

▶ Variceal diameter greater than 5 mm is associated with an increased risk of bleeding.

REFERENCES

Biecker E. Portal hypertension and gastrointestinal bleeding: diagnosis, prevention and management. *World J Gastroenterol.* 2013;19:5035-5050.

Kim BSM, Li BT, Engel A, et al. Diagnosis of gastrointestinal bleeding: a practical guide for clinicians. *World J Gastrointest Pathophys.* 2014;5:467-478.

Singra E, Perricone G, D'Amico M, Tine F, D'Amico G. Systematic review with meta-analysis: the hemodynamic effects of carvedilol compared with propranolol for portal hypertension in cirrhosis. *Aliment Pharmacol Ther.* 2014;39:557-568.

Tripathi D, Stanley AJ, Hayes PC, et al. UK guidelines on the management of variceal haemorrhage in cirrhotic patients. *Gut.* 2015;0:1-25.

A 53-year-old woman presented with atrial fibrillation and the sudden-onset of abdominal pain 8 days ago. She was taken to surgery for an exploratory laparotomy after the initial work-up suggested intestinal perforation. During the operation, she was discovered to have superior mesentery artery (SMA) embolism resulting in infarction of significant portions of the distal small bowel and right colon. She underwent SMA embolectomy and resection of the necrotic intestinal segment with a primary jejunum-transverse colon anastomosis. On postoperative day 7, enteral feeding using a polymeric formula was initiated through a nasogastric (NG) tube. With tube feeding, she began to produce a large amount of liquid stools. Her physical examination is unremarkable except for postoperative changes. Her stool sample was analyzed and found to be negative for fecal leukocytes and *Clostridium difficile*.

► What is the most likely diagnosis?
► How is this problem defined?
► What is the best therapy?

ANSWERS TO CASE 21:
Short Bowel Syndrome

Summary: A 53-year-old woman presented 8 days ago with atrial fibrillation and SMA embolism, right colon and small bowel infarction, required resection of the right colon and large portion of her small bowel. The patient develops severe diarrhea after the initiation of tube feedings. Her fecal leukocyte and C. *difficle* toxin titers are negative.

- **Diagnosis:** Malabsorption and diarrhea related to short bowel syndrome (SBS).

- **Definition:** SBS refers to the malabsorptive state caused by physical or functional loss of a significant portion of the small intestine. There is no set definition or length of bowel loss that is associated with the process.

- **Best therapy:** Bowel rest, parenteral nutrition, and pharmacologic therapy until bowel adaptation takes place.

Considerations

A 53-year-old woman with a history of an SMA embolism and small bowel necrosis underwent resection of significant portions of her small bowel. She develops diarrhea with the initiation of postoperative enteral tube feeding. The SMA provides blood supply to the small bowel a short distance distal to the ligament of Treitz to the right colon. An SMA embolus typically lodges in the distal artery and is associated with ischemia of the right colon, ileum, and the distal portion of the jejunum. For this patient with diarrhea, the absence of fecal leukocytes and C. *difficile* toxin makes infectious causes of diarrhea less likely. Her surgical history and the negative laboratory test results strongly suggest that her current problem is malabsorption related to SBS.

The most important therapeutic objective at this time is to maintain her nutritional status and fluid/electrolyte balances. The long-term prognosis of any patient with SBS is influenced by the length, location, and function of the residual (remnant) bowel, age of the patient, and the supportive care that the patient receives. This patient lost her distal small bowel and proximal colon. Theoretically, with appropriate nutritional and pharmacological support, she should have enough residual intestines to meet her long-term nutritional needs. A period of adaptation will be required before she fully recovers her bowel functions.

APPROACH TO:
Short Bowel Syndrome and Malnutrition

DEFINITIONS

ILEOCECAL VALVE: This is the anatomic sphincter between the small bowel and colon and regulates the flow of small bowel contents into the colon and the flow of colonic contents into the small bowel. The loss of the ileocecal valve seems to have some negative effects nutritionally on patients with SBS. Some people believe that loss of the terminal ileum where the ileocecal valve resides is the real cause of the nutritional dysfunction following loss of ileocecal valve.

ILEAL BRAKE: Nutrients entering the ileum elicit this physiologic feedback mechanism causing slowing of small bowel peristalsis and delays in gastric emptying, which allows for increased nutrient absorption. The ileal brake is one of the major reasons that preservation of the ileum helps maintain nutritional status following small bowel resection. The loss of the ileal brake can result in rapid gastric emptying, decreased intestinal transit time that is similar to dumping syndrome.

TOTAL PARENTERAL NUTRITION (TPN): Nutrition that is delivered directly into the central venous system. This route of delivery permits the delivery of hyperosmolar solutions. TPN can be administered to the patients in the hospital or at home. Adverse effects of TPN include catheter and vascular-related complications, toxicities, biliary effects including cholestasis, hepatic effects including steatosis and fibrosis, renal effects such as hyperoxaluria and kidney stones, and osteoporosis.

PERIPHERAL PARENTERAL NUTRITION (PPN): Nutrition delivered to the peripheral veins through normal intravenous catheters. This route does not allow the delivery of hyperosmolar solutions, therefore limiting the amount of calories and proteins that can be provided. Because this mode of nutritional support is neither sustainable nor effective in providing sufficient nutrition, there is extremely limited role for PPN in the acute or chronic setting.

"WORKLOAD HYPOTHESIS": This is the working hypothesis regarding intestinal adaptation following resection. The hypothesis states that delivery of complex nutrients to the intestinal lumen has beneficial trophic effects on the intestinal remnant. For instance, the administration of polysaccharides and disaccharides are preferable to monosaccharides.

FERMENTATION: This is the process where colonic bacteria convert unabsorbed carbohydrates to short-chain fatty acids to utilize as energy source. In individuals with extensive small bowel losses, colonic fermentation of carbohydrates to short-chain fatty acids (butyrate) also helps to produce substances promoting mucosal proliferation and nutrient transport in the remnant small bowel (small bowel adaptation).

CLINICAL APPROACH

Pathophysiology

SBS is a rare and complex clinical condition that results from the loss of normal intestinal absorptive capacity. Since the normal small bowel absorptive capacity far exceeds the normal nutritional needs, most individuals do not have any clinical manifestation of SBS until more than half of the normal small bowel absorptive surface/function is lost. Most cases of SBS are caused by surgical resections, traumatic injuries, or functional defects such as radiation enteritis and severe inflammatory bowel disease. Patients with SBS often suffer from diarrhea, dehydration,

Table 25–1 • INTESTINAL NUTRIENT ABSORPTION BY SITES	
Intestinal site	Nutrients/Micronutrients/Fluid absorption
Duodenum/Jejunum	Protein, carbohydrate, fat (requires bile acid production by liver), water-soluble vitamins, mineral (calcium, iron, folate)
Ileum	B_{12}, bile acids (enterohepatic circulation), magnesium
Colon	Water, magnesium, sodium, fermentation of carbohydrates to short-chain fatty acids

electrolytes abnormalities, malabsorption, and progressive weight loss, with many of these symptoms being aggravated by oral intake. Under normal physiologic conditions, the ileum and jejunum are the primary sites of absorption of fluids and most nutrients. Most nutrients taken by mouth are digested in the small bowel and absorbed through the mucosal lining.

The normal adult small bowel length is usually over 600 cm (~240 in or 20 ft). Most adults with <200 cm of (or less than one-third) of small bowel will experience symptoms of SBS. Most adults with <100 cm (39.4 in) of small bowel and no functional colon will need some long-term parenteral nutritional/fluid support. Similarly, an adult with <50 cm of small bowel connected to a functional colon may also become dependent on long-term parenteral nutritional support. Clearly, the colon is important for the absorption of fluids and some nutrients. (For the absorption of various nutrients by site, please refer to Table 25–1.)

In addition to the length of residual small bowel following resection, the location of the remaining small bowel that is retained also has important implications on long-term nutritional outcomes. For example, as the ileum is able to adapt both functionally and structurally and the jejunum can only adapt functionally after surgery; thus, **preservation of the ileum is associated with better nutritional outcomes in comparison to preservation of the jejunum.** Because the terminal ileum is the site of absorption of intrinsic factor-bound B_{12} and bile salts, extensive resection of the ileum can lead to disruption of the enterohepatic-bile salt circulation and produce fat malabsorption and steatorrhea.

Intestinal Adaptation

Functional recovery of the remnant intestines occurs after partial intestinal resections, but usually requires time (weeks, months, to years). The most significant adaptation process begins almost immediately and can continue up to 2 years; 95% of the patients with SBS who ultimately regain nutritional independence do so within this time frame. During adaptation, the remnant small bowel will dilate, the intestinal villi and crypt depth will increase to expand the small bowel absorptive surface area. Oral intake during intestinal adaptation plays an important role in stimulating a multitude of endogenous GI hormone releases to upregulate the adaptive process; some of the important stimulatory/regulatory hormones include glucagon-like peptide 2 (GLP-2), epidermal growth factor (EGF), growth hormone, gastrin, cholecystokinin (CCK), insulin, and neurotensin. In general, adaptation processes are more robust in younger individuals without significant comorbidities, and in individuals with remnant distal small bowel.

Parenteral nutrition plays an important role for many individuals during their intestinal function recovery process. Parenteral nutrition is often started early postoperatively to help patients meet their nutritional requirements while intestinal recovery and adaptation are taking place. As the patients' intestinal functions improve, parenteral nutrition can be weaned. Long-term parenteral nutrition has clear benefits but is also associated with many complications, including vascular complications, catheter-related complications, and hepatic and renal complications. The benefits of parenteral nutritional and alternatives to parenteral nutrition need to be clearly delineated to justify the initiation and/or continuation of parenteral nutritional support. In patients with intestinal failure, in whom the remnant small bowel does not provide sufficient absorptive surface to sustain the individual, indefinite parenteral nutritional support and small bowel transplantation are sometimes the only viable life-sustaining options.

MANAGEMENT OF PATIENTS WITH SHORT BOWEL SYNDROME AND INTESTINAL INSUFFICIENCY OR INTESTINAL FAILURE

Patients with SBS can be further categorized as having **intestinal insufficiency or intestinal failure**, the major difference being the level of parenteral nutritional support that individuals need. Intestinal failure is a term applied to individuals requiring prolonged parenteral nutritional support to meet their nutritional needs (Grades 1–5 differentiates the level of parenteral support needed), and intestinal insufficiency refers to individuals with sufficient absorptive surfaces but require some temporary parenteral or fluid support during the postoperative intestinal adaptation periods.

PHARMACOLOGIC TREATMENTS

Two peptide analogs targeting intestinal absorptive functions are currently approved for pharmacological support of SBS. The glucagon-like-peptide (GLP) analog Teduglutide was shown in preclinical trials to increase intestinal absorption while decreasing gastric motility and gastric emptying. In clinical trials, Teduglutide administration to SBS patients reduced their parenteral nutritional requirements and promoted more rapid enteral nutrition independence in the treated patients. The limitation of this treatment is cost, which is estimated at $295,000 per year in the United States. Human growth hormone analog (somatropin) is a non-GI tract specific growth stimulant, and its administration is associated with excess fluid retention and glucose intolerance. Because of these adverse effects, somatropin is only used for temporary nutritional support.

SURGICAL TREATMENTS

Surgery plays a role in the treatment of patients with SBS. For some patients, the reversal of small bowel stoma with reconnection of small bowel to the colon can help improve fluid and nutritional retention. For selected patients with SBS with dilated small bowel, intestinal lengthening procedures including longitudinal lengthening or serial transverse enteroplasty may help increase the absorptive surface of the existing small bowel. In rare cases of patients with SBS and nondilated small bowel, creation of a reverse segment can help slow down intestinal transit and help improve absorption. Small bowel transplantation is a salvage procedure reserved for patients with SBS-related intestinal failure who have either TPN-related liver insufficiency or a history of TPN-line related severe complications. In some patients with intestinal failure and hepatic failure due to TPN-related toxicities, liver and small bowel transplantation is indicated. In the United States, the national average survival following small bowel transplantation is 87% at 1 year and 71% at 3 years.

CASE CORRELATION

- See also Case 18 (Small Bowel Obstruction) and Case 22 (Obesity [Morbid]).

COMPREHENSION QUESTIONS

21.1 A 46-year-old woman with hypercoagulable state underwent resection of all of her jejunum and ileum from the Ligament of Treitz to the cecum and her right colon up to the mid-transverse colon after she developed intestinal infarction due to SMA thrombosis. Which of the following is the most appropriate therapy for her?

A. Oral diet

B. Feeding gastrostomy

C. Short-term TPN with progression to oral diet in 3 to 6 months

D. Oral elemental diet

E. Long-term TPN

21.2 A 50-year-old woman has undergone multiple small bowel resections for severe Crohn disease. She has weight loss, diarrhea, and electrolyte disturbances with regular oral diet. Which of the following therapies is most appropriate for her?

A. Complete bowel rest and long-term TPN

B. Small bowel transplantation

C. Continue limited modified diet, begin temporary TPN support with progression to complete weaning of TPN and transition back to oral diet

D. Perform a calorie count and observe

E. Place a colostomy

21.3 Which of the following statements is most accurate regarding the role of the colon in patients with short bowel syndrome?

A. The colon absorbs short-chain fatty acids

B. The colon absorbs water only

C. The colon remodels to assume the role of small bowel absorptive roles

D. The colon contributes to bacterial overgrowth and should be resected

E. The colon produces growth factors for small bowel regeneration

21.4 Which of the following is a beneficial effect of parenteral nutrition in the treatment of short bowel syndrome?

A. TPN provides nutritional support and fluid hydration when GI absorption is inadequate

B. TPN along with bowel rest promotes GI adaptation

C. TPN results in lower infectious complication

D. TPN improves liver functions

E. TPN should not be used while patient is able to eat

21.5 Which of the following patients with short bowel syndrome is the best candidate to regain nutritional independence?

A. A 58-year-old man with strangulated small bowel obstruction requiring removal of 320 cm of distal small bowel and cecum followed by primary anastomosis

B. A 34-year-old man with traumatic injuries resulting in the resection of 320 cm of jejunum followed by primary anastomosis

C. A 58-year-old man after having undergone a prior total colectomy 2 years ago presents with strangulated small bowel obstruction requiring resection of 320 cm of his distal small bowel. He is left with an end-jejunostomy

D. A 58-year-old woman with prior history of cervical cancer treated with radiation therapy and recurrent bowel obstructions requiring resection of 320 cm of her distal small bowel. Her jejunum containing radiation enteritis is anastomosed to her right colon

E. A 34-year-old man with Crohn disease and chronic small bowel obstruction with resection of 320 cm of his distal small bowel. He also had stricturoplasty at several sites in his jejunum that is narrowed by Crohn disease

ANSWERS

21.1 **E.** This patient has lost all of her jejunum, ileum, and her right colon. She has essentially no small bowel absorptive surface remaining; therefore, she would not be able to gain nutritional independence. Long-term TPN is the best treatment choice for her, with possible small bowel transplantation after appropriate evaluations.

21.2 **C.** This patient has diarrhea and fluid/electrolytes complications related to SBS. At this time, it is best to help manage some of the metabolic complications with supplemental parenteral nutrition/fluids. At the same time, we should explore why she developed diarrhea and try to modify her diet to see if we can develop a strategy for her to not have these complications related to her oral diet.

21.3 **A.** The colon absorbs water and electrolytes, and also converts carbohydrates to short-chain fatty acids and absorbs the fatty acids.

21.4 **A.** Parenteral nutrition provides the needed nutrients and fluids for patients whose GI absorptive functions are inadequate. Nutrients in the gut lumen help stimulate intestinal adaptation. Parenteral nutrition and bowel rest are detrimental to the intestinal adaptation process. TPN is associated with increasing infectious complications and can cause liver injury. Parenteral nutrition can be supplemented for patients with functional GI tracts but are unable to meet their nutritional goals with enteral nutritional support only.

21.5 **B.** SBS patients who are younger and without significant systemic diseases do better in terms of intestinal adaptation and recovery. In addition, extensive loss of ileum is associated with worse recovery potential than the loss of same length of jejunum. The length of the remnant small bowel is important for functional recovery; in addition, small bowel that is not diseased (eg, Crohn disease or radiation enteritis) tends to have better functional recovery.

CLINICAL PEARLS

▶ Adults with less than 200 cm (one third of normal) of small bowel are at risk of developing diarrhea and malabsorption.

▶ The most common causes of short bowel syndrome in adults are Crohn' disease and mesenteric infarction.

▶ The goal of treating patients with SBS is to increase absorptive functions and this can be accomplished by increasing the amount of time that the intraluminal contents stay within the small bowel before passing through.

▶ Selective patients with short bowel syndrome and intestinal failure are candidates for small bowel transplantation.

▶ Teduglutide is a human glucagon-like-petide 2 (GLP-2) analog that is FDA approved for patients with SBS. It improves absorptive function of the remnant small bowel and promotes mucosal growth in the remnant small bowel.

▶ Surgical lengthening operations can improve the absorptive surface area in selective patients with SBS.

REFERENCES

Abu-Elmagd K. The concept of gut rehabilitation and the future of visceral transplantation. *Nat Rev Gastroenterol Hepatol.* 2015;12:108-120.

Jeppesen PB. Spectrum of short bowel syndrome in adults: intestinal insufficiency to intestinal failure. *J Parenteral Enterl Nutri.* 2014;38(suppl 1):8S-13S.

Kim HB, Jasic T. The management of short bowel syndrome. In: Cameron JL, Cameron AM, eds. *Current Surgical Therapy.* 11th ed. Philadelphia, PA: Elsevier Saunders; 2014:137-142.

A 38-year-old woman is referred to a bariatric clinic for surgical evaluation and management of morbid obesity. She tells you that she has been extremely over-weight ever since childhood. She has tried numerous dietary modifications, exer-cise regimens, and medications, but has not been able to achieve sustained weight loss. She is concerned about her health status because of obstructive sleep apnea, a recent diagnosis of type 2 diabetes mellitus, and a history of coronary artery dis-ease in several immediate family members. Her current medications are an oral hypoglycemic agent and insulin. On examination, she is found to be 5 ft 3 in and weighs 280 lb. Her body mass index (BMI) is 47 kg/m^2. Her pulse is 95 beats/minute and her blood pressure is 168/96 mm Hg. The findings from her cardiopulmonary examination and abdominal examination are unremarkable. The patient states interest in additional therapy and would like your opinion regarding operative interventions for management of her obesity.

▶ Is surgical therapy a reasonable treatment option in this patient?
▶ What are the complications associated with morbid obesity?

ANSWERS TO CASE 22:
Obesity (Morbid)

Summary: A 38-year-old morbidly obese woman (BMI 47 kg/m^2) with obesity-associated complications (diabetes and obstructive sleep apnea) is inquiring about the surgical treatment of obesity.

- **Surgical therapy:** Surgical therapy is a reasonable option in this patient.

- **Complications associated with morbid obesity:** Diabetes mellitus, hypertension, hyperlipidemia, atherosclerosis, cardiomyopathy, sleep apnea syndrome, gallstones, arthritis, and infertility are disease processes associated with morbid obesity.

ANALYSIS

Objectives

1. Become familiar with the complications associated with morbid obesity and the effectiveness of bariatric operations on metabolic syndrome.

2. Become familiar with the short-term and long-term outcomes in weight reduction achieved with operative treatment.

Considerations

This patient falls within the National Institutes of Health (NIH) class III (Table 22–1) category of clinically severe obesity. On the basis of weight-to-height ratio alone, she is a candidate for surgical therapy. Her comorbidities, diabetes, and obstructive sleep apnea add further evidence of the advanced nature of her disease. She is at high perioperative risk for complications including respiratory compromise, infection, and venous thrombosis. Her blood

Table 22–1 • NIH CLASSIFICATION OF OBESITY (REVISED)			
Description	BMI (kg/m^2)	Obesity class	Disease risk
Normal	18.5-24.9		
Overweight	25.0-29.9		Increased

Obesity
  Mild
  Moderate
  Severe
	
	30.0-34.9
	35.0-39.9
	>40
		
		I
		II
		III
			
			High
			Very high
			Extremely high

Superobese	>50		Extremely high

Data from NIH Conference on Gastrointestinal Surgery for Severe Obesity: Consensus Development Conference Panel. *Ann Intern Med.* 1991;115:956-961.

glucose level should be carefully monitored during the postoperative period, and she should be treated prophylactically during surgery with heparin and sequential compression stockings.

APPROACH TO:
Surgical Treatment of Morbid Obesity

DEFINITIONS

BODY MASS INDEX: The ratio of weight to height, which is used to estimate appropriate patient size. It is calculated by dividing the weight (in kg) by the height (in m^2).

CLINICALLY SEVERE OBESITY: BMI greater than 40 kg/m^2.

OBESITY-RELATED COMORBIDITIES: Various diseases are considered to be caused due to obesity: hypertension, diabetes, coronary and hypertrophic heart disease, gallstones, gastroesophageal reflux disease (GERD), sleep apnea, asthma, reactive pulmonary disease, osteoarthritis, lumbosacral disk disease, urinary incontinence, infertility, polycystic ovarian syndrome, and cancer. This list attests to the serious nature of this problem.

GASTRIC RESTRICTIVE PROCEDURES: These are operations which involve reduction in the size of the gastric conduit to limit weight gain.

MALABSORPTIVE PROCEDURES: Surgeries that decrease the contact of food with the digestive juices and the absorptive surface of the small intestine to limit weight gain.

METABOLIC SYNDROME: A disorder of energy utilization and storage which includes a constellation of comorbidities including hypertension, diabetes mellitus, and hyperlipidemia. Metabolic syndrome is associated with morbid obesity, and puts the patient at risk for cardiovascular disease and health-related complications.

CLINICAL APPROACH

Obesity has reached epidemic proportions and qualifies as one of the leading medical problems among Americans. The adverse health effects associated with obesity may reduce the affected patient's quality of life and longevity. The treatment goals of any patient with morbid obesity should be focused on weight loss as well as on the reduction in comorbidities (Tables 22–2 to 22–4). Numerous studies have shown that the surgical treatment of morbid obesity provides better long-term weight loss results and clinically significant improvement of obesity-related complications over diet and exercise alone. It is important for the patient and physician to have realistic expectations about surgical treatment outcome. Most successfully treated patients achieve a reduction in weight that is sustainable. Because patients rarely achieve the ideal body weight, results of regimens are quantified

Table 22–2 • OPERATIONS USED TO TREAT CLINICALLY SEVERE OBESITY	
Operation	Description
Adjustable lap band	Silastic band around upper stomach with circumferential balloon accessible by subcutaneous port
Sleeve gastrectomy	Reduction of stomach conduit size by resection of the greater curvature
Roux-en-Y gastric bypass	Small proximal gastric pouch to Roux limb of jejunum
Duodenal switch	Stomach reduction with division of duodenum at the pylorus. The distal small bowel is attached to the gastric tube, and the proximal small bowel is attached to the lower ileum

by percentage of excess body weight loss. Most of the patients additionally experience an improvement in obesity-related complications following a successful surgery. The American Society for Metabolic and Bariatric Surgery recommends adjustable gastric band (Figure 22–1), sleeve gastrectomy (Figure 22–2), roux-en-Y gastric bypass (Figure 22–3), and duodenal switch (Figure 22–4) procedures in selected patients. Durable weight loss has been shown with each of these bariatric procedures, but the success and the patient satisfaction associated with surgical therapy are further augmented when patients receive proper preoperative counseling and undergo modifications in their dietary habits and lifestyle.

PATIENT SELECTION

All surgical candidates must have failed supervised weight-loss programs by diet, exercise, or medications, and fulfill minimum weight criteria that include BMI of 35 to 40 kg/m^2 with comorbidity or BMI of greater than 40 kg/m^2 without comorbidity. In addition, all patients must pass a psychological evaluation and be willing to comply with postoperative lifestyle changes and dietary restrictions, exercise, and follow-up programs. Because the majority of current procedures are performed laparoscopically with vastly decreased complication rates, indications for surgery have expanded to more extremes of age and health, including appropriately selected adolescents.

Table 22–3 • TREATMENT RESULTS AND COMPLICATIONS		
Method	Results	Complications
Gastric banding	Loss of 33%-64% of excess weight at 3-5 y	Up to 23% rate of band slippage, resulting in reoperation
Sleeve gastrectomy	Loss of 35%-75% of excess weight	GERD. Insufficient long-term data supporting durable weight loss
Roux-en-Y gastric bypass	Sustained results are good; loss of 50%-60% of excess weight	B$_{12}$ deficiency in 15%-20%; iron deficiency anemia in 20%; marginal ulcer 2%-10%; osteoporosis
Duodenal switch	Excellent long-term results; loss of 60%-80% of excess weight	Highest rates of nutritional deficiencies with malabsorption in up to 39%

Table 22–4 • EFFECTS OF SURGERY ON OBESITY COMORBIDITY	
Diabetes mellitus	82% of patients cured of type 2 diabetes at 15-y follow-up
Sleep apnea	Up to 93% of patients have improvement
Hypertension	Success correlated with the amount of weight loss
Serum lipid abnormalities	Successful gastric bypass is associated with a sustained reduction in triglycerides and low-density lipoproteins and an increase in high-density lipoproteins

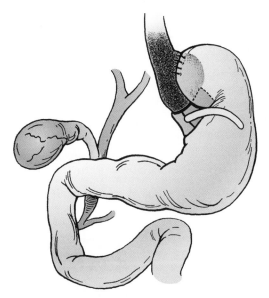

Figure 22–1. Adjustable gastric band. (Reproduced, with permission, from Brunicardi FC, Andersen DK, Dunn DL, et al., eds. *Schwartz's Principles of Surgery*. 8th ed. New York, NY: McGraw-Hill; 2005:1004.)

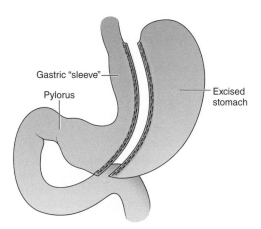

Figure 22–2. Sleeve gastrectomy. (Reproduced, with permission, from Brunicardi FC, Andersen DK, Dunn DL, et al., eds. *Schwartz's Principles of Surgery*, 8th ed. New York: McGraw-Hill, 2005:1007.)

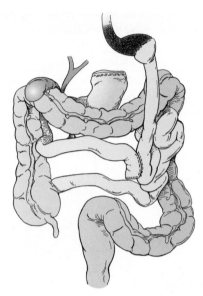

Figure 22–3. Roux-en-Y gastric bypass. (Reproduced, with permission, from Brunicardi FC, Andersen DK, Dunn DL, et al., eds. *Schwartz's Principles of Surgery*. 8th ed. New York, NY: McGraw-Hill; 2005:1007.)

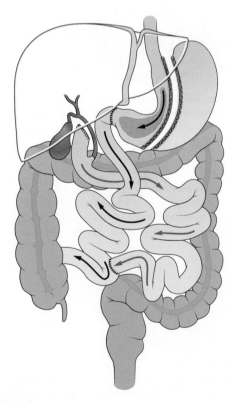

Figure 22–4. Duodenal Switch.

> **CASE CORRELATION**
>
> • See also Case 21 (Short Bowel Syndrome).

COMPREHENSION QUESTIONS

22.1 A 23-year-old woman is referred for an opinion regarding the advisability of surgical treatment for obesity. The patient is 5 ft tall and weighs 210 lb. She has no known comorbidities and is free of symptoms. Which of the following would be your best advice?

A. A small-pouch gastric bypass

B. A Vertical banded gastroplasty (VBG) procedure

C. A Lap-Band procedure

D. Further efforts at medical therapy

E. Pharmacologic therapy

22.2 A 45-year-old woman, the mother of two adolescents, presents with long-standing, clinically severe obesity (BMI 50 kg/m²) that is refractory to medical therapy. Which of the following surgical procedures is most likely to provide the best chance of long-term weight reduction with the least morbidity?

A. VBG

B. Small-pouch gastric bypass

C. Adjustable Lap-Band

D. Duodenal switch

E. Jejunal–ileal bypass

22.3 Which of the following explains the mechanism whereby gastric restrictive procedures lead to weight loss?

A. Increasing the basal metabolic rate

B. Enhancing maldigestion and absorption

C. Producing early satiety

D. Inducing nausea and vomiting

E. Altering glucose metabolism

22.4 Which of the following is the most common, most serious postoperative complication associated with small-pouch gastric bypass?

A. Pneumonia

B. Leakage of intestinal contents from the gastrojejunal anastomosis

C. Intestinal obstruction

D. Pulmonary embolus

E. Insufficient weight loss

22.5 Which of the following is the most likely late sequelae from gastric restrictive procedures?

A. Anemia

B. Osteoporosis

C. Vitamin deficiencies

D. Marginal ulcer

E. All of the above

22.6 Which of the following bariatric procedures offers durable weight loss and improvement of diabetes control while leaving an option for a more aggressive future surgical modification?

A. Vertical band gastroplasty

B. Adjustable gastric band

C. Sleeve Gastrectomy

D. Roux-en-Y gastric bypass

E. Duodenal switch

ANSWERS

22.1 **D.** The patient is young, free of comorbid medical problems, and has a BMI less than 40. Her BMI is calculated as $210 \times 704 / 64 \times 64 = 36.1 \, kg/m^2$. Further attempts at medical management should be made; however, if significant complications such as hypertension and diabetes are already present, a surgical approach might be appropriate.

22.2 **B.** This patient has strong indications for a surgical approach (BMI > 50, superobese). A small-pouch gastric bypass performed by either an open or a laparoscopic technique will provide the best long-term weight reduction with minimal early and late long-term morbidity.

22.3 **C.** Gastric restrictive operations help people lose weight by producing early satiety and decreasing their appetite. To be successful, the patient must simultaneously restrict caloric intake.

22.4 **B.** Leakage from the attachment of the stomach to the intestine can be a devastating complication. It is usually characterized by fever, leukocytosis, and left shoulder pain on postoperative days 3 to 5.

22.5 **E.** A small-pouch gastric bypass can be accompanied by anemia, osteoporosis, and vitamin deficiencies in view of the marked decrease in food intake. Patients need supplemental vitamins, calcium, and oral iron and vitamin B_{12} following the procedure. In addition, marginal ulcer is a complication that can occur following RYGB procedure, where patients present with epigastric pain that is not affected by eating; the treatment for this complication is proton pump inhibitor administration.

22.6 **C.** The sleeve gastrectomy can be performed as the first stage of the two-stage duodenal switch procedure. It was developed as an first surgery in patients who initially may not tolerate the duodenal switch.

CLINICAL PEARLS

▶ The BMI represented in kilograms per meter squared body surface area is a common tool in assessing obesity.

▶ Many diseases are considered to be obesity-related comorbidities such as hypertension, diabetes, coronary heart disease, gallstones, and sleep apnea.

▶ In general, surgical weight-reduction surgeries should be reserved for severe obesity or those obese individuals with comorbidities.

REFERENCES

Clinical guidelines on the identification, evaluation, and treatment of overweight and obesity in adults. National Institute of Health (NIH), Lung, and Blood Institute; 2012.

Richards WO, Schirmer BD. Morbid obesity. In: Townsend CM Jr, Beauchamp RD, Evers BM, eds. *Sabiston Textbook of Surgery*. 18th ed. Philadelphia, PA: Elsevier Saunders; 2008:399-430.

Schirmer BD, Schauer PR. The surgical management of obesity. In: Brunicardi FC, Andersen DK, Dunn DL, et al., eds. *Schwartz's Principles of Surgery*. 9th ed. New York, NY: McGraw-Hill; 2010:949-978.

Scortino C, Schweitzer MA, Magnuson T. Morbid obesity. In: Cameron JL, Cameron AM, eds. *Current Surgical Therapy*. 10th ed. Philadelphia, PA: Elsevier Saunders; 2011:88-92.

A 73-year-old man presents to the emergency center after having had eight bloody bowel movements during the previous day. The patient described that his symptoms began with the urge to defecate, followed shortly by several voluminous bowel movements containing maroon-colored stool mixed with blood clots. Following these events, the patient felt light-headed and only felt better after lying down in his bed. His past medical history is significant for hypertension and type II diabetes mellitus. His surgical history is significant for having had a right knee replacement for severe degenerative joint disease 2 years ago. He denies any prior history of GI bleeding episodes. His current medications include a diuretic for hypertension and an oral medication for glycemic control. His blood pressure is 100/80 mm Hg, pulse is 114 beats/minute, and respiratory rate is 22 breaths/minute. His abdomen is nontender and nondistended. The rectal examination revealed no rectal masses and a large amount of maroon-colored stool in the rectal vault.

▶ What is your next step?
▶ What are some important goals in the management of this patient?
▶ What are the major causes associated with this process?

ANSWERS TO CASE 23:
Lower Gastrointestinal Hemorrhage

Summary: A 73-year-old man presents with apparent acute lower GI bleeding. The patient's history suggests that the bleeding has been significant. His symptoms are compatible with orthostatic hypotension.

- **Next step:** Resuscitation with crystalloids and blood products as needed.

- **Goals in management:** Treat hemorrhage as needed. Localize the bleeding site and stop the bleeding if the bleeding persists.

- **Major causes associated with lower GI hemorrhage:** Most common sources of lower GI bleeding are diverticulosis, arteriovenous malformations, and neoplasms in this age group. Meckel's diverticulum, polyps, neoplasms, and inflammatory bowel disease are the common bleeding sources in younger adults.

ANALYSIS

Objectives

1. Learn to recognize bleeding from the lower GI tract and be able to develop diagnostic and treatment strategies for these patients.

2. Learn the limitations and advantages of the various diagnostic modalities for GI bleeding evaluations.

Considerations

This patient presented with passage of maroon-colored stools and blood clots per rectum. The maroon-colored stools means that there had been sufficient mixing of blood and fecal material prior to evacuation, which suggests that the bleeding source is likely a lower GI source (distal to the ligament of Treitz) but proximal to the anorectal segment (which generally will present as blood coating of normal-appearing, formed stools and/or blood dripping into the toilet during a normal appearing bowel movement). It is important to recognize that brisk bleeding from the upper GI tract can sometimes present as hematochezia; therefore, efforts should be made to rule out an upper GI bleeding source at the onset.

Patient monitoring and resuscitation are important prior to localization of the bleeding source. Monitoring of vital signs, CBC, and monitoring of the volume of blood or bloody stools per rectum are important to gauge the severity of bleeding. Careful placement of an NG tube is valuable to rule out an upper GI bleeding source. If the NG aspirate is bilious, nonbloody, and does not contain "coffee-ground" material, upper GI bleeding can generally be ruled out; however, if there is any uncertainty regarding a potential upper GI bleeding source, an EGD should be performed to fully evaluate sites of potential upper GI bleeding.

During the history and physical examination, it is important to inquire about symptoms such as abdominal pain and weight loss which suggest the possibility of colonic neoplasms. Medication usage, including NSAIDS, anti-platelet agents, and anticoagulants, may contribute to GI bleeding. For a GI bleeding patient, it is not only important to know if the patient is on these medications but also to know the indications for the medications, because we need to understand the risks and benefits of continuing or stopping these medications. As part of the H&P, we need to determine whether the patient has had prior surgery for GI malignancies, history of prior abdominal aortic surgeries, and recent history of colonoscopies with polypectomies, as these circumstances can be associated with unique bleeding scenarios. A history of trauma to the liver can also be a rare source of GI bleeding. In these cases, the bleeding from the liver can communicate with the biliary system producing hemobilia and upper GI bleeding.

The most common lower GI bleeding causes in a 73-year-old man are diverticulosis, arteriovenous malformation, and neoplasms. In contrast to upper GI bleeding, lower GI bleeding episodes are generally slower in rate and do not usually cause hypotension unless it is not recognized or neglected. Once the patient's condition is stabilized, we should obtain a CT scan with intravenous contrast to try to localize the bleeding site. If this does not demonstrate the bleeding site, a colonoscopy should be performed.

APPROACH TO:
Lower Gastrointestinal Hemorrhage

DEFINITIONS

OCCULT GI BLEEDING: Slow bleeding originating from anywhere along the GI tract. This presentation is most commonly associated with bleeding from GI neoplasms, gastritis, and esophagitis. Patients are not generally aware of the bleeding because there are often no striking changes in their bowel habits or appearances of the stools. Most patients will present with iron-deficiency anemia, fatigue, and hemoccult-positive stools.

OVERT LOWER GI BLEEDING: Presentation is often hematochezia, melena, or bright red blood per rectum. The common causes by age groups are listed in Table 23–1.

CT SCAN WITH INTRAVENOUS CONTRAST: CT scan performed with intravenous contrast is being more commonly applied in many centers as an

Table 23–1 • COMMON CONDITIONS CAUSING HEMATOCHEZIA	
Age group	Lower GI bleeding sources
Children, adolescents, and young adults	Meckel's diverticulum Inflammatory bowel disease Juvenile polyps
Adults up to 60 years old	Diverticulosis Inflammatory bowel disease Neoplasms
Adults over 60 years old	Arteriovenous malformations Diverticulosis Neoplasms

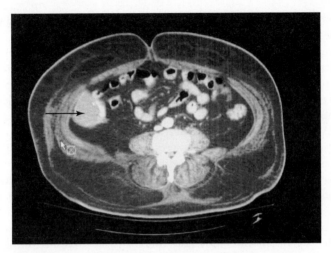

Figure 23–1. CT angiography in patient with cecal bleeding. (The dark arrow points to intravenous contrast extravasation at the medial aspect of the cecum due to active bleeding from an arteriovenous malformation)

initial screening modality for patients with lower GI bleeding. The CT is generally done without contrast first to identify any hyper-attenuating materials in the GI tract that may cause false positive studies, and then following intravenous contrast administration, CT is again performed to look for intra-luminal pooling of contrast material that signifies active bleeding sites. This modality can detect bleeding that exceeds **0.3–0.5 mL/min** (Figure 23–1).

TAGGED RBC SCAN: This is a nuclear medicine imaging study using technetium 99-m-labeled RBC. This modality is highly sensitive in identifying active bleeding as slow as **0.1 mL/min**; however, the images obtained may not help localize the exact anatomic site of bleeding. Some centers use this modality to screen for patients who might benefit from mesenteric angiography to further characterize the bleeding site.

MESENTERIC ANGIOGRAPHY: Selective angiography of the superior and inferior mesenteric arteries can be done to localize active bleeding from the midgut and hindgut. This modality is invasive but highly specific in localizing the site of bleeding. In addition, angiographic embolization or selective vasopressin injections can be performed to stop the bleeding. To be visualized by this modality, the bleeding has to be active and exceeding a rate of **0.5–1.0 mL/min**.

COLONOSCOPY: Flexible endoscopy that is performed in hemodynamically stable patients with lower GI bleeding. The sensitivity of colonoscopy has been reported to be as high as 70% to 90%. An added advantage of colonoscopy is that therapeutic interventions can be applied when bleeding sources are visualized. The disadvantages of this diagnostic modality include requirement for sedation and requirement for pre-procedural mechanical cleansing of the colon to help improve visibility. Another disadvantage is the need for sedation during the procedure, which may be poorly tolerated by older patients and hypovolemic patients.

VIDEO CAPSULE ENDOSCOPY: A small capsular video camera can be swallowed to help visualize the mucosal surface of the entire GI tract. This study is most useful for the evaluation of obscured bleeding in patients who have no obvious bleeding sources in the upper GI tract and colorectal regions. The process is time-consuming and does not work well when there is significant overt bleeding.

RIGID PROCTOSIGMOIDOSCOPY: A simple bedside procedure that can often be done with or without sedation medications. This procedure is useful to identify anorectal bleeding source and pathology within the most distal 20 to 25 cm of the GI tract.

ANGIODYSPLASIA: This term has often been used interchangeably with arteriovenous malformation (AVM). This is a common and acquired degenerative vascular condition leading to the formation of small, dilated, thin-walled veins in the submucosa of the GI tract. It occurs most commonly in the cecum and ascending colon of individuals older than 60 years old. **Approximately 50% of the patients with angiodysplasia have associated cardiac diseases, and up to 25% of the patients have aortic stenosis.** Most patients with angiodysplasia have low-grade, chronic, self-limiting bleeding, and ~15% of the patients can present with acute bleeding.

CLINICAL APPROACH

A patient presenting with overt lower GI bleeding needs immediate assessment of hemodynamic stability and intravascular volume status. Patients with lower GI bleeding are often individuals greater than 60 years of age and have cardiovascular comorbidities; consequently, lower GI bleeding patients frequently require close monitoring and meticulous fluid and blood products management, even without overt signs of instability. It is important to determine if the patient has medical causes of bleeding (such as coagulopathy, thrombocytopenia, and platelet dysfunction). A patient who presents with GI bleeding and a previous abdominal aortic vascular reconstruction would require rapid assessment to rule out the possibility of an aorto-duodenal fistula, which can be assessed with either a CT scan of the abdomen or upper GI endoscopy that includes direct visualization of the 3rd and 4th portions of the duodenum.

Key points in the history should include detailed descriptions of the patient's stools. Melena (tarry stool) indicates degradation of hemoglobin by bacteria and this appearance is associated with intra-luminal contents remaining in the GI tract for more than 14 hours; therefore, melena is generally encountered in patients with upper GI bleeding that is not brisk. The passage of maroon-colored stools usually excludes anorectal bleeding sources. Bleeding from an anorectal bleeding source is associated with the passage of formed stools streaked with blood or passage of normal stools followed by blood dripping into the toilet.

Most episodes of lower GI bleeding resolve spontaneously without specific treatment. It is important in patients with a history of GI bleeding to rule out GI neoplasm as the sources of bleeding even after the bleeding has stopped. Surgeons are often asked to help manage patients with lower GI bleeding, and it is important that we understand that the natural history of this problem is often self-limiting. **As surgeons, the primary goal in management of these patients is to localize** the anatomic site of bleeding, so that surgical resection can be applied for individuals when the bleeding does not stop. Over-aggressive surgical approaches for patients prior to the precise localization of bleedings sites seldom benefit the patients and can turn into unnecessary operations that do not address the bleeding problems. Figure 23–2 provides a simplified algorithm for the management of patients with overt lower GI bleeding.

Over the past decade, angiographic techniques have improved with the development of smaller catheters that allows for greater precision in accessing smaller vessels and for the deployment of gelfoam particles and microcoils. These improvements have resulted in improvement in the success of stopping the bleeding (approximately 90% success) and lowered risk (approximately 3%-5%) of colonic ischemia related to angiographic embolizations.

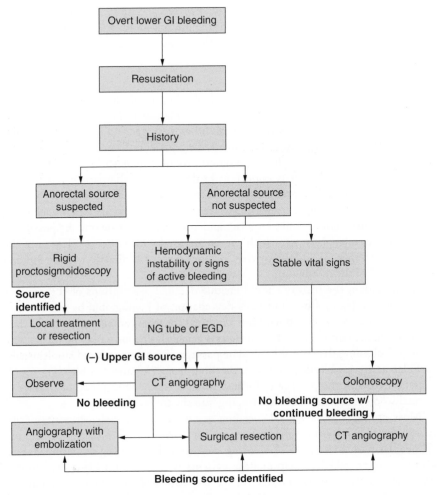

Figure 23–2. Algorithm for the management of hematochezia.

The majority of patients with lower GI bleeding do not need surgery. Only 10% to 20% of the lower GI bleeding patients need surgical interventions. The rate of bleeding correlates with the need for surgery, as 50% of patients who with transfusion requirements of four or more units of PRBCs during the first 24 hours of presentation require surgical interventions. In the past, some surgeons have performed total abdominal colectomy for patients with lower GI bleeding and unclear bleeding sites. Following these procedures, the rate of re-bleeding has been reported to be less than 4%. Unfortunately, some groups have reported postoperative mortality rates of up to 27% for patients undergoing emergency total abdominal colectomy for lower GI bleeding. These observations suggest that it is preferable to identify the site of bleeding so that a limited resection could be performed to help minimize the complications associated with the operation.

CASE CORRELATION

- See also Case 19 (Upper GI Tract Bleeding [Nonvariceal]) and Case 20 (Upper GI Tract Bleeding [Variceal]).

COMPREHENSION QUESTIONS

23.1 A 78-year-old man develops hematochezia and presents with a blood pressure of 92/60 mm Hg and a heart rate of 120 beats/minute. His vital signs improve transiently with crystalloid and packed RBC infusion. Which of the following choices is the most appropriate for this patient's management?

A. Proctosigmoidoscopy followed by total abdominal colectomy

B. EGD and colonoscopy

C. NG tube, mesenteric angiography

D. NG tube, CT angiography, and angiographic embolization

E. EGC and capsular endoscopy

23.2 Which of the following conditions is most likely to be associated with painless hematochezia?

A. Ulcerative colitis

B. Aorto-enteric fistula 3 years following abdominal aortic aneurysm repair

C. Superior mesenteric artery embolus

D. Bleeding duodenal ulcer

E. Ischemic colitis

23.3 Which of the following approaches has the best specificity in identifying the site of lower GI tract bleeding?

A. Mesenteric angiography

B. Tagged RBC scan

C. Surgical exploration

D. Barium enema

E. CT scan with oral and intravenous contrast

23.4 A 62-year-old man with history of hypertension presents with hematochezia. He is admitted to the hospital for observation. During the first 24 hours in the hospital, he has two more small maroon-colored stools and remains hemodynamically stable without requiring blood transfusions. The EGD reveals no abnormality, and a colonoscopy reveals scattered diverticulosis throughout the colon but no identifiable source of bleeding. Which of the following is the best treatment strategy at this time?

A. Mesenteric angiography

B. Total abdominal colectomy

C. Barium enema

D. Repeat colonoscopy

E. Observation

23.5 A 63-year-old man presents with two bouts of hematochezia. He characterized his bleeding as bloody, maroon-colored stools. His past medical history is significant for hypertension and abdominal aortic aneurysm that was repaired with placement of a tube graft 2 years ago. He remains stable without additional bleeding during his initial 8 hours of in-hospital observation. Which of the following is the best course of action in the management of this patient?

A. Continue in-hospital observation

B. Colonoscopy

C. Mesenteric angiography

D. Upper GI endoscopy

E. Tagged RBC scan

23.6 A 73-year-old woman presents to the emergency center with abdominal pain and passage of bloody stools. Her past medical history is significant for hypertension and noninsulin-dependent diabetes mellitus. Her blood pressure is 94/64 mm Hg, pulse rate is 114 beats/minute, and her temperature is 38.8°C. Palpation of the abdomen reveals diffuse tenderness on the left side of the abdomen. There is no evidence of peritonitis. Which of the following is the most appropriate next step?

A. EGD

B. CT of the abdomen without contrast

C. Colonoscopy

D. Tagged RBC scan

E. Exploratory laparotomy

23.7 A 58-year-old woman with history of hypertension and osteoarthritis presents to the emergency center with a history of having several tarry stools. She complains of feeling light-headed following these events. Her home medications include metoprolol for hypertension and ketorolac for arthritic knee pain. Her physical examination reveals heart rate of 90 beats/minute and blood pressure of 100/86. NG tube placement was attempted in the emergency center and resulted in a nosebleed with unsuccessful placement. High-dose proton-pump inhibitor drip was started in the emergency center by the emergency medicine physician. Which of the following is the most appropriate treatment course at this time?

A. Colonoscopy and capsular endoscopy

B. Attempt placement of NG tube

C. EGD followed by colonoscopy

D. CT with intravenous and oral contrast

E. Mesenteric angiography

ANSWERS

23.1 **D.** This 78-year-old man presents with GI bleeding and initial hemodynamic instability that responds only transiently to resuscitation. At this point, we are uncertain whether his bleeding is from the upper or lower GI tract. Placement of an NG tube can help us identify clearly whether the bleeding is upper GI tract in origin. CT angiography is helpful at this time because it could help us identify a site of active contrast extravasation either in the upper or lower GI tract, and once a site of contrast extravasation is seen, angiographic catheter-directed treatment can be carried out to stop the bleeding. Proctosigmoidoscopy and total abdominal colectomy is not a good choice for this patient because we are not certain that this bleeding is not an upper GI source, and emergency "blind" total abdominal colectomy is a strategy that is associated with potentially significant morbidity and mortality. EGD and colonoscopy are good diagnostic strategies for a stable patient with GI bleeding, but for this patient who is actively bleeding and unstable, endoscopy with sedation may not be well-tolerated by the patient. NG tube and mesenteric angiography is a reasonable strategy; however, given the intermittent pattern of most GI bleeding patients, angiography without knowing an anatomic site of contrast extravasation and active bleeding, the angiography often will need to perform 3-vessel angiography (celiac, superior mesenteric, and inferior mesenteric arteries) that is more time consuming and involving significantly greater amount of intravenous contrast injection. Capsular endoscopy is a time-consuming process and is not appropriate in a patient with active overt bleeding and unstable.

23.2 **B.** Aorto-enteric fistula 3 years after abdominal aortic aneurysm repair. The cause of bleeding in this case is related to the close proximity between the aortic graft and the overlying 3rd or 4th portion of the duodenum and erosion of the graft into the duodenum followed by chemical/bacterial involvement causing a leak from the aorta. Bleeding associated with this process is painless and often intermittent before exsanguination occurs. The intermittent nature of the bleeding is described as "herald bleeding." Ulcerative colitis, duodenal ulcer, and ischemic colitis are often associated with pain. Superior mesenteric artery embolus causes the sudden-onset of ischemic pain, and bleeding is generally a secondary complaint that sets in after ischemic necrosis occurs.

23.3 **A.** Mesenteric angiography is the most specific modality in identifying the site of lower GI bleeding. This modality is less sensitive for bleeding identification because in order to visualize contrast extravasation, the patient has to be actively bleeding at a rate greater than 0.5 to 1.0 mL/min during the angiographic study. Tagged RBC scan is highly sensitive in visualizing bleeding (rate > 0.1 mL/min); however, this study is not very specific in identifying the anatomic site of bleeding. Surgical exploration is frequently unable to identify the bleeding site, because the bleeding sites are often not associated with gross findings that can be seen during an operation. Barium enema is not useful at all for identification of bleeding because most lower GI bleeding etiologies are not associated with specific mucosal contour abnormalities. CT scan with oral and intravenous contrast is not helpful for lower GI bleeding identification, because intraluminal contrast interferes with visualization of contrast extravasation into the lumen.

23.4 **E.** This 62-year-old man has lower GI bleeding of unknown source. His bleeding at this point does not appear life-threatening. Upper GI endoscopy is negative, and the colonoscopy reveals only diverticulosis and no bleeding source. Observation is the most appropriate choice for this patient. If his bleeding remains resolved, he should probably have a capsular endoscopy performed as an outpatient to rule out possible small bowel bleeding sources such as small bowel gastrointestinal stromal tumors (GIST).

23.5   **D.** This 63-year-old man with prior history of abdominal aneurysm repair comes in with GI bleeding. Even though the probability is low that an aorto-duodenal fistula is the source of bleeding, unrecognized and untreated bleeding from aorto-enteric fistula is uniformly lethal. The location of the fistula in the GI tract is most commonly in the 3rd or 4th portion of the duodenum. An upper endoscopy to evaluate this area is the best choice listed. Some groups have advocated doing a CT scan to try to identify inflammation or air near or around the aortic graft. Angiography is not as useful because it only visualizes intra-arterial anatomic abnormalities and contrast extravasation that may not be active during the angiography.

23.6   **C.** A 73-year-old woman presents with fever, abdominal pain, and passage of bloody stools. Her physical examination reveals nonfocal tenderness of the left side of the abdomen. There is no evidence of peritonitis. This patient most likely has ischemic colitis, which is the most common form of intestinal ischemia. The process is most common in patients over the age of 65. The disease can range from mild, self-limiting mucosal ischemia, to severe transmural infarction that requires surgical resection. Fortunately, only about 20% of the patients with ischemic colitis require surgical resection. This patient's clinical presentation does not suggest that surgical intervention is needed at this point. A colonoscopy to assess the severity of ischemic changes in the colon is appropriate at this time. If pale mucosa with superficial ulcerations is visualized during colonoscopy, the patient can then be treated with non-operative treatment that includes bowel rest, intravenous antibiotics, and intravenous fluids. However, if colonoscopy reveals transmural necrosis, the patient will need exploratory laparotomy with colectomy. A CT scan can be performed to look for signs of perforation, such as free air and pneumatosis, but this study is most useful with the administration of intravenous and intraluminal contrast.

23.7   **C.** A 58-year-old woman with history of hypertension, osteoarthritis and NSAID usage presents with melena (or passage of tarry stools), which is most suggestive of relatively slow upper GI bleeding as melena represents degradation of hemoglobin by bacteria in the GI tract. NSAID use in women is associated with a significant increase in risk of gastritis and gastric ulcerations; therefore, EGD followed by colonoscopy is the most appropriate choice in this situation.

CLINICAL PEARLS

▶ The primary goals in the treatment of a patient with acute and continued lower bleeding are maintaining hemodynamic stability with resuscitation and then localizing the bleeding site.

▶ The ability to localize the bleeding site during an abdominal exploration is greatly compromised. Exploration of the abdomen should be avoided prior to precise localization of the bleeding site.

▶ CT angiography and colonoscopy are the two most commonly used initial diagnostic studies in patients with overt lower GI bleeding.

▶ Visceral angiography and selective embolization techniques have evolved greatly during the past decade, and this has become the preferred treatment modality in some institutions.

▶ Surgery is rarely needed for patients with acute lower GI bleeding, and it is most useful after a bleeding site has been localized. It remains unclear whether surgical resection or angiographic embolization is the better treatment option for patients with localized lower GI bleeding.

▶ Whenever a patient with a history of prior abdominal aortic reconstruction presents with GI bleeding, the priority is to rule out an aortic-enteric fistula as the source of bleeding.

REFERENCES

Ghassemi KA, Jensen DM. Lower GI bleeding: epidemiology and management. *Curr Gastroenterol Rep.* 2013;15. DOI: 10.1007/s11894-013-0333-5.

Raphaeli T, Menon R. Current treatment of lower gastrointestinal hemorrhage. *Clin Colon Rectal Surg.* 2012;25:219-227.

Shanmugan S, Stein SL. Lower gastrointestinal bleeding. In: Cameron JL, Cameron AM, eds. *Current Surgical Therapy.* 11th ed. Philadelphia, PA: Elsevier Saunders; 2014:302-306.

A 20-year-old woman with abdominal pain is being evaluated in the emergency department. She describes a gradual onset of pain 24 hours previously, which has been persistent in its location in the lower abdomen. She denies any diarrhea or abnormal urinary symptoms. Her last menstrual period was approximately 12 days ago, and she denies any abnormal pattern in her menses. The patient is sexually active with one partner. Her past medical and surgical history is unremarkable. She takes no medications and consumes alcohol socially. On physical examination, her temperature is 38.2°C (100.8°F) and her blood pressure, pulse rate, and respiratory rate are normal. The cardiopulmonary examination is unremarkable. Her abdomen is soft, nondistended, and tender to palpation in the suprapubic and right lower quadrant. No peritonitis nor masses are detected. The bowel sounds are hypoactive. The rectal examination is unremarkable. Pelvic examination reveals no purulent discharge; however, there is tenderness in the right adnexal region. Laboratory studies reveal a white blood cell count of 14,000/mm³, normal hemoglobin and hematocrit values, and normal serum electrolyte and amylase levels. The urinalysis reveals concentrated urine with 3 to 5 red blood cells per high-power field, 3 to 5 white blood cells per high power field, and negative for leukocyte esterase. The serum pregnancy test is negative.

▶ What is your next step?
▶ What are the differential diagnoses?
▶ What are the treatment options, and what are the advantages and disadvantages of the treatment options?

ANSWERS TO CASE 24:

Abdominal Pain (Right Lower Quadrant)/Acute Appendicitis

Summary: A 20-year-old woman has 24-hour history of lower abdominal pain of undetermined etiology. She has low-grade fever, lower abdominal tenderness, and leukocytosis.

- **Next step:** Obtain a CT scan of the abdomen and pelvis.

- **Differential diagnosis:** Acute appendicitis, infectious colitis and enteritis, Crohn disease, ovarian cyst rupture/torsion, pelvic inflammatory disease (PID), urinary tract infection (UTI), renal calculus.

- **Treatment options for appendicitis:** Surgical treatment or nonoperative management that includes antibiotic treatment.

- **Advantages and disadvantages of treatment options:** Surgical treatment is effective but associated with complications and costs of surgery. Antibiotic treatment is associated with some delayed responses and has the potential of failure; however, antibiotic management avoids surgery-related complications in those who are successfully treated.

ANALYSIS

Objectives

1. Learn about the clinical presentation of acute appendicitis.

2. Learn the diagnostic and treatment approaches for patients with possible acute appendicitis.

3. Learn the outcomes associated with operative and nonoperative treatment of acute appendicitis.

Considerations

This young woman presents with a history of lower abdominal pain, low-grade fever and leukocytosis. Although her history and physical findings are not typical for acute appendicitis, this possibility has to be strongly considered. At this time, the options are to admit the patient for observation, obtain imaging studies, or simply proceed to diagnostic laparoscopy and possible appendectomy. Observation is often a reasonable option, especially if the patient has abdominal pain but no physical findings to suggest that there is infectious or inflammatory process that are ongoing in the abdomen. In this patient's case, she already has fever, leukocytosis, and abdominal tenderness, which are parameters that we can help establish the diagnosis. Observation for her is less desirable because it would mean that we are waiting worsening of the infectious parameters and could lead to delayed treatment. Performing a diagnostic laparoscopy is a reasonable choice, if the patient has clear surgical indications such as localized peritonitis or strong indications of other processes

Table 24–1 • DIAGNOSTIC OPTIONS FOR ACUTE APPENDICITIS			
	Advantages	Disadvantages	Recommended Use
CT imaging	Identifies appendicitis changes or other pathology (~95% accuracy)	Limited sensitivity for early appendicitis and pelvic pathology	Inflammatory process not related to pelvic pathology
Ultrasonography	Greater sensitivity and specificity for gynecologic pathology than CT	Limited by body habitus; appendicitis signs less well defined	Suspected gynecologic pathology; young children
Clinical observation with serial laboratory studies	Allows the natural history of disease evolution	Limited application if localized pain, fever, and leukocytosis are already present	Possible early appendicitis and without localized signs
Diagnostic laparoscopy	Allows accurate assessment of pathology	Invasive; some morbidities	Inflammatory or pathology of uncertain source

Abbreviation: CT, computed tomography.

that would require surgical intervention. Given her current presentation, a CT scan of the abdomen and pelvis would be helpful to confirm or rule out the diagnosis of acute appendicitis. If the CT scan demonstrates findings suggestive of ovarian pathology and no evidence of appendicitis, a pelvic ultrasound can be obtained to help further evaluate the abnormalities, and she can be referred for appropriate care of her gynecologic pathology (see Table 24–1 for diagnostic options).

APPROACH TO:
Suspected Acute Appendicitis

DEFINITIONS

CHRONIC OR RECURRENT APPENDICITIS: This entity describes the milder forms of appendicitis that has traditionally been overlooked. Patients with this process often are not severely ill and may describe recurrent pain that is often self-limiting. Appendectomy will improve the patients' quality of life but it is unclear whether operations are always necessary.

INTERVAL APPENDECTOMY: This is an operation for the treatment of appendicitis typically complicated by abscess or phlegmon. The patients are classically treated with antibiotics with or without CT-guided drainage. Following resolution of symptoms, the appendectomy is performed. Cohort studies suggest that without interval appendectomy, some patients may develop recurrent appendicitis; however, it remains unknown which of the patients with this process would benefit from interval appendectomy. It is acceptable to take a "wait and see" approach rather than proceeding with routine interval appendectomies for all patients.

MESENTERIC ADENITIS: An inflammatory condition occurring with a viral illness, resulting in painful lymphadenopathy in the small bowel mesentery, and clinically "mimics" appendicitis. This process can be associated with right lower quadrant pain and tenderness and is more common in children.

CLINICAL APPROACH

The pathophysiologic process leading to acute appendicitis was initially described by Dr. Reginald Fitz in 1886, where appendicitis was described as a process that began with appendiceal luminal obstruction that led to secondary bacterial infection, ischemia, necrosis, and perforation. Based on these descriptions, the goals of treatment are to diagnose the process early so that timely removal of the appendix can take place. Over the past 130 years, our understanding of the pathogenesis and clinical spectrum of acute appendicitis has changed significantly. Our current understanding of appendicitis is that appendicitis can be produced by a number of different causes with only some forms of appendicitis having the potential to progress to develop gangrenous changes and perforations. There is evidence to suggest that dietary changes, trauma, foreign body reactions, ischemia, and allergic reactions can all produce inflammation of the appendix. However, unlike the variant of acute appendicitis described originally by Fitz, the other varieties of appendicitis can be mild and self-limiting.

Previously, research efforts regarding appendicitis had been primarily directed toward the development of diagnostic and operative strategies for timely treatment of the process; however, much of the recent investigational efforts have evolved toward disease severity stratification and the identification of patients who would be best treated with surgery and those who can be treated nonoperatively.

Management Based on the Alvarado Scores

The diagnosis of acute appendicitis is frequently made on the basis of clinical history, physical findings, and laboratory data. The "classic" or "textbook" history of acute appendicitis begins with vague pain in the peri-umbilical area, with nausea, vomiting and urge to defecate. T symptoms are then followed by localization of the pain to the right lower quadrant with associated peritonitis. In reality, many patients with appendicitis do not have the "classic" presentation due to atypical locations of the appendix in some people (such as retro-cecal or pelvic locations). **The Alvarado Score is a 10-point scoring system initially introduced in 1986 to help clinicians in making the diagnosis** (see Table 24–2). Patients with Alvarado scores of 0 to 4 have "low probability" of having appendicitis; patients with scores of 5 to 6 are "compatible" with appendicitis; patients with scores of 7 to 8 have "probable" appendicitis, and those with scores of 9 to 10 are "highly probable." Various groups have developed treatment strategies based on the Alvarado scores. In general, there is agreement among the practitioners that patients with Alvarado scores of 0 to 4 have low probability and may be safely observed. For patients with Alvarado scores of 5 to 8, some groups have proposed diagnostic imaging such as CT scan to further determine whether the patients truly have appendicitis; alternatively, some practitioners have proposed that these patients have mild appendicitis and should be treated with antibiotics rather than imaging. Many practitioners agree that patients

Table 24–2 • ALVARADO SCORE	
Parameter	Score
Migratory pain to RLQ	1
Anorexia	1
Nausea/or vomiting	1
Tenderness in RLQ	2
Rebound tenderness in RLQ	1
Fever (temperature > 37.5°C or 99.5°F)	1
White blood cell count >10,000	2
Shift to the left in WBC	1
Total	10

with Alvarado scores of 9 to 10 have very high likelihood of having severe appendicitis and should be managed with operative treatment without the need for further imaging.

The Role of Imaging

Because gynecologic processes can cause pain in the lower abdomen, the list of differential diagnosis is far more complex for female patients. Consequently, misdiagnoses and delays in diagnosis tend to occur more often in women of child-bearing. Accordingly, most clinicians will rely heavily on diagnostic imaging modalities during the assessment of lower abdominal pain in female patients. Imaging studies are also particularly useful when patient present with atypical symptoms or atypical physical examination findings. Over the past 15 years, imaging has been applied more liberally in the diagnosis of acute appendicitis. Computed tomography and ultrasonography are the two imaging modalities that are most commonly applied for children and adults with potential diagnosis of acute appendicitis. The sensitivity of CT scan for the diagnosis of acute appendicitis is significantly better than that of the ultrasound. The pooled sensitivity and specificity of CT is reported at ~94% for adult patients. CT sensitivity and specificity are reported at 94% and 95%, respectively for children. Alternatively, pelvic ultrasonography is a more sensitive diagnostic modality than the CT scan for evaluation and characterization of ovarian and other gynecologic processes.

Approach to Pregnant Patients

Appendectomy is the most common non-obstetrical surgical procedure performed in pregnant women. The diagnosis of appendicitis can be particularly challenging in pregnant women because some of the findings associated with appendicitis are also common during pregnancy, including leukocytosis, nausea, vomiting, and abdominal discomfort. In addition, the appendiceal location can be displaced by the enlarged uterus during pregnancy. CT imaging can be used in pregnant women for the diagnosis of appendicitis when ultrasound or MRI results are inconclusive. The estimated fetal radiation exposure from CT scan can range from 19.9 to 43.6 mGy, depending on the trimester of exposure. A radiation exposure dose of 50 mGy is generally considered acceptable to the fetus; however, it should be clearly understood that there is probably no "safe" radiation dose for the infant, and exposure should be weighed against the risks of alternative management strategies. Due to the limitation associated with appendicitis diagnosis during pregnancy, some groups have advocated for a more aggressive approach in pregnant women; however, it is important to note that negative appendectomies can also cause premature labor and fetal losses.

Treatment of Patients with Appendicitis

Appendectomy is currently the primary treatment for acute appendicitis in North America. In some developing countries, patients with acute appendicitis are routinely managed with antibiotics treatment initially, and appendectomy is performed only for patients who fail medical treatment and for those with appendiceal complications. Appendectomies are generally performed by a laparoscopic approach, which has been shown to be associated with less pain and more rapid recovery in comparison to open appendectomies. Patients with perforated appendicitis and/or gangrenous acute appendicitis benefit from a prolonged course (5-7 days) of antibiotics treatment following appendectomy. The purpose of postoperative antibiotics treatment in patients with complicated appendicitis is to reduce the occurrence of intra-abdominal abscesses.

CASE CORRELATION

- See also Case 17 (Peptic Ulcer Disease).

COMPREHENSION QUESTIONS

24.1 A 19-year-old woman presents with 2-day history of lower abdominal pain and no fever. She has a tender left adnexal mass, a normal WBC count, negative pregnancy test, and normal urinalysis. Which of the following is the most appropriate management?

A. CT of the abdomen and pelvis

B. Discharge the patient after giving her reassurance

C. Diagnostic laparoscopy

D. Observation with serial abdominal examination and laboratory testing

E. Pelvic ultrasonography

24.2 A 24-year-old man complains of colicky intermittent peri-umbilical and right lower quadrant pain of 24-hour duration. He complains of anorexia and nausea. His temperature is 36.6°C (98°F). Which of the following is the most likely diagnosis?

A. Acute appendicitis

B. Chronic appendicitis

C. Peptic ulcer

D. Acute pancreatitis

E. Gastroenteritis

24.3 An 18-year-old woman has 1-day history of worsening lower abdominal pain, nausea, vomiting, and low-grade fever. Her temperature is 38.5°C (101.3°F), and she has lower abdominal tenderness and no rebound. She has right adnexal tenderness and cervical motion tenderness. Which of the following approaches will definitively differentiate pelvic inflammatory disease from acute appendicitis?

A. CT of the abdomen and pelvis

B. MRI of the abdomen and pelvis

C. Ultrasonography of the abdomen and pelvis

D. Laparoscopy

E. Clinical response to broad-spectrum antibiotics

24.4 A 43-year-old woman presents with 1-day history of right flank and right lower quadrant pain. She has a history of nephrolithiasis and indicates that the pain she experiences now is not the same as what she has experienced before. Her temperature is 38.5°C (101.5°F), and her abdomen and right flank are tender to deep palpation. Her urinalysis shows 10 to 20 WBC/hpf and 5 to 10 RBC/hpf. Which of the following is the best management strategy?

A. Intravenous fluid, analgesics, antibiotics for urinary tract infection

B. Perform pelvic ultrasound to rule out ovarian torsion

C. Perform CT of the abdomen

D. Diagnostic laparoscopy

E. Cystoscopy, retrograde ureteroscopy, and ureteral stent placement

24.5 A 14-year-old boy presents with right lower quadrant abdominal pain of 2 days duration. He indicates that he has been ill for the past 10 days with a cough, runny nose, fever. Over the past 2 days, he has been having pain in his right lower quadrant. Over the past 12 hours, his abdominal pain has improved slightly. His temperature is 37.8°C (100.4°F). His abdomen is tender in the right lower quadrant, without masses or signs of peritonitis. His WBC count is 11,000/mm^3 and urinalysis is normal. CT of the abdomen reveals no inflammatory changes around the cecum. There are several enlarged lymph nodes in the mesentery of the ileum. The appendix is not visualized. What is your diagnosis and treatment?

A. Mesenteric adenitis. Discharge home with outpatient follow-up

B. Probably mesenteric adenitis. Perform diagnostic laparoscopy for confirmation

C. Crohn disease. Consult the gastroenterologist for initiation of medical therapy

D. Mesenteric adenitis. Admit the patient for antibiotics treatment

E. Perform CT-guided biopsy of the mesenteric lymph nodes for definitive diagnosis

24.6 A 20-year-old college student had perforated appendicitis with periappendiceal abscess treated by CT-guided drainage and antibiotics 4 weeks ago. She is currently doing well and has returned to school and normal activities, but she is concerned that her appendicitis might recur. Which of the following statements regarding interval appendectomy is TRUE?

A. Interval appendectomy should be performed in all cases because it eliminates the possibility of recurrence

B. Interval appendectomy is indicated following the resolution of appendicitis because the appendiceal abnormality will produce recurrences in most patients

C. Recurrent appendicitis can develop in some patients; performing routine interval appendectomy results in over-treatment in some individuals

D. Interval appendectomies should be performed in all female patients because it will help reduce diagnostic confusions in the future

E. Interval appendectomies are rarely indicated because fibrotic changes from the initial bout of appendicitis eliminate possibilities of recurrence

ANSWERS

24.1 **E.** This young woman has 2-day history of lower abdominal pain, no fever, and no leukocytosis. She has a tender adnexal mass on pelvic examination. Pelvic ultrasonography may be the best choice to evaluate her ovaries and pelvic organs. Diagnostic laparoscopy is not yet indicated, because her current condition has not yet been fully evaluated, and there is no urgency in her care that prompts surgery at this time. CT scan could help rule out appendicitis but her presentation is more consistent with gynecologic pathology.

24.2 **E.** The colicky nature of his pain is not compatible with acute appendicitis, chronic appendicitis, peptic ulcer disease, or acute pancreatitis. Colicky or intermittent pain associated with the GI tract is generally caused by mechanical obstruction or excessive peristaltic activities that can be associated with gastroenteritis.

24.3 **D.** Diagnostic laparoscopy is the approach that will provide us with the definitive diagnosis of either acute appendicitis, pelvic inflammatory disease, or other alternative disease process. Even though this will provide a definitive answer regarding her condition, it is not necessarily indicated in this patient.

24.4 **C.** This woman has flank pain, lower abdominal pain, and fever. Her urinalysis reveals WBCs and RBCs. These findings are highly suggestive of infected kidney or ureteral stones, or pylonephritis. CT scan without contrast in this patient may help us identify kidney stones or ureteral stones. If no stones are demonstrated, CT with contrast may help us identify appendicitis, pylonephritis, or other abdominal pathology. Without knowing whether she has an obstructing ureteral stone, cystoscopy and ureteral stent placement is not indicated.

24.5 **A.** This patient's clinical picture (symptoms, physical findings, laboratory findings, and CT findings) is consistent with mesenteric adenitis, which is process related to viral illnesses and self-limiting. Given his findings and his work-up that has been completed, discharge with outpatient follow-up is acceptable. Antibiotic treatment, diagnostic laparoscopy, and biopsy are not necessary at this time.

24.6 **C.** Recurrent appendicitis can happen in some individuals after an occurrence of perforated appendicitis with peri-appendiceal abscess. The frequency of occurrence is unknown, and treatment can be a "wait and see" approach or "routine appendectomy" approach. With the routine appendectomy approach, there is the potential of performing unnecessary surgery in some patients, but the possibility of untimely recurrences is eliminated. In general, the current trend in the medical and surgical community is toward the "wait and see" approach.

CLINICAL PEARLS

▶ The options in the management of patients with atypical presentations of appendicitis include imaging studies, clinical observation with serial laboratory testing, and diagnostic laparoscopy.

▶ The "classic" history of acute appendicitis begins with vague pain in the peri-umbilical region, nausea, vomiting, and the urge to defecate; these symptoms are followed by localization of pain in the right lower quadrant with associated localized peritonitis.

▶ Only 50% of patients with acute appendicitis have the "classic" presentation.

▶ The clinical picture of appendicitis can be produced by a variety of pathologic processes in the appendix; consequently, the clinical picture and natural history can be highly variable.

▶ Ultrasonography is generally the best modality to assess pelvic pathology; whereas, a CT scan is the best way to assess for nongynecological processes.

▶ The Alvarado score is a 10-point scoring system that is useful to diagnose appendicitis, and this scoring system also helps to stratify the severity of disease in individuals with appendicitis.

▶ Antibiotics treatment is an acceptable option for patients with acute appendicitis.

▶ Randomized controlled trials comparing appendectomy to antibiotics in patients with acute appendicitis showed that roughly two-thirds of the patients can be successfully treated with antibiotics. Approximately, 15% of patients do not respond completely and 15% of patients recur.

▶ Interval appendectomy is not necessary for patients whose appendicitis is successfully treated with antibiotics.

REFERENCES

Carr NJ. The pathology of acute appendicitis. *Ann Diagnos Pathol.* 2000;4:46–58.

Stewart D. The management of acute appendicitis. In: Cameron JL, Cameron AM, eds. *Current Surgical Therapy.* 11th ed. Philadelphia, PA: Elsevier Saunders; 2014:252-255.

Teixeira PGR, Demetriades D. Appendicitis: changing perspectives. *Adv Surg.* 2013;47:119-140.

Thurston F, Flum DR. Improvement in the diagnosis of appendicitis. *Adv Surg.* 2013;47:299-328.

A 63-year-old man complains of dyspnea and chest pain on exertion. His current symptoms have been present for approximately 3 to 4 weeks. Over approximately the same period of time, the patient has noted post-prandial bloating in his abdomen. His past medical history is significant for hypertension and stable angina. On physical examination, he appears well-nourished and in no acute distress. The abdominal examination reveals an obese abdomen without masses or tenderness. The rectal examination reveals no rectal masses, a smooth and mildly enlarged prostate gland, and strongly Hemoccult-positive stool in the rectal vault. His complete blood count reveals normal WBC count, hemoglobin 8.2 g/dL, hematocrit 28.5%, and mean cell volume 72 fL (normal range, 76-100 fL). The electrolytes and liver function tests are within normal limits. A 12-lead ECG reveals normal sinus rhythm with mild left ventricular hypertrophy. A chest x-ray reveals normal cardiac silhouette, no pulmonary infiltrations, no pleural effusion, and no pulmonary masses.

▶ What is the most likely cause of his current condition?
▶ How would you confirm the diagnosis?

ANSWERS TO CASE 25:
Colorectal Cancer and Polyps

Summary: A 63-year-old man presents with a recent onset of dyspnea on exertion, chest pain, and nonspecific gastrointestinal tract complaint related to occult GI blood loss and possibly mild mechanical obstruction symptoms.

- **Most likely cause:** The combination of anemia and post-prandial bloating are compatible with symptoms produced by colorectal (CRCs) cancers.

- **Confirmation of diagnosis:** GI endoscopy, with esophagogastroduodenoscopy (EGD) to evaluate the upper GI tract and colonoscopy to evaluate the lower GI tract. Biopsies of abnormalities are important for tissue diagnosis.

ANALYSIS
Objectives

1. Learn the clinical presentation and management of CRCs.

2. Know the risk factors for CRC and surveillance and screening strategies for patients based on risk factors.

3. Learn the evolving trend in the treatment of patients with advanced stages of CRC.

Considerations

This 63-year-old man presents with new-onset angina, dyspnea with exertion, post-prandial bloating, and guaiac-positive stool. His laboratory studies indicate micro-cytic anemia. It is highly probable that his angina and dyspnea are caused by the severe anemia. Because he is quite symptomatic at point, addressing the anemia should be one of our initial priorities in management. We should treat the anemia with iron supplementation and then resort to RBC transfusion if he does not improve with iron therapy. The rationale behind limiting transfusional treatment is that blood transfusions have been known to adversely affect immune functions and can independently affect cancer-related outcome in the transfused patients. A thorough GI evaluation will need to be done once his cardiopulmonary symptoms improve, and this work-up will include colonoscopy with biopsies and EGD. Once CRC is identified and confirmed by biopsy, we need to stage the disease and formulate a multimodality treatment strategy best suited for this patient and his stage of disease.

APPROACH TO:
Colorectal Cancer (CRC) and Polyps

DEFINITIONS

HYPERPLASTIC POLYPS: These types of polyps are commonly found in the distal colon and rectum. These are often small, smooth, and pale in appearance. In the past, these polyps were believed to be of no clinical relevance; however, with the recognition of serrated adenomas/polyps, there has been increased interest in hyperplastic polyps.

SESSILE POLYP: This is a description of the appearance of the polyp. A sessile polyp has a flat-appearance with a broad base and complete resection endoscopically can be technically more challenging.

PEDUNCULATED POLYP: This describes a polyp that has a stalk and has the appearance of a mushroom. Complete resection endoscopically is technically easier.

SERRATED ADENOMAS/POLYPS: This variant of mucosal lesion has only been recognized over the past 10 years as a precursor to CRC. Phenotypically, these lesions appear flat or sessile and are easy to overlook during colonoscopy. Histologically, these lesions appear architecturally similar to hyperplastic polyps. Most serrated adenomas or polyps are larger than 5 mm and are found in the right colon. Serrated adenomas are high-risk lesions with approximately 15% of the lesions progress to become cancers. Epidemiologically, these lesions occur more commonly in females, and cancers arising from these lesions tend to occur later in life with peak incidences in the mid-to-late 1970s.

MECHANICAL BOWEL PREPARATION FOR ELECTIVE COLON SURGERY: These are solutions that consist of polyethylene glycol solution or phosphor soda solutions to try to clear the colon of solid stool prior to surgery. The use of mechanical preparations is controversial.

ANTIBIOTIC PREPARATIONS FOR ELECTIVE COLON SURGERY: The administration of oral poorly absorbed antibiotics for patients prior to elective colon surgery appears to be associated with the reduction in infectious complications, therefore should be strongly considered.

ABDOMINAL PERINEAL RESECTION (APR): This involves resection of the rectum and anus thus leaving the patient with a permanent colostomy. This procedure can be done by open surgery or laparoscopically and is often applied when the patient has a low-lying invasive rectal cancer that is at the level of the levator and rectal sphincter muscles.

LOW ANTERIOR RESECTION: This describes surgery for resection of the rectum and lower sigmoid colon. This can be done when the cancer is above the levator muscles and the anal sphincters. This operation preserves the patient's continence and anal sphincter mechanisms.

CLINICAL APPROACH

Epidemiology

Colorectal cancer is the third most common cancer in men and the second most common cancer in women in the United States. The estimated lifetime probability of CRC development for persons residing in the US is approximately 5% (1 in 20) for males and 4.6% (1 in 22) for females, with a reported median age of 68 at diagnosis. In the US, sporadic CRCs account for the majority of CRC (75%) cases, hereditary syndromes such as familial polyposis syndrome (FAP) and hereditary nonpolyposis cancer (HPNNC) account for about 5% of the CRCs, and the remaining 20% of CRCs occur in familial clusters. Screening is an effective strategy for the prevention and early diagnosis of CRC, and screening and surveillance guidelines based on patient risk factors have been proposed by a number of professional organizations (see Tables 25–1 and 25-2 for summary of surveillance screening).

Biology

The development and progression of CRCs follow the **adenoma–carcinoma sequence, de novo cancer sequence, serrated polyp to cancer sequence,** and the **dysplasia–carcinoma sequence.** By far **the most common CRC development pathway is the adenoma–carcinoma pathway,** which validates colonoscopies and polyp removal as an effective strategy in CRC prevention. The recent discovery of serrated polyps suggests that these are variants of hyperplastic polyps that carry the genetic signatures for CRC development (eg, BRAF mutation, KRAS mutation, and microsatellite instability).

Table 25–1 • SCREENING AND SURVEILLANCE GUIDELINES
Average-Risk Individuals Age 50 or Older (~60%-65% of US population)
• Annual fecal occult blood testing
• Flexible sigmoidoscopy every 5 years
• Colonoscopy every 10 years or double contrast barium enema every 5 years
• For patients who cannot tolerate colonoscopy, CT colography can be applied
Moderate-Risk Individuals (~25% of US population)
Based on personal history
• Patients with 3 to 10 adenomatous polyps, one polyp >1 cm, or polyps with high-grade dysplasia needs clearance of all polyps and then repeat colonoscopy in 3 years
Based on family history
• Patients with first-degree relative with CRC diagnosed before age 60 should have first colonoscopy at age 40 or 10 years before the youngest diagnosed family member; the patients need surveillance colonoscopy every 5 years
High-Risk Individuals (FAP, HNPCC, or IBD)*(6%-8% of US population)
• FAP patients need sigmoidoscopy or colonoscopy starting at age 10 to 12 years and continued until proctocolectomy
• HNPCC patients need colonoscopy every 1 to 2 years beginning at age 20 to 25 or 10 years before the youngest family member's age of CRC diagnosis
• IBD patients need colonoscopy with biopsies every 1 to 2 years starting at 8 years after diagnosis of pancolitis or 12 to 15 years after diagnosis of left-sided colitis

*FAP: familial adenomatous polyposis syndrome; HNPCC: hereditary nonpolyposis colon cancer; IBD: inflammatory bowel disease (ulcerative colitis patients have much higher CRC risk than Crohn colitis patients).

Table 25–2 • AGA 2012 RECOMMENDATIONS FOR SURVEILLANCE AND SCREENING INTERVALS IN INDIVIDUALS WITH BASELINE AND MODERATE RISKS

Findings at colonoscopy	Recommended surveillance interval (years)
No polyps	10
Small (<10 mm) hyperplastic polyps	10
1-2 small tubular polyps (< 10 mm)	5-10
3-10 tubular adenomas	3
> 10 adenomas	<3
One or more tubular adenoma ≥ 10 mm	3
One or more villous adenoma	3
Adenoma with high-grade dysplasia	3
Serrated lesion	
Sessile serrate <10 mm without dysplasia	5
Sessile serrated >10 mm or serrated dysplasia	3
Serrated polyposis syndrome	1

Screening

Disease screening and surveillance are effective in the prevention of CRC, and screening and surveillance are best accomplished by complete colonoscopy. Prior to initiating a screening or surveillance plan for any patient, it is important to classify the patient based on risk (average-risk, moderate-risk, or high-risk). See Table 25–1 for summary of guidelines.

Clinical Presentation

Symptoms of colorectal cancer vary depending on the location of the tumor. **The most common presenting symptom is bleeding per rectum that is either occult or gross.** Change in bowel habit is also common and is reported in 77% to 92% of patients. Only 6% to 16% of patients present with intestinal obstruction, and 2% to 7% of patients present with colonic perforation. Some of the bowel habit changes reported by patients with left-sided tumors include change in stool caliber and diarrhea whereas patients with right-sided colon cancers tend to present more often with anemia.

Cancer Staging

The TNM (tumor-node-metastasis) system is the most commonly applied staging system for CRC (Table 25–3).

Treatment

Polyps

Patients with colonic polyps are best treated with endoscopic resection. Endoscopic treatment is definitive when polyp is completely removed. The risk of cancer within a polyp increases as the polyp size increases. For polyps less than 1 cm in size, the risk of cancer is 1.3%; polyps measuring 1 to 2 cm have 9.5% risk of cancer,

Table 25–3 • UICC/AJCC STAGING OF COLORECTAL CANCER		
Stage	TNM	5-year Survival with Rx
Stage 0	Tis, N0, M0	Normal life expectancy
Stage I	T1-T2, N0, M0	92%
Stage IIA	T3, N0, M0	87%
Stage IIB	T4a, N0, M0	63%
Stage IIC	T4b, N0, M0	50%
Stage IIIA	T1-T2, N1, M0 or T1, N2a, M0	89%*
Stage IIIB	T3-T4a, N1, M0 or T2-T3, N2a, M0 or T1-T2, N2b, M0	69%
Stage IIIC	T4a, N2a, M0 or T3-T4a, N2b, M0 or T4b, N1-N2, M0	53%
Stage IVA	Any T, any N, M1a	16%
Stage IVB	Any T, any N, M1b	11%

Tis: mucosa involvement only;
T1: invades submucosa;
T2: invades muscularispropria;
T3: invades subserosa;
T4a: invades past the visceral peritoneum;
T4b: invades adjacent structure;
N0: no lymph node involvement;
N1: up to 3 regional lymph nodes involved;
N2a: 4-6 regional lymph nodes involved;
N2b: 7 or more regional lymph nodes involved;
M1a: cancer spread to 1 distant organ or nonregional lymph node;
M1b: cancer spread to more than 1 distant organ or to the peritoneum;
*Stage III patients have better survival than stage II patients because systemic chemotherapy is a part of the treatment for Stage III patients.

and polyps > 2 cm have 46% risk of containing cancers. Roughly, 65% to 80% of colon polyps are tubular adenomas, 10% to 25% are tubulovillous adenomas, and 5% to 10% are villous adenomas. **Villous adenomas are associated with the greatest cancer risk.** When the cancer within the polyp does not penetrate the submucosa, polypectomy with clear margins is considered sufficient treatment. However, with submucosa penetration by the cancer, the spread of tumor to the regional lymph nodes become possible, and treatment should include resection of the involved area of the colon/rectum.

Colon Cancer

For patients with colon cancers identified by colonoscopy and confirmed by biopsy, CT scans of the abdomen/pelvis and chest x-rays should be obtained to define the local extent of disease as well to look for metastases. The most common site of distant metastasis for colon cancer is the **liver**, which makes CT a valuable imaging tool. Serum CEA levels should be obtained so that levels can be followed during the course of the disease treatment and follow-up. For the majority of patients with invasive colon cancers, the treatment begins with resection of the colon segment that contains the cancer. **During the operation, strong efforts should be made to**

harvest >12 lymph nodes so that the regional disease would be appropriately staged. The length of colon that is removed is generally dictated by the blood supply to the cancer-involved segment of colon (see Figure 25–1). For example, resection for a patient with cancer in the cecum involves a right colectomy that removes a segment of intestine including the distal ileum, cecum, ascending, and right side of the transverse colon (ileocolic artery, right colic artery, and right branch of the middle colic artery distribution) (see Figure 25–1). Elective colon resection are commonly performed by the laparoscopic approach, which has been shown to be associated with less postoperative pain, shorter hospitalization, and earlier return to work in comparison to open colectomies. Patients with stage III or stage IV colon carcinoma benefit from adjuvant chemotherapy following their colectomies. The principle in the management of patients with stage IV disease is to address the site that causes the most significant symptoms first. For example, for a patient with cancer in the right colon that is minimally symptomatic but has significant tumor burden in the liver, we would treat the metastatic disease first with systemic chemotherapy and/or targeted biologic agents. In some cases, the primary tumor would not be addressed at all if it remains asymptomatic. On the other hand, if the patient with the right colon cancer is profoundly anemic from bleeding or has obstructive symptoms, the patient will undergo resection of the colon prior to systemic adjuvant therapy. Patients with advanced colorectal cancers are most optimally managed by a multispecialty team made up of surgeons, medical oncologists, radiation oncologists, radiologists, nurses, and social workers. Nearly all patients with colon cancers with lymph node involvement will benefit from adjuvant systemic therapy following colon resections. The two most common regimens currently used are **FOLFOX4** (oxaliplatin, 5-fluorouracil, and leucovorin) and **FOLFIRI** (irinotecan, 5-fluorouracil, leucovorin). The duration of adjuvant therapy is generally 6 months or longer. In patients with metastatic disease, the use of biologic therapy targeting the KRAS has been shown to provide increased survival. When considering this treatment, the patient's tumor needs to be analyzed for KRAS mutation. If the patient's tumor is KRAS wild-type (nonmutated), the patient is then likely to respond to the anti-epidermal growth factor antibody (cetuximab).

Rectal Cancer

The rectum is generally defined as the last 12 to 15 cm of the most distal end of the large bowel. From the oncologic standpoint, the rectum differs from the colon in that it is extraperitoneal in location, it is not covered by the visceral peritoneum, and it is in close proximity to neighboring structures. For these reasons, **invasive rectal cancers have a much greater risk of local recurrences following treatment.** Another important difference between the rectum and colon is the difference in venous drainage. Venous drainage of the colon and upper part of the rectum is portal venous, therefore making the liver the most common site of distant metastasis. For the lower rectum the venous, drainage eventually ends up in the vena cava, making the lung a common site of distant metastases.

Due to the increased risk of local recurrence, patients with rectal cancers not only benefit from resection of the rectum with total mesorectal resection, most patients also seek benefit from adjuvant radiation therapy. Local staging of low rectal cancers can be best accomplished with endoscopic ultrasound or MRI of the

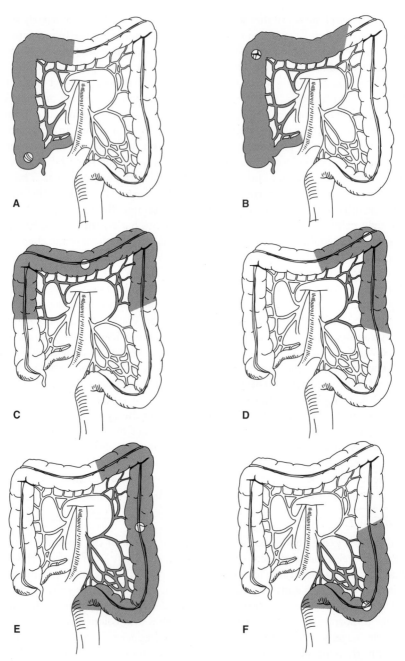

Figure 25–1. Resection of colon cancer. Right colectomy (**A**), right hemicolectomy with division of middle colic pedicle (**B**), transverse colectomy (**C**), resection of splenic flexure sparing left colic artery (**D**), left hemicolectomy (**E**), sigmoid colectomy sparing left colic artery (**F**). *(Reproduced, with permission, from Niederhuber JE, ed. Fundamentals of Surgery. Stamford, CT: Appleton & Lange; 1998:322 as modified from Schwartz SI, Ellis H. Maingot's Abdominal Operations. 10th ed. Norwalk, CT: Appleton & Lange; 1989:1053.)*

pelvis. While receiving their radiation therapy, patients are usually given adjuvant chemotherapy to increase the effectiveness of radiation treatments. In selective cases when the tumor is locally advanced, chemoradiation therapy is given before surgery to help improve the probability of having a complete resection.

Similar to patients with colon cancers, patients with node-positive rectal cancers also benefit from systemic chemotherapy using the regimens that have been described for colon carcinoma. An important difference regarding rectal cancer is that aggressive local resection with radiation therapy can frequently cause sexual and urinary dysfunction in male patients, and urinary and fertility dysfunction in female patients. These potential complications should be discussed and addressed with each patient prior to the initiation of treatments. An important issue regarding the treatment of low-lying rectal cancers (1-5 cm from the anal verge) is that complete resections in these patients sometimes require removal of the rectal sphincter complex leaving the patients with a permanent colostomy (Abdominal perineal resection or APR). Because of these additional concerns, rectal cancer patients should be provided with extensive counseling and appropriate support before, during, and after treatment.

Metastatic Disease

The presence of metastases in the liver or lungs in a patient with CRC generally indicates disseminated disease, and the focus is to treat the systemic disease. However, there are small subsets of patients with hepatic or pulmonary metastases who benefit from local treatments such as surgical resection or ablation of the metastases. Metastases are classified as **synchronous** (identified the same time as the primary tumor) or **metachronous** (identified after the primary had been treated). Prognostically, the patients with metachronous metastases do better than patients with synchronous metastases.

CASE CORRELATION

- See also Case 23 (Lower GI Tract Hemorrhage) and Case 24 (Abdominal Pain [Right Lower Quadrant]).

COMPREHENSION QUESTIONS

25.1 Which of the following patients has the highest risk of developing colorectal cancer?

    A. A 46-year-old man whose younger brother is just diagnosed with colon cancer

    B. A 46-year-old woman with BRCA1 mutation

    C. A 46-year-old man with 12-year history of ulcerative colitis

    D. A 46-year-old man who had two 1-cm adenomatous polyps removed 1 year ago

    E. A 46-year-old man with familial adenomatous polyposis (FAP) syndrome

25.2   Which of the following is the most appropriate treatment for a 40-year-old man with a T3N1 carcinoma of the ascending colon?

   A.   Preoperative chemoradiation therapy followed by right hemicolectomy

   B.   Right colectomy and postoperative adjuvant therapy with oxaliplatin, 5-FU, and leucovorin

   C.   Endoscopic removal of the tumor followed by chemoradiation therapy

   D.   Right hemicolectomy and postoperative raditation and tamoxifen therapy

   E.   Definitive treatment with six cycles of FOLFOX4 and remove the colon only if symptoms develop

25.3   Which of the following is the most appropriate surveillance strategy for a 60-year-old man who recently had complete endoscopic removal of a 1-cm-pedunculated polyp from the transverse colon?

   A.   Annual colonoscopy

   B.   Repeat colonoscopy in 5 years, and if negative, repeat every 5 to 10 years

   C.   CT scan of the chest, abdomen, pelvis, repeat colonoscopy at 3 years, and if negative, repeat every 5 years

   D.   Repeat colonoscopy every 2 years

   E.   Fecal occult blood testing every 6 months

25.4   A 58-year-old man with a history of stage III colon cancer that was treated by colectomy and adjuvant FOLFOX4 regimen develops a sudden rise in his serum CEA level and is found on CT scan to have a 2-cm lesion in the greater omentum. A CT-guided biopsy of this mass revealed metastatic adenocarcinoma. Which of the following is the most appropriate treatment?

   A.   Radiation therapy

   B.   Operative resection of the mass

   C.   Systemic therapy with chemotherapy and biologic agents

   D.   Immunotherapy

   E.   Comple colectomy and omentectomy

25.5   A 43-year-old woman presents with blood per rectum and is found to have a circumferential but nonobstructing adenocarcinoma located at 7 cm from the anal verge. Which of the following is the best treatment approach for this patient?

   A.   Surgical resection, chemotherapy if node positive, and surveillance

   B.   Surgical resection, radiation therapy, and chemotherapy if node positive

   C.   Radiation therapy followed by systemic chemotherapy

   D.   Endoscopic resection followed by radiation therapy

   E.   Surgical resection and targeted biologic therapy

25.6 Which of the following colon polyps carries the worse prognosis?

A. A 0.8 cm hyperplastic polyp without evidence of serrated adenomatous changes

B. A man with a 20-year history of ulcerative colitis involving the left colon with pseudopolyps in the rectum

C. A 1.5 cm serrated adenomatous polyp

D. A 48-year-old woman with a pedunculated adenomatous polyp in the sigmoid colon measuring 1.5 cm in diameter

E. A 45-year-old man FAP with multiple colonic polyps

25.7 A 53-year-old man undergoes his initial colonoscopy and was found to have a 1.9-cm pedunculated polyp in the sigmoid colon. This polyp was completely resected endoscopically. The pathology of the polyp reveals well-differentiated, invasive adenocarcinoma extending into the submucosa, and the stalk and the margin of resection are not involved with cancer. A subsequent CT scan of the abdomen and pelvis reveals no abnormalities. Which of the following is the most appropriate treatment?

A. Observation with repeat colonoscopy every 3 years

B. Radiation therapy and repeat colonoscopy every 3 years

C. Sigmoid colectomy and repeat colonoscopy every 3 years

D. Sigmoid colectomy, radiation therapy, and repeat colonoscopy every 3 years

E. Sigmoid resection and repeat colonoscopy every 10 years

25.8 An asymptomatic 63-year-old woman undergoes her initial colonoscopy and is found to have a nonobstructing adenocarcinoma in the descending colon. A staging CT scan reveals extensive metastatic disease in the liver involving approximately 45% of the liver distributed in both the right and left lobes. Which of the following is the most appropriate treatment for her?

A. Laparoscopic sigmoid colectomy and systemic chemotherapy treatment

B. Systemic chemotherapy

C. Laparoscopic colectomy, radiation therapy, and systemic chemotherapy

D. Sigmoid colectomy followed by resection, and ablative therapy for the liver metastases followed by systemic chemotherapy

E. Ablative therapy for the liver metastases followed by colon resection and systemic chemotherapy

ANSWERS

25.1 **E.** Statistically, the risk of CRC associated with FAP is 7% cancer risk by age 21, 87% by age 45, and 93% risk by age 50; therefore, the risk of CRC in a 46-year-old man with untreated FAP is roughly 90%. The patient who had two 1-cm adenomatous polyps removed has slightly increased CRC risk from the baseline population which is ~6% lifetime risk. BRCA mutation is not a risk factor for CRC. The patient with one first-degree relative with CRC has CRC lifetime risk that is 2-3 times the baseline risk of 6%, therefore lifetime risk of 12% to18%.

25.2 **B.** The most appropriate treatment for a 40-year-old man with T3N1 CRC involving the ascending colon is right colectomy and adjuvant therapy with FOLFOX4 (Oxaliplatin, 5-FU, and leucovorin).

25.3 **B.** The 60-year-old man with a single small pedunculated polyp without cancer resected should receive a repeat colonoscopy in 5 years followed by another colonoscopy in 5 to 10 years. Roughly 30% to 50% of the population has polyps. Patients with cancerous polyps, on the other hand, need to have earlier and more intensive follow-up with a colonoscopy at 1 year, and then the colonoscopy can be scheduled every 5 to 10 years depending on the findings.

25.4 **C.** Intraperitoneal recurrence of CRC in a patient following curative resection and adjuvant therapy for stage III CRC is considered to have distant metastasis(stage IV). The treatment of an asymptomatic patient with stage IV CRC is systemic chemotherapy and/or biologic therapy.

25.5 **B.** This 43-year-old woman has a nonobstructing rectal cancer located 7-cm from the anal verge. The best treatment choice for her is surgical resection, radiation therapy, followed by systemic chemotherapy if the disease is node positive.

25.6 **E.** A 45-year-old man with FAP who still has the at-risk colon and rectum has approximately 85% to 90% risk of harboring CRC. Roughly, the FAP cancer risk is 7% by age 21, 87% by age 45, 93% by age 50%, and nearly 100% lifetime risk. The individual with a 20-year history of ulcerative colitis has approximately 8% risk of having CRC, and this risk increases to 18% by 30 years. The average cancer risk associated with the history of serrated adenoma is approximately 5%. The history of a hyperplastic polyp does not confer increased CRC risk.

25.7 **A.** This 53-year-old man has a 1.9 cm pedunculated cancerous polyp removed completely by colonoscopy. The tumor is well differentiated and extends into the submucosa. The stalk and resection margin are uninvolved. Because the cancer is described as not through the submucosa or involving the stalk and margins, excision of the polyp alone is sufficient given the low risk of regional lymph node metastasis and low risk of local recurrence. This patient should not require additional treatments for this cancerous polyp. Observation and repeat colonoscopy in 3 years should be appropriate.

25.8 **B.** This 63-year-old woman has an asymptomatic carcinoma in the descending colon and has hepatic metastases occupying both liver lobes and replacing approximately 45% of the liver volume. Since she is asymptomatic from the primary tumor, the treatment strategy should be directed toward the treatment of the systemic disease process first, and then proceed with surgical resection of the colon only if it becomes symptomatic (bleeding, obstruction, or perforation).

CLINICAL PEARLS

▶ Many of the symptoms associated with CRC are nonspecific, including postprandial bloating, distension, and constipation.

▶ Patients with FAP syndrome are not only at risk for CRC, some individuals are at risk for duodenal adenomas, duodenal carcinomas, and desmoid tumors.

▶ FAP-related cancer risk is 7% by age 21, 87% by age 45, 93% by age 50, and nearly 100% lifetime.

▶ CRC risks related to ulcerative colitis is related to duration of disease: 10 years, 2%; 20 years, 8%; 30 years, 18%.

▶ Total proctocolectomy is the prophylactic surgery recommend for FAP patients prior to the age of 20 to 25 years.

▶ Chemoprevention of adenomatous polyps has been found effective with long-term intake of sulindac or celcoxib (COX-2 inhibitors). Intake is also associated with the regression of small polyps.

▶ CRC development pathways include polyp to cancer progression, de novo formation, dysplasia progression, and serrated progression pathways.

REFERENCES

Hechenbleikner E, Wick E. Colon cancer. In: Cameron JL, Cameron AM, eds. *Current Surgical Therapy.* 11th ed. Philadelphia, PA: Elsevier Saunders; 2014:213-218.

Roses R, Rodriguez-Biagas M. The management of rectal cancer. In; Cameron JL, Cameron AM, eds. *Current Surgical Therapy.* 11th ed. Philadelphia, PA: Elsevier Saunders; 2014:218-224.

Sun Z, Thacker JM. Contemporary surgical options for metastatic colorectal cancer. *Curr Oncol Rep.* 2015;17:1-7.

A 26-year-old man with a 3-year history of Crohn disease presents to the emergency department with postprandial abdominal pain and vomiting of 2 days' duration. He has been receiving infliximab (Remicade) infusions at 5 mg/kg every 8 weeks for the past 8 months. Before that time, he had taken prednisone 40 mg/d for several weeks intermittently for disease flare-ups. In addition, he had received Asacol (a 5-aminoslicylate: 5-ASA derivative), 2.4 g/d. The patient reports a 15-lb (6.8 kg) weight loss over the past 2 months. His past surgical history is significant for an appendectomy 4 years ago. On examination, his temperature is 38.0°C (100.4°F), pulse rate 96 beats/minute, and blood pressure 130/70 mm Hg. His abdomen is moderately distended and tender in the right lower quadrant. There are no masses or evidence of peritonitis. A rectal examination reveals no perianal disease or abnormalities. The remainder of his physical examination is unremarkable. The complete blood count reveals a WBC count of 14,000 mm^3, and his hemoglobin level is 10.5 g/dL. The results from the serum electrolyte studies and urinalysis are within the normal ranges.

▶ What is the most likely diagnosis?
▶ What is the next step?

ANSWERS TO CASE 26:

Crohn Disease

Summary: A 26-year-old man presents with a history of Crohn disease with disease exacerbation. Despite infliximab therapy, the patient's symptoms have not improved. Currently, he has nausea, vomiting, abdominal pain, distension, low-grade fever, and leukocytosis, which are suggestive of chronic small bowel obstruction and low-grade inflammatory or infectious process.

- **Most likely diagnosis:** Crohn disease, likely ileocolic, complicated by obstruction and possibly an intra-abdominal infectious process.

- **Next step:** Define the extent of disease involvement, the site of obstruction, and presence or absence of intra-abdominal abscesses. A computed tomography (CT) scan of the abdomen and pelvis and small bowel follow-through radiography (SBFT) should be performed. If these initial radiographic findings are suspicious for colonic involvement, then colonoscopy should be considered.

ANALYSIS

Objectives

1. Know the clinical features, diagnosis, and natural history of Crohn disease.

2. Be familiar with the medical therapy and the role of surgery in the care of patients with Crohn disease.

Considerations

A 26-year-old man presents with a 3-year history of Crohn disease that appears to be refractory to maintenance therapy with 5-ASA derivative and recent course of infliximab (anti-TNF-alpha therapy). Despite these treatments, the patient has had disease progression as evident by his weight loss and worsening symptoms. His clinical picture associated with Crohn disease can be due to **inflammation, fibrosis, penetration (fistulization)**, or combination of these processes. Inflammatory obstructions and certain fistulizing diseases are more likely to resolve with medical treatment regimens, whereas strictures that are primarily fibrotic in nature are less likely to respond to medications and may need operative treatment. The initial management of any patient with a known history of Crohn disease needs to start with a conversation between the surgeon and the patient's gastroenterologist. This discussion may help us appreciate prior treatments, responses to treatments, and long-term treatment plans that have been formulated and previously discussed with the patient and his family. Coordination of care between medical providers and surgical providers are especially important for the optimal and timely treatment of patients with Crohn disease.

APPROACH TO:
Crohn Disease

DEFINITIONS:

DISEASE ACTIVITY: Severity of disease can be assessed by histology, endoscopy, radiography, symptoms, or surgical findings. The histologic, radiographic, and surgical criteria do not always correlate with the clinical criteria and may not reflect the physiologic impact of the disease on the patient. It is always more important to know how the disease is affecting the patient rather than where or how extensive the disease is. The histologic finding of granulomas is pathognomonic for Crohn disease.

DISEASE PATTERNS: Crohn disease can be intra-abdominal, perianal, or both. Intra-abdominal Crohn disease is usually associated with one of three disease patterns: stricture, penetration, or inflammation. Perianal diseases can be associated with anal strictures, fistula-in-ano, or perirectal abscesses.

MEDICAL THERAPY FOR CROHN DISEASE: Pharmacologic therapy can be categorized as maintenance therapy (to maintain disease remission) or therapy for active disease (flare-ups). Medication prescribing approaches are described either as a "step-up" approach that begins treatment with the least aggressive medication and then add or change to "bigger guns" as needed or a "top-down" approach that begins treatment with the "biggest guns" and then de-escalate the treatment if the initial responses are favorable.

STEP-UP	TOP-DOWN
5-ASA/Sulfasalazine (First-line)	Biologic (First-line)
Corticosteroids	AZA/MTX
Azathioprine (AZA)/ methotrexate (MTX)	Combination therapy
Biologic (Last-line)	Corticosteroids (Last-line)

STRICTUREPLASTY: A surgical option that may be effective for patients with intestinal strictures from Crohn disease. The strictured segment of the intestine is opened longitudinally and then closed transversely, thus increasing the diameter of the bowel segment without having to remove that segment. This approach may help preserve bowel length and function for patients with involvement of multiple sites by fibrotic strictures.

CLINICAL APPROACH

Crohn disease is a complex, multifactorial disease with a strong genetic component that likely influences disease location, disease phenotype, age of onset, biologic behaviors, and responses to therapy. Most of the patients with Crohn disease exhibit distinct anatomic distribution of disease that is usually stable over time, with ileum and right colon involvement in 35% to 50% of patients, ileum involvement in

30% to 35% of patients, colon involvement in 25% to 35% of patients, and stomach and duodenal involvement in 0.5% to 4% of the patients. Anorectal involvement is common, especially among patients with small bowel Crohn disease. In 10% of patients with Crohn disease, anorectal disease is the initial manifestation of their disease; therefore, it is important to consider Crohn disease in the differential diagnosis whenever we encounter a patient with complex anorectal fistulizing disease. Some of the other symptoms can be nonspecific, and these may include chronic abdominal pain, postprandial crampy pain, weight loss, and fever. It is not uncommon for patients to present with these nonspecific complaints several months prior to their diagnosis.

The **Vienna Classification of Crohn disease** has been developed in the attempt to group and predict disease behaviors in patients. This system takes into account the age of diagnosis, anatomic location of disease, and disease type (inflammatory, fibrostenosis, or penetrating). Observations using this classification system have shown that disease locations for most patients remain stable over time. In contrast, the inflammatory components often diminish with disease progression, while the frequency of fibrostenosing and penetrating patterns increases.

The goals of management are to relieve symptoms and optimize the patient's quality of life. Medical and surgical therapies should be viewed as complementary therapeutic options rather than competing modalities. Thus, when medical therapy becomes ineffective or treatment significantly compromises the patient's quality of life, surgical options should be considered. The role of surgery in Crohn disease treatment is for palliation of symptoms and not to cure the disease. Therefore, surgical treatments should be directed toward symptom relief without exposing patients to excessive short-term and long-term morbidity. To optimize outcomes, the surgeons should discuss and coordinate surgical treatment plans with the patients' gastroenterologists, primary care physicians, and other members of the treatment team before proceeding with operative interventions.

Medical Therapy

The etiology of Crohn disease remains unknown, but it is in part caused by stimulation of an intestinal immune cascade in genetically susceptible individuals. The severity of disease dictates medical treatment, and many gastroenterologists use a sequential approach, using more aggressive medications for more aggressive manifestations, or so called a "bottom-up" approach. Categories of disease severity are broadly grouped as mild, moderate, and severe (Table 26–1). The commonly applied medical therapy can be grouped as nutritional, antimicrobial, anti-inflammatory, immunomodulatory, and antitumor necrosis factor (TNF) (see Table 26–2). Nutritional therapy includes bowel rest with total parenteral nutritional support, elemental feeding, or omega-3 fatty acid supplementation. Nutritional therapy has shown to improve symptoms and in some cases cause disease remission, but the major drawback is they are generally short-term treatments that are not sustainable. The first-line therapy for mild-to-moderate disease is usually either antimicrobial or anti-inflammatory modalities. Antimicrobial treatments, such as metronidazole or ciprofloxacin, are effective in resolving active intestinal and/or perianal diseases. Long-term metronidazole maintenance therapy is effective in preventing disease recurrence.

Table 26–1 • DISEASE SEVERITY OF CROHN DISEASE

Disease Severity	Clinical Presentation
Mild to moderate disease	Ambulatory, eating and drinking without dehydration, toxicity, abdominal tenderness, painful mass, obstruction or >10% weight loss
Moderate to severe disease	Failure of response to mild medical therapies or fevers, significant weight loss, abdominal pain or tenderness, intermittent nausea and vomiting (without obstructive findings) or significant anemia
Severe to fulminant disease	Persistent symptoms despite use of corticosteroids as outpatient or high fevers, persistent vomiting, evidence of intestinal obstruction, rebound tenderness, cachexia, evidence of abscess

Data from Friedman S. General principles of medical therapy of inflammatory bowel disease. Gastroenterol Clin North Am. 2004;33:191-208.

The mechanisms of action of antimicrobial therapy are largely unknown and may be in part based on its immunosuppressive effects. Long-term metronidazole treatment is poorly tolerated because of its associated nausea, metallic taste, disulfiram-like reactions, and peripheral neuropathies. Aminosalicylates (5-ASA) are effective in maintenance therapy and in the treatment of mild active disease. Limitations of 5-ASA derivatives include GI tract and systemic side effects, and hypersensitivity reactions.

Moderate to severe disease refractory to antimicrobials and inflammatory medications are typically treated with corticosteroids. Corticosteroids are

Table 26–2 • THERAPY FOR CROHN DISEASE

Agents	Indications	Adverse Effects
5-Aminosalicylate derivatives (sulfasalazine, Asacol, Pentasa)	Mild to moderate disease: maintenance therapy	Sperm abnormalities, folate malabsorption, nausea, dyspepsia, headache
Metronidazole	Mild to moderate disease: maintenance therapy	Nausea, metallic taste, peripheral neuropathy, disulfiram-like reaction
Corticosteroids	Moderate to severe disease: induce remission during acute flares	Multiple metabolic side effects
Azathioprine and 6-mercaptopurine	Moderate to severe disease: maintenance of remission after flare	Nausea, rash, fever, hepatitis, bone marrow suppression, B-cell lymphoma
Methotrexate	Moderate to severe disease: induce and maintain remission	Nausea, hepatotoxicity, bone marrow suppression, stomatitis
Cyclosporin A	Severe to fulminant disease	Hypertension, tremors, opportunistic infections, nephrotoxicity, paraesthesias, hepatotoxicity, gingival hyperplasia
Anti–tumor necrosis factor	Moderate to severe disease or severe perianal fistulizing disease	Abdominal pain, myalgias, lymphoma, teratogenic effects, delayed hypersensitivity reactions, nausea, fatigue

nonspecific anti-inflammatory agents that are effective in controlling small bowel and ileocolic diseases. Steroids are most commonly applied for disease flare-ups and then tapered or discontinued to avoid their long-term major side effects. Budesonide is a newer corticosteroid agent that is being utilized as it is metabolized more rapidly than prednisone and is associated with fewer side effects.

In patients with moderate to severe disease in remission after a course of corticosteroids treatment, immunomodulators are sometimes prescribed for maintenance therapy. **Azathioprine (AZT) and 6-mercaptopurine (6-MP)** are the most commonly used medications of this class. The major side effects of these medications are bone marrow suppression, nausea, fever, rash, hepatitis, and pancreatitis. Methotrexate is also used in the treatment of active disease, and this medication can cause nausea, headache, stomatitis, bone marrow suppression, hepatitis, and pneumonitis. Methotrexate is generally reserved for patients who are not able to take AZT or 6-MP.

Cyclosporine A (CSA) is another potent immunosuppressive medication that often produces disease improvements in patients with severe fistulizing diseases. CSA use is associated with some serious side effects, including hypertension, hyperesthesias, tremor, and nephrotoxicity. CSA use has been largely replaced by infliximab (a chimeric monoclonal antibody targeting the TNF receptor).

Infliximab is highly effective in the treatment of patients whose disease is refractory to all other treatments. Studies suggest that it may delay or obviate operative treatments for some patients with severe disease. It can also be used as the first-line treatment of patients with severe perianal fistulizing diseases. The major side effects and complications associated with this treatment include opportunistic infections and B-cell lymphoma development.

Recently, there has been some debate within the gastroenterology circle regarding the optimal strategy in the medical management of Crohn disease patients. Some practitioners believe that the "top-down" approach that initiates treatments with the most potent medication, and transitioning to the less potent medications after the patients response is a better approach than the traditional "treatment escalation" approach.

Surgical Management

The two most common reasons that surgeons are consulted for Crohn disease patients are medical treatment failures (unable to maintain employment, schooling, dietary intake, or maintain sufficient body weights due to failure to thrive or medical refractory disease), or when the medical treatment side effects affect quality of life. At other times, surgeons are asked to help treat disease complications including obstruction, fistulization, and neoplastic transformation. Adenocarcinoma of the small bowel is an unusual disease in the general population. However, the disease incidence is approximately 100 times greater in Crohn disease patients. Surgical treatment options include intestinal resection, strictureplasty, and intestinal bypass. Endoscopic dilatation of intestinal strictures is a new technique that is being applied for some patients with Crohn disease related intestinal obstructions. **When considering intestinal resections, the initial operations should be conservative** because 50% of patients will eventually require a second operation. One of the potential long-term complications associated with reoperative treatments for patients with Crohn disease is the loss of bowel length to maintain normal nutritional functions (short bowel syndrome); this complication is reported in less than 1% of patients with Crohn disease.

Postoperative Strategies

The initiation of medical therapies early during the postoperative periods has been suggested to reduce disease recurrences. Because these medications can affect wound healing and increase surgical complications, most practitioners recommend a slight delay before initiation of pharmacologic treatments after a surgical operation (10 days). The decision regarding timing and the types of medical treatments should be determined by a multidisciplinary team. Life-style modifications can affect the natural history of Crohn disease, and it has been well documented that **the use of nonsteroidal anti-inflammatory drugs (NSAIDs) and/or tobacco smoking have been linked to disease flare-ups and recurrences; therefore, the patient should be counseled regarding these risks.** For smokers, smoking cessation has been demonstrated to be associated with up to a 50% reduction in disease recurrences. Studies comparing the postoperative pharmacological treatments suggest that the anti-TNF strategy to be most effective in reducing recurrences after surgical therapy.

CASE CORRELATION

- See also Case 24 (Abdominal Pain [Right Lower Quadrant]) and Case 27 (Ulcerative Colitis).

COMPREHENSION QUESTIONS

26.1 Which of the following statement regarding Crohn disease behavior pattern is true?

A. The disease manifestation is consistent in terms of being inflammatory, stricturing, or penetrating

B. The anatomic locations remain fairly stable over the course of disease progression in most individuals

C. The penetrating disease never occurs as the initial manifestation

D. The disease commonly occurs in the esophagus

E. Anorectal disease is the initial presentation in 60% of patients

26.2 Which of the following anatomic distributions is most common for Crohn disease?

A. Stomach and duodenum

B. Colon

C. Ileum

D. Esophagus

E. Terminal ileum and right colon

26.3 Which of the following statements regarding surgery for Crohn disease is true?

A. Repeat operations are needed for 25% of the patients who require one operation

B. Surgical resection often cures patients with Crohn disease

C. Medical refractory disease is the most common indication for surgical treatments

D. Surgical therapy rarely improves the patient's quality of life

E. Surgical treatments should be avoided at all costs in this patient population

26.4 Four weeks following appendectomy for presumed acute appendicitis, a 23-year-old man returns to the emergency center with a small amount of drainage of enteric content-appearing fluid from his right lower quadrant incision. The patient is afebrile and has been tolerating a normal diet. The CT scan of the abdomen revealed postoperative inflammatory changes and no abscess. A review of the pathology report from his operation reveals involvement of the appendix base with transmural inflammation and granulomatous changes. Which of the following is the most appropriate treatment at this time?

A. Exploratory laparotomy to identify and remove the segment of intestine involved in the leakage of enteric contents

B. CT of the abdomen followed by injection of thrombogenic agent to plug the leakage

C. Corticosteroids

D. Infliximab

E. Exploration and cecectomy

26.5 A 22-year-old woman is newly diagnosed with Crohn disease of the terminal ileum. She complains of significant abdominal pain. Her temperature is 36.7°C (98.0°F) and heart rate is 90 beats/minute. Which of the following is the best management for this patient?

A. Exploratory celiotomy to assess for bowel perforation

B. Medical management and reassess

C. Radionucleotide-tagged leukocyte imaging study to assess the location of disease

D. Intravenous morphine for pain control

E. Exploratory laparotomy and strictureplasty

26.6 For which of the following symptoms of Crohn disease is medical treatment the best initial option?

A. Partial small bowel obstruction

B. Enterocolonic fistula

C. Abdominal pain related to an inflammatory mass

D. Perianal disease

E. All of the above

26.7 Which of the following has been found to be associated with Crohn disease recurrences?

A. Initial surgical treatment

B. Smoking

C. Narcotic analgesics

D. Protein/calorie malnutrition

E. Age

26.8 Which of the following medical treatments has been shown to be most effective in reducing recurrences of Crohn disease following surgical treatments?

A. Corticosteroids

B. Nutritional therapy

C. Anti-inflammatory therapy

D. Anti-TNF therapy

E. Immunosuppressive therapy

ANSWERS

26.1 **B.** Crohn disease anatomic locations remain fairly stable in most patients over the patient's lifetime. The disease characteristics can vary during the lifetime of the patient with Crohn disease, but the inflammatory pattern is the most common initial presenting pattern. Anorectal presentation is the initial presentation in 10% of patients. Crohn disease rarely affects the esophagus.

26.2 **E.** Terminal ileum/right colon disease is seen in 35% to 50% of patients; ileal disease is seen in 30% to 35% of patients; colonic disease is seen in 25% to 35% of patients; stomach/duodenal disease is seen in 0.5% to 4% of patients.

26.3 **C.** Medical refractory disease is the most common indication for surgery in Crohn disease patients. The role of surgery is to improve the patient's quality of life, and surgery has no impact on the disease itself. Repeat operations are required in up to 50% of surgical patients. Surgery is indicated when medical therapy is not working or if medical treatment side effects are compromising the patients' quality of life significantly.

26.4 **D.** This patient's presentation is compatible with enterocutaneous fistula presumably related to Crohn disease. Enterocutaneous fistula formation in the setting of Crohn disease does not always require surgical treatment, especially when it is associated with minimal amount of systemic systems. A trial of conservative treatment including infliximab may be helpful to promote spontaneous closure of the fistula. The rate of enteric fistula closure using infliximab has been reported to range from 6% to 70%.

26.5 **B.** Medical therapy is the appropriate choice for this patient with uncomplicated and newly diagnosed Crohn disease. A CT scan might be helpful during the initial evaluation to help rule-out the presence of intra-abdominal abscess and to rule out appendicitis.

26.6 **E.** Medical management may be effective for all of the findings/complications listed. Surgery is also indicated for these same complications if a patient does not respond to medical therapy, or if medical therapy compromises the patients' quality of life significantly.

26.7 **B.** Cigarette smoking has been linked to Crohn disease recurrences. Smoking cessation among postoperative patients is associated with 50% reduction in reoperation rates.

26.8 **D.** All of the medical therapies listed have been shown to help reduce the recurrence of Crohn disease following surgical therapy; however, anti-TFN treatment appears to have been the most effective.

CLINICAL PEARLS

▶ With the exception for the treatment of toxic colitis, emergency, unplanned operative treatment for patients with Crohn disease is rare.

▶ Fibrotic strictures cannot be resolved with medical therapy and generally require operative treatments to resolve the obstruction.

▶ Crohn disease may involve both the small bowel and colon; therefore, a complete evaluation should include colonoscopy and small bowel follow-through study to visualize the location and severity of the disease.

▶ Repeat resection of the GI tract for Crohn disease can result in the short bowel syndrome that requires long-term total parenteral nutrition (TPN) support in less than 1% of the patients with Crohn disease.

▶ In general, the role of surgery in Crohn disease is to relieve symptoms that are refractory to medical treatments (eg, pain, obstruction, weight loss) and to improve the quality of life of patients who experience severe medication-related side effects.

▶ Whether the initial medical treatment strategy for patients with severe Crohn disease should be a "bottom-up" or "top-down" approach is currently controversial.

REFERENCES

Howley I, Gearhart SL. The management of Crohn's disease of the small bowel. In Cameron JL, Cameron AM, eds. *Current Surgical Therapy*. 11th ed. Philadelphia, PA: Elsevier Saunders; 2014:113-117.

Michelassi F, Sultan S. Surgical treatment of complex small bowel Crohn disease. *Ann Surg.* 2014;260:230-235.

Singh S, Garg SK, Pardi DS, et al. Comparative efficacy of pharmacologic interventions in preventing relapse of Crohn's disease after surgery: a systematic review and network met-analysis. *Gastroenterol.* 2015;148:64-76.

A 45-year-old man with a 15-year history of ulcerative colitis (UC) is evaluated in the outpatient office because of chronic bloody diarrhea over the past 6 weeks. The patient's vital signs are normal. His hemoglobin level is 11.0 g/dL. His current medications consist of prednisone and mesalamine (a 5-aminosalicylate derivative), and he recently completed a course of cyclosporine therapy 2 months ago for another bout of disease flare-up. The patient has been unable to maintain full-time employment as an accountant over the past year because of UC exacerbations. Previous colonoscopy has shown that his disease extends from the rectum to the cecum.

▶ What should be your next step?
▶ What is the best therapy?

ANSWERS TO CASE 27:
Ulcerative Colitis

Summary: A 45-year-old man with pancolonic chronic UC that has become refractory to medical management and is causing him significant disability.

- **Next step:** The option of surgical therapy should be presented to this patient. The discussion should explain the benefits, risks, and limitations of surgery versus those of continued medical therapy.

- **Best therapy:** Proctocolectomy with ileal pouch-anal anastomosis.

ANALYSIS

Objectives

1. Learn with the clinical presentation, natural history, medical management, and complications of UC.

2. Learn the indications for urgent and elective operations for the treatment of UC.

3. Describe the surgical options and their outcomes for the treatment of UC.

Considerations

UC is a chronic disease with variability in severity and anatomic involvement. The symptoms associated with UC often respond to medicated enemas and systemic pharmacologic therapies. In this case, a 45-year-old man presents with a 15-year history of pancolitis that is producing disabling symptoms that appear to be refractory to medical therapy. The discussion regarding treatment should include medical treatment options as well as surgical options. Surgical resection of diseased colon and rectal segments would drastically improve the gastrointestinal (GI) symptoms associated with UC. However, the operation would result in permanent changes in bowel functions and body image. It is essential to convey to the patient that surgical removal of the bowel may improve some of the extraintestinal manifestations of UC, especially erythema nodosum, arthritis, and eye changes. Another important reason to consider surgical resection in this patient has to do with reducing the risk of colorectal cancer (CRC). The risk of CRC increases with the extent of UC involvement as well as the duration of disease. Proctocolectomy with ileal pouch reconstruction is an operation that would improve this patient's quality of life and reduce his risk for CRC development.

APPROACH TO:
Ulcerative Colitis

DEFINITIONS

FULMINANT COLITIS AND TOXIC MEGACOLON: Fulminant colitis is a condition characterized by abdominal pain, fever, and sepsis that develops in the setting of UC but may also occur with Crohn colitis and pseudomembranous colitis. Toxic megacolon occurs when these clinical findings are associated with radiographic evidence of significant colonic distension (transverse colon >8 cm diameter). The cecum is the most frequent site of involvement. Patient can become extremely ill with clinical signs of sepsis, and this condition is highly lethal if not promptly recognized and treated. When identified with either condition, the patient requires prompt fluid resuscitation, broad-spectrum antibiotics administration, and maximal supportive therapy. Roughly one-third of the patients affected will go on to require colectomies.

EXTRACOLONIC MANIFESTATIONS ASSOCIATED WITH UC: The extracolonic manifestations may include skin, joints, eyes, and liver. *Skin*-erythema nodosum and pyoderma gangrenosum are the two most common, and others include psoriasis stomatitis. *Joint*-peripheral and axial arthritis can occur. Type I peripheral arthropathy is acute and flares with the colitis. Type 2 arthropathy is chronic and typically involves more than six joints and can be migratory. Axial arthropathy manifestation includes ankolysing spondylitis and sacroiliitis, and these conditions can lead to decreased mobility and chronic disability. *GI*-primary sclerosing cholangitis, autoimmune hepatitis, and pancreatitis can occur. *Eyes*-uveitis, scleritis, and optic neuritis.

DYSPLASIA: A premalignant transformation of the mucosa caused by chronic UC. The risk of cancer associated with dysplasia varies depending on the severity of the dysplastic changes. Roughly 40% of the patients with high-grade dysplasia harbor synchronous cancers, and 20% of patients with low-grade dysplasia harbor synchronous cancers.

DYSPLASIA ASSOCIATED LESIONS OR MASS (DALM): This is a sessile pseudopolyp arising from dysplastic mucosa affected by chronic UC. Fifty percent of patients with DALM have carcinomas within these lesions. Patients with these findings should be recommended to undergo proctocolectomy.

PANCOLITIS: This refers to UC involvement extending from the rectum to the distal small bowel. Patients with this disease pattern have a significantly greater risk of developing cancers in comparison to individuals with shorter segments of colonic involvement. Prophylactic proctocolectomies are generally recommended for patients with pancolitis of significant durations.

UC SURVEILLANCE RECOMMENDATIONS: The current recommendation from the American Gastroenterological Association recommends that patients with at least one-third of their colon involved with UC undergo initial screening colonoscopy and multiple quadrants biopsies 8 years after disease diagnosis, followed by subsequent surveillance colonoscopies with biopsies every 1 to 3 years.

ILEAL-J-POUCH: A neorectum constructed from the terminal ileum in the shape of a J. This pouch can then be attached to the anus to form an ileal-j-pouch to anal anastomosis.

CONTINENT ILEOSTOMY (KOCH POUCH): This is a surgical reconstruction option following total proctocolectomy when there is no remaining anus or rectal sphincters left remaining. The terminal ileum is fashioned to create a pouch with 500 to 1000 mL capacity and invagination of the ileum just below the fascia is constructed to provide continence. The pouch is emptied with the placement of a drainage catheter. Because the drainage mechanisms are prone to failure in a high percentage of patients, this procedure is rarely done today.

TOTAL PROCTOCOLECTOMY WITH ILEAL–RECTAL ANASTOMOSIS: The resection involves removal of the entire colon and the majority of the rectum except for the last few cm segment of the distal rectum. The procedure has the advantage of being technically easier to reconstruct; however, the major disadvantage is that cancer-prone mucosa is left behind and requires close surveillance.

POUCHITIS: Idiopathic inflammatory process involving the ileal pouch that can develop following J-pouch formations. Patients may present with any number of symptoms, including increased stool frequencies, fecal urgency, fecal incontinence, watery diarrhea, bleeding, abdominal cramps, fever, and malaise. Bacterial overgrowth can be a contributing factor for pouchitis. Therefore, most patients with pouchitis improve with a course of antibiotic treatment. Approximately 50% of patients following ileal-pouch reconstructions will have at least one episode of pouchitis, and 10% to 15% of patients will develop chronic pouchitis.

CLINICAL APPROACH

UC is a chronic, inflammatory condition of unknown etiology. Patients typically present with bloody diarrhea, abdominal pain, urgency, and tenesmus of varying severity with episodes of remissions and flare-ups. Gastrointestinal infections, nonsteroidal inflammatory drugs (NSAIDs), and antibiotics have all been implicated in the development of UC. Enteric infections by *Salmonella* or *Campylobacter* species have been shown to correlate with disease development. Similarly, the chronic use of NSAIDs in women is associated with increased risk of UC. Antibiotic exposure, particularly tetracyclines, has also been linked to UC development. UC appears to follow a familial distribution; however, the risk of first-degree relatives of a patient with UC developing the disease is only 10% to 25%. Unlike Crohn disease, cigarette smoking appears to confer a protective effect against UC development, and smoking cessation seems to be associated with disease development. **Histologically, UC differs from Crohn disease in that the disease is limited to the mucosa as opposed to transmural in Crohn disease.**

The diagnosis of UC is based on typical symptoms and endoscopic evidence of continuous colonic inflammation beginning in the rectum. Occasionally, UC may

Table 27–1 • UC DISEASE SEVERITY

Disease severity	Clinical picture
Mild	<4 stools/day; no systemic signs; normal inflammatory markers
Moderate	>4 but <6 stools/day; minimal signs of toxicity
Severe	>6 but <10 stools/day; demonstrates systemic signs of toxicity; elevated inflammatory markers
Fulminant	>10 stools/day; with clinical signs of toxicity; abdominal distension; blood transfusion requirement; dilated colon by imaging

Inflammatory markers: Erythrocyte sedimentation rate, C-reactive protein.
Systemic toxicity: Fever, tachycardia, anemia, and elevated inflammatory markers.

present with skipped areas of inflammation in the colon. The anatomic extent of UC can be described as proctitis (rectal involvement only), proctosigmoiditis (rectum and sigmoid colon), left-sided disease (disease does not extend beyond the splenic flexture), extensive colitis (disease extends beyond the splenic flexture), and pancolitis (disease extends all the way to the ileal–cecal valve). See Table 27–1 for description of severity of UC.

Treatment of UC

Treatments generally follow a "step-up" approach that is similar to that described for Crohn disease treatment. Patients with mild-to-moderate disease are often treated with 5-ASA by oral, rectal, or both routes. Flare-ups or bouts of disease exacerbations can be controlled with short courses of corticosteroids treatment (induction therapy), with transition to nonsteroidal agents once the patient's disease is under control. Immunosuppressive agents such as thiopurines and anti-TNF antibody (infliximab) are also effective in inducing and maintaining remissions. Recent observations suggest that the combination of infliximab and azathioprine may be more effective than either agent alone.

Patients who present with fulminant colitis associated with UC need to be closely monitored in hospital settings and treated with intravenous steroids. Generally two-third of the patients will respond to this treatment; however, for the one-third of patients who do not respond to intravenous steroids, rescue therapy with infliximab, intravenous cyclosporine, or surgical resection will need to be expeditiously implemented.

UC is a chronic inflammatory disease that is typically treated with medical management; however, 10% to 15% of patients with the disease may require colectomy either due to refractory disease or complications. Operative treatments for patients under these circumstances generally consist of total abdominal colectomy with end ileostomy formation, and with the removal of significant portions of the diseased burden. The patient's conditions generally improve. Preservation of the rectal segment during the initial operation gives patients the opportunity to undergo completion proctectomy and ileal–anal J-pouch reconstruction when the patient's conditions stabilizes. See Table 27–2 for surgical options.

Table 27–2 • SURGICAL OPTIONS FOR ULCERATIVE COLITIS			
Surgical Procedure	**Indication**	**Advantages**	**Disadvantages**
Abdominal colectomy with ileostomy	Acute toxic colitis; less frequently for other indications	Less morbidity under urgent settings	Cancer risk in rectum up to 15%-20% at 25-30 y
Abdominal colectomy with ileorectal anastomosis	For intractability or cancer or dysplasia	Preservation of bowel functions with acceptable results in patients with limited rectal disease	Cancer risk in rectum up to 15%-20% at 25-30 y; patients can have continued symptoms
Total proctocolectomy with permanent ileostomy	For intractability or cancer or dysplasia	All colorectal diseases removed with symptom resolution	Permanent ileostomy
Total proctocolectomy with ileal pouch-anal anastomosis	For intractability or cancer or dysplasia	All colorectal diseases removed with symptom resolution and maintenance of transanal continence	4-12 bowel movements per day; some have day or nighttime incontinence; pouchitis (7%-40%)
Total proctocolectomy with continent ileostomy	For intractability or cancer or dysplasia	All colorectal diseases removed with symptom resolution; patients do not require external stoma appliance	High malfunction rate associated with the nipple valve requiring revision or urgent cannulation for drainage

Selective Adhesion Molecule Inhibitors

In 2014, the Food and Drug Administration (FDA) approved the use of **vedolizumab** for use in patients with moderate to severe UC when standard treatments fail. Vedolizumab is the first selective adhesion molecule inhibitor developed. It blocks leukocyte migration that, which is believed to be a cause of inflammation associated with UC. Early observations suggest that this drug is associated with few adverse reactions and does not lead to the increase in infectious risks.

Colorectal Cancer Risks Associated with UC

Patients with long-segment UC have increased risks of developing adenocarcinoma of the colon and rectum. These cancers are different from the usual colorectal cancers in that these cancers generally do not develop from polyps. A patient with a UC history for more than 8 years should undergo initial surveillance colonoscopy with biopsies from multiple quadrants, and subsequent surveillance colonoscopies every 1 to 3 years. If a surveillance program is not instituted or not feasible, then a prophylactic proctocolectomy should be considered. The classic report of colorectal cancer risks associated with UC stated up to 5% to 10% risk at 20 years, and up to 12% to 30% risk after 30 to 35 years of disease; however, recent data suggests that the risks have been generally over-estimated. Factors associated with an increased risk of CRC include diagnosis of UC prior to age 15, duration of disease, anatomic extent of disease, family history of colorectal cancers, history of sclerosing cholangitis, male sex, shortened colon, and the presence of strictures or pseudopolyps.

Surgery for UC Patients

The main indications for surgical therapy in UC are for treatment of fulminant colitis or toxic megacolon, the treatment of dysplasia and cancers, and the treatment of medically refractory disease. The most commonly performed operation for the treatment of fulminant colitis is total abdominal colectomy with end ileostomy formation. This operation gives patients the opportunity to recover from their acute disease, with the possibility for a second operation where completion proctectomy with ileal–anal J-pouch reconstruction can restore continence. If a patient does not have functional nalsphincters, permanent end ileostomy or continent-ileostomy (Koch Pouch) are the remaining long-term options. Following proctocolectomy and J-pouch reconstruction, most patients experience 4 to 6 bowel movements a day and have occasional minor soilage. Preoperative patient counseling and patient education, and proper patient selection are critical factors for long-term patient satisfaction.

COMPREHENSION QUESTIONS

27.1 Which of the following statements regarding UC-related colorectal cancer is true?

    A. Surveillance colonoscopy every 1-3 years is recommended for patients with UC involving the rectal-sigmoid segment

    B. Colorectal cancer risk of UC patients is not influenced by family history of colorectal cancers

    C. Women have increased risk

    D. UC patients with more than one-third of their colons involved by UC and sclerosing cholangitis should undergo yearly colonoscopy once surveillance begins

    E. There is no evidence to support yearly surveillance colonoscopies in UC patients

27.2 Which of the following patients can be described as having moderately severe UC?

    A. 3 bloody bowel movements a day, no systemic signs, and normal C-reactive protein level

    B. 12 bloody bowel movement a day, fever of 39.0°C (102.2°F), elevated C-reactive protein level

    C. 8 bloody bowel movements a day, temperature of 38.3°C (100.9°F), mildly elevated C-reactive protein level

    D. 5 bloody bowel movements a day, temperature of 38.0°C (100.4°F), normal C-reactive protein level

    E. 5 bloody bowel movements a day, temperature of 39.0°C (102.2°F), and elevated C-reactive protein level

27.3 Which of the following statements regarding UC is true?

A. Proctocolectomy is associated with improvements in some extracolonic manifestations associated with UC

B. The risk of colorectal cancer in UC patients has been markedly underestimated

C. The peak age at diagnosis is the 6th decade

D. Tobacco smoking is associated with disease exacerbation

E. The rectum is typically spared from disease in most patient with UC

27.4 A 46-year-old woman underwent total abdominal colectomy and ileostomy formation for a severe bout of colitis associated with sepsis one year ago. She has recovered and now desires restoration of GI tract continuity. Which of the following findings would be considered a contraindication for completion proctectomy and ileal pouch-anal anastomosis?

A. The finding of high grade dysplasia in the rectal segment at 10 cm from the anal verge

B. The finding of high grade dysplasia with carcinoma in situ in the previously resected colon

C. The finding of granulomatous changes and transmural inflammatory changes in the previously resected colon

D. A prior history of alcohol induced pancreatitis

E. Presence of mucosal ulcerations without dysplasia in the remaining rectum

27.5 A 40-year-old woman with 15-year history of chronic diarrhea and diagnosis of UC is referred for consideration for total proctocolectomy with ileal–anal J-pouch reconstruction to reduce future risks of developing cancer. During the colonoscopy, you notice that the disease involves the entire colon and terminal ileum, with sparing of the rectum. Which of the following is the most appropriate treatment?

A. Proctocolectomy with ileal pouch-anal anastomosis

B. Total abdominal colectomy with ileal–rectal anastomosis

C. Repeat biopsy of the rectum and the involved colon and ileum

D. Total proctocolectomy with construction of continent ileostomy

E. Total colectomy and ileal pouch-rectal anastomosis

27.6 A 35-year-old woman with ulcerative colitis for approximately 15 years undergoes colonoscopy, revealing an area of colonic dysplasia described as high-grade. Which of the following is the best management for this patient?

A. Surgical resection of the colon and rectum

B. Intensive medical therapy and re-evaluation with colonoscopy in 3 months

C. Shorten the interval between screening colonoscopies to 3 months

D. Add an immunosuppressive agent to her medical therapy

E. Initiate chemoprevention with a COX2 inhibitor

ANSWERS

27.1 **D.** Screening and surveillance colonoscopy with biopsies is recommended in patients with at least left-sided disease (>one-third of colon involvement) or pancolitis. The recommendation of initial screening is at 8 years after disease diagnosis. The associated finding of sclerosing cholangitis further increases the risk of colorectal cancers, and these patients are recommended to have yearly colonoscopy and biopsy. Men have higher risk for cancers. Patients with proctitis or protosigmoiditis do not have significantly increased risk of colorectal cancers. A family history of colorectal cancer in a first-degree relative confers an additional 2-fold to 3-fold increase in cancer risk.

27.2 **D.** Moderate disease severity is defined by more than four but less than six stools/day, minimal signs of systemic toxicity, normal or minimally increased inflammatory markers. The patient described in "A" has mild disease. The patient described in "B" has fulminant disease. The patient described in "C" has severe disease.

27.3 **A.** Proctocolectomy is associated with some improvements in extracolonic disease manifestations, particularly erythema nodosum, arthritis, and some eye changes. The risk of colorectal cancers in UC patients had been over-estimated in the past; currently the high-risk groups are believed to be patients with greater than one-third colon involvement for greater than 8 years. The peak age at diagnosis is during the second and third decades of life.

27.4 **C.** The findings of granulomatous changes and transmural inflammatory changes suggest the diagnosis of Crohn colitis, and proctocolectomy with ileal J-pouch to anal reconstruction is not an appropriate operation for treatment in a patient with Crohn disease.

27.5 **C.** The colonoscopy finding of rectal sparing disease with terminal ileum involvement raises the question that ulcerative colitis is not the correct diagnosis, and the patient may actually have Crohn disease. Repeat biopsies are indicated at this time.

27.6 **A.** High-grade dysplasia found on colonic surveillance in a patient with UC needs to be treated with proctocolectomy because of the risk of cancers being present already and the risk for future cancer development.

CLINICAL PEARLS

▶ The main indications for surgical therapy in UC are fulminant colitis, toxic megacolon, dysplasia or cancer, and intractable disease.

▶ Extra-intestinal manifestations of UC include ankolysing spondylitis, uveitis, erythemasnodosum, sclerosing cholangitis, and dermatomyositis. Proctocolectomy is associated in improvements in some of the extra-clonic processes.

▶ Surgical and medical therapy for UC are complementary and not competing modalities.

▶ The term "refractory to medical management" is not strictly defined and should refer to failure of appropriate medical therapy as well as patient intolerance to the adverse effects of medical therapy.

▶ Transmural inflammation and sparing of the rectum should raise suspicion of Crohn disease rather than UC.

▶ Vedolizumab is a newer selective adhesion molecule inhibitor that is effective for the treatment of UC.

▶ Approximately, 10% to 15% of patients with UC will develop complications or refractory disease to medical management and will need surgical treatments.

REFERENCES

Fang SH, Efron JE. The management of chronic ulcerative colitis. In: Cameron JL, Cameron AM, eds. *Current Surgical Therapy*. 11th ed. Philadelphia, PA: Elsevier Saunders; 2014:154-160.

Feurstein JD, Cheifetz AS. Ulcerative colitis: epidemiology, diagnosis, and management. *Mayo Clin Proc.* 2014;89:1553-1563.

Kedia S, Ahuja V, Tandon R. Management of severe ulcerative colitis. *World J Gastrointest Pathophysiol.* 2014;5:579-588.

Lowenberg M, D'Haens G. Next-generation therapeutics for IBD. *Curr Gastroenterol Rep.* 2015;17:21-29.

A 62-year-old man presents to the emergency center with a 1-week history of left lower quadrant abdominal pain. He complains of increased pain, mild nausea, and subjective fever. The patient indicates a prior similar episode that was milder and lasting several days once before. The previous episode resolved with oral antibiotics as an outpatient. The patient is otherwise healthy and without risk factors for cardiac or pulmonary diseases. On examination, his temperature is 38.2°C (100.8°F). Blood pressure is 140/80 and pulse rate is 106 beats/minute. His abdomen is soft and mildly distended, with localized tenderness to palpation in the left lower quadrant. He does not have evidence of generalized peritonitis. His white blood cell (WBC) count is 17,000/mm³.

▶ What is the most likely diagnosis?
▶ How would you confirm the diagnosis?
▶ What are the complications associated with this disease process?

ANSWERS TO CASE 28:
Diverticulitis

Summary: A 62-year-old man presents with signs and symptoms compatible with recurrent acute diverticulitis.

- **Most likely diagnosis:** Acute sigmoid diverticulitis.

- **Confirmation of diagnosis:** A CT scan of the abdomen and pelvis will help with radiographic confirmation and identify complications; however, this patient will need endoscopy to rule out colon cancer after the acute inflammation resolves.

- **Associated complications:** Perforation, abscess formation, bowel obstruction, and fistula development are potential complications.

ANALYSIS

Objectives

1. Learn the pathophysiology of diverticulitis.

2. Learn the work-up and management of patients with diverticulitis.

3. Learn the severity-grading of diverticulitis.

4. Be aware of the current controversies in the management.

Consideration

This patient's history of repeated episodes of left lower quadrant pain and fever are highly suggestive of recurrent acute diverticulitis. Although it is somewhat reassuring that he does not have generalized peritonitis, his fever, tachycardia, and leukocytosis are nevertheless concerning to us. **A CT scan of the abdomen would be helpful to differentiate between uncomplicated diverticulitis and complicated diverticulitis (disease associated with perforation, abscess, phlegmon, stricture, obstruction, or fistula).** The CT scan findings will help us determine if the additional therapeutic interventions such as percutaneous drainage or operative treatment will be needed. Most of the patients with localized diverticulitis can be managed with antibiotic treatments alone, even when small (<2 cm) mesenteric abscesses are present. For this patient, it is reasonable to initiate broad-spectrum intravenous antibiotics, obtain the CT scan, and admit the patient for in-patient observation. Patients with uncomplicated diverticulitis may be managed with outpatient antibiotics; however, in this case, because the patient exhibits some systemic signs of sepsis (fever and tachycardia), it is safer to treat him initially as an in-patient and then transition him to outpatient care when these systemic signs of infection resolve. A number of antibiotics options are available, and the principle behind antibiotic treatment is to select broad-spectrum coverage targeting Gram-negative organisms and anaerobes (eg, second-generation or third-generation cephalosporin + metronidazole, fluoroquinolone + metronidazole, or single agent such as meropenem).

APPROACH TO:
Diverticulitis

DEFINITIONS

DIVERTICULOSIS: These are defined as outpouchings of the colon that do not contain all layers of the colonic wall musculature. Diverticulosis most frequently occurs in the sigmoid colon. The location of the diverticulum is usually on the mesenteric side of the colon at anatomically weakened areas where blood vessels enter the colon. The formation of colon diverticuli is believed to be contributed by the consumption of lower-fiber and higher fat western-type diets.

DIVERTICULITIS: Inflammation of the diverticulum caused by obstruction of the "neck" of the outpouching leading to localized infection. This process can occur with or without microperforation.

DIVERTICULAR PHLEGMON: This describes an inflammatory mass related to diverticulitis. Clinically and radiographically, this clinical entity is difficult to differentiate from a colorectal cancer; therefore, patients with diverticular phlegmon will need to have colonoscopy to evaluate the area after the acute inflammation has resolved (usually in 4 to 6 weeks).

COLOVESICULAR FISTULA: This describes a fistula communication between the lumen of the colon and the urinary bladder. Most commonly, the condition is recognized when a patient complains of pneumaturia (air passage during urination), fecaluria (passage of stool in urine), or recurrent urinary infections. A small percentage of the patients with colovesicular fistulas have complex infections of the bladder or bladder cancer as the primary cause, and in these cases, the bladder is the "offending organ" and the colon is the "victim organ".

HINCHEY CLASSIFICATION OF COMPLICTED DIVERTICULITIS	
Class I	Colonic inflammation with peri-colic abscess confined by the colon mesentery
Class II	Colonic inflammation with localized retroperitoneal or pelvic abscess
Class III	Colonic inflammation with generalized purulent peritonitis
Class IV	Colonic inflammation with generalized fecal peritonitis

Hinchey I–II diverticulitis can generally be treated with nonoperative treatment by antibiotic alone or antibiotics + drainage.

Hinchey III–IV diverticulitis patients are associated with high failure rates and recurrences when managed nonoperatively.

CT-CLASSIFICATION OF DIVERTICULITIS SEVERITY		
Mild	Moderate	Severe
Thickening of the colonic wall with inflammation	Thickening of the colonic wall with inflammation of colon and pericolic fat, localized edema with fat stranding in the mesentery	Pericolic abscess or remote abscess; colonic stenosis; extravasation of contrast; free air; abscess; nonlocalized peritoneal stranding and inflammation

CLINICAL APPROACH

The clinical diagnosis of diverticulitis can be made on the basis of history and physical examination. Most cases of diverticulitis are located in the sigmoid colon; however, diverticulitis of the cecum can occasionally occur. A cecal diverticulum is a true diverticulum that contain all layers of the colon.

When the diagnosis is uncertain, the patient exhibits systemic toxicity, or when there is lack of improvement with initial treatment, a CT scan of the abdomen and pelvis can be helpful to confirm the diagnosis and stage the disease. In the acute setting, barium enema and colonoscopy are contraindicated, since these procedures involve increasing colonic pressure and can exacerbate the diverticulitis, and don't provide additional information to help direct the acute management.

Uncomplicated Diverticulitis

Antibiotic treatment is the mainstay of therapy for patients with diverticulitis. Outpatient treatment is as effective as in-patient therapy with uncomplicated disease. Oral antibiotics are generally prescribed in outpatient settings, even though there is no clear evidence to support their use as hastening resolution or preventing recurrences. Commonly prescribed outpatient antibiotics include quinolone + metronidazole, or amoxicillin/clavulanate. The optimal duration of antibiotics therapy is unknown. Patients who are immune-compromised, exhibiting signs of sepsis, frail, or unreliable should be managed initially with intravenous antibiotics and in-patient monitoring. See Figure 28–1 for management of uncomplicated diverticulitis.

Follow-Up Care for Patients with Diverticulitis

Four to six weeks after the resolution of diverticulitis episodes, patients should undergo colonoscopy to rule out colon malignancy, as colon cancers with local perforations can mimic the clinical and radiographic findings of diverticulitis. Traditionally, high-fiber diet has been recommended for patients to prevent diverticulitis recurrences. Unfortunately, there is no clinical evidence to prove that dietary modification helps to prevent recurrences. Randomized trials suggest that the oral antibiotic rifaximin or rifaximin + fiber administration following bouts of diverticulitis improved patients' symptoms; however, these treatments were not associated with reduction in recurrences. Mesalazine (an anti-inflammatory agent) and probiotics have been applied for the treatment of diverticulitis, and clinical trial

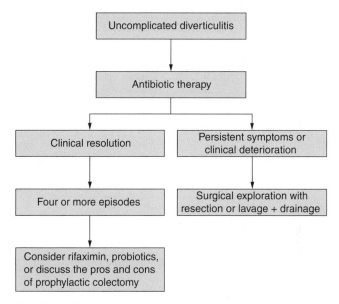

Figure 28–1. Algorithm for the management of uncomplicated diverticulitis.

findings suggest that these treatments are associated with the reduction in symptoms recurrences.

Complicated Diverticulitis and Indications for Surgery

Surgery for the treatment of diverticulitis can be broadly divided into surgery for complications and surgery for the prevention of diverticulitis recurrence (see Figure 28-2). Patients who present with Hinchey class III or class IV disease frequently require urgent operations to control the sources of sepsis. In most cases, the operations consist of segmental colon resection with formation of a temporary end-colostomy (Hartmann's procedure). The reason for the colostomy rather than primary anastomosis in the acute setting is that healing of the anastomosis under these less than ideal conditions can predispose to high rates of anastomotic complications. After the patients recover from their infectious process, these colostomies can be reversed. To avoid the inconveniences and complications associated with colostomies, some surgeons have advocated an initial operation consisting of laparoscopic peritoneal lavage with placement of drains to minimize the intraperitoneal infections. The laparoscopic lavage and drainage approach has been reported to be effective in small, single-center patient populations.

Patients with recurrent bouts of diverticulitis can develop signs and symptoms of large bowel obstruction that require surgical treatments. For these patients, it is important to attempt to determine if the obstruction is related to a cancer or diverticulitis, which is helpful in the planning of the operation. Because resections for patients with colonic obstructions often required the formation of temporary colostomies, some groups have attempted to relieve the obstructive processes with the endoscopic placement of colonic stents prior to attempting colon resections.

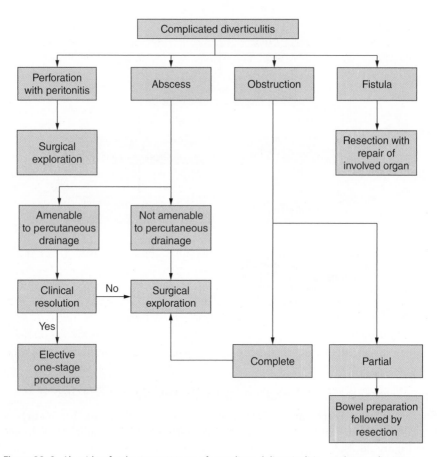

Figure 28–2. Algorithm for the management of complicated diverticulitis—early complications.

Patients with complicated diverticulitis associated with colovesicular fistulas should undergo resection of the segment of colon involved with the fistula. At this operation, the opening in the bladder can be primarily repaired. Prior to the operation, it is helpful to identify the "offending organ" and the "victim organ." In most cases, CT scan, preoperative colonoscopy, and cystoscopy will help to rule out primary bladder pathology such as bladder cancer as the cause of the condition.

In the past, elective surgical resections with primary anastomoses have been suggested for patients who present with recurrent bouts of diverticulitis. The rationale for elective resection in these patients is to prevent the morbidity and mortality associated diverticulitis recurrence. At one time, the standard recommendation was to offer elective colectomy after the second bout of diverticulitis. Based on a decision tree cost-effective analysis published in 2004, many practitioners shifted toward a strategy of elective colectomies for patients after four episodes of diverticulitis. More recently, based on the observations that recurrence rates are lower than previously described, and that conservative treatment outcomes are significantly improved with modern medical management, many surgeons no longer perform prophylactic-colon resections for this disease. **Rather than operating after a set number of episodes of diverticulitis, the current recommendations are to discuss the pros and cons of elective resections and expectant management with patients so that a rational decision can be made for each individual patient.**

CASE CORRELATION

- See also Case 23 (Lower GI Tract Hemorrhage), Case 24 (Abdominal Pain [Right Lower Quadrant]), Case 26 (Crohn Disease), and Case 27 (Ulcerative Colitis).

COMPREHENSION QUESTIONS

28.1 A 57-year-old man presents to his primary care physician with left lower quadrant abdominal pain of 5 days duration, nausea, and vomiting. He is not able to maintain normal oral intake at home. On presentation, he has mild tenderness to palpation in the left lower quadrant without peritoneal signs. His WBC is 14,000/mm³. He denies ever having these symptoms in the past. Which of the following is the most appropriate treatment for this patient?

A. Hospitalize for bowel rest, administer intravenous fluids and antibiotics, and monitor patient

B. Begin a course of outpatient antibiotics and encourage fluid intake

C. Obtain a barium enema to rule out diverticulitis

D. Consult a surgeon for discussions regarding colectomy to prevent future episodes of the process

E. Immediate operative treatment with segmental colectomy and formation of temporary colostomy

28.2 A 61-year-old woman presents to the emergency department with left-sided abdominal pain of 10 days' duration. She has been constipated over this period of time and had her last bowel movement 2 days ago. She also complains of fever up to 38.9°C (102°F) at home. Over the past 24 hours, the patient has vomited several times. On examination, her abdomen is diffusely tender to palpation. Plain films demonstrate dilated loops of small bowel and dilated air-filled right, transverse, and proximal descending colon, and no air in the rectum. Her WBC count is 26,000/mm³. Which of the following is the most appropriate treatment for this patient?

A. Obtain a barium enema to confirm diverticulitis and colonic obstruction

B. Flexible sigmoidoscopy to evaluate the source of obstruction

C. Admission to the hospital for observation and intravenous hydration, and repeat the abdominal films in 24 hours

D. Admission for intravenous antibiotics, intravenous hydration

E. Surgical exploration of the abdomen

28.3 A 53-year-old woman presents to her primary care physician with complaints of pneumaturia and recurrent bouts of urinary tract infections. She has a prior history of diverticulitis 6 months ago that required hospitalization for antibiotics treatment. Which of the following tests is most likely to lead to the diagnosis?

A. CT scan of the abdomen and pelvis

B. Urinalysis

C. Intravenous pyelogram (IVP)

D. Colonoscopy

E. Cystography

28.4 Which of the following is the most common cause of gastrointestinal tract fistulas?

A. Appendicitis

B. Ulcerative colitis

C. Crohn disease

D. Diverticulitis

E. Colon cancer

28.5 For which of the following patients is sigmoid colectomy most indicated?

A. 30-year-old man with two bouts of sigmoid diverticulitis that were successfully treated with antibiotics, and he is currently asymptomatic

B. A 56-year-old man with a recent bout of diverticulitis that was treated successfully with antibiotics as an outpatient. He subsequently underwent colonoscopy that revealed diverticula and no mucosal abnormalities. The patient is highly concerned about having colon cancer because his brother was just recently diagnosed with colon cancer

C. A 57-year-old man with a history of diverticulitis that has required three prior hospitalizations for localized phlegmon of the sigmoid colon. Even though the inflammation has mostly resolved, he continues to have significant pain

D. A 66-year-old woman with five prior episodes of diverticulitis, requiring hospitalization on two occasions. Her symptoms have resolved, and she has been symptoms-free for the past 8 months

E. A 60-year-old otherwise healthy man was hospitalized 2 months ago for diverticulitis with an abscess. He was successfully treated with antibiotics and CT-guided drainage of the abscess. He has remained without symptoms for the past 5 weeks

28.6 Which of the following statements is TRUE regarding diverticulitis?

    A. Patients with diverticulitis diagnosed prior to 40 years of age should have sigmoid colectomy performed to prevent future occurrences

    B. Patients with four or more bouts of diverticulitis should have elective colectomy to prevent future occurrences

    C. High-fiber diet has been shown to prevent diverticulitis recurrences

    D. Rifaximin is effective in improving symptoms related to diverticulitis

    E. Colectomies performed for patients with diverticulitis complications should target the removal of all diverticula within the colon

ANSWERS

28.1 **A.** Hospitalization for hydration, antibiotics therapy, and monitoring is the most appropriate choice given this patient is not able to tolerate oral intake at home. Surgical resection may be indicated if the patient develops further complications related to his diverticulitis, however the operation will not be done to prevent further episodes of diverticulitis.

28.2 **E.** This patient has signs and symptoms of large bowel obstruction and evidence of ongoing infectious process in the abdomen. Given these findings, surgical exploration is the most appropriate approach listed. CT scan would be helpful to obtain prior to abdominal exploration, however that is not a given option here.

28.3 **A.** A CT scan of the abdomen and pelvis is the best choice given here for identifying the colovesicular fistula. Most of these fistulas related to diverticulitis will involve the dome of the bladder. CT scan will demonstrate the bladder proximity to the colon and often demonstrate air within the bladder and associated bladder thickening at the location. Surprisingly, colonoscopies often do not help identify the location of the fistula.

28.4 **D.** All of the choices listed can be associated with the formation of fistulous tracts from the GI tract to an adjacent organ, with diverticulitis being the most common cause of fistula formation.

28.5 **C.** The main reason for performing colectomies in patients with diverticulitis is to relieve symptoms related to the process or help control a source of sepsis or obstruction. The patient in choice C has ongoing pain related to his diverticulitis, and colectomy may help improve his symptoms. All of the patients presented in the other choices have had significant history of diverticulitis but have become free of symptoms following nonoperative management; therefore, they are not likely to benefit from colon resections.

28.6 **D.** Rifaximin administration for patients with uncomplicated diverticulitis has been shown to control pain and symptoms related to their disease. High-fiber diet is a common recommendation given to patients, however this strategy has not been shown to help prevent diverticulitis recurrences or improve symptoms. Removal of all colon containing diverticula during operations for complications of diverticulitis has not been found to help reduce the risk of recurrence; in fact, this approach can lead to increased complications.

CLINICAL PEARLS

▶ CT imaging is helpful in identifying and guiding percutaneous drainage of diverticular abscesses.

▶ Diverticulitis is the most common cause of GI tract fistulas.

▶ Observations suggest that only 10% to 15% of patients with diverticulitis ultimately require surgical therapy.

▶ Hinchey classification helps categorize complicated diverticulitis severity.

▶ Most patients with Hinchey I and II disease can be managed without operative treatments.

▶ Surgical treatment of diverticulitis is directed toward the management of complications related to the disease and not to prevent future diverticulitis episodes.

REFERENCES

Biondo S, Lopez Borao J, Kreisler E, Jaurrieta E. Current status of the treatment of acute colonic diverticulitis: a systematic review. *Colorectal Dis.* 2011;14:e1-e11.

Ferrada P, Ivatury RR. The management of diverticular disease of the colon. In: Cameron JL, Cameron AM, eds. *Current Surgical Therapy.* 11th ed. Philadelphia, PA: Elsevier Saunders; 2014:149-153.

Medina-Fernandez FJ, Diaz-Jimenez N, Gallardo-Herrera AB, et al. New trends in the management of diverticulitis and colonic diverticular disease. *Rev Esp Enferm Dig.* 2015;107:162-170.

Wieghard N, Geltzeiler CB, Tsikitis VL. Trends in the surgical management of diverticulitis. *Ann Gastroenterol.* 2015;28:25-30.

A 35-year-old man presents with a 3-week history of perianal pain. He describes having excruciating pain and bleeding associated with defecation. These episodes of pain generally last for 15 to 30 minutes. Because of this pain, he has been unable to defecate for the past 3 days. He denies any fever, difficulty with urination, or previous episodes of pain. His past medical history is unremarkable. He does not take any medications. On physical examination, his temperature is 37.7°C (99.9°F), pulse rate is 100 beats/minute, and blood pressure is 140/90 mm Hg. Examination of the perianal region is difficult due to pain. There is a small posterior midline anal skin tag (sentinel pile). There are no masses, erythema, or tenderness over the buttock or perianal region. During an attempted digital rectal examination (DRE), the patient developed exquisite tenderness resulting in an aborted DRE. The laboratory evaluations reveal a normal WBC, normal hemoglobin and hematocrit values, and normal platelet count.

▶ What is the most likely diagnosis?
▶ What is the most likely mechanism for this condition?
▶ What are your next steps?

ANSWERS TO CASE 29:
Anorectal Diseases

Summary: A 35-year-old man presents with severe anorectal pain associated with defecation. He has no fever. The examination is incomplete due to discomfort and has revealed a posterior sentinel pile at the anal verge and no erythema, mass, swelling, or drainage.

- **Most likely diagnosis:** Anal Fissure.

- **Most likely mechanism:** Causes include trauma to the anal canal mucosa from the passage of hard stool, regional mucosal ischemia, and non-healing related to hypertonic internal sphincter.

- **Next step:** Complete anorectal examination is important to confirm the diagnosis. Discomfort related to manipulation is limiting the extent of our evaluation; thus, the patient will need sedation and topical, regional, or general anesthesia for us to complete this important evaluation.

ANALYSIS
Objectives

1. Learn the differential diagnosis for anorectal pain and common anorectal complaints.

2. Learn the approach to the diagnosis and treatment of common anorectal diseases.

Considerations

This patient's history and clinical presentation are typical of an anal fissure. Anal fissure, hemorrhoids, fistula-in-ano, perirectal abscess, and anorectal neoplasms comprise of the list of the most common anorectal-related complaints. The first step to the diagnosis is to elicit detailed history regarding pain, discomfort, constipation, diarrhea, normal bowel habits, and in relevant cases, sexual practices. The presentation of a fissure is typically pain that begins with the initial passage of a hard stool bowel movement. The patients most commonly describe no pain until the next bowel movement, which reproduces severe and excruciating perianal pain. Often, the patient will also describe having small amount of bright red blood with the bowel movement or noted on the toilet paper. The underlying problem is non-healing of the skin or mucosal tear at the anal verge secondary to hypertonic (spasms) anal sphincter muscles. In this patient's case, the condition has only gone on for 3 weeks; therefore, it is classified as an acute anal fissure (<6-8 weeks in duration). A patient with acute fissure is managed with increase dietary fiber supplements, increase fluid intake, warm sitz baths, and topical analgesic ointment as needed. It is helpful to initiate conversations about long-term dietary changes and bowel habits modifications to promote long-term colorectal health.

APPROACH TO:
Anorectal Complaints

DEFINITIONS

PHYSIOLOGIC FUNCTIONS OF HEMORRHOIDS: Hemorrhoids are fibrovascular cushions that are normal parts of the anal canal near the dentate line. The locations of the three cushions are **right-anterior, right-posterior,** and **left-lateral.** The hemorrhoidal cushions contribute to 15% to 20% of the anal resting pressure. Hemorrhoidal engorgement during valsalva maneuvers or coughing also helps to maintain fecal continence. Additionally, sensory functions of the hemorrhoids allow differentiation of liquid from solid stools and help in the maintenance of continence.

HEMORRHOIDAL DISEASE: Abnormal enlargement of the hemorrhoidal venous plexus can occur due to diarrhea, constipation, obesity, and increased abdominal pressure. Hemorrhoidal diseases include **itching, pain** (mostly associated with thrombosis), **bleeding,** and **prolapse.**

PROLAPSED HEMORRHOID GRADES:

Grade I: Prominent hemorrhoids on external inspection or anoscopy only.

Grade II: Hemorrhoids that prolapse but reduce spontaneously.

Grade III: Hemorrhoids that prolapse and require manual reduction.

Grade IV: Prolapsed hemorrhoids that are irreducible.

ANORECTAL (PERIRECTAL) ABSCESS: Common infections that originate in the cryptoglandular area above the dentate line, within the rectum. The subsequent abscess that develops from tracking of the infection to several locations between the rectal sphincter muscles, and these categories include **perianal** (superficial at the anal verge), **submucosal** (just under the mucosa in the rectum), **intersphincteric** (between the internal and external sphincters), **ischiorectal** (lateral to the rectal sphincter muscles and in the ischiorectal fat), **supralevator** (deep above the levator muscles). Deep abscesses tend to cause the most problems because diagnoses are often delayed and deep perirectal space infections (with polymicrobial organisms) can produce sepsis. **Treatment is prompt recognition and drainage.**

FISTULA-IN-ANO: Approximately 50% of patients with perirectal abscesses will develop fistula-in-ano after resolution of the abscesses. This is generally due to the failure of healing after spontaneous drainage or surgical drainage of the abscess. The fistula in most cases will remain open due to epithelialization of the fistulous tract, which prevents it from healing. Fistula types include: (1) **Intersphincteric**—between the internal and external sphincters. (2) **Transphincteric**—through the internal and external sphincter muscles. (3) **Extrasphincteric** (suprasphincteric)—this can be a rectal opening above the sphincter muscles to an opening lateral to the sphincters.

GOODSALL RULE: This is a rule that can be helpful to identify the internal opening of fistulous tracts. With a transverse line drawn between the anterior half and posterior half of the anus, external openings anterior to this line track radially, straight into the rectum; posterior openings track in curvilinear fashion to the posterior midline.

SETON: A loop of plastic or silicone (commonly a "vessel loop") that can be placed into the fistula-in-ano. A seton can be helpful as mechanism of drainage (draining seton), or it can serve as a marker (marking seton), or to cause chronic granulation/fibrosis along the fistula. Seton placement can be helpful as the initial stage procedure when a subsequent ligation of intersphincteric fistula tract (LIFT) procedure is anticipated.

FISTULOTOMY: Simple unroofing and removal of the epithelial lining of the fistula to allow for secondary healing. This should not be done in a single stage or the entire or majority of the rectal sphincter complex will be disrupted. Under those circumstances, a partial fistulotomy with completion fistulotomy after healing of the initial procedure can be an option. Alternatively, a LIFT procedure can be done.

LIGATION OF INTERSPHINCTERIC FISTULA TRACT (LIFT) PROCEDURE: This is a procedure for the treatment of a mature trans-sphincteric fistula tract (6-12 weeks after initial seton placement). The tract in this case should be easily identifiable by palpation. An incision in the perineum at the intersphincteric space is made, and the dissection is carried deeper in this location without disrupting the sphincter muscles, to identify the chronic fistula. The fistula is then ligated distally and proximally and divided, with excision or unroofing of the external segment of the fistula.

MEDICAL MANAGEMENT OF HEMORRHOIDAL DISEASES: Treatments include dietary modifications to increase fiber and water intake, dietary fiber supplementation, modification of bowel habits (no scheduled, forced bowel movements), increase physical activity/exercise, decrease in fatty food intake.

HEMORRHOIDECTOMY: This is surgical removal of the hemorrhoids (most often combination of enlarged internal and external hemorrhoids). Hemorrhoidectomies are reserved for patients with grade 3 or grade 4 hemorrhoids, or bleeding/symptomatic hemorrhoids that are refractory to appropriate medical management.

HEMORRHOID BANDING OR ABLATION: These are office-based procedures directed at the treatment of **internal hemorrhoids**. Because these areas are insensate, rubber band ligation can be performed to cause ischemia and subsequent fibrosis. Alternatively, ablation of the internal hemorrhoids with injections of sclerosant agents or application of infrared energy can be accomplished.

STAPLED HEMORRHOIDECTOMY: For circumferentially prolapsed internal hemorrhoids, a stapled hemorrhoidectomy can be performed by using a circular stapler inserted into the rectum.

CLINICAL APPROACH

Many patients with perianal, anal, or rectal diseases self-medicate with over-the-counter products. They consult a physician only when the symptoms have worsened or become complicated. It is therefore imperative to obtain a thorough, detailed history regarding symptom duration and prior treatments. An anorectal examination can be performed with the patient either in the left lateral decubitus position with knees flexed and drawn toward the chest or in the prone jackknife position. The key is to provide the most privacy and comfort for the patient. This examination begins with an inspection of the perianal area followed by a digital rectal examination and circumferential anoscopy. In some anxious patients, these maneuvers require time to build trust and in some cases office-based sedation and/or topical analgesics. During the evaluation, it is important to look for skin lesions, mucosal lesion, submucosal lesion, discharges, and indurations. (Table 29–1) Malignancies and unusual inflammatory/infectious conditions should always be considered in the differential diagnosis when patients present with chronic and or recurrent processed in the anorectal areas. Anoscopy is important to visualize anal tears, mucosal abnormalities, and to inspect and evaluate palpable lesions and hemorrhoids. Care should be taken to note the dentate line, which is the dividing line between rectal mucosal and anal epithelium. The lack of somatic innervation above the dentate line helps with manipulation and biopsy of structures above this area.

Symptom Complexes Associated with Common Anorectal Complaints

Anal fissure: Severe anal pain and minor bleeding only with defecation. Some patients complain of baseline itching. Usually patients have minimal drainage.

Hemorrhoids: Swelling and sensation of fullness in the anal area throughout the day, with symptoms worsening with bowel movements. Patients can have bleeding with defecation that is usually more significant bleeding than associated with fissures. The problem is often chronic or recurrent.

Perirectal abscess: The patient describes onset of pain over days with increasing swelling and pain. Most patients can localize the exact area of pain that corresponds to the abscess location. Some patients complain of associated fever and severe abscess with pelvic sepsis can be associated with the inability to urinate normally.

Table 29–1 • EXAMINATION FINDINGS AND TREATMENT			
Source	Appearance	Palpation	Anoscopy
Anal fissure	Superficial tear in anoderm, sentinel tag	Tear; increased sphincter tone, hypertrophic anal papilla	Tear, bleeding, hypertrophic anal papilla
Hemorrhoids	Blue or purple mass at anus	Enlarged soft mass	Prominent veins above or below dentate line
Fistula-in-ano	Purulent drainage, erythema, ulcer, fluctuant mass	Fluctuant mass, induration	Small rough areas in anus

Table 29-2 • ANORECTAL DISEASES AND TREATMENT			
	Symptoms	Findings	Treatment
Fissure-in-ano	Anal pain with defecation, bleeding, itching, drainage	Tear in anoderm, spastic sphincter tone sentinel tag, hypertrophic anal papilla	Sitz baths, stool softeners, suppositories, nitroglycerin; partial internal sphincterotomy
Hemorrhoids:			
Grade I	Painless bleeding	Engorged hemorrhoids	Diet changes
Grade II	Bleeding, pruritus, mild pain	Hemorrhoid prolapses	Diet, band ligation, infrared coagulation
Grade III	Pain, bleeding	Prolapsing hemorrhoids, manual reduction	Rubber band ligation hemorrhoidectomy
Grade IV	Nonreducible hemorrhoids, severe pain	Bleeding, strangulation	Hemorrhoidectomy
Fistula-in-ano	Ulcer, painful fluctuant mass, purulent	Scarred tract from dentate line to external opening	Draining and/or fistulotomy

Fistula-in-ano: This is often seen in patients with clear history of prior spontaneous drainage of perirectal abscesses or surgical drainage of abscesses. The symptoms at presentation are often just soilage of the perineum with mucous discharge.

Treatments

Anal fissure:

Sitz baths, stool softeners, suppositories, increase dietary fiber intake, stool bulking agents. Topical nitroglycerine ointment or topical nifedipine ointment can be prescribed to reduce sphincter spasm for some patients with acute or chronic fissures. For patient symptoms >6 to 8 weeks (chronic fissures), botulinum toxin injection or lateral internal sphincterotomy can be helpful (Table 29–2).

Hemorrhoids:

Grade I: Diet modifications (increase fiber and fluids), bowel habit modification (no scheduled, forced BMs).

Grade II: Same as above + rubber band ligation, infrared coagulation if symptoms are severe and refractory to modification.

Grade III: Same as above + rubber band ligation or surgical hemorrhoidectomy.

Grade III: Same as above + surgical hemorrhoidectomy.

Fistula-in-ano:

Fistulotomy for superficial fistulas and fistulas not involving a large portion of the sphincter muscles. Seton placement if significant sphincters are involved.

Abscess:

Treatment consists of drainage of abscess and counseling regarding 50% possibility of subsequent fistula-in-ano development.

> ## CASE CORRELATION
> - See also Case 25 (Colorectal Cancer and Polyp) and Case 27 (Ulcerative Colitis).

COMPREHENSION QUESTIONS

29.1 A 39-year-old man comes to your office with the complaint that he has noticed mucous-like discharge on his underwear; he denies any pain associated with this process. He indicates that the problem has been ongoing for 2 to 3 weeks. When questioned regarding past history of anorectal complaints, the man indicates that several years ago, he had some severe pain in his anal area that spontaneously resolved after several days. Which of the following is the most likely current problem for this patient?

    A. Crohn disease

    B. Chronic perirectal abscess

    C. Anal fissure

    D. Prolapsed hemorrhoids

    E. Fistula-in-ano

29.2 Which of the following is the best treatment option for this patient?

    A. Repeat drainage of the abscess

    B. Lateral internal sphincterotomy

    C. Botulinum toxin injection

    D. Seton placement and delayed LIFT

    E. Photocoagulation

29.3 Which of the following is considered the most appropriate treatment for acute anal fissure?

    A. Infrared coagulation, sitz baths, and oral antibiotics

    B. Rubber band ligation, suppositories, and topical antibiotics

    C. Increased dietary fiber, sitz baths, and nitroglycerin ointment

    D. Infrared coagulation and fissurectomy

    E. Excision of the fissure

29.4 Which of the following is the most appro for a patient suspected of having chronic anal fissure based on clinical history?

    A. Obtain a barium enema, followed by a colonoscopy

    B. Anorectal examination under sedation, anoscopy, and proctoscopy

    C. Anal biopsy, anoscopy in the office, and barium enema

    D. Anorectal examination in the office with sedation, anal biopsy, fissurectomy

    E. Prescribe stool bulking agents

29.5 A 44-year-old man is being evaluated for possible anal fissure. Which of the following findings are suggestive of anal fissure?

    A. Fever, fluctuant mass

    B. Painless rectal bleeding, purple perianal mass,

    C. Presence of a sinus tract with discharge and local fluctuance

    D. History of nighttime incontinence of gas and liquid stool

    E. Severe anal pain, with a tear in the posterior anoderm

29.6 Which of the following is the most appropriate treatment of a man with a 1.5 cm, prolapsed circumferential mucosal mass that occurs during defecation and requires manual reduction with some effort?

    A. Dietary modification and stool bulking agents

    B. Lateral internal sphincterotomy

    C. LIFT procedure

    D. Stapled hemorrhoidectomy

    E. Rubber band ligation

ANSWERS

29.1 **E.** This patient's history of a perirectal abscess that likely spontaneously resolved several years ago and new onset of mucous discharge not associated with pain and active infection suggests that the problem is a fistula-in-ano. Chronic abscesses often have induration and chronic pain. A fissure is not associated with mucous drainage but with pain upon defecation with small amount of blood.

29.2 **D.** Seton placement followed by delayed LIFT procedure is a good treatment option for patients with suprasphincteric or trans-sphincteric fistula-in-ano. The other treatment choices listed are not appropriate for treatment of fistula-in-ano.

29.3 **C.** The initial treatment of anal fissure includes sitz baths, increase dietary bulking agents, and nitroglycerin ointment application.

29.4 **B.** For patients suspected of having chronic anal fissure, the approach can include examination under anesthesia, anoscopy, and proctoscopy to evaluate for other potential causes. Once the diagnosis is confirmed, treatment can range from dietary modifications, nitroglycerin ointment, Botox injection, to lateral internal sphincterotomy depending on the chronicity and severity of symptoms.

29.5 **E.** Severe anal pain associated with bowel movements, a tear in the posterior anoderm, bleeding, and increased sphincter tone are findings compatible with anal fissure.

29.6 **D.** The description of a circumferential mucosal mass prolapsing during defecation can be consistent with prolapsed circumferential hemorrhoid that only involves prolapsed mucosal components or rectal prolapse that has full-thickness rectum prolapsed. The treatment of circumferential prolapsed hemorrhoid is stapled hemorrhoidectomy.

CLINICAL PEARLS

▶ Patients may be reluctant to volunteer information regarding bowel habits and duration of symptoms; therefore, it is important to be specific in questioning the patient during the interview.

▶ Anorectal carcinoma may manifest as severe perianal pain and tenderness and must be considered part of the differential diagnosis.

▶ Hemorrhoids are almost never palpable on digital rectal examination (DRE), and everything palpable on DRE is a neoplasm until proven otherwise.

▶ Patients with anal fissure characteristically have severe anal pain, a tear in the posterior anoderm, bleeding, and increased rectal sphincter tone.

▶ A thrombosed external hemorrhoid not responding to medical therapy should be treated by excision rather than incision and drainage because drainage alone is associated with a high rate of recurrence.

REFERENCES

Blumetti J, Cintron JR. Anorectal abscess and fistula. In: Cameron JL, Cameron AM, eds. *Current Surgical Therapy*. 11th ed. Philadelphia, PA: Elsevier Saunders; 2014:265-273.

Chaudhry V, Abcarian H. Hemorrhoids. In; Cameron JL, Cameron AM, eds. *Current Surgical Therapy*. 11th ed. Philadelphia, PA: Elsevier Saunders; 2014:255-261.

Gearhart SL. Anal fissure. In: Cameron JL, Cameron AM, eds. *Current Surgical Therapy*. 11th ed. Philadelphia, PA: Elsevier Saunders; 2014:262-265.

Following recovery from an exploratory laparotomy and repair of a colon injury caused by a gunshot wound to the abdomen, a 26-year-old man developed a soft tissue infection in the superior portion of his midline incision that required local wound care. He was discharged from the hospital on postoperative seven and returns today approximately 2 weeks later for a follow-up visit in the out-patient clinic. The patient indicates that he has been doing well except for fluid drainage from his midline abdominal wound for the past several days. On examination, his temperature is 37.5C (99.5F), pulse rate is 70 beats/minute, blood pressure is 130/80 mmHg, and respiratory rate is 18 breaths/minute. His cardiopulmonary examinations are within normal limits. The examination of his abdomen reveals a small amount of serosanguinous fluid seeping from the superior aspect of his midline incision. A close inspection of this area shows a 4-cm fascia defect at this site without signs of evisceration.

▶ What are the complications associated with this condition?
▶ What are the risk factors for this condition?
▶ What is the best treatment?

ANSWERS TO CASE 30:

Fascial Dehiscence and Incisional Hernia

Summary: A 26-year-old man presents with a stable abdominal fascia dehiscence 3 weeks following exploratory laparotomy for the treatment of traumatic injuries.

- **Complications:** Abdominal fascial dehiscence can lead to the evisceration of intrabdominal contents, the development of enterocutaneous fistula, and development of incisional hernia.

- **Risk factors:** The occurrence of wound infection is the most significant contributor to poor fascial healing, with many defined comorbidities and risk factors contributing to wound infections, and these include *smoking, diabetes, COPD, CAD, malnutrition, immunosuppression, low serum albumin, chronic steroid use, obesity,* and *advanced age.* Less common contributing factors include failure of surgical techniques, failure of suture material, and insufficient anesthetic relaxation.

- **Best treatment:** For this patient who does not exhibit active infectious concerns, local wound care with elective repair of the incisional hernia at a later date is the preferred approach.

ANALYSIS

Objectives

1. Recognize contributing/risk factors and preventive measures for wound dehiscence and incisional hernias.

2. Learn the treatment options and basis for application of the treatment options for patients with wound dehiscence or incisional hernias.

Considerations

Disruption of fascial closure following an abdominal operation is referred to as fascial dehiscence. The two important principles guiding this patient's care at this time are: assessment of stability of the intra-abdominal contents (whether or not evisceration is present or imminent) and assessment/management of ongoing infections. At this time, the dehiscence appears stable without evisceration (extrusion of intestines through the fascia). Our initial assumption of a stable fascial dehiscence is based on the timing of this event (3 weeks postoperatively), which provides some reassurance that some adhesions have developed to prevent the evisceration of intra-abdominal contents. During inspection of the wound and fascial defect, it is very important to note whether omentum or intestine is underneath the fascial defect. The presence of intestines directly under the fascial opening would greatly increase the likelihood of intestinal perforation due to tearing as the fascial edges further separate, or as the result of desiccation associated with exposure to the external environment. On the other hand, if omentum is present directly underneath the defect, the likelihood of intestinal perforation and the development of an enterocutaneous fistula are reduced given this added protective layer. Our initial opinion that this patient's wound dehiscence is stable and is at lower risk for progression to evisceration is largely based on the timing of the dehiscence diagnosis. At approximately 3 weeks after the initial laparotomy, we expect that adhesion formation has already occurred within the peritoneal cavity, and this process should help minimize the extrusion of intra-abdominal contents. It is important at this time to assess the patient for active intra-abdominal infections (deep space infections), which requires initial screening laboratory studies such as CBC with differentials in addition to the review of vital signs for fevers and other signs of infections. If ongoing infections are suspected, a CT scan of the abdomen should be obtained for further evaluation.

If no active infections are identified, the patient can be managed with wound care and close observation. The patient needs to be informed that the treatment of his condition can be a long and drawn out process. In addition, the patient needs to know that a ventral hernia will eventually develop and may require additional operative repair at a later date. Early reoperation is indicated if the patient has evisceration or if he has uncontrolled sepsis due to intra-abdominal infections that are not amendable to nonoperative treatments.

APPROACH TO:
Fasical Dehiscence and Incisional Hernias

DEFINITIONS

FASCIA DEHISCENCE: This refers to the disruption of abdominal fascia closure within days of an operation. This complication may occur with or without evisceration.

INCISIONAL HERNIA: This is the delayed development of fascial defect due to inadequate healing of the fascia. For some patients, this process may not become apparent for up to 5 years.

EVISCERATION: This is the protrusion of abdominal viscera (bowel or omentum) through a fascial dehiscence or traumatic defect in the abdominal wall.

ENTEROCUTANEOUS FISTULA: This is defined as an opening between the small bowel lumen and the skin opening. It can be due to intestinal leakage leading to wound dehiscence or this problem can develop following wound dehiscence and exposure of the intestines to the external environment producing intestinal injury and fistula formation.

CARE OF PATIENTS WITH ENTEROCUTANEOUS FISTULAS: Overall care plans require a stepwise approach: (1) control sepsis; (2) stabilize fluid/electrolyte abnormalities; (3) nutritional support (given as enteral, parenteral, or combined); (4) control of spillage including wound care, skin care, and pharmacologic control; (5) definitive repair (if necessary).

ENTEROCUTANEOUS FISTULA OUTPUT: Enterocutaneous fistula output volume affects the fluid/electrolyte and nutritional status of patients and their prognosis. *Low-output fistulas* are defined as those with <200 mL/day. *Moderate-output fistulas* are defined as those with 200 to 500 mL/day. *High-output fistulas* are fistulas with >500 mL/day output.

"HOSTILE ABDOMEN": Generally between 7 days to 28 days after an abdominal operation, there are a combination of inflammatory changes and fibrosis in the peritoneal cavity, and as the result of these processes, surgical dissections tend to be bloody and injuries to intestines can occur more easily. This is the time period when reoperations are most likely to cause complications such as enterocutaneous fistulas.

ABDOMINAL WALL COMPONENT SEPARATION: This is a technique often applied in the repair of complex incisional hernias. The technique involves separation of the anterior and posterior oblique muscle layer with lateral release and advancement of the anterior layer. The advantage of this type of repair is tissue-to-tissue approximation of the reconstructed abdominal wall. Generally, the medialized anterior muscle layer and the lateral posterior muscle layers are reinforced with prosthetic mesh or biologic material for added strength.

CENTER FOR DISEASE CONTROL (CDC) SURGICAL WOUND CLASSIFICATIONS: Surgical wounds are classified from class I–IV. Class I wounds are clean (wound infection rate of 1%-5%), Class II wounds are clean-contaminated (wound infection rate of 3%-11%), Class III wounds are contaminated (wound infection rate of 10%-17%, Class IV wounds are dirty or infected (wound infection rate of 27%).

CLINICAL APPROACH

Physiology of Wound Healing as it Relates to Fascial Healing

Fascia dehiscence and incisional hernias often develop because of insufficient healing of the fascia after surgery. Understanding wound healing and factors that affect wound healing are helpful to prevent these complications. Wound healing is generally subdivided into three phases, including the inflammatory phase, proliferation phase, and the remodeling (maturation) phase. Table 30–1 lists the phases of

Table 30–1 • PHASES OF WOUND HEALING	
Inflammatory phase	Begins immediately and ends within 5-6 days. Inflammatory cells help sterilize the wound and secrete growth factors and stimulate fibroblasts and keratinocyte activities
Proliferation phase	Extends from 3-15 days postinjury. Deposition of fibrin-fibrinogen matrix and collagen occurs with formation of the wound matrix resulting in the increase in wound strength
Remodeling (Maturation) phase	Extends from one week to several months postinjury. Capillary regression leads to a less vascularized wound. Along with collagen cross-linking the wound gradually increases in tensile strength

Table 30–2 • CLINICAL FACTORS AFFECTING WOUND HEALING	
Infections	Leads to delays in fibroblast proliferation, wound matrix synthesis, and deposition
Malnutrition	**Vitamin C** deficiency causes inadequate collagen production; **vitamin A** deficiency causes impaired fibroplasia, collagen synthesis, cross-linking, and epithelialization; **vitamin B6** deficiency causes impaired collagen cross-linking
Poor oxygenation	Collagen synthesis is impaired by hypoxia and augmented with oxygen supplementation
Corticosteroids	Reduces wound inflammation, collagen synthesis, and wound contraction. In addition, corticosteroids predispose to hyperglycemia and its adverse effects
Diabetes mellitus (Hyperglycemia)	Diabetes is associated with microvascular occlusive disease leading to poor wound perfusion; impairment in keratinocyte growth factor and platelet-derived growth factor functions in the wound
Advanced age	Aging is associated with delayed wound healing. Aging produces qualitative and quantitative changes in collagen production and deposition
Smoking	Smoking is associated with multiple factors that affect wound healing, including hypoxia, vasoconstriction, and increase susceptibility to infections
Low serum albumin	May reflect poor nutritional state and contributes to tissue edema and poor wound healing
Obesity	Contributes to increase in wound infection
Immunosuppression	Poor inflammatory response and poor wound healing
COPD	Contributes to hypoxia and increased wound stress related frequent coughing

wound healing and the corresponding timing of these activities. Table 30–2 lists some clinical factors that impair wound healing.

TREATMENT

Fascial defects develop in 2% to 20% of patients who undergo abdominal surgery. The incidence of postoperative fascial complications increases four-fold in patients who develop wound infections; accordingly, wound infections after abdominal operations are the most common cause of incisional hernia formation. Table 30–2 lists some of the patient factors that affect wound healing and Table 30–3 lists some of the technical factors that contribute to failure of abdominal fascial closures. For the majority of patients, patient factors are the major causes of fascial closure complications, and technical failures are causative in only a small subset of the patients. Unfortunately, the patient factors or conditions often persist in some patients and ultimately contribute to failures of incisional hernia repairs in these same patients.

Table 30–3 • TECHNICAL FACTORS RELATED TO ABDOMINAL CLOSURE FAILURE
Inadequate tissue incorporation
Inappropriate suture size or suture material
Excessive tension
Inadequate patient relaxation
Inappropriate suture placement

Management

Fascial defects can present early in the postoperative course as serous or sero-sanguinous fluid drainage from an otherwise normal-appearing wound or may present as a soft tissue protruberance under the incision. When excessive fluid drainage is encountered from an abdominal incision, the skin wound may need to be opened so that the fascia can be examined. Depending on the precise timing and circumstances associated with the fascial dehiscence, the treatment may require emergent return to the operating room for repair. Alternatively, the fascial defect can be addressed months later after the patient recovers. Several factors may favor delayed surgical treatment, including a stable dehiscence with no exposed bowel, a low-risk wound for evisceration, and the anticipation of a "hostile" abdominal environment.

Open Abdomen

The "open-abdomen" is a condition that has developed following the introduction of damage-control laparotomies for trauma and complex intra-abdominal infectious processes. In these situations, the initial operation is done to control life-threatening conditions in unstable patients; during these initial operations, only essential steps such as controlling bleeding and enteric spillage are accomplished. After improvement in the patients' conditions a few days later, they are returned to the operating room for definitive treatments. In some cases, patients may require several return trips to the operating room, the abdomens are left open and become uncloseable. Ultimately in these patients, absorbable meshes are placed over the abdominal contents for temporary closure, and once the contents granulate, split-thickness skin grafts are placed over the abdominal contents. Following healing, the patients are left with large fascial defects or "open abdomens." Open abdomens have a high risk of producing enterocutaneous fistulas, when the intestines are exposed to the atmosphere or the absorbable mesh. The end results are giant abdominal fascial defects in many of these patients. Abdominal wall repairs in these patients generally require reconstruction either with the placement of prosthetic material or by component separation.

Incisional Hernia Repair

Unlike the repair of a groin hernia, the repair of incisional hernia is associated with a significant risk of wound infections (7%-20%) and high-recurrence rate (20%-50%). In 2010, a hernia grading system was introduced to stratify the surgical site complication risks and guide decisions on the type of repairs that should

Table 30–4 • INCISIONAL HERNIA GRADING SYSTEM REPAIR RECOMMENDATIONS			
Grade 1 Low Risk	Grade 2 Comorbidities	Grade 3 Potentially Contaminated	Grade 4 Infected
• Low risk of complications • No history of wound infections	• Smoker • Obese • COPD • Immuno-suppressed	• Prior wound infection • GI stoma present • GI tract violation	• Infected mesh • Septic dehiscence
Choice of repair material by surgeon preference	High-risk with permanent prosthetics placement, should consider biologic material or component separation	Permanent prosthetic material not recommended, should place biologic material or component separation	Permanent prosthetic material not recommended, should place biologic material or component separation

be performed in patients with incisional hernias. This grading scheme divided incisional hernias into four separate grades (1-4), with grade 1 being low-risk hernias and grade 4 being the highest risk hernias. Table 30–4 contains the incisional hernia grades and the respective repairs that are recommended.

In general, primary repair of fascial defects greater than 2 cm in diameter is associated with high recurrences; therefore, placement of either prosthetic material, biologic material, or component separations are recommended for the larger hernias. Repair of incisional hernia with prosthetic mesh placement can be done either by an open approach or a laparoscopic approach. Randomized controlled trials comparing these techniques have shown little difference in hernia recurrences, but the laparoscopic approach is associated with lower rate of wound infection in comparison to open repairs. Component separation is a technique that was introduced in the 1980s, and this approach has the advantage of allowing apposition of natural tissue for defect closure.

CASE CORRELATION

- See also Case 22 (Obesity [Morbid]).

COMPREHENSION QUESTIONS

30.1 Which of the following conditions is known to have detrimental effects on wound healing?

A. Obesity

B. Hyperthyroidism

C. C-reactive protein deficiency

D. Diabetes mellitus

E. Hyperthyroidism

30.2 Twelve days following abdominal surgery, a patient noted drainage of 20 mL of fluid from her midline abdominal wound. Which of the following is the most appropriate management?

A. Reinforce the wound dressing and reassure the patient that the seroma will stop draining spontaneously

B. Initiate antibiotics therapy targeting enteric flora

C. Perform an immediate laparotomy

D. Obtain a CT scan

E. Open the skin wound to inspect the fascia

30.3 A 23-year-old nursing student undergoes a laparotomy for perforated appendicitis and asks about the possibility of incisional hernia occurrence. Which of the following statements is TRUE regarding incisional hernias?

A. The incidence may reach upwards of 20% in infected wounds

B. Repairs are associated with less than 1% recurrence rate

C. Primary repair is associated with less infections and is the preferred method of repair for the majority of patients

D. Formation of an incisional hernia can always be recognized within 3 months of surgery

E. Incisional hernias do not develop in healthy individuals without predisposing risk factors

30.4 A 40-year-old man undergoes a laparotomy and lysis of adhesions for small bowel obstruction. He was discharged from the hospital on postoperative day 5 and returns for follow-up. On examination, his wound is covered with gauze that is soaked with fluid from the wound. Which of the following would be helpful to differentiate fascial dehiscence from an enteral-cutaneous fistula?

A. Abdominal CT scan

B. Wound inspection for fascial defect

C. Blood sample for complete blood count analysis

D. Visual inspection of the drainage fluid

E. Bacterial culture of the fluid

30.5 Which of the following statements is most accurate regarding incisional hernias?

A. Laparoscopic repairs are associated with lower risk of wound infections

B. The results of incisional hernia repairs are more favorable in comparison to outcomes associated with inguinal hernia repairs

C. Incisional hernia occurrence is the same for patients with and without wound infections

D. Early occurrence of fascial dehiscence is always associated with fevers and leukocytosis

E. Incisional hernias are rarely found in patients with open abdomens

30.6 Which of the following is a TRUE statement regarding open abdomen?

A. Open abdomens are the result of inappropriate patient care

B. Fluid management following damage-control laparotomy can impact the rate of development of open abdomens

C. Enteral-atmospheric fistulas rarely occur in patients with open abdomens

D. Open abdomens are the result of diabetes and poor wound healing

E. The failure of anesthetic management during abdominal surgery is a common contributor to the formation of open abdomens

30.7 Based on the Incisional Hernia Grading Scores, what is the best repair method for a 43-year-old man with diabetes mellitus and a prior ventral hernia repair that failed following wound infection and prosthetic mesh infection? The current size of the fascial defect is 8 × 6 cm.

A. Primary repair

B. Repair placement of permanent prosthetic material

C. Repair with placement of absorbable prosthetic material

D. Repair by component separation and re-enforcement with biologic material

E. No repairs should be attempted due to high risk

ANSWERS

30.1 **D.** Diabetes mellitus is associated with poor wound healing due to microvascular occlusion and impairment in certain growth factor functions in the wound. Obesity is associated with an increased risk of wound infections but is not associated with known detrimental effects on wound healing.

30.2 **E.** The description of the patient here is highly suggestive of fascial dehiscence, but infection of the wound is also possible. Opening the skin incision to inspect the subcutaneous space and fascia is the most helpful choice listed here. Simple observation is not appropriate because if there is fascial disruption, evisceration may occur, and early diagnosis can prevent that from occurring. At 12 days following her abdominal operation, a fascial dehiscence can be managed nonoperatively, therefore returning to the operating room may not be necessary.

30.3 **A.** The incidence of incisional hernia may reach 20% in infected wounds. Up to 50% of complex incisional hernia repairs can fail and result in recurrences. Primary repairs of incisional hernias are not usually performed due to increased risk of recurrences. The development of incisional hernias are due to a number of patient-related factors (ie, patient disease or conditions) and technical factors. Incisional hernias occur less commonly in young, healthy individuals in comparison to older individuals with comorbidities.

30.4 **D.** This patient presents with fluid drainage from his laparotomy incision. The concerns at this point are for fascial dehiscence or enterocutaneous fistula. Inspection of the fluid can be helpful to differentiate these two possibilities. Enterocutaneous fistula drainage has the gross appearance of enteric contents; in contrast, dehiscence is associated with the drainage of serous or serosanguinous fluid.

30.5 **A.** Incisional hernias can be repaired either by open or laparoscopic approaches. The laparoscopic approach is associated with lower wound infection rate and shorter length of hospitalization; however, no significant difference in recurrence rates is reported between the two different approaches. Fascial dehiscence can be associated with fever and WBC elevation when wound infection is an associated problem. Fever and leukocytosis are not always present. Patient outcomes associated with inguinal hernia repairs are significantly better than those associated with incisional hernia repairs.

30.6 **B.** Avoidance of excessive fluid administration can improve the fascial closure rates for patients following damage-control laparotomies. Enteral-atmospheric fistula is a known complication associated with open abdomens. Host comorbidities have not been identified for patients at risk for having open abdomens.

30.7 **D.** The patient described here is a 43-year-old man with diabetes and a prior failed ventral hernia repair that was associated with wound infection and prosthetic mesh infection. This patient falls into grade 4 with very high risk for wound complications. Based on this grading, the most appropriate choice listed is repair by component separation with biologic material reinforcement. The recommendation of no repair is also possible based on his high-risk status, but this is less desirable for a reasonably young individual.

CLINICAL PEARLS

▶ The tensile strength of uncomplicated wounds steadily increases for approximately 8 weeks reaching 75% to 80% of the original tissue tensile strength. The tensile strength will continue to increase thereafter, but it never returns to the preinjury level.

▶ The use of braided, nonabsorbable suture material is associated with the trapping of tissue debris within the suture material, and this type of suture material is less than ideal in a heavily infected operative field.

▶ The 4:1 ratio refers to the ratios of the running closure suture length to the length of the wound. Using sutures shorter than this ratio may result in excessive tension on the suture or inadequate tissue incorporation in the fascia closure.

▶ Reclosoure of a previously healed fascia incision is associated with lower strength of healing and higher rate of wound breakdown.

▶ The avoidance of excess fluid administration in a patient following damage-control laparotomy can help improve the probability of fascial closure during the subsequent operation(s).

▶ A potentially "hostile" abdominal condition exists during the wound healing phase when there is residual inflammatory process and ongoing fibrosis (~ postoperative days 7 to 28).

▶ Factors that have found to influence wound infection rates include duration of operation (>2 hours associated with higher infections), condition of the tissue at the completion of surgery, and host susceptibility.

REFERENCES

Curcillo II PG. Incisional, epigastric, and umbilical hernias. In: Cameron JL, Cameron AM, eds. *Current Surgical Therapy*. 11th ed. Philadelphia, PA: Elsevier Saunders; 2014:539-545.

Diaz JJ, Dutton WD, Miller RS. The difficult abdominal wall. In; Townsend CM Jr, Beauchamp RD, Evers BM, Mattox KL, eds. *Sabiston Textbook of Surgery: The Biological Basis of Modern Surgical Practice*. 19th ed. Philadelphia, PA: Elsevier Saunders; 2012:471-479.

Leong M, Phillips LG. Wound healing. In: Townsend CM Jr, Beauchamp RD, Evers BM, Mattox KL, eds. *Sabiston Textbook of Surgery: The Biological Basis of Modern Surgical Practice*. 19th ed. Philadelphia, PA: Elsevier Saunders; 2012:151-177.

The Ventral Hernia Working Group. Incisional ventral hernias: review of the literature and recommendations regarding the grading and technique of repair. *Surgery*. 2010;148:544-558.

A 36-year-old man presents with a 1-day history of groin pain. The patient states that the pain developed during a tennis match the previous evening. On his way home, he noticed swelling in the area. His past medical history is unremarkable. The patient denies any history of medical problems or similar complaints. He has not undergone any previous operations. The physical examination reveals a well-nourished man. The results of the cardiopulmonary examination are unremarkable, and the abdominal examination reveals a nontender and nondistended abdomen. Auscultation of the abdomen reveals normal bowel sounds. Examination of the inguinal areas reveals no inguinal masses. There is a 3-cm nonerythematous bulge on the medial thigh just below the right inguinal ligament. Palpation reveals localized tenderness. The lower extremities are otherwise unremarkable. Laboratory findings reveal a WBC count of 6,500/mm^3 and normal hemoglobin and hematocrit levels. Electrolyte concentrations are within normal ranges as are the results of the urinalysis. Radiographs of the abdomen reveal normal findings.

▶ What is the most likely diagnosis?
▶ What are the complications associated with this disease process?
▶ What is the best therapy?

ANSWERS TO CASE 31:

Hernias

Summary: A 36-year-old active man presents with complaints of a new-onset painful mass in the infra-inguinal region that developed during tennis match the previous day.

- **Most likely diagnosis:** Incarcerated femoral hernia.

- **Complications:** Strangulation of the hernia sac content with associated sequelae.

- **Best therapy:** Operative exploration of the area to evaluate hernia, reduce the hernia sac contents, and repair the femoral hernia.

ANALYSIS

Objectives

1. Know the presentations of inguinal, femoral, and umbilical hernias.

2. Recognize the anatomic landmarks of the different types of hernias.

3. Learn the pros and cons of hernia repairs, and the outcomes associated with the different approaches to hernia repairs.

Considerations

This patient presents with the sudden onset of pain and a mass in his right infra-inguinal area. The differential diagnosis of groin pain and/or mass includes inguinal hernia, femoral hernia, muscle strain, and adenopathy. This patient provides a history of being well until the sudden onset of pain during his tennis match. While it is not uncommon for many individuals to believe that the sudden development of pain or mass in the groin is the classic presentation of hernias, the story described by this individual is actually very atypical for hernia presentation. Inguinal hernia patients will often describe intermittent groin discomfort or "heaviness" that is more prominent with activity and after standing for prolonged periods of time. The mass that is identified in his right infra-inguinal area along with his description of the events suggests that he has an acutely incarcerated right femoral hernia. Because a femoral hernia is an unusual hernia, and this patient's story is not entirely straight forward, imaging should be performed to confirm the diagnosis. In this case, a CT scan of the pelvis should be able to help us establish the diagnosis. Once the diagnosis is confirmed, we should proceed with expeditious exploration and repair of the hernia. The repair can be approached using an open incision placed above the inguinal ligament that allows the surgeon to go through the inguinal floor to identify the femoral canal and address the contents in the incarcerated hernia. Once the hernia is reduced, a McVay-type repair (Cooper's ligament repair) can be carried out with placement of prosthetic mesh.

APPROACH TO:
Hernias

DEFINITIONS

INDIRECT INGUINAL HERNIA: This is an inguinal hernia in which the abdominal contents protrude through the internal inguinal ring through a patent processus vaginalis into the inguinal canal. In men, the hernia sacs follow the spermatic cord and may descend into the scrotum, whereas the indirect inguinal hernia in women may present as labial swelling.

DIRECT INGUINAL HERNIA: This refers to an inguinal hernia that protrudes through the Hesselbach triangle and medial to the ipsilateral inferior epigastric vessels.

FEMORAL HERNIA: This is a hernia that protrudes through the femoral canal, which is bound by the inguinal ligament superiorly, the femoral vein laterally, and the pyriformis and pubic ramus medially. The subtle difference between femoral hernia and inguinal hernia is that the femoral hernia is located **below** the inguinal ligament. Care should be taken to verify the location of the inguinal ligament during the examination of patients with hernias in that region of the body.

UMBILICAL HERNIA: This is a hernia that results from the improper closure of the abdominal wall defect where the umbilical cord was in utero. Eighty percent of these defects close spontaneously by 2 years of life. Umbilical hernias can also be acquired hernias, where subclinical defects increase in size due to increased intra-abdominal pressures (eg, pregnancy, ascites, or excess weight gain).

LITTRE HERNIA: This refers to any type of hernia that contains a Meckel diverticulum.

AMYAND'S HERNIA: This refers to an inguinal hernia that contains the appendix.

DE GARENGEOT'S HERNIA: This is a femoral hernia that contains the appendix.

RICHTER'S HERNIA: This is herniation of part of the bowel wall through any hernia defect. What is unique about this type of hernia is that it may or may not be associated with intestinal obstruction, and that this type of hernia is often smaller and can be more difficult to diagnose. The area of incarcerated intestine can develop ischemia and necrosis when the process goes undiagnosed.

SPIGELIAN HERNIA: This is a hernia just lateral to the rectus sheath and located at the semilunar line, or the lower limits of the posterior rectus sheath.

OBTURATOR HERNIA: This is herniation along the obturator canal alongside the obturator vessels and obturator nerve. This hernia occurs most commonly in women, particularly multiparous women with history of recent weight loss. A mass can be palpable in the medial thigh, particularly with hip flexed, externally rotated, and abducted. The Howship–Romberg sign is associated with approximately 50%

of the patients with obturator hernias, and this is pain along the inner thigh produced by hip flexion, abduction, internal rotation, or external rotation.

SLIDING HERNIA: This term describes an indirect inguinal hernia with a hernia sac containing either sigmoid colon (left) or cecum (right). The indirect hernia sac in this type of hernia will contain the attachment of the intestines. High-ligation of the sac without clearly identifying a hernia as a sliding hernia can cause ischemic injury to the intestine within the sac.

CLINICAL APPROACH

Abdominal wall hernias are protrusion of abdominal contents through defects in the abdominal wall. **Incarceration** involves the trapping of the abdominal content within the hernia sac (failure for the contents to spontaneously reduce). **Strangulation** occurs when the blood supply to the trapped intra-abdominal contents becomes compromised, leading to ischemia, necrosis, and ultimately perforation. Intestinal obstruction can occur in association with either incarcerated or strangulated hernias. Abdominal wall defects that develop following abdominal operations not related to hernia repairs are referred to as incisional hernias and are addressed elsewhere in this text.

Anatomy

Knowledge of the regional anatomy is essential for the diagnosis and repair of hernias. In the groin region, the inguinal ligament separates inguinal hernias from femoral hernias. Inguinal hernias are further divided into direct and indirect hernias based on the relationship of the defects to the inferior epigastric vessels. **The Hesselbach's triangle, is defined by the edge of the rectus muscle medially, the inguinal ligament inferolaterally, and inferior epigastric vessels superiolaterally, and is the site of direct hernia occurrence.** An indirect inguinal hernia originates lateral to Hesselbach's triangle. Direct inguinal hernias develop initially as tears in the abdominal wall within Hesselbach's triangle, and this area is sometimes referred to by some surgeons as the "inguinal floor." Direct inguinal hernias are the result of tears in the transversus abdominal musculature that makes up the inguinal floor. Cooper's ligament or the pectineal ligament is a fibrous structure that extends from the pubic tubercle medially and extending posteriorly to the femoral vessels; **the femoral canal is between the inguinal ligament, Cooper's ligament, and the femoral vein.** Because this area is a small space bordered by touching structures, femoral hernias have a higher rate of incarceration and/or strangulation than inguinal hernias (see Figure 31–1).

Indications for Elective Inguinal Hernia Repairs

Symptoms produced by hernias are related to the size and location of the defects and the activity level of the individuals with the hernias. It is not uncommon for individuals with small hernias to have little or no associated discomfort. Until approximately 10 years ago, it was the general opinion within the surgical community that all patients with inguinal hernias should undergo repair unless the patient's life expectancy is limited. The common belief that inguinal hernias in all

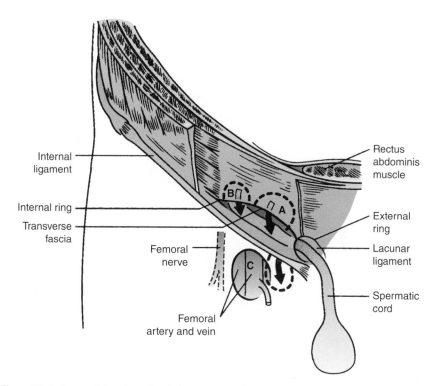

Figure 31–1. Anatomic location of groin hernias. Direct hernia (**A**), indirect hernia (**B**), femoral hernia (right groin from an anterior view) (**C**).

patients needed repairs was based on the premise that all hernias left alone will produce symptoms, and that some of the hernias can become acutely incarcerated or strangulated if managed expectantly. In 2006, the "watchful waiting vs repair" trial was published suggesting that the rate of hernia complications (incarceration) was only 0.18% over 2 years with no strangulations occurring. Based on these observations, it was determined that it was safe and cost-effective to observe individuals with minimally symptomatic or asymptomatic inguinal hernias. In contrast, nearly one-third of the patients with femoral hernias developed acute events requiring emergency repairs: therefore, a watchful-waiting strategy may not be an acceptable recommendation for patients with femoral hernias.

Open Inguinal Hernia Repair Versus Laparoscopic Repair

The standard open inguinal hernia repairs are performed with the placement of prosthetic material mesh ± plug. In comparison to open repairs with suture repairs of native tissue, repairs with prosthetic material have produced lower recurrence rates. With introduction of laparoscopic preperitoneal inguinal hernias repairs approximately 15 years ago, many patients and surgeons have embraced the laparoscopic approach. The advantages of the laparoscopic approach include less pain and discomfort during the initial postoperative period. A randomized controlled trial comparing open to laparoscopic inguinal hernia

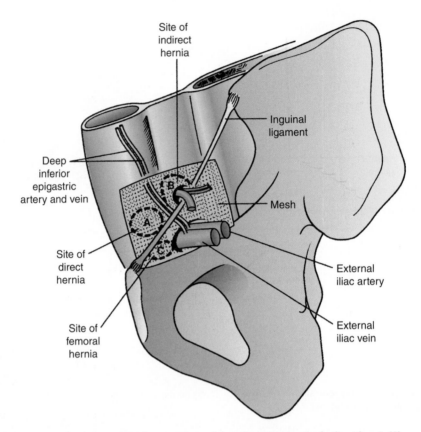

Figure 31–2. Right groin anatomy by preperitoneal view. Operative repair of a direct hernia (**A**), an indirect hernia (**B**), and a femoral hernia using a prosthetic mesh in a posterior (preperitoneal) approach (**C**).

repairs published in 2004 suggests that laparoscopic repair outcomes are highly dependent on surgeon experience, and this study suggested that the learning curve to develop competence in this operative approach is 250 or more cases (see Figure 31–2 for surgical anatomy).

Postoperative Pain Following Hernia Repairs

Quality of life is the most important reason most individuals seek treatment for inguinal hernias. For this reason, the patient should be given clear expectations of possible outcomes following inguinal hernia repairs. While most patients have improvements in quality of life, chronic pain can occur following repairs. Chronic pain is defined as pain persisting for more than 3 months after a hernia repair, and **this problem has been reported most commonly in young adults and women.** Outcomes reported over the past 10 years suggest that chronic pain is reported in 15% to 30% of the patients following inguinal hernia repairs, with approximately 3% of the postoperative patients reporting severe and excruciating chronic pain. There are a number of causes of chronic postoperative pain following inguinal hernia repairs, and these include **hernia recurrence** (generally 1%-5%), **mesh-related**

pain, nerve irritation, and **infections.** Many practitioners believe that nerve irritation-related pain can be minimized with routine excision of the ilioinguinal and the genitofemoral nerves. Mesh-related pain can be recognized as pain associated with activities requiring hip flexion, such as driving, sitting, and bending. This is believed to be related to abnormal inflammation and fibrosis that develop in some individuals, and treatments such as anti-inflammatory agents can help reduce the discomfort. In some patients with severe pain from mesh reactions, mesh removal is necessary for pain relief. Discussion regarding the possibility of chronic postoperative pain prior to surgery is important. If these symptoms develop, early treatments are important to prevent worsening of the disability related to psychosocial components of chronic pain syndrome.

Approach to an Incarcerated Hernia

Manual reduction of an incarcerated hernia should be attempted unless there are concerns that the hernia contents are ischemic and/or necrotic. When there is concern about possible compromised hernia contents, it is important to visually inspect the tissue rather than blindly pushing the contents back into the abdomen. Suggestions of possible compromised contents include hernias with local skin changes such as edema and/or erythema. In addition, a hard and tender hernia is more concerning for strangulation. Most surgeons, dealing with acutely incarcerated hernias will perform surgical repairs with the intention of visually inspecting the contents during the operation. When ischemic bowel is identified during the hernia repair, the hernia defect can often be extended slightly to allow for resection of the ischemic bowel and primary reanastomosis of the intestine. When contamination or spillage of intestinal contents occur, permanent prosthetic material is usually avoided in the repair.

CASE CORRELATION

- See also Case 30 (Fascial Dehiscence and Incisional Hernia).

COMPREHENSION QUESTIONS

31.1 A 63-year-old man has a small and asymptomatic right femoral hernia that was detected during an annual physical examination. Which of the following statements regarding this hernia is false?

A. Femoral hernias are found inferior to the inguinal ligament

B. Anterior approach to femoral hernia repair requires opening of the inguinal floor

C. The "watchful waiting" approach to femoral hernias is reported with the same success rate as the approach for inguinal hernias

D. Femoral hernias can be repaired by laparoscopic or open approaches

E. Expertise of laparoscopic repair of groin hernias requires surgeon experience with greater than 250 cases

31.2 Which of the following is true of Hesselbach's triangle?

A. This was named after a German actor

B. The borders are the lateral border of rectus muscle, inguinal ligament, and inferior epigastric vessels

C. Indirect inguinal hernias are found here

D. Femoral hernias are found lateral to the triangle

E. The borders are the linea alba, femoral vessels, and inferior epigastric vessels

31.3 An 80-year-old woman who resides in a nursing home has a several-pound weight loss over the past several months. She presents with a 3-day history of vomiting and anorexia. Her abdominal examination reveals distension and tympany. On examination of the groin and lower extremities, there are no masses seen or palpated, but the patient complains of pain along the medial thigh upon abduction, internal rotation, and external rotation of the right hip and leg. CT scan of the abdomen reveals dilated loops of small bowel with air-fluid levels. Which of the following is the most appropriate treatment for this patient?

A. Exploratory laparotomy and repair of the sliding inguinal hernia

B. Exploratory laparotomy and repair of the femoral hernia

C. Exploratory laparotomy and repair of the obturator hernia

D. Exploratory laparotomy and reduction of the small bowel intus-susception

E. Nasogastric tube (NGT) decompression and nonoperative management

31.4 A 70-year-old man presents with intermittent nausea and vomiting of 6-hour duration that he noticed coinciding with his long-standing right inguinal hernia becoming hard and painful. On physical examination, he is noted to have temperature of 38.3C (101F). His abdomen is distended and tympanic. Examination of his groin reveals a right scrotal hernia that is tender and firm. The overlying skin is tender and edematous. The patient has received intravenous fluid and NG decompression. Which of the following is the best next step to be taken?

A. Attempt manual reduction of the incarcerated right inguinal hernia

B. Exploration of the right inguinal hernia with inspection and repair of the hernia

C. Continue NG suction for 24 hours before proceeding with surgical treatment

D. Perform manual reduction of the hernia and laparoscopy to repair the hernia

E. Perform bilateral inguinal exploration and repair of both hernias

31.5 A 40-year-old man presents with recurrent bulge in the left groin 2 years after open left inguinal hernia repair with mesh. The physical examination showed a moderately dilated external inguinal ring with a small bulge produced by Valsalva maneuver. Which of the following is the most appropriate treatment approach?

A. Obtain a CT scan to rule out a femoral hernia, followed by elective repair

B. Schedule the patient for a left groin exploration and hernia repair with mesh placement

C. Advise the patient to limit his physical activities and re-evaluate in 6 months

D. Send the patient to an immunologist for management of collagen dysfunction

E. Schedule the patient for bilateral inguinal exploration

31.6 A 20-year-old construction worker complains of pain and an intermittent bulge in his left groin. He indicates that the symptoms have been worsening over the past 3 months and are beginning to affect his activities. On examination, he appears to have a small indirect inguinal hernia. Which of the following is the appropriate management?

A. Discuss with the patient regarding potential benefits of "watchful waiting" and re-evaluate him in 3 months

B. Advise the patient to undergo laparoscopic inguinal hernia repair, because the large randomized trials showed lower recurrence rates

C. Perform an open left inguinal hernia repair with primary sutured repair

D. Perform left inguinal hernia repair with prosthetic mesh and ilioinguinal neurectomy

E. Advise the patient to not have the hernia repaired

31.7 Which of the following is true of chronic pain after inguinal hernia repairs?

A. The most common cause of this problem is hernia recurrence

B. Chronic pain has become a rare occurrence with the introduction of mesh implantation during repairs

C. Young adults and women are the least susceptible to this problem

D. Causes of this condition include hernia recurrence, mesh-related reactions, nerve irritation, and infections

E. This problem can be virtually eliminated when hernia repairs are performed by expert surgeons

ANSWERS

31.1 **C.** While watchful waiting for femoral hernias has not been evaluated in a large prospective randomized fashion, limited observations suggest that femoral hernias are subjected to high rates of incarceration and strangulation and should not be managed by a "watchful waiting" approach. Femoral hernias are found inferior to the inguinal ligament and are amendable to both laparoscopic and open repair approaches. Open anterior femoral hernia repair require opening of the inguinal floor to identify the femoral canal and Cooper's ligament. Expertise for laparoscopic groin hernia repair is associated with greater than 250 cases.

31.2 **B.** Hesselbach's triangle is bordered by the rectus muscle medially, the inguinal ligament inferiorly, and the inferior epigastric vessels laterally. Direct inguinal hernias are found within Hesselbach's triangle. Indirect inguinal hernias are found lateral to Hesselbach's triangle.

31.3 **C.** Pain along the medial thigh with hip abduction, internal rotation, and/or external rotation is a finding consistent with the Howship–Romberg sign, which is associated with an obturator hernia.

31.4 **B.** This patient exhibits signs and symptoms of intestinal obstruction and findings of incarcerated right scrotal hernia. He also has fever and edema over the skin covering the hernia, which are findings suspicious for strangulation. No attempt at manual reduction of this hernia should be made, and the best treatment is resuscitation, followed by groin exploration to evaluate the hernia contents and repair of the hernia.

31.5 **B.** This patient has a history and physical findings compatible with recurrent left inguinal hernia. If the hernia affects the patient's quality of life, he should be offered the opportunity to have the hernia repaired again.

31.6 **D.** This is a young and active patient with a symptomatic inguinal hernia that is interfering with his work and activities. Based on these factors, the patient should be offered the opportunity to have his hernia repaired, and the repair that has been shown to work well is open repair with prosthetic mesh placement. Given the increased rate of nerve irritation from mesh placement, ilioinguinalneurectomy should be discussed with the patient.

31.7 **D.** Chronic postoperative pain following inguinal hernia repairs is defined as pain lasting longer than 3 months and is reported by 15% to 30% of patients. The cause of chronic pain is multifactorial and can include hernia recurrence (rare), nerve irritation, mesh-related responses, and infections.

CLINICAL PEARLS

▶ Recent evidence suggests that inguinal hernia incarcerations and strangulation rates are quite low for patients with small, asymptomatic inguinal hernias, therefore an initial trial of observation should be considered.

▶ The Howship–Romberg sign refers to the obturator neuralgia produced by nerve entrapment by an obturator hernia. This sign can be reproduced with hip abduction, internal rotation, extension, and external rotation.

REFERENCES

Fitzgibbons RJ Jr, Giobbie-Hurder A, Gibbs JO, et al. Watchful waiting vs repair of inguinal hernia is minimally symptomatic men: a randomized clinical trial. *JAMA*. 2006;295:285-292.

Neumayer L, Giobbie-Hurder A, Jonasson O, et al. Open mesh versus laparoscopic mesh repair of inguinal hernia. *N Engl J Med*. 2004;350:1819-1827.

Towfigh S, Neumayer L. Inguinal hernia. In: Cameron JL, Cameron AM, Eds. *Current Surgical Therapy*. 11th ed. Philadelphia, PA: Elsevier Saunders; 2014:531-536.

A 51-year-old woman presents with a 24-hour history of abdominal pain that began approximately 1 hour after dinner. This pain initially began as a dull ache in the upper abdomen but then later localized in the right upper abdomen. Associated with the pain, the patient had nausea without vomiting. While in the emergency department, her symptoms have improved somewhat after receiving a dose of parenteral analgesia. She describes having had similar pain episodes over the past several months, but the current episode is the worst. Her history is significant for type 2 diabetes controlled with diet only. Her temperature is 37.8°C (100°F), with the remaining vital signs being normal. Her abdomen is non-distended, with some focal tenderness in the right upper quadrant. Her WBC count is 13,000/mm³, her serum glucose is 212 mg/dL, and the remainder of her laboratory studies including chemistries, liver function tests, urinalysis, and amylase are within normal limits. The ultrasound of the right upper quadrant (RUQ) demonstrates multiple stones in the gallbladder, a thickened gallbladder wall, a small amount of fluid around the gallbladder, and a common bile duct (CBD) diameter of 4.5 mm (normal < 5 mm).

▶ What is the most likely diagnosis?
▶ What is the best therapy for this patient?
▶ What are the complications associated with this disease process?

ANSWERS TO CASE 32:
Gallstone Disease

Summary: A 51-year-old woman with type 2 diabetes presents with 1-day history of upper abdominal pain that began after a meal. Her history, physical examination, laboratory findings, ultrasound findings are suggestive of gallstone disease.

- **Most likely diagnosis**: Acute cholecystitis.

- **Best therapy**: Admission, IV fluids, IV antibiotics, followed rather quickly by laparoscopic cholecystectomy (LC). Surgery is the preferred treatment for a patient with normal life expectancy and no prohibitive risk for general anesthesia and abdominal surgery.

- **Complications**: Gallstone disease can include complications associated with the gallbladder (acute and/or chronic cholecystitis); complications related to the passage of stones from the gallbladder into the biliary duct (choledocholithiasis, cholangitis, and biliary pancreatitis); or stone passage into the GI tract (gallstone ileus).

ANALYSIS

Objectives

1. Learn the causes of gallstone disease and learn to differentiate and treat biliary colic, acute cholecystitis, and chronic cholecystitis.

2. Learn the diagnostic and therapeutic strategies for patients presenting with gallstone diseases.

3. Learn the complications that can develop from gallstone disease.

Consideration

This patient's history of recurrent upper abdominal pain occurring following meals suggests that she may have been experiencing recurrent bouts of biliary colic over the past year. Currently, she indicates that the pain has been persistent for 1 day, and more severe than prior episodes. Given her 24-hour duration of pain, low-grade fever, focal tenderness over the gallbladder, laboratory finding of leukocytosis, and sonographic findings of thickened gallbladder wall with peri-cholecystic fluid, her current clinical picture is most consistent with acute cholecystitis. With this diagnosis, the patient needs to be admitted to the hospital for monitoring, intravenous fluids, antibiotic treatment, and cholecystectomy during this hospitalization. A factor that should prompt us to proceed with cholecystectomy as early as feasible is her history of type II diabetes mellitus. Diabetic patients are highly susceptible to develop stress-induced hyperglycemia, and with hyperglycemia, her leukocyte functions are compromised, thus increasing her risk of infectious complications from acute cholecystitis.

APPROACH TO:
Gallstone Disease

DEFINITIONS

BILIARY COLIC: This describes the waxing and waning, poorly localized post-prandial upper abdominal pain that patients may have when their gallbladders are stimulated to contract but are unable to empty either because there is a gallstone obstruction at the gallbladder neck or cystic duct. Rarely, biliary colic can also be produced by cholecystokinin (CCK) stimulation of a dysfunctional gallbladder, such as in the case of biliary dyskinesia.

ACUTE CHOLECYSTITIS: In most patients, this infectious process occurs as the result of persistent obstruction of the cystic duct by a gallstone. When the obstructive process does not resolve spontaneously, bacterial infection can occur via the lymphatic channels. The most common organisms involved in acute cholecystitis are *Escherichia coli, Klebsiella, Proteus,* and *Steptococcus faecalis.* Patients present with persistent RUQ pain, with or without fever, focal gallbladder tenderness, mild leukocytosis or normal WBC count, and normal LFTs or nonspecific abnormalities in the LFTs. Treatment is NPO, intravenous antibiotics, and cholecystectomy during the hospitalization.

ACALCULOUS CHOLECYSTITIS: This condition involves gallbladder inflammation and infection secondary to biliary stasis. This type of cholecystitis is responsible for <5% of all patients with acute cholecystitis. Most often, affected individuals are hospitalized patients undergoing other medical treatments. Patients who are susceptible to this condition often have low perfusion states and are not taking an oral diet (classically, ICU patients receiving mechanical ventilation who are NPO and receiving vasoactive agents for blood pressure support). The NPO status contributes to GB distension, and with decrease perfusion, ischemic injury of the GB occurs along with bacterial infection.

CHRONIC CHOLECYSTITIS: This is produced by recurrent bouts of biliary colic and acute cholecystitis, which causes fibrosis and chronic inflammation of the GB. Most patients complain of long-standing history of postprandial RUQ pain with pain becoming more tolerable as the process continues over time. This change in pain pattern probably correlates with increasing fibrotic changes and decreasing inflammatory changes in the GB over the course of disease. Ultrasound findings may reveal gallstones, thickened GB wall, and possibly a small, contracted GB.

CHOLANGITIS: This is a very serious infection within the bile ducts. It most commonly occurs in the setting of stones within the CBD causing either partial or completed obstruction of the CBD. Classically, **Charcot's Triad (fever, RUQ pain, and jaundice)** is seen in about 70% of the patients. This condition can be serious and associated with sepsis, septic shock, and distant-organ dysfunction. Systemic manifestations of this illness occur because ascending infections in the biliary tree can cause activation of the Kupffer cells (hepatic macrophages) and produce systemic proinflammatory responses and multiple-organ-dysfunction syndrome. Patients suspected of having cholangitis should be hospitalized. Early treatments for these patients include close monitoring, resuscitation, early broad-spectrum antimicrobial therapy, and biliary decompression. **Reynolds pentad** refers to the clinical picture produced by severe cholangitis (**fever, abdominal pain, jaundice, shock,** and **altered mental status**), and patients presenting with this picture need aggressive supportive care, antibiotics, and urgent biliary decompression.

RIGHT UPPER QUADRANT ULTRASONOGRAPHY: This imaging modality possesses 98% to 99% sensitivity in identifying gallstones in the GB. The examination also helps identify the diameter of the CBD, which has a high negative-predictive value for common bile duct stones (CBDS) when the CBD is small (<5 mm).

BILIARY SCINTIGRAPHY: This is a nuclear medicine study involving intravenous injection of nuclear tracer that is taken up by the liver and excreted into the biliary system. Becase the patient with acute cholecystitis generally has obstruction of the cystic duct, this study can be used to determine if a patient has acute cholecystitis. Therefore the tracer will visualize the liver and extrahepatic biliary tree with subsequent visualization of the duodenum, but the gallbladder is never visualized.

MAGNETIC RESONANCE CHOLANGIOPANCREATOGRAPHY (MRCP): This is an MRI study using a set of sequences that allows for imaging of the biliary ducts and pancreatic ducts. With this technique, stones and masses within these ducts will cause signal void and thus can be demonstrated. The sensitivity and specificity of MRCP is nearly identical to that of **endoscopic retrograde cholangiopancreatography** (ERCP), but this technique cannot be utilized for intervention when CBDS are seen.

LAPAROSCOPIC CHOLECYSTECTOMY (LC): This is a laparoscopic approach to the removal of the gallbladder. LCs are performed under general anesthesia in most cases. Commonly, three or four ports are placed with the introduction of a camera and instruments. Postoperatively, the majority of patients either go home the same day or the next day. Most patients are able to return to work or normal daily activities within a few days. During LC, cholangiography can be performed by inserting a catheter through the cystic duct and injecting contrast to visualize stones or abnormalities in the biliary tree.

ENDOSCOPIC RETROGRADE CHOLANGIOPANCREATOGRAPHY (ERCP): Using the side-viewing flexible endoscope, the ampulla of Vater can be visualized and canalized, thus allowing for contrast injection and visualization of the CBD and pancreatic duct. Through the working channel of the scope, baskets, balloons, and snares can be inserted to help with the extraction of stones and biopsy of tissue.

COMMON BILE DUCT EXPLORATION (CBDE): This is a direct exploration of the CBD by either open surgery or the laparoscopic approach. The goal in most cases is to remove CBDS in the bile ducts. CBDE is not commonly done unless less invasive means to remove the CBDS (such as by ERCP) are unsuccessful or unavailable.

CLINICAL APPROACH

Pathophysiology

At least 16 million Americans have gallstones, and 800,000 new cases occur each year. Gallstone types are categorized as **cholesterol stones, black pigment stones, and brown pigment stones.** Cholesterol stones make up majority of the gallstones (80%) in Western populations. Cholesterol stone development is predisposed by an imbalance of cholesterol to bile acid ratio in the bile. When this biochemical imbalance exists in the bile, the bile is lithogenic and the patient is susceptible to cholesterol stone formation in the gallbladder. Stone formation requires an activation process that is contributed to by defects within the gall bladder mucosa; therefore, cholesterol stones only form in the gallbladder when there is underlying GB dysfunction. For patients with cholesterol stone disease, if the GB is removed with all the stones, the patient should become free from further stone recurrences.

There are many people with gallstones who remain asymptomatic but for reasons that are unknown, approximately 15% to 20% of patients with gallstones will develop symptoms (biliary colic). Once a patient develops symptoms, he/she is then at risk for subsequent complications related to the gallstones (eg, cholecystitis, biliary pancreatitis, choledocholithiasis, and cholangitis).

Patient Evaluation and Treatment

The evaluation for every patient suspected of gallstone disease should include a history, physical examination, a complete blood count, liver function studies, serum amylase, and a RUQ ultrasound. If the patient with gallstones does not have symptoms or complications that can be attributed to the stones, no treatment is necessary. For patients with symptoms, it is important to differentiate whether the patient has simply biliary colic or GB complications (ie, cholecystitis, choledocholithiasis, biliary pancreatitis, or cholangitis). Frequently, those with gallstone complications need hospitalization, antibiotics, and possibly additional diagnostic studies, and/or interventions such as ERCP with endoscopic sphincterotomy. As outlined in Table 32–1, there are subtle differences in the history and physical examinations, laboratory findings, and ultrasound findings that may suggest that a patient may have a CBDS. The frequency of finding CBDS concurrently in a patient under evaluation for cholecystectomy is reported to range from 8% to 20%, and the probability of concurrent CBDS varies greater depending on the patient's clinical presentations. Dilatation of the CBD (>5mm) with elevation in LFTs (eg, bilirubin, alkaline phosphatase, AST, and ALT) should raise the concern for common bile duct stones. When the suspicion is high, the patients should undergo an ERCP to evaluate the CBD prior to or after the completion of cholecystectomy. For patients in whom there is a moderate suspicion (30%-50% probability) for CBDS (such as a patient with cholecystitis or biliary pancreatitis with CBD >5 mm and LFT elevations), an MRCP can be performed to rule out CBDS; if CBDS are visualized then an ERCP can be performed for duct clearance. It is important to consider that because stones can pass from the GB to the CBD at any time. Whenever a patient with cholelithiasis develops new symptoms or a change in the clinical picture, laboratory and ultrasound reassessment are needed to make sure that there

Table 32–1 • GALLSTONE DISEASE PRESENTATIONS

Disease	Symptoms	Physical Examination	Ultrasonography	Laboratory Studies
Biliary colic	Postprandial pain, usually <6 h in duration	Afebrile, mild tenderness over gallbladder	Gallstones in gallbladder but no wall thickening, no CBD dilation	Normal WBC count, normal LFT values, normal serum amylase level
Acute cholecystitis	Persistent epigastric or RUQ pain lasting >8 h	May be febrile or afebrile; usually localized gallbladder tenderness	Gallstones in gallbladder; may have pericholecystic fluid; may or may not have CBD dilation	Normal or elevated WBC count; may have normal or mildly elevated LFT values
Chronic cholecystitis	Persistent recurrent RUQ pain	Afebrile; may have localized tenderness over a palpable gallbladder	Stones in gallbladder, thickened gallbladder wall; in advanced cases contracted gallbladder	Normal WBC count; may have mild elevation in LFT values
Choledocholithiasis	Postprandial abdominal pain that improves with fasting	May or may not be clinically jaundiced; nonspecific RUQ abdominal tenderness	Gallstones in gallbladder; CBD usually dilated	Elevation in LFT values; the pattern of elevation is dependent on the chronicity and partial vs complete obstruction
Biliary pancreatitis	Persistent epigastric and back pain	Epigastric tenderness to deep palpation is present	Gallstones in gallbladder; CBD dilation may occur because of pancreatitis (does not always indicate CBD stones)	Leukocytosis, serum amylase level frequently >1000 U/L, LFT values may be transiently elevated, but persistence may indicate CBD stones

Abbreviations: CBD, common bile duct; LFT, liver function test; RUQ, right upper quadrant; WBC, white blood cell.

are no CBDS present. Complications of undiagnosed and untreated CBDS include cholangitis, pancreatitis, and biliary cirrhosis.

Whether a routine intraoperative cholangiogram should be done during every LC has been a controversial topic among surgeons. The proponents for routine cholangiography believe that this procedure helps to clarify the biliary tract anatomy, and minimizes inadvertent operative injuries. Opponents to routine intraoperative cholangiography believe that because the rate of injuries is so low during elective cases (0.2%-0.5%) that cholangiography during every LC contributes to extended operating times and wasted resources.

Biliary Pancreatitis

Priorities for patients who present with acute biliary pancreatitis include the determination of pancreatitis severity, and the provision of monitoring and supportive care. The majority of patients with biliary pancreatitis have a short disease course and recover within hours to days. Biliary pancreatitis patients with sonographic CBD measurements <5 mm and rapid clinical resolution have only a 1-2% risk of CBDS therefore no additional diagnostic studies to look for CBDS are necessary. When patients present with biliary pancreatitis, they should have cholecystectomy performed during the same hospitalization, because delayed LC for these patients is associated with recurrent pancreatitis, greater morbidity, and increased treatment costs. Clinical evidence suggests that patients presenting with mild cases of biliary pancreatitis (<3 Ranson's criteria) can safely undergo LC within 48 hours of admission. Furthermore, for patients with biliary pancreatitis, it is safe to proceed with LC once their pain and symptoms resolve, and it is unnecessary to wait for normalization of the serum amylase and lipase. The optimal timing for LC in patients presenting with severe pancreatitis with complications remains unclear, and those patients should be managed on a case by case basis.

CASE CORRELATION

- See also Case 33 (Peri-Ambullary Tumor), Case 34 (Liver Tumor), and Case 35 (Pancreatitis).

COMPREHENSION QUESTIONS

32.1 A 65-year-old woman presents to the emergency department with postprandial RUQ pain, nausea, and emesis over the past 12 hours. The pain is persistent and radiates to her back. She is afebrile, and her abdomen is tender to palpation in the RUQ. An ultrasound demonstrates cholelithiasis, gallbladder wall thickening, and a CBD of 12 mm. Her laboratory studies reveal WBC count of 13,000/mm^3, AST 220 U/L, ALT 240 U/L, alkaline phosphatase 385 U/L, and direct bilirubin 4.1 mg/dL. Which of the following is the most appropriate management at this time?

A. Admit her to the hospital, start intravenous fluids, and check her hepatitis serology

B. Admit her to the hospital and perform laparoscopic cholecystectomy as soon as possible

C. Admit the patient to the hospital, provide intravenous hydration, begin antibiotics therapy, and recommend ERCP

D. Provide pain medication in the emergency room and ask the patient to follow-up in the outpatient clinic

E. Schedule the patient for laparoscopic cholecystectomy and liver biopsy

32.2 A 28-year-old woman undergoing an obstetric ultrasound during the second trimester of pregnancy is found to have gallstones in her gallbladder. She claims that she has had indigestion and frequent belching throughout her pregnancy. Which of the following is the most appropriate treatment for her?

A. Recommend a low-fat diet until the end of pregnancy and then a postpartum laparoscopic cholecystectomy

B. Schedule her laparoscopic cholecystectomy during the second trimester of her pregnancy

C. Perform an open cholecystectomy during the second trimester

D. Prescribe chenodeoxycholate

E. Recommend no treatment

32.3 A 45-year-old man is seen in the emergency center for abdominal pain. A presumptive diagnosis of acute cholecystitis is made. Which of the following findings are most consistent with this diagnosis?

A. Fever, intermittent RUQ pain, and jaundice

B. Persistent upper abdominal pain, RUQ tenderness, and leukocytosis

C. Intermittent abdominal pain, minimal tenderness over the gallbladder, normal LFTs

D. Persistent epigastric pain and back pain, temperature of 100.5°F (38.1°C)

E. Afebrile, jaundice, with palpable and nontender gallbladder

32.4 A 69-year-old man presents with confusion, abdominal pain, shaking chills, a temperature of 34°C (95°F), and jaundice. An abdominal radiograph demonstrates air in the biliary tree and normal bowel gas pattern. Which of the following is the most likely diagnosis?

A. Acute pancreatitis

B. Acute cholangitis

C. Acute cholecystitis

D. Acute viral hepatitis

E. Gallstone ileus

32.5 A 33-year-old otherwise healthy woman presents to the emergency center with RUQ pain. Her temperature is 38.1°C. Her abdomen is focally tender in the RUQ. Her WBC is 11,000/mm^3, and the liver function studies demonstrate mild elevation of the bilirubin, alkaline phosphatase, AST, and ALT. An ultrasound reveals stones in the GB, and CBD diameter of 4 mm. Which is the most appropriate management for this patient?

A. Prescribe pain medication and oral antibiotics and then schedule her for laparoscopic cholecystectomy in 6-8 weeks

B. NPO, antibiotics, ERCP followed by laparoscopic cholecystectomy

C. NPO, antibiotics, and laparoscopic cholecystectomy

D. NPO, antibiotics, repeat her laboratory studies and ultrasound in 24-48 hours

E. Viral hepatitis panel and inquire regarding travel history

32.6 A 30-year-old woman presents with recurrent postprandial abdominal pain for the past 6 months. She has undergone two ultrasound studies that revealed a normal appearing gallbladder without gallstones. Her liver function studies, serum amylase and lipase studies are normal. Which of the following is the best management for this patient?

A. Obtain a CCK-stimulated HIDA (hepatobiliaryiminodiacetic acid) scan

B. Proceed with laparoscopic cholecystectomy

C. Provide empiric treatment for *H. pylori*

D. Repeat the gallbladder ultrasound study

E. Obtain a hepatitis panel to rule out viral hepatitis

32.7 A 26-year-old woman presents with epigastric pain. Her temperature and vital signs are normal. Her WBC count is 11,000/mm³, and her LFTs and urinalysis are within normal limits. Her serum amylase is 1200 mg/dL. Her ultrasound revealed cholelithiasis and a CBD diameter of 3.8 mm. One day after admission, her pain resolves. Her serum amylase remains elevated at 985 mg/dL. Which of the following is the best treatment for her?

A. Continue to observe patient and repeat her laboratory studies, and proceed with laparoscopic cholecystectomy when labs normalize

B. Discharge the patient and schedule her for elective laparoscopic cholecystectomy in 6 weeks

C. Proceed with laparoscopic cholecystectomy

D. Recommend dietary modification and prescribe ursodeoxycholate to help dissolve her gallstones

E. Perform an ERCP to clear her CBD prior to laparoscopic cholecystectomy

32.8 A 63-year-old woman presents to the emergency center after being found confused at home by her neighbors. Her temperature is 39.0°C (102.2°F), blood pressure is 96/50 initially and improved to 105/60 after 2000 mL of IV normal saline. Her abdomen is mildly tender diffusely in the upper abdomen. The laboratory findings are significant for a WBC count of 18,000/mm³, total bilirubin to 4.8 mg/dL, amylase of 45 mg/dL, and alkaline phosphatase value of 385 mg/dL. Her ultrasound demonstrates a gallbladder filled with small stones, mild-moderate intrahepatic ductal dilatation, and CBD diameter of 9.0 mm. Which of the following is the best management plan for this patient?

A. Initiate broad-spectrum antibiotics treatment, administer intravenous fluid and admit the patient to the ICU

B. Initiate broad-spectrum antibiotics treatment, administer intravenous fluid, and proceed with urgent cholecystectomy and common bile duct exploration

C. Initiate broad-spectrum antibiotics, administer intravenous fluids, perform an ERCP to decompress her bile ducts

D. Initiate broad-spectrum antibiotics, administer intravenous fluids, obtain a CT scan to rule out intra-abdominal abscess or other infectious sources

E. Initiate broad-spectrum antibiotics, administer intravenous fluids, proceed with immediate operative CBD exploration

ANSWERS

32.1 **C.** This 65-year-old woman has upper abdominal pain, leukocytosis, and marked abnormalities in her LFTs, specifically marked elevation of the total bilirubin and alkaline phosphatase values. Her picture is consistent with cholangitis. Treatment for a patient with cholangitis includes close monitoring, intravenous antibiotics, and biliary decompression. This condition should not be confused with cholecystitis, because the treatment priority for a patient with cholecystitis is antibiotics and cholecystectomy. The reason that the LFT elevations are more likely related to CBD obstruction rather than hepatitis or other hepatic abnormalities is because her common bile duct is markedly dilated at 12 mm.

32.2 **E.** This 28-year-old pregnant woman with incidental gallstones seen during her obstetrics sonography has belching and some indigestion during her pregnancy. Her symptoms are more likely related to physiologic changes related to pregnancy than her gallstones. It is likely that she has asymptomatic gallstones and would not need any specific treatment. It is important to educate the patient regarding symptoms related to gallstones so that she can undergo early evaluation and treatment if symptoms should develop.

32.3 **B.** Persistent upper abdominal pain, RUQ tenderness, and leukocytosis are most consistent with acute cholecystitis. Fever, intermittent RUQ pain, and jaundice listed in "A" are most consistent with symptomatic choledocholithiasis. Intermittent abdominal pain, minimal tenderness over GB, and normal LFTs best describe biliary colic. Persistent epigastric pain, back pain, and fever suggest with acute pancreatitis. A patient who is afebrile with palpable and nontender gallbladder describes Courvoisier's sign, which points to malignant obstruction of the biliary tree such as from a peri-ampullary tumor.

32.4 **B.** The patient described here has confusion, abdominal pain, shaking chills, fever, and jaundice. These findings are most indicative of acute cholangitis.

32.5 **C.** This patient presents with fever, RUQ pain, and has focal tenderness over her gallbladder. The liver function studies are mildly elevated and her CBD diameter is 4 mm by ultrasound imaging. Given these findings, she most likely has acute cholecystitis. Liver function test abnormality is not uncommon in patients with acute cholecystitis, and the possible causes include common bile duct stone obstruction of the common bile duct or nonspecific hepatitis due to gallbladder inflammation. For this patient, whose bile duct is 4 mm in diameter, the probability that a CBD stone is obstructing her CBD is very low; therefore, ERCP is not indicated. The best course of treatments for this patient is NPO, antibiotics, and laparoscopic cholecystectomy as soon as feasible.

32.6 **A.** This is a woman with 6 months-history of postprandial abdominal pain that is consistent with biliary colic; however, ultrasound reveals no stones in her gallbladder. It is possible that she has biliary dyskinesia, which is due to functional defects of the gallbladder causing ineffective gallbladder contractions producing pain patterns that are nearly identical to those associated with biliary colic. To determine whether biliary dyskinesia is the problem, a CCK-stimulated HIDA scan should be obtained. If she has biliary dyskinesia, her CCK-stimulated HIDA scan will demonstrate inadequate emptying (gallbladder ejection fraction that is less than one-third of normal) following CCK injection, and CCK should also reproduce her symptoms.

32.7 **C.** This young woman with gallstones presents with a mild bout of acute biliary pancreatitis. Her symptoms improve one day after admission. Cohort observation studies have shown that it is safe to proceed with laparoscopic cholecystectomy when patients with acute biliary pancreatitis show improvement in symptoms, and it is not necessary to follow her serum amylase or lipase as those values do not reflect pancreatitis severity, and do not help determine the optimal timing for cholecystectomy.

32.8 **C.** The 63-year-old woman described here has cholangitis with septic shock. Since this process is caused by obstruction of the CBD and cholangitis, treatment priorities are to provide supportive care, start broad-spectrum antibiotics, and arrange for urgent decompression of the biliary tree by ERCP. Even though the gallbladder is the source of the common bile duct stones and needs to be removed, the patient's current primary concern is with her common bile duct obstruction and cholangitis.

CLINICAL PEARLS

▶ Cholecystitis is generally not present unless there is a clear link between the patient's symptoms and gallstones or if there is objective evidence of gallbladder dysfunction or pathology (eg, a thickened gallbladder wall on ultrasound, nonvisualization of the gallbladder by HIDA scan) or gallstone-related complications (choledocholithiasis, cholangitis, cholecystitis, or biliary pancreatitis).

▶ In general, the treatment of cholecystitis involves hospitalization, NPO, intravenous antibiotics, and laparoscopic cholecystectomy prior to hospital discharge.

▶ Choledocholithiasis should be suspected when patient present with gallstone-related disease, elevated liver enzymes (especially bilirubin and alkaline phosphatase) and CBD diameter greater than 5 mm based on ultrasound.

▶ Cholangitis should be suspected when patients with gallstones present with nonfocal upper abdominal pain, liver enzyme elevation, dilated CBD, and fever.

▶ Gallstone ileus should be suspected when patients present with pneumobilia (air in the biliary system) and small bowel obstruction.

▶ Acute cholecystitis should be suspected when patients with gallstones present with biliary colic-like symptoms that fail to resolve after more than 6-8 hours.

▶ Biliary colic symptoms and choledocholithiasis symptoms are nearly identical. Only patients with biliary colic do not have abnormalities in their liver enzymes, whereas choledocholithiasis patients have LFT elevations that can be nonspecific.

REFERENCES

Aboulian A, Chan T, Kaji AH, et al. Early cholecystectomy safely decreases hospital stay in patients with mild gallstone pancreatitis: a randomized prospective study. *Ann Surg*. 2010;251:615-619.

Ahmed R, Duncan MD. The management of common bile duct stones. In: Cameron JL, Cameron AM, eds. *Current Surgical Therapy*. 11th ed. Philadelphia, PA: Elsevier Saunders; 2014:391-395.

Jackson PG, Evans SRT. Biliary system. In: Townsend CM Jr, Beauchamp RD, Evers BM, Mattox KL, eds. *Sabiston Textbook of Surgery: The Biological Basis of Modern Surgical Practice*. 19th ed. Philadelphia, PA: Elsevier Saunders; 2012:1476-1514.

A 58-year-old woman presents to your office complaining of generalized itching. On examination, she appears jaundiced. During your interview, you learn that she has experienced a 10-lb (4.5-kg) weight loss over the past several months and recently has noted the passage of tea-colored urine. Her past medical history is significant for type 2 diabetes mellitus that was diagnosed 5 months previously, and she denies any history of hepatitis. She smokes one pack of cigarettes a day but does not consume alcohol. Her temperature and the remainder of her vital signs are within normal limits. The abdomen is soft and nontender. The gallbladder is palpable but without tenderness. Her stool is hemoccult negative. The laboratory evaluation reveals a normal complete blood count. Other laboratory findings include a total bilirubin 14.5 mg/dL, direct bilirubin 10.8 mg/dL, aspartate aminotransferase (AST) 120 U/L, alanine aminotransferase (ALT) 190 U/L, alkaline phosphatase 448 mg/dL, and serum amylase 85 IU/L.

▶ What it the cause of the biochemical abnormalities?
▶ What is the most likely diagnosis?
▶ How would you confirm the diagnosis?

ANSWER TO CASE 33:
Peri-Ampullary Tumor

Summary: A 58-year-old woman presents with painless obstructive jaundice, weight loss, recent onset diabetes mellitus, and generalized pruritis.

- **Cause of the biochemical abnormalities:** Obstruction of the biliary tree.

- **Most likely diagnosis:** Obstructive jaundice caused by a peri-ampullary cancer.

- **Confirmation of the diagnosis:** Start with an ultrasound of the biliary system to rule-out biliary stones as the cause of obstruction. A CT scan of the abdomen is helpful to visualize obstructive lesions along the intrahepatic and extrahepatic biliary system and determine the location of the obstruction. If a peri-ampullary mass is seen on CT, endoscopic ultrasonography can be helpful to visualize the local extent of the lesion and can be utilized to obtain biopsies of the lesion.

ANALYSIS

Objectives

1. Be familiar with the diagnostic approach for obstructive jaundice.

2. Be familiar with the roles and outcomes of surgical and palliative therapies in the treatment of patients with peri-ampullary cancers.

Considerations

Mechanisms contributing to jaundice can be broadly categorized as disorders of bilirubin metabolism, hepatocellular dysfunction, and biliary tract obstruction. The pattern of this patient's liver functions tests strongly suggests an obstructive pattern with hyperbilirubinemia contributed by a predominance of direct bilirubin elevation. Her alkaline phosphatase elevation and mild AST and ALT elevations are consistent with obstructive jaundice of some chronicity leading to mild hepatocellular injury. Her physical examination is consistent with this diagnosis, as she is noted to have a palpable and nontender gallbladder (known as **Courvoisier sign**). The recent history of type 2 diabetes mellitus and weight loss further suggest that this patient's current picture of obstructive jaundice is secondary to a peri-ampullary cancer that may be a pancreatic adenocarcinoma, ampullary carcinoma, duodenal carcinoma or distal cholangiocarcinoma.

Even though biliary stone disease is by far the most common cause of biliary obstruction, most patients with common bile duct stones (CBDS) do not have the level of bilirubinemia that is exhibited by this patient (total bilirubin 14.5 mg/dL). The reason that obstructive jaundice from CBDS usually does not produce hyperbilirubinemia to this level is because the obstruction is usually intermittent in nature rather than a persistent obstruction; therefore, the total bilirubin elevations from gallstones rarely exceed 6 to 8 mg/dL.

Ultrasonography of the liver, gallbladder, and biliary tree is a good imaging study to assess for stones in the gallbladder and measure the CBD diameter. In all likelihood, a CT of the abdomen will also be needed to evaluate the pancreas, the liver, biliary ductal dilatations, and mass lesions in the liver and/or near the extrahepatic biliary tree and peri-ampullary region.

If the imaging studies confirm a peri-ampullary tumor, then evidence of distant disease should be sought. The next step of the evaluation is to determine if the tumor is curable by surgical resection. Localized peri-ampullary cancer without significant invasion/involvement of the superior mesenteric vein/portal vein area is potentially curable with surgical resection and adjuvant chemotherapy. Prior to surgical exploration, most surgeons will obtain an endoscopic retrograde pancreatography (ERCP) and/or an endoscopic ultrasound (EUS). The ERCP in this case can be helpful to see if there are obstructing lesions involving the ampulla of Vater or duodenum. In addition, ERCP can be used to place a biliary stent to help relieve the patient's biliary obstruction and help treat her pruritis. The EUS is particularly helpful to assess whether tumor invasion of the superior mesenteric vessels has occurred. In addition, needle biopsies can be obtained during EUS for tissue diagnosis. If all diagnostic studies suggest that the lesion is a localized and potentially resectable peri-ampullary carcinoma, operative treatment by pancreaticoduodenectomy (PD) should be offered to the patient as potentially curative treatment.

APPROACH TO:
Peri-Ampullary Tumors

DEFINITIONS

PERI-AMPULLARY CANCERS: Common cancers in this location are pancreatic ductal adenocarcinoma, distal CBD cancers (cholangiocarcinomas), adenocarcinomas of the ampulla of Vater, and duodenal adenocarcinomas. Mucinous cystic tumors of the pancreas and pancreatic lymphomas are two of the less commonly found tumors in this region.

PANCREAS PROTOCOL CT: This is a dedicated CT designed to provide high-quality images to help determine the resectability of tumors in head of the pancreas cancers. Generally, this is CT takes 1-mm thin sections after intravenous contrast administration. CT image acquisitions are timed to depict arterial and portal venous phases to help visualize the structures adjacent to the superior mesenteric vein, superior mesenteric artery, and portal vein.

PANCREATICODUODENECTOMY (PD): This is an operation involving resection of the duodenum, the head of pancreas, distal common bile duct, gallbladder, and sometimes the distal stomach. PD can be performed with an open abdominal approach or laparoscopic approach. PD is indicated for the treatment of patients with tumors and benign conditions localized in the area immediately surrounding the ampulla of Vater. The classic form of this operation is called a Whipple resection. The operative outcomes of PD have improved significantly over the past two decades with reported 30-day mortality rates of 0% to 2% by some groups; however, the procedure is still associated with high rates of postoperative complications (20%-40%). With improvements in the operative outcomes of PDs, many groups now will perform PD with en-bloc resections of superior mesenteric vein/portal vein and vascular reconstructions.

PERI-AMPULLARY CARCINOMA RESECTABILITY: Given that PD with venous resection and reconstruction has become feasible, involvement of the superior mesenteric vein is no longer a contraindication to attempted tumor resection. Most surgical centers feel that with <90-degree circumferential involvement of the SMV, tumor resection with vascular reconstruction is feasible, while other groups feel that a greater amount of venous involvement does not necessarily contraindicate surgical resection. Involvement of the SMA is a contraindication to resection because the prognosis is poor even after resection of all gross disease. Presence of distant metastases and intraperitoneal metastases are considered contraindications to resection.

GEMCITABINE: This is a chemotherapeutic agent (deoxycytidine analogue) that appears to prolong the survival of patients with pancreatic ductal carcinoma and other peri-ampullary carcinomas. Gemcitabine is an effective radiation sensitizer, and are often given in conjunction with external beam radiation therapy. In addition to its oncologic benefits, gemcitabine helps to relieve pain related to pancreatic cancers.

CLINICAL APPROACH

Peri-ampullary cancers are a set of neoplasms that can originate from the **pancreatic duct, the ampulla, duodenum**, or **bile duct epithelium**. These tumors have different biological behaviors but are grouped together because patients with these lesions often present with clinical presentations that are quite similar (obstructive jaundice is the most common).

Pancreatic ductal carcinoma is the most common of the peri-ampullary cancers. Pancreatic cancers make up only 2% of the newly diagnosed cancers in the United States, but are the fourth leading cause of cancer deaths. Five to ten percent of patients who develop pancreatic cancer have familial forms of pancreatic cancers related to *BRCA2*, hereditary nonpolyposis colorectal cancer (HNPCC), or other germ line defects. Surgical resection is possible in 20% to 30% of patients with pancreatic cancer, with 5-year survival rates of 15% to 25% reported following resections. **CA19-9 is a tumor marker that is highly sensitive for the diagnosis of adenocarcinoma of the pancreas.** Unfortunately, *CA19-9* elevation is not specific for pancreatic cancers. This tumor marker can become elevated as the result of biliary obstruction from other causes, or as the result of blood Lewis-antigen negative status. *CA19-9* can be useful for post-treatment surveillances. Two-thirds of pancreatic cancers arise from the head and uncinate process, 15% originate in the body, and 10% originate from the tail. See Table 33–1 for staging.

Cholangiocarcinoma of the distal CBD is the second most common peri-ampullary cancer. These lesions typically are found in patients in their sixties. Risk factors

Table 33–1 • TNM STAGING OF PANCREATIC ADENOCARCINOMA	
Tumor status (T)	
Tis:	Carcinoma in situ (tumor is confined to top layer of pancreatic ductal cells)
T1:	≤2 cm and confined to the pancreas
T2:	>2 cm and confined to the pancreas
T3:	Tumor extending beyond pancreas but not into surround major structures
T4:	Tumor extending beyond pancreas and involves surrounding structures
Nodal status (N)	
NX:	Regional lymph nodes cannot be assessed
N0:	No regional lymph node involvement
N1:	Regional lymph node involvement present
Metastasis status (M)	
M0:	No evidence of distant spread
M1:	Cancer has either spread to distant lymph nodes and/or distant sites
Stage 0	Tis, N0, M0
Stage IA **Stage IB**	T1, N0, M0 T2, N0, M0
Stage IIA **Stage IIB**	T3, N0, M0 T1-3, N1, M0
Stage III	T4, any N, M0
Stage IV	Any T, Any N, M1

described for cholangiocarcinoma include sclerosing cholangitis, choledochal cysts, hepatolithiasis, and liver flukes. Surgical resections for patients with distal cholangiocarcinomas are associated with a 20% to 40% 5-year survival.

Adenocarcinoma of the Ampulla of Vater is the third most common peri-ampullary cancer. These lesions are rare and appear to be the peri-ampullary cancer associated with the best prognosis. Because of the origin of this cancer, patients generally present with jaundice earlier than patients with other forms of peri-ampullary cancers. The reported 5-year survival after resection is 35% to 55%.

Peri-ampullary duodenal carcinoma makes up only about 5% of the peri-ampullary cancers. These lesions tend to be larger than the other types of peri-ampullary cancers at diagnosis. The biological behavior of duodenal carcinoma is better than the other types of peri-ampullary cancers, and the 5-year survival after resection is in the range of 40% to 60%.

Adjuvant and Neoadjuvant Therapy

Surgery alone for peri-ampullary cancers can be associated with up to 80% disease recurrences, thus suggesting that surgery alone is not sufficient for most patients (see Figure 33–1 for treatment algorithm). One of the most difficult issues involving the treatment of this patient population is that effective adjuvant treatment options currently do not exist. Current adjuvant chemotherapy and chemoradiation

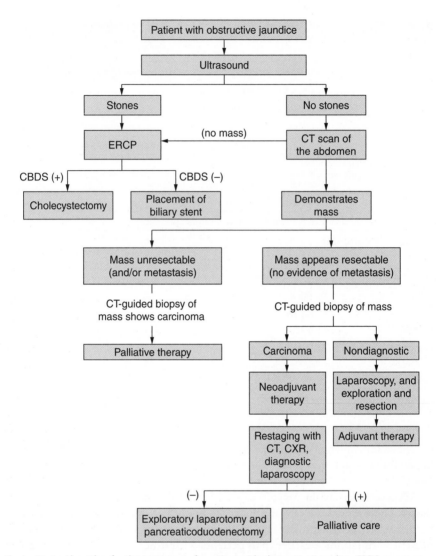

Figure 33–1. Algorithm for the treatment of a patient with obstructive jaundice. CBDS, common bile duct stone; CT, computed tomography; CXR, chest radiograph; ERCP, endoscopic retrograde cholangiopancreatography.

therapy provide additional survival that is often measured in term of months. At this time, adjuvant radiation therapy is offered to patients with close or involved resection margins, and adjuvant chemotherapy is offered to most patients with good functional status and recovery following surgical resection. Some investigators have developed neoadjuvant chemotherapy regimens and have reported that patients with resectable pancreatic cancers who underwent (neoadjuvant) chemoradiation therapy prior to resection had improved survival in comparison to patients who underwent resection followed by adjuvant therapy. Unfortunately, the real benefits of neoadjuvant therapy in these patients remain unclear because it is difficult to sort out whether observed improved survival may be due to selection bias, by selection of patients with more favorable tumor biology for surgical resections.

Palliative Therapy for Peri-Ampullary Cancers

Survival of patients with pancreatic cancers and other peri-ampullary cancers is often in the range of several weeks up to 2 years, when the tumors are not amendable to curative resections. Unfortunately, most of these individuals will develop biliary obstruction, duodenal obstruction, and/or pain prior to death. The biliary obstructions in patients with peri-ampullary cancers are most often located in the distal bile duct, and these types of obstructions can be addressed with placement of intraluminal stents to bypass the biliary obstructions. Stent placement can be performed endoscopically in some cases or by a percutaneous transhepatic route, depending whether the biliary tree can be accessed through the Ampulla of Vater. When prolonged survival (>6 months) is anticipated, a metal mesh stent can be placed. Otherwise, in patients who are expected to have shorter survival, a plastic stent can be inserted for short-term palliation. For patients who undergo operative explorations and are subsequently found to have unresectable disease, surgical bypass of the biliary tree and the duodenum can be performed with the creation of a cholecystojejunostomy or choledochal-jejunostomy. Similarly, duodenal obstruction can be relieved surgically with formation of a gastrojejunostomy. Duodenal obstruction by peri-ampullary tumors can be palliated endoscopically with the placement of self-expanding metal stents when the obstructive process is not complete.

When considering palliative procedures for patients with peri-ampullary cancers, it is important to determine the severity of the biliary obstruction, its effects on the quality of life, and assess whether GI tract obstruction has occurred or will likely occur. The greatest uncertainty for these patients is estimation of their life-expectancies, as we do not want to over-treat individuals with limited survival or under-treat individuals with longer than expected survival. Palliative chemotherapy or palliative chemoradiation therapy can be also considered for some individuals and have been demonstrated to extend survival. Over the past decade, palliative chemotherapy and chemoradiation treatments have become more effective in prolonging patient survival, thereby increasing the need for palliative surgical and endoscopic procedures in patients with unresectable peri-ampullary cancers.

Palliation of Pain

Pain associated with peri-ampullary cancers can be excruciating; for some patients, this pain can be alleviated or partially alleviated with percutaneous celiac plexus nerve blocks or nerve ablation in addition to standard narcotic analgesia. These procedures can often be accomplished under CT guidance. Alternatively, endoscopic/endo-ultrasound-guided celiac plexus blocks can also be performed in some patients for pain relief.

CYSTIC NEOPLASMS OF THE PANCREAS

Cystic tumors of the pancreas are the second most common exocrine pancreatic neoplasms; pancreatic pseudocysts are by far the most common cystic lesions

Table 33–2 • CYST FLUID ANALYSES RESULTS FOR PANCREATIC CYSTIC LESIONS				
Cystic Entity	Amylase	Choreal embryonic antigen (CEA)	Mucin Stain	Cytology
Pseudocyst	Very high	Low	Negative	Inflammatory cells
Serous cystic neoplasm	Low	Low	Negative	Scant glycogen rich cells
Mucinous cystic neoplasm	Low	High	Positive	Clusters or sheets of mucin-containing cells
Intraductal papillary mucinous neoplasm (IPMN)	High	High	Positive	Tall columnar mucin containing cells

associated with the pancreas. The assessment of patients with cystic lesions of the pancreas begins with a good history and examination, followed by imaging studies, and cyst fluid analyses. (Please see Table 33–2 for details of cyst fluid analyses.) Cyst fluid analyses are helpful to differentiate the various cystic pancreatic lesions. Cyst fluid from pancreatic pseudocysts will reveal very high amylase values, low CEA, and negative mucin staining.

Mucinous cystic neoplasms (MCNs) include a wide variety of tumors ranging from benign to frankly malignant lesions. What the MCNs have in common are mucin-secreting epithelial cells lining the exocrine ducts. MCN development is believed to be hormonally stimulated, since MCNs are nearly always discovered in women. Cyst fluid analyses generally reveal low amylase, high CEA, and positive mucin stain.

Intraductal papillary mucinous neoplasm (IPMN) is a mucous producing neoplasm that can involve the main pancreatic duct or one of its side branches. IPMNs are often recognized as incidental cystic masses by imaging such as CT. Once identified, it is important to further determine the anatomic origin of the IPMN, because IPMN arising from the **main duct has a 30% to 50% probability of harboring pancreatic ductal adenocarcinoma.** Side-branch IPMNs have low malignant potential and can be simply observed. IPMNs often become clinically apparent as causes of abdominal pain and pancreatitis; these lesions often appear on CT imaging as cystic masses in the pancreas. Magnetic resonance cholangiopancreatography (MRCP) can be useful to determine whether the lesion is associated with the main duct of side branches. IPMNs are identified with equal distributions in males and females, usually in their sixties and seventies. Fluid analysis from IPMN will generally reveal high amylase and CEA values and be positive for mucin staining.

Serous cystic neoplasms have a predilection for the head of the pancreas and do not have a potential for malignant transformation. Surgical resection is indicated only when the lesions become symptomatic or in cases of diagnostic uncertainty. Fluid analyses from these lesions will generally reveal low amylase values, low CEA, and negative for mucin staining.

> **CASE CORRELATION**
>
> • See also Case 32 (Gallstone Disease), Case 34 (Liver Tumor), and Case 35 (Pancreatitis).

COMPREHENSION QUESTIONS

33.1 A 50-year-old man is noted to have painless jaundice, and the CT scan reveals a peri-ampullary tumor. Which of the following is the most likely peri-ampullary cancer?

A. Cholangiocarcinoma

B. Ampullary carcinoma

C. Pancreatic ductal carcinoma

D. Pancreatic lymphoma

E. Duodenal carcinoma

33.2 A 45-year-old woman is diagnosed with pancreatic cancer, and the histology appears to be adenocarcinoma. Which of the following is most accurate statement regarding this type of malignancy?

A. Most of these cancers are located in the head and uncinate process of the pancreas

B. Right upper quadrant pain, fever, and jaundice are the most common findings associated with tumor

C. Most of these cancers are located in the tail of the pancreas

D. Curative surgery is typically obtainable when the malignancy is located in the body of the pancreas

E. This tumor is highly chemosensitive

33.3 A 33-year-old man has been diagnosed with widely metastatic pancreatic cancer originating from the head of the pancreas. He has severe itching and hyperbilirubinemia. Which of the following is best treatment?

A. Administration of cholestyramine

B. Radiation therapy directly to the head of the pancreas

C. Pancreaticoduodenectomy (Whipple procedure)

D. Operative decompression of the biliary tract

E. Endoscopic biliary stent placement

33.4 Pancreaticoduodenectomy is indicated for which one of the following patients?

A. A 55-year-old man with a history of alcoholism who presents with jaundice and an isolated mass in the head of the pancreas. Biopsy of the mass is nondiagnostic

B. A 60-year-old man with Child Class C cirrhosis and cancer of head of the pancreas. He has diffuse ascites

C. A 40-year-old man with carcinoma of the head of the pancreas with tumor invasion of the superior mesenteric vein and artery

D. A 50-year-old man with Gardner syndrome and a 2-cm adenoma of the second portion of the duodenum

E. A 38-year-old woman with an 8-cm pseudocyst involving the head of the pancreas

33.5 A 42-year-old woman is evaluated and diagnosed with probable adenocarcinoma of the pancreas. Which of the following is most accurate regarding this diagnosis?

A. A majority of the patients have unresectable tumors at presentation

B. Anemia is a common presenting symptom

C. Patients with isolated liver metastasis can often be cured with surgical resection

D. It is usually associated with predominantly elevated indirect serum bilirubin levels

E. Smoking is not a risk factor for this disease

33.6 Which of the following statements regarding pancreatic ductal carcinoma is TRUE?

A. This cancer is an uncommon cancer making up of 2% of all cancers diagnosed in the United States, and it is responsible for 2% of deaths due to cancer in the United States

B. More than 50% of patients in the United States with pancreatic cancers have distant metastases at the time of diagnosis

C. Complete resection is associated with a high rate of cure

D. Surgical palliation for pancreatic cancer is directed at reducing the tumor burden

E. Pancreaticoduodenectomy with venous resection and reconstruction is associated with a 5-year survival rate of 1%

33.7 Which of the following statements regarding pancreaticoduodenectomy (Whipple procedure) is TRUE?

A. Whipple procedures are being applied more liberally in the treatment of patients with head of the pancreas cancers because long term survival has significantly improved following this operation

B. Whipple procedure can provide the opportunity for cure for patients with peri-ampullary carcinoma

C. Whipple procedure with arterial and venous reconstruction is indicated for patients with tumor invasion of the superior mesenteric artery and vein

D. This operation is not indicated because of the high rate of postoperative complications

E. This operation is now done by endoscopic/endoluminal approach

33.8 Which of the following statements regarding IPMN is TRUE?

A. IPMN is most often asymptomatic and clinically irrelevant

B. 30% to 50% of main duct IPMN harbor pancreatic cancers

C. Side-branch and main duct IPMN have similar biologic behaviors

D. Patient with IPMNs can be monitored with surveillance of CA19-9

E. Operative resections are indicated for all patients with IPMNs

33.9 A 63-year-old woman has an incidentally identified cystic lesion in the head of the pancreas. She has no prior history of pancreatitis. The fluid analysis revealed normal amylase value, low CEA, negative mucin stain, and scant cells. Which of the following is the most likely diagnosis associated with this lesion?

A. IPMN

B. Pancreatic pseudocyst

C. Mucinous cystic neoplasm

D. Serous cystic neoplasm

E. Pancreatic duplication

ANSWERS

33.1 **C.** Adenocarcinoma of pancreatic ductal origin is the most common of the peri-ampullary cancers. Cholangiocarcinomas arising from the distal common bile duct is the second most common, and adenocarcinoma of the Ampulla of Vater is the third most common. Duodenal carcinoma is the least common peri-ampullary cancer.

33.2 **A.** Roughly two-thirds of pancreatic adenocarcinomas are located in the head or uncinate process of the pancreas; 15% are located in the body; 10% are located in the pancreatic tail, and the remaining lesions are diffuse in location. Pancreatic cancers located in the head and unicinate process are the most likely to be curable because of earlier symptom onset.

33.3 **E.** For this patient with obstructive jaundice and severe itching secondary to widely metastatic pancreatic cancer originating from the pancreatic head, endoscopic stent placement can help relieve his jaundice and improve his quality of life. With metastatic disease, there is no indication for surgical resection.

33.4 **A.** This patient has obstructive jaundice and a localized mass of unknown nature in the head of the pancreas and is a candidate for pancreaticoduodenectomy. The procedure can be both diagnostic and therapeutic for this gentleman providing that he is healthy enough to withstand the surgical procedure. The patient with Childs Class C cirrhosis is a poor surgical candidate for this operation. Treatment of an isolated duodenal adenoma is local resection. Treatment of a large symptomatic pseudocyst in the head of the pancreas is internal drainage.

33.5 **A.** The majority of patients with pancreatic cancers present with unresectable disease either because of local advancement or the presence of distant metastases. The prognosis of patients with distant metastasis is extremely poor; therefore, there is no indication to perform liver resections for patients with metastases to the liver. Obstructive jaundice is associated with elevations in total bilirubin with predominant elevations in **direct** bilirubin values.

33.6 **B.** Greater than 50% of patients with pancreatic cancers present with locally advanced disease or distant metastases. Complete resections of pancreatic cancers are associated with approximately 15% 5-year survival.

33.7 **B.** Whipple procedures with complete resections (R0) can provide patients with the opportunity for cure; however, it is only associated with 10% to 15% 5-year survival. The postoperative mortality associated with Whipple resections has improved significantly over the past 20 years owing to improvements in operative and supportive care; however, the long-term survival has not change dramatically.

33.8 **B.** Thirty to fifty percent of main-duct IPMNs harbor adenocarcinomas; therefore, pancreatic resection is indicated with this diagnosis. The goal of surgical resection for IPMN is to prevent cancer occurrence. On the other hand, IPMNs arising from minor ducts have a low probability of becoming malignant and do not require surgical removal.

33.9 **D.** A cystic mass in a patient without a prior history of pancreatitis and with fluid analysis revealing low amylase, low CEA, negative mucin stain, and scant cells most likely represents a serous cystic neoplasm. This is a benign finding with low malignant potential.

CLINICAL PEARLS ·

▶ The classic presentation of malignant extrahepatic biliary obstruction is painless jaundice and a palpable nontender gallbladder.

▶ The majority of patients with pancreatic cancers have locally-advanced diseases or metastases at the time of diagnosis.

▶ In general, pancreaticoduodenectomy should be reserved for patients with resectable malignancies near the Ampulla of Vater.

▶ Patients with pancreatic cancers directly invading the superior mesenteric artery are not considered candidates for surgical resection because of poor disease prognosis even after resection.

▶ High amylase values, low CEA, and negative mucin stain during fluid analysis of a cystic pancreatic lesion rules out malignancy or lesions with malignant transformation potentials.

▶ Endoscopic ultrasound is the most reliable diagnostic modality to evaluate the relationship between a pancreatic adenocarcinoma in the head or uncinate process and the superior mesenteric vessels.

REFERENCES

Conrad C, Lillemoe KD. Palliative therapy for pancreatic cancer. In: Cameron JL, Cameron AM, eds. *Current Surgical Therapy.* 11th ed. Philadelphia, PA: Elsevier Saunders; 2014:481-487.

Edil BH, McCarter M, Gajdos C, Schulick RD. *Periampullary carcinoma.* In: Cameron JL, Cameron AM, eds. *Current Surgical Therapy.* 11th ed. Philadelphia, PA: Elsevier Saunders; 2014:471-477.

Fong VF, Tan WP, Lavu H, et al. Preoperative imaging for resectableperi-ampullary cancer: clinico-pathological implications of reported radiographic findings. *J Gastrointest Surg.* 2013;17:1098-1106.

Jesus-Acosta A, Laheru D. Neoadjuvant and adjuvant therapy of pancreatic cancer. In: Cameron JL, Cameron AM, eds. *Current Surgical Therapy.* 11th ed. Philadelphia, PA: Elsevier Saunders; 2014:487-491.

A 41-year-old woman presents with a sudden onset of abdominal pain that began 1 hour prior to coming to the emergency center. She denies previous abdominal complaints, history of recent trauma, weight loss, a change in bowel habits, hematochezia, or hematemesis. She is otherwise healthy and takes an oral contraceptive medication. Her systolic blood pressure is 98 mm Hg during her initial evaluation but drops to 76 mm Hg after getting up from the supine position. Following the infusion of 1000 mL of intravenous fluid, the systolic blood pressure improves to 100 mm Hg. Her abdominal examination reveals no peritoneal signs, her bowel sounds are hypoactive, and there is mild tenderness diffusely in the right upper quadrant. Her hematocrit value is 28%. A computed tomography (CT) scan of the abdomen demonstrates free-intraperitoneal blood and a 5-cm solid mass in the right lobe of her liver with evidence of recent hemorrhage into the lesion.

▶ What are your next steps?
▶ What is the most likely diagnosis?

ANSWERS TO CASE 34:
Focal Liver Lesion

Summary: A 41-year-old woman who takes an oral contraceptive presents with acute abdominal pain, hypotension, and anemia. The CT scan reveals a focal liver lesion with evidence of recent hemorrhage, including hemoperitoneum.

- **Next steps:** Admit the patient to the intensive care unit for close monitoring and frequent reassessments for ongoing bleeding. Once the patient stabilizes, we need to perform additional imaging studies and laboratory studies to better characterize the lesion. This lesion will likely require resection to prevent further hemorrhage.

- **Most likely diagnosis:** Hepatic adenoma with hemorrhage.

ANALYSIS
Objectives

1. Learn to develop an appropriate differential diagnosis for hepatic lesions based on patient characteristics, risk factors, and radiographic imaging characteristics.

2. Know the pertinent differences in the management of primary and secondary liver masses.

3. Know the natural history and imaging characteristics of primary and secondary liver tumors to avoid unnecessary investigations, biopsies, and operations.

4. Learn the evolving management for patients with colorectal cancers with metastases to the liver.

Considerations

Most of the individuals with liver masses are asymptomatic or minimally symptomatic. This patient's presentation is dramatic but typical for a patient with a ruptured liver tumor. Ruptures or spontaneous bleeding related to liver tumors are most commonly associated with hepatic adenomas and hepatocellular carcinomas (HCC). The history of a young woman who takes exogenous hormone pills for contraception and presents with bleeding into a solid liver lesion is more compatible with a ruptured hepatic adenoma. At this point where the bleeding appears to have stopped, it is helpful to consider angiographic embolization to prevent further/recurrent bleeding. Following the initial cessation of bleeding, additional imaging studies are ideally obtained to help plan the elective resection of this tumor at a later time.

APPROACH TO:
Focal Liver Lesions

DEFINITIONS

FOCAL LIVER LESIONS: Focal liver lesions are solid masses, cystic masses, or areas of tissue that are identified as abnormal parts of the liver. Included are *primary benign liver tumors* (hemangioma and focal nodular hyperplasia), *primary potentially malignant tumors* (adenomas), and *primary malignant tumors* (hepatocellular carcinomas). Focal liver lesions also include *secondary tumors* that by definition are malignant, including metastases from GI adenocarcinomas, neuroendocrine tumors, carcinoid tumors, melanomas, and breast carcinomas.

PRIMARY LIVER TUMORS: These originate from the hepatocytes, bile duct epithelial cells, or mesenchymal cells within the liver. Primary liver tumors can follow a benign course, have the potential for malignant transformation, or can be frankly malignant. The most common primary hepatic benign tumors are focal nodular hyperplasia (FNH) and hemangiomas. The most common tumor with the potential to undergo malignant transformation is hepatic adenoma. The most common primary malignant liver tumors are hepatocellular carcinoma and cholangiocarcinoma.

SECONDARY LIVER TUMOR: These originate from tissues outside of the liver and spread to the liver by the hematogenous route. They are by definition malignant. The most common metastatic tumor found in the liver is colorectal carcinoma. Other metastatic lesions include neuroendocrine tumors of the GI tract, breast carcinomas, and adenocarcinomas from other parts of the GI tract (stomach and pancreas are some of the other common ones).

BENIGN TUMORS: Tumors that do not spread to distant sites but can cause problems by direct spread or impingement.

HEMANGIOMA: This is the most commonly encountered benign liver tumor. Most of these lesions are asymptomatic; however, large hemangiomas can cause vague abdominal pain, nausea, and loss of appetite. Spontaneous rupture of liver hemangiomas is rare. Hemangiomas can be identified with properly obtained T_2-weighted MRI or 3-phase CT. The "light bulb sign" is classically seen on T_2 MRI or 3-phase CT. During the early arterial phase the lesion demonstrates peripheral enhancement, and with continued gradual filling of the lesion during portal phase and the equilibrium phase. Biopsy is contraindicated because it can lead to life-threatening bleeding. Surgical resection or embolization may be indicated for palliation of symptoms related to these lesions.

KASABACH–MERRITT SYNDROME: This is a rare syndrome associated with highly vascularized liver tumors, most commonly large liver hemangiomas. The syndrome describes a consumptive process related to the tumors resulting in thrombocytopenia, low clotting factors, and low fibrinogen levels.

FOCAL NODULAR HYPERPLASIA (FNH): This is the second most common benign liver tumor. FNH occurs most commonly in women in their forties and fifties. Most FNH (60%-80%) are asymptomatic and identified incidentally during medical imaging. An FNH is truly benign and without any malignant potential. FNH typically has a "central scar" appearance on CT scan. Some FNH are difficult to differentiate from hepatic adenomas on the basis of imaging alone and may require biopsies to make that differentiation. In the past, a telangiectactic variant of FNH was observed with malignant degeneration potentials; however, this lesion has been reclassified as a hepatic adenoma.

NODULAR REGENERATIVE HYPERPLASIA: This is a focal regeneration that is believed to be related to obstructed blood flow to liver regions resulting in injury with subsequent regeneration. This lesion is more common in older individuals where the prevalence in individuals over 80 is ~5.5%. No treatment is necessary for this entity.

TRIPLE-PHASE CT SCAN: This CT scan technique with intravenous contrast acquires images during the early arterial phase (30 seconds), portal-venous phase (60 seconds), and the equilibrium phase (90 seconds). It allows improved characterization of liver lesions.

CLINICAL APPROACH

Initial Approach

Liver tumors may be identified incidentally during medical imaging, during evaluation of nonspecific complaints, during follow-up of unrelated tumors (eg, staging or surveillance of a patient with colorectal cancer), or during surveillance of an at-risk individual (eg, HCC identified during surveillance of a cirrhotic patient). The approach to any patient with a liver mass begins with a thorough history and physical examination focusing on identifying risk factors, history of primary malignancy at another site, and symptoms possibly attributable to the liver mass. The physical examination is directed at identifying stigmata of liver dysfunction and the evaluation of potential cancer sources (eg, breast examination and skin examination for melanoma). The information gained from the history and physical examination can be useful to characterize liver lesions as either primary or secondary.

Imaging of Liver Tumors

Selection of the imaging modality is one of the most crucial aspects of the evaluation. Proper selection of imaging studies helps establish the diagnosis for many liver tumors and can reduce unnecessary biopsies and operations for patient with incidentally discovered lesions. Characterization of a liver lesion as cystic or solid is the first goal of imaging. Simple cysts with water-density fluid and no wall irregularities are most likely benign whereas complex cysts with septations, nodularity, or thickened walls may suggest hydatid cysts, biliary cystadenomas, or cystadenocarcinomas, which require additional diagnostic studies for characterization (see Table 34–1 for details regarding imaging). It is important to keep in mind that the sensitivity and specificity of the imaging studies are negatively affected when focal

Table 34–1 • IMAGING MODALITIES FOR LIVER TUMORS

Modality	Hemangioma	Focal Hyperplasia	Adenoma	Hepatocellular Carcinoma	Metastatic Adenocarcinoma
Triple-phase CT (Triphasic CT)	High sensitivity and specificity, early contrast enhancement with peripheral outlining of tumor	Low specificity (central scar is characteristic finding)	Low specificity	Low specificity	High sensitivity and specificity; gold standard
Magnetic resonance imaging	High sensitivity and specificity	Low specificity (central scar is characteristic finding)	Low specificity	Low specificity	High sensitivity and specificity
Angiography	Gold standard test with high sensitivity and specificity, but invasive	High sensitivity and specificity, but invasive	Low specificity	Low specificity	Infrequently used
Laparoscopic ultrasound	Poor	Poor	Helpful when combined with laparoscopic biopsy	Gold standard test	Highly sensitive when combined with laparoscopic biopsy
Biopsy	Contraindicated because of high risk for bleeding	Rarely useful	Helpful	Mandatory	Mandatory

liver lesions occur in a background of cirrhosis. In studies of explanted livers from individuals undergoing liver transplantation, it has been demonstrated that CT scans done prior to explantation identified only 68% to 77% of the hepatocellular carcinomas that were present in the recipients' livers.

Primary Liver Tumors

Common primary liver tumors include *benign lesions* (FNH and hemangiomas), *potentially malignant lesions* (adenomas), and *malignant lesions* (cholangiocarcinomas and hepatocellular carcinomas). Asymptomatic and minimally symptomatic benign lesions can generally be observed and followed. For patients with FNH or hemangiomas, surgical resections are rarely performed for tissue diagnosis, and resections are uncommon to address symptoms produced by the lesions.

Many patients with hepatic adenomas will require resections due to either concerns for hemorrhage (11%-29%) or malignant transformations. Patients with **adenomas <5 cm in size can be observed because the risk of rupture and malignant transformation is low.** Patients who are taking oral birth control (OCP) or anabolic steroids should be advised to stop these medications. Pregnancy is not contraindicated for women with adenomas less than 5 cm. **Patients with adenomas >5 cm should be considered for tumor resection or ablation to reduce bleeding and malignant transformation risks.** Frequent and long-term imaging follow-up is recommended for individuals with lesions > 5cm who do not wish to undergo therapeutic interventions. Recently, molecular characterization of hepatic adenomas has been introduced. Based on biopsy results, it is possible to subcategorize these lesions into *inflammatory, hepatocyte nuclear factor-1 (HNF-1) mutated,* and *beta-catenin activating* subtypes. The subtypes of adenomas also are associated with some characteristic MRI findings that may allow differentiation by MRI. Clinically, an adenoma with **inflammatory subtype and >5cm in size is at high risk for bleeding and low risk for malignant transformation.** The **HNF-1 mutated type has no risk of bleeding or malignant transformation,** and **the beta-catenin activated type has increased risk of malignant transformation when its size exceeds 5 cm.** Based on these characteristics, lesions can be observed without specific treatment if biopsy of an asymptomatic hepatic adenoma reveals the HNF-1 variant.

Hepatocellular Carcinoma

Hepatocellular carcinoma (HCC) is the most common primary malignancy of the liver and is one of the most commonly occurring malignancies worldwide. HCC is particularly common in Sub-Saharian Africa and parts of Asia where hepatitis B is endemic. HCC development in patients with hepatitis B can happen without cirrhotic changes, as hepatitis B virus can cause HCC by incorporating viral DNA into the host genome. In western, developed countries, HCC is most commonly associated with cirrhosis from fatty liver changes, alcoholism, or chronic hepatitis C infections. Surgical resection can be curative for patients with HCC; however, the procedure is often associated with excess morbidity and mortality when underlying liver cirrhosis is present. Some patients with small HCCs are good candidates for liver transplantation, and patient selection for transplantation should follow either of the two defined sets of published criteria (Milan Criteria, UCSF Criteria).

Secondary Tumors

The liver is a frequent site for the deposit of metastatic tumors, especially malignancies from the GI tract. For patients with liver metastases and unknown primary, tumor markers can be helpful for primary tumor identification (Table 34–2). **Colorectal cancer metastases are the most commonly encountered liver metastases in the United States.** The following are some of the conditions that should raise the clinical suspicion that the liver lesions are metastatic: (1) Focal liver lesions identified in individuals with history of malignancy treated within the past 5 years. (2) Liver lesion identified in individuals with advanced untreated primary malignancy (such as individual with a large obstructing colon cancer). (3) Individuals with miliary or diffuse distributions of hepatic lesions. (4) Patients with colorectal cancers with marked (>10-fold) elevation in serum CEA values.

In individuals presenting with secondary liver tumors with unknown primaries, strong efforts should be made to identify the primary site of disease. In the past, patients diagnosed simultaneously with colorectal cancers with liver metastases were routinely treated with surgical resections of the primary colorectal cancers before addressing the metastatic processes. There has been a recent shift to treat the patients' systemic disease with systemic therapy first, when minimally symptomatic patients present with newly diagnosed colorectal cancer and liver metastases. For these patients, surgical resections of the primary cancers are performed only when significant symptoms related to the primary tumors are present.

Table 34–2 • TUMOR MARKERS POTENTIALLY USEFUL FOR IDENTIFYING THE ORIGIN OF SECONDARY LIVER TUMORS

Tumor Marker	Type of Cancer
CEA	Colon cancer
AFP	Hepatocellular carcinoma
CA 19-9	Pancreatic cancer
CA 125	Ovarian cancer
β-hCG	Testicular cancer
PSA	Prostate cancer
CA 50	Pancreatic cancer
Neuron-specific enolase	Small cell lung cancer
CA 15-3	Breast cancer
Ferritin	Hepatocellular carcinoma

Abbreviations: AFP, α-fetoprotein; CA 15-3, carbohydrate antigen 15-3; CA 19-9, carbohydrate antigen 19-9; CA 50, carbohydrate antigen 50; CA 125, carbohydrate antigen 125; CEA, carcinoembryonic antigen; β-hCG, β-human chorionic gonadotropin; PSA, prostate-specific antigen.

Occasionally, patients with stable liver metastases are candidates for curative resections of their metastatic lesions. In general, ideal candidates for curative liver resections have fewer metastases, smaller metastases, lower CEA (<200), or disease-free intervals of >12 months since resection of the primary cancers. In addition to resection, some smaller metastatic lesions can be treated with radiofrequency ablation for curative intent.

CASE CORRELATION

- See also Case 32 (Gallstone Disease), Case 33 (Periampullary Tumor), and Case 35 (Pancreatitis).

COMPREHENSION QUESTIONS

34.1 A 30-year-old woman is noted to have a hepatic mass during laparoscopy for acute appendicitis. This lesion is biopsied and reveals focal nodular hyperplasia. Which of the following is the most accurate statement regarding this condition?

A. This lesion has a potential for malignant transformation when it exceeds 5 cm

B. Surgical excision is indicated

C. Radiolabeled sulfur colloid scintigraphy is highly specific for confirming the diagnosis

D. Oral contraceptive is a risk factor

E. These lesions generally pose problems during pregnancy

34.2 During an ultrasound for his gallbladder, a 65-year-old man is found incidentally to have a 6-cm liver mass. He has a history of hepatitis B but his liver transaminase levels are within normal limits. Which of the following is the most appropriate treatment for this patient?

A. Superior mesenteric artery embolization

B. Interferon alpha treatment

C. Metronidazole treatment for amebic abscess

D. Biopsy and resection

E. Repeat the ultrasound in 6 months

34.3 A 73-year-old woman presents with new-onset jaundice and is noted to have multiple lesions replacing approximately 70% of the liver parenchyma. Which of the following is the most likely primary site of her malignancy?

A. Stomach

B. Lung

C. Colon

D. Cervix

E. Ovary

34.4 A 47-year-old man with vague abdominal discomfort is noted to have adeno-carcinoma of the cecum that was causing mild obstructive symptoms. A CT scan for cancer staging reveals 6 separate lesions distributed throughout both lobes of the liver, in addition to an 8-cm cecal cancer. Which of the following is the most appropriate treatment approach for this patient?

A. Proceed with colon resection followed by chemotherapy

B. Resect the colon cancer then refer the patient for liver transplantation

C. Treat the patient with systemic chemotherapy

D. Resect the colon and liver lesions then treat with systemic chemotherapy

E. Radiation therapy to the liver and colon followed by resection and chemotherapy

34.5 A 46-year-old woman underwent an abdominal CT for evaluation of nephrolithiasis, and this study revealed a 5-cm focal lesion in the right lobe of the liver. A 3-phase CT of the abdomen was then obtained that revealed early rim enhancement during the portal-venous phase with late filling during the arterial and the equilibrium phases. Which of the following is the most appropriate management?

A. Obtain a serum alpha fetoprotein level and then perform a CT-guided biopsy to rule-out cancer

B. Perform colonoscopy to identify the primary colorectal cancer

C. Refer the patient for liver transplantation

D. Perform a right hepatic resection

E. Observe the patient clinically and obtain imaging if the patient becomes symptomatic

34.6 A 35 year-old woman underwent an ultrasound of the right upper quadrant for the evaluation of indigestion that was thought to be related to gallstones. No gallstones were seen, but a 3-cm mass was noted in the right lobe of the liver. During a subsequent 3-phase CT, a solid 6-cm mass was visualized and biopsied. The biopsy revealed hepatic adenoma containing hepatocyte nuclear factor 1 (HNF-1) mutation. Which of the following is the best management for this patient?

A. Observe the patient clinically and repeat imaging as needed

B. Perform liver resection of the mass

C. Refer the patient for liver transplantation

D. Initiate exogenous estrogen treatment

E. Initiate antiestrogen therapy

34.7 A 33-year-old woman has symptoms suggestive of gallstone disease. She undergoes an ultrasound evaluation that reveals gallstones and a 3-cm cystic mass in the left lobe of the liver. A CT scan of the abdomen reveals a fluid-filled mass with smooth edges and no heterogeneity. Which of the following is the best treatment for this liver lesion?

A. Aspiration of the cyst

B. Resection of the cyst

C. Repeat CT imaging every 6 months to monitor growth

D. No specific treatment for the mass

E. Only resect the mass if it grows to >5cm

ANSWERS

34.1 **C.** Radiolabeled sulfur colloid scintigraphy is very helpful to differentiate hepatic adenomas from FNH. The isotope applied is taken up by the Kupffer cells that are present in FNH but not in adenomas. Although rarely performed for the diagnosis of FNH, angiography is also useful to help differentiate FNH from other focal liver lesions. Specifically, FNH is associated with bland vascular features as opposed to the other commonly seen solid liver lesions. FNH has no potential for malignant transformation, and surgical excision is only indicated when the lesion is symptomatic. Even though it is more common in women, FNH development is not linked to oral contraceptive use.

34.2 **D.** This patient has a history of hepatitis B but without biochemical values that suggest cirrhosis. In this individual, a solid focal liver lesion is highly suspicious for hepatocellular carcinoma (HCC). HCC can occur in patients with hepatitis B even without the onset of cirrhosis, because the hepatitis B virus is a DNA virus that can cause direct cancer transformation. Antibiotic treatment, mesenteric embolization, interferon therapy, or observation with repeat imaging is not appropriate for this patient.

34.3 **C.** This patient presents with apparent extensive metastatic disease in her liver. Cancers from all of the sources listed can produce metastatic disease to the liver. Statistically, colorectal carcinoma is the most likely cancer to cause this clinical presentation. Confirmation would require tissue biopsy and/or evaluation of the primary sites.

34.4 **C.** There has been a paradigm shift in the treatment of asymptomatic or minimally symptomatic patients with stage 4 colorectal cancers. The current approach is to address the systemic disease in these patients, because the metastatic diseases are the more important issues in these patients. Resections of the colorectal primary cancers are performed initially only in patients who present with severe symptoms related to their primary cancers (eg, obstruction, severe bleeding, perforation). In a series of patients managed systemically at the Memorial Sloan-Kettering Cancer Center, the patients had less morbidity and a better quality of life, and only a small percentage of patients actually required surgical resection prior to death from their metastatic disease.

34.5 **E.** The early contrast appearance at the periphery of the liver lesion with later filling of the mass by contrast is also referred to as the "light bulb sign." This finding is characteristic of liver hemangiomas. Hemangiomas do not have malignant potential. Surgical resections or angio-embolizations are only indicated if these lesions are symptomatic.

34.6 **A.** A hepatic adenoma containing the HNF-1 mutation has a low potential for spontaneous rupture or for malignant degeneration. If this subtype is confirmed by molecular studies and MRI, the asymptomatic patient with this lesion can be observed without additional therapy. It is important to stop the patient's use of oral contraceptive pills (OCP) use, if the patient is taking OCP.

34.7 **D.** No specific treatment is needed for this lesion because it is a 3-cm simple cyst. Observation with or without repeat imaging with ultrasound is most appropriate for a patient with an asymptomatic and small simple cyst of the liver.

CLINICAL PEARLS

▶ Hemangiomas are the most common benign solid liver lesions.

▶ Hepatic adenomas are associated with exogenous estrogen or anabolic steroids use.

▶ The most common metastatic disease in the liver comes from colorectal cancers.

▶ Because of the risk of bleeding, hemangiomas should be ruled-out before attempting needle biopsies.

▶ Hepatic adenomas greater than 5 cm in size have increased risk of bleeding or undergoing malignant transformation, with the exception of adenomas with HNF-1 mutations.

▶ Hemangiomas can be easily recognized by the contrast filling of the periphery during the initial or portal-venous phase of the triple phase CT or contrast-enhanced MRI (Light bulb sign).

▶ Patients who present with stage IV colorectal cancer with liver metastases should have initial systemic treatment directed toward the systemic disease unless the primary tumor is causing significant symptoms related to obstruction, bleeding, or perforation.

REFERENCES

Chiche L, Adam J-P. Diagnosis and management of benign liver tumors. *Semin Liver Dis.* 2013;33: 236-247.

Hirose K. The management of benign liver lesions. In: Cameron JL, Cameron AM, eds. *Current Surgical Therapy.* 11th ed. Philadelphia, PA: Elsevier Saunders; 2014:322-327.

Melstrom LG, Fong Y. *The management of malignant liver tumors.* In: Cameron JL, Cameron AM, eds. *Current Surgical Therapy.* 11th ed. Philadelphia, PA: Elsevier Saunders:2014:328-335.

Morrero JA, Ahn J, Reddy R, et al. ACG clinical guideline: the diagnosis and management of focal liver lesions. *Am J Gastroenterol.* 2014;109:1328-1347.

A 26-year-old man is seen in the emergency department for abdominal pain that began after he returned home from a party, where he consumed pizza and eight cans of beer. The pain is constant, located in the upper part of his abdomen, and radiates to his back. Approximately 3 to 4 hours after the onset of pain, he vomited a large amount of undigested food, but the emesis did not resolve his pain. His past medical history is unremarkable, and he consumes alcohol only on weekends when he attends parties with his friends. On examination, the patient appears uncomfortable. His temperature is 38.8C (101.8F), heart rate is 110 beats/minute, blood pressure is 110/60 mm Hg, and respiratory rate is 28 breaths/minute. The abdomen is distended and tender to palpation in the epigastric and periumbilical areas. Laboratory studies reveal a WBC count of 18,000/mm^3, hemoglobin 17 g/dL, hematocrit 47%, glucose 210 mg/dL, total bilirubin 3.2 mg/dL, aspartate aminotransferase (AST) 380 U/L, alanine aminotransferase (ALT) 435 U/L, lactate dehydrogenase (LDH) 300 U/L, and serum amylase 6800 IU/L. Arterial blood gas on room air reveals pH 7.37, PaCO$_2$ 33 mm Hg, PaO$_2$ 68 mm Hg, and HCO$_3$ 21 mEq/L. Chest radiography reveals the presence of a small left pleural effusion.

▶ What is the most likely diagnosis?
▶ What are your next steps?
▶ What are the complications associated with this disease process?

ANSWERS TO CASE 35:

Pancreatitis (Acute)

Summary: A 26-year-old man presents with acute abdominal pain radiating to his back, nausea, and vomiting following binge drinking. The clinical presentation of fever, abdominal pain, leukocytosis, hemoconcentration, elevated serum amylase, and hypoxemia suggests that the patient has severe acute pancreatitis.

- **Most likely diagnosis:** Acute alcoholic pancreatitis.

- **Next steps:** Resuscitation measures including administration of supplemental oxygen and intravenous fluids.

- **Complication of disease:** Acute pancreatitis can cause local complications including hemorrhage, necrosis, fluid collection, and infection. Pancreatitis can also lead to systemic complications such as pulmonary, cardiac, and renal dysfunction.

ANALYSIS

Objectives

1. Be familiar with the diagnosis and initial management of patients with acute pancreatitis.

2. Recognize the value and limitations of clinical prognosticators and computed tomography (CT) scans in evaluating patients with acute pancreatitis.

3. Describe the diagnosis and management of the regional and systemic complications of acute pancreatitis.

Considerations

This patient presents with the sudden onset of abdominal and back pain after a binge drinking episode. He has the history and clinical findings that support a diagnosis of acute pancreatitis due to alcohol ingestion. The elevated serum amylase further supports the diagnosis of acute pancreatitis. It is important to keep in mind that the degree of amylase elevation (far greater than 3× normal value) is helpful in establishing the diagnosis, but does not correlate with pancreatitis severity. There are several details provided in his initial presentation that are concerning: fever, tachycardia, tachypnea, WBC of 18,000/mm^3, elevation in LDH, elevations in AST and ALT, and low PaO$_2$ demonstrated on arterial blood gas. Currently, this patient does not have any definable organ dysfunction, but the hypoxemia and tachypnea are worrisome signs that he may be on his way to developing respiratory failure. Given these early concerns, the patient should be admitted to the ICU for close monitoring and resuscitation. The cornerstone of acute pancreatitis management is aggressive and appropriate volume resuscitation. Based on the results of a prospective randomized trial, it is reasonable to provide this patient with an **initial bolus of Lactated Ringers at 20 mL/kg** in the emergency department followed by a **continuous infusion of 3 mL/kg/hour**, with **interval assessment of vital signs, laboratory values, and urine output in 6 to 8 hours**. Patients whose BUN levels do not decrease during reassessments are given a repeat fluid bolus, whereas patients whose BUN levels decrease can have the fluid infusion rate reduced to 1.5 mL/kg/hour. For this patient, the likelihood of developing respiratory failure is extremely high during the initial 24 hours, given his level of hypoxemia at presentation. Because the patient's respiratory status is expected to worsen and his airways are likely to become more edematous following fluid resuscitation, it is not unreasonable to semielectively intubate the patient to secure his airway before the onset of florid respiratory failure. Once the patient's intravascular volume is improved with fluid resuscitation, a CT scan of the abdomen should be performed to further assess the severity of pancreatitis. Monitoring of end-organ functions is important during the early course of his disease. The degree of respiratory dysfunction can be measured using the PaO_2/FiO_2 ratios; cardiac dysfunction can be quantified based on blood pressure and the need for pressors; renal dysfunction can be measured by quantifying urine output and serum creatinine values; neurologic dysfunction can be measured by Glasgow Coma Score (GCS). Based on information available at this point, it is clear that his pancreatitis is not mild, and whether his disease will be moderate or severe remains unknown because moderate and severe disease is differentiated by transient organ dysfunction (<48 hours in duration) or prolonged organ dysfunction.

An important intervention to consider after the completion of the patient's resuscitation is nutritional support. Patients with acute pancreatitis experience severe catabolism associated with rapid loss of lean body mass; therefore, nutritional support should be initiated to counteract this process as soon as the patient is no longer requiring resuscitation. For most patients, intragastric tube feeding can be initiated once the patient stabilizes from the resuscitation standpoint. In the past, prophylactic antibiotic administration had been routine for patients with severe pancreatitis with pancreatic necrosis; however, they are no longer indicated because the practice did not reduce peripancreatic infectious complications.

APPROACH TO:
Acute Pancreatitis

DEFINITIONS

MILD ACUTE PANCREATITIS: Acute pancreatitis that is not associated with distant organ failure, local complications (eg, peripancreatic fluid collection, necrosis), or systemic complications. The process is self-limiting and carries less than 1% mortality. Approximately 80% to 85% of patients with acute pancreatitis have mild pancreatitis.

MODERATELY SEVERE ACUTE PANCREATITIS: This describes acute pancreatitis associated with transient organ failure (<48 hours). These patients may have local complications or systemic complications. These patients may have prolonged hospitalization, but the process is associated with low mortality.

SEVERE ACUTE PANCREATITIS: Defined as acute pancreatitis with persistent organ dysfunction (>48 hours), which carries an overall mortality rate of 4%. Many of these patients may have pancreatic necrosis, which is associated with an even worse prognosis (mortality rate of 10%). Some patients with pancreatic necrosis will develop infected pancreatic necrosis, which confers a mortality rate of 40% to 70%.

PERIPANCREATIC LOCAL DISEASE PROGRESSION: Severe acute pancreatitis may produce pancreatic and peripancreatic necrosis during the first few days of disease onset. This process may or may not be associated with peripancreatic fluid collections, which are different from pancreatic pseudocysts. In this process, the fluid is walled off by surrounding tissue rather than a fibrous pseudocapsule. As the severe pancreatitis improves, areas of pancreatic necrosis undergo liquefaction producing a combination of solid and liquid structures that is commonly referred to as pancreatic phlegmon. With continued improvement of the pancreatitis, the solid components of the phlegmon may breakdown, and at the same time, the local inflammatory response produces a fibrous response around the fluid collections to form pseudocysts.

INFECTED PANCREATIC PSEUDOCYSTS: Usually occur several weeks following the onset of severe acute pancreatitis. Most patients with this problem can be treated by percutaneous drainage.

PANCREATIC ABSCESS: This describes secondary infection involving the pancreatic phlegmon. The timing of this formation is generally 3 to 6 weeks after the onset of severe acute pancreatitis. Since the phlegmon contains both solid and liquid material, pancreatic abscesses also contain infected solid and liquid material. Drainage is the preferred initial approach for this problem, but some patients need surgical drainage/debridement.

CLINICAL APPROACH

In North America and Europe, gallstones and alcohol consumption are the leading causes of acute pancreatitis in adults. The diagnosis of acute pancreatits in most patients is made on the basis of upper abdominal pain, with or without radiation to the back, nausea, vomiting, and fever. Serum amylase and/or lipase elevations are helpful to confirm the diagnosis in patients with symptoms; however, elevation in serum amylase by itself is not diagnostic because other pathologic conditions cause serum amylase elevations.

Acute pancreatitis severity can be classified as mild, moderate, or severe, where 85% of patients have mild disease. Mild pancreatitis is a disease that is not associated with local or systemic complications or with organ dysfunction, and the process is usually self-limiting and does not require specific treatment. Patients with moderately severe disease generally have either transient organ dysfunction and/or local complications of disease. Quite often, patients with moderate disease may require prolonged hospital care without a significant increase in risk of mortality.

Individuals with severe acute pancreatitis have persistent organ dysfunction lasting greater than 48 hours and experience an increased risk of pancreatitis-related mortality.

Prognostication of Acute Pancreatitis

Given the wide clinical spectrum and outcome differences associated with acute pancreatitis, many risk-stratification systems have been introduced to gauge disease severity and help predict patient outcomes. One of the oldest but most commonly applied models for disease severity stratification is the Ranson Criteria (see Table 35–1). This system takes into account 11 patient characteristics, clinical factors, and laboratory parameters that can be easily obtained within the first 48 hours of hospitalization. Observations suggest that patients exhibiting three or more of Ranson's criteria may develop severe disease and may benefit from close monitoring and CT imaging. Other disease severity evaluation systems that have been applied to acute pancreatitis patients include the Acute Physiologic and Chronic Health Evaluation (APACHE) scoring systems and the multiple organ failure scores. In general, most scoring systems have been found to have excellent negative predictive values (eg, low Ranson or APACHE scores are associated with low complication and mortality rates).

Diagnosis of Acute Pancreatitis

The diagnosis of acute pancreatitis is initially a presumptive one. Patients presenting with acute abdominal symptoms require careful clinical, biochemical, and radiographic evaluation to exclude other intra-abdominal processes such as bowel obstruction, perforated viscus, mesenteric ischemia, and biliary tract diseases. Once the diagnosis of acute pancreatitis is established, it is important to determine the cause. Patients who still have their gallbladders in place should undergo ultrasound evaluation of the right upper quadrant to rule out gallstones as a potential cause of pancreatitis. The typical presentation of acute biliary pancreatitis involves an individual with no other risk factors for pancreatitis who presents with the sudden onset of epigastric and back pain that resolves quite rapidly (usually less than 24-48 hours) and have small gallstones identified in the gallbladder on ultrasound. The laboratory findings usually demonstrate transient, marked elevation of serum amylase and lipase, with nonspecific elevations in other liver function studies.

Table 35–1 • RANSON CRITERIA	
On Admission	**Subsequent 48 h**
White blood cell count >16,000/mm3	Hematocrit fall of 10%
Glucose >200 mg/dL	Calcium <8 mg/dL
Age >55 y	Serum urea nitrogen increase of 5 mg/dL
Aspartate aminotransferase >250 U/L	Fluid requirement of >6 L
Lactate dehydrogenase >350 U/L	Base excess of >4 mEq/L PO_2 <60 mm Hg

Role of Computed Tomography Imaging

Contrast-enhanced CT scan of the abdomen is not necessary for the diagnosis of acute pancreatitis. However, this imaging modality is valuable to identify peripancreatic complications in patients who do not improve clinically after 3 to 5 days of treatment. In addition, CT imaging is valuable in identifying the presence and degree of pancreatic necrosis, which are closely related to disease severity clinical course. For example, **patients with two or more extrapancreatic fluid collections or necrosis (nonenhancement) involving >50% of the pancreas have significantly increased risk of complications and mortality.** It is important to note that 15% to 20% of the patients with pancreatic necrosis can develop infected pancreatic necrosis. In the past, antibiotics were routinely given to prevent infected pancreatic necrosis; however, two double-blind randomized trials showed that prophylactic antibiotics did not reduce the rate of infected necrosis. The current practice is to withhold antibiotic therapy until an infection is clearly identified.

Pancreatic CT scan scores have been developed to quantify the pancreatitis severity. The score is based on the presence and percentage of pancreatic necrosis identified, as well as the presence and the extent of peripancreatic inflammatory changes. CT scores range from 1 to 10, and patient scores have been shown to correlate with clinical outcomes.

Treatment

Treatment of acute pancreatitis is mainly supportive. Maintenance of hydration is important to prevent secondary organ injuries. At one time, oral food intake was thought to be detrimental to patients with acute pancreatitis; however, more recent evidence suggests that maintaining an NPO status is not necessary. In fact, **recent research evidence suggests that oral diet or enteral nutritional administration is helpful in reducing the complications associated with acute pancreatitis.** If the patient is ill and not able to tolerate oral intake, the delivery of enteral nutrition into the stomach is safe and has significant benefits for critically ill patients with acute pancreatitis. The trend in surgical treatment of patients with severe pancreatitis with pancreatic necrosis has shifted over the past decade. Currently, surgical debridement for patient with severe pancreatitis is delayed for several weeks whenever possible, because clinical observations have shown that delayed surgical treatment is associated with better patient outcomes when compared to early interventions.

For individuals with biliary pancreatitis, strong efforts should be made to perform cholecystecomies during the patients' hospitalization. Clinical observations have shown that early recurrences are common, when cholecystectomies are delayed. Often, additional imaging studies such as magnetic resonance cholangiographies may be helpful to identify common bile duct stones in this patient population.

> **CASE CORRELATION**
>
> • See also Case 32 (Gallstone Disease), Case 33 (Peri-Ampullary Tumor), and Case 34 (Liver Tumor).

COMPREHENSION QUESTIONS

35.1 A 29-year-old, 70 kg man with a 5-day history of worsening abdominal pain, nausea, and vomiting is diagnosed with acute pancreatitis. Which of the following is the best treatment for this patient?

A. NPO and fluid administration at 75 mL/hour

B. Intravenous broad-spectrum antibiotics to prevent infectious complications

C. Hypertonic glucose solution to prevent hypoglycemia

D. Laparoscopy to help identify complications related to the pancreas

E. Monitoring, maintenance intravenous fluid, parenteral analgesic, and oral diet

35.2 A 22-year-old man with alcoholism has a history of recurrent bouts of acute pancreatitis over the past several years. He appears well clinically and is noted to have a nontender and palpable epigastric mass, and a slight elevation in serum amylase. Which of the following is the most likely diagnosis?

A. Pancreatic cancer

B. Pancreatic necrosis

C. Pancreatic divisum

D. Pancreatic pseudocyst

E. Hepatic abscess

35.3 A 63-year-old woman is hospitalized with gallstone pancreatitis and noted to have significant abdominal pain, emesis, tachycardia, and tachypnea. Her amylase level is 3100 IU/L, glucose is 120 mg/dL, and calcium is 13 mg/dL. Which of the following is most likely to correlate with poor prognosis in disease outcome?

A. The patient's age

B. The high amylase level

C. The glucose level being less than 140 mg/dL

D. Hypercalcemia

E. Body mass index of 22

35.4 A 41-year-old woman has been hospitalized for 15 days due to worsening pancreatitis associated with multiple organ dysfunction syndrome. She now has developed fever and leukocytosis, and is diagnosed with extensive infected pancreatic necrosis. Which of the following is the most appropriate treatment option for this patient?

A. Broad-spectrum antibiotics

B. Percutaneous drainage

C. Surgical debridement and drainage

D. Endoscopic drainage

E. Antifungal therapy

35.5 A 38-year-old man presents with acute onset of epigastric and back pain one hour after eating dinner, which consisted of steak, mashed potatoes with gravy, and a glass of red wine. His WBC is 12,000/mm³, amylase is 2400 IU/L, and the remaining laboratory studies are normal. The patient was admitted to the hospital for observation with a diagnosis of acute pancreatitis. His pain and hyperamylasemia resolve within 12 hours of hospital admission. The patient indicates that he has had prior episodes of upper abdominal pain after meals, but never as severe. His ultrasound of the gallbladder demonstrates numerous small gallstones within the gallbladder. Which of the following is the most appropriate treatment for this patient?

A. Advise the patient to stop all alcohol consumption

B. Advise the patient to lose weight

C. Advise the patient to change to a vegan diet

D. Advise the patient to undergo a laparoscopic cholecystectomy

E. Advise the patient to have a laparoscopic cholecystectomy if he has another episode of pancreatitis

35.6 A 26-year-old man was involved in an altercation, and was kicked in the abdomen several times. He presents to the hospital with persistent abdominal pain and back pain. His vital signs are normal. The WBC count is 13,000/mm³ and his serum amylase is 800 IU/L. A CT scan of the abdomen reveals inflammation of the head and body of the pancreas with some peripancreatic inflammation and no peripancreatic fluid. Which of the following is the best treatment for this man?

A. Admit the patient, start intravenous fluids, keep him NPO until pain resolves

B. Admit the patient for observation, start intravenous fluid, give him a low fat diet

C. Admit the patient for observation, start intravenous fluid and antibiotics, give him a regular diet

D. Admit the patient for observation, start intravenous fluids, and give him a regular diet

E. Send the patient home and advise him to stay on a low fat diet for 6 weeks

35.7 Which of the following is NOT one of the Ranson's criteria?

A. Age > 55

B. Calcium > 8 mg/dL

C. WBC count > 16,000/mm³

D. Fluid requirement > 6000 mL over first 48 hours

E. Hematocrit drop > 10%

35.8 Which of the following strategies has been shown to correlate with improved outcomes in patients with severe pancreatitis and pancreatic necrosis?

A. Prophylactic antibiotics therapy

B. Prophylactic antifungal therapy

C. Delayed surgical intervention

D. NPO and total parenteral nutrition

E. Cholecystectomy within 48 hours of pancreatitis onset

ANSWERS

35.1 **E.** Supportive care is the mainstay of treatment for patients with acute pancreatitis. Treatments include maintenance intravenous fluid if the patient is unable to tolerate sufficient oral intake, oral diet, and analgesia for pain control. Maintenance intravenous fluid for a 70 kg man can be calculated by the "4-2-1" approach; that is 4 mL/kg for first 10 kg, 2 mL/kg for second 10 kg, and 1 mL/kg for each kg above 20 kg. For this 70 kg man, the hourly rate is 40 + 20 + 50 = 110 mL/hour.

35.2 **D.** This 22-year-old patient has a history of recurrent bouts of acute pancreatitis and presents with a painless palpable mass in the epigastrium. Based on the history of recurrent pancreatitis and an asymptomatic epigastric mass, this mass is most likely a pancreatic pseudocyst, and a CT scan is indicated for further evaluation. Pancreatic cancer is possible, but is generally seen in patients who are in their fifties and seventies. Pancreas divisum refers to aberrant pancreatic ductal anatomy causing recurrent pancreatitis, and this process is not usually associated with a mass. Patient with pancreatic necrosis generally will have some systemic manifestations such as fever and hyperdynamic picture.

35.3 **A.** The patient's age being >55 is a poor prognostic factor based on the Ranson criteria. The level of amylase elevation does not correlate with pancreatitis outcomes. Her glucose value of less than 140 is not an indicator of poor outcome. Hypercalcemia does not correlate with poor pancreatitis outcome, whereas hypocalcemia (<8 mg/dL) correlates with poor outcome. High body mass index (BMI > 28) is a poor prognosticator for pancreatitis outcomes.

35.4 **C.** Patients with infected pancreatic necrosis generally are critically ill and will need ICU monitoring, supportive care, broad-spectrum antibiotic therapy, and most importantly debridement of the infected necrosis.

35.5 **D.** This patient presents with acute pancreatitis while at dinner where wine is also served. The past history of frequent postprandial upper abdominal pain is suggestive of biliary colic; therefore, the cause of his pancreatitis is most likely related to the gallstones that are visualized in his gallbladder. He would benefit from laparoscopic cholecystectomy prior to his hospital discharge.

35.6 **D.** The patient described here most likely has pancreatitis secondary to trauma. Patients with traumatic pancreatitis can have more complicated disease courses. Admission to the hospital for observation, intravenous fluids, and a regular diet are appropriate initial treatments for this patient. There is no indication for antibiotics treatment for him. Low-fat diet has not been demonstrated to benefit patients with pancreatitis.

35.7 **B.** A calcium value greater than 8 mg/dL is not one of Ranson's criteria. Age >55, calcium <8 mg/dL, fluid requirement >6000 mL during the initial 48 hours, and hematocrit drop of >10% are all components of Ranson Criteria.

35.8 **C.** Patients with infected pancreatic necrosis have been studied in a randomized prospective trial comparing early surgical intervention to delayed surgical intervention, and the results showed that patients treated with delayed surgical interventions had lower complication rates and lower mortality rates.

CLINICAL PEARLS

▶ The most important element in preventing multiple organ dysfunction syndrome is fluid resuscitation.

▶ Serum amylase and lipase elevations are useful in diagnosing acute pancreatitis, but these values correlate poorly with disease severity.

▶ The primary indication for surgery for acute pancreatitis is to treat local complications such as symptomatic pseudocysts, infected pancreatic necrosis, and pancreatic abscess.

▶ Patients with biliary pancreatitis should have their cholecystectomy performed prior to hospital discharge because randomized controlled trials have demonstrated that patients randomized to delayed cholecystectomy in 6 weeks experienced higher rates of disease relapse and readmissions for pancreatitis.

▶ Pancreatic pseudocyst occurs as the result of pancreatic duct disruption with subsequent leakage of exocrine pancreatic fluid excretion.

▶ Oral diet does not worsen the course of acute pancreatitis and is beneficial in preventing infectious complications related to the pancreatitis.

▶ Delaying surgical debridement beyond 30 days after disease onset in patients with pancreatic necrosis is associated with improved outcomes in comparison to patients treated with early surgical interventions.

REFERENCES

Stern JR, Mathews JB. Pancreas necrosis. In: Cameron JL, Cameron AM, eds. *Current Surgical Therapy.* 11th ed. Philadelphia, PA: Elsevier Saunders; 2014:450-454.

Valsangkar N, Thayer SP. Acute pancreatitis. In: Cameron JL, Cameron AM, eds. *Current Surgical Therapy.* 11th ed. Philadelphia, PA: Elsevier Saunders; 2014:431-439.

Working Group IAP/APA Acute pancreatitis Guidelines. IAP/APA evidence-based guidelines for the management of acute pancreatitis. *Pancreatology.* 2013;13:e1-e15.

Wu BU, Banks PA. Clinical management of patients with acute pancreatitis. *Gastroenterol.* 2013; 144:1272-1281.

A 23-year-old man presents with the sudden onset of left chest pain and shortness of breath that occurred while he was working in his yard. He denies any trauma to his chest, cough, or other respiratory symptoms prior to the onset of pain. His past medical history is unremarkable, and he takes no medications. He consumes a half a pack of cigarettes a day and two to three beers a day. On physical examination, he appears anxious. His temperature is normal and his pulse rate is 110 beats/minute. The pulmonary examination reveals diminished breath sounds on the left and normal breath sounds on the right. The cardiac examination demonstrates no murmurs or gallops. Results of the abdominal and extremity examinations are unremarkable. The laboratory examination reveals a normal complete blood count and normal serum electrolytes. The chest radiograph shows a 60% left pneumothorax, without effusions or pulmonary lesions.

▶ What is your next step?
▶ What are the risk factors for this condition?

ANSWERS TO CASE 36:

Spontaneous Pneumothorax

Summary: An otherwise healthy 23-year-old-man presents with a large primary spontaneous pneumothorax.

- **Next step:** Perform either tube thoracostomy or needle aspiration to allow re-expansion of the left lung.

- **Risk factors for this condition:** Primary spontaneous pneumothorax is caused by the rupture of subpleural blebs. Secondary spontaneous pneumothorax may be caused by bullous emphysematous disease, cystic fibrosis, primary and secondary cancers, and necrotizing infections with organisms such as Pseudocystis jiroveci (formerly known as P carinii).

ANALYSIS

Objectives

1. Learn to distinguish between primary and secondary spontaneous pneumothorax.

2. Learn the treatments and diagnostic strategies for patients presenting with spontaneous pneumothorax.

Considerations

This is an otherwise healthy young man who presents with a symptomatic and sizeable (>50%) spontaneous left pneumothorax. Primary spontaneous pneumothorax is most commonly caused by rupture of subpleural bullae (found in 76% to 100% of the surgical specimen during videoscopic-assistant thoracic surgery or VATS performed for this condition). This patient does not have any risk factor for secondary spontaneous pneumothorax such as malignancy, tuberculosis, sarcoidosis, or chronic obstructive pulmonary disease. Because this patient is symptomatic from the condition, the best treatment would be to either aspirate the pneumothorax or place a chest tube to help re-expand the left lung and improve his symptoms.

APPROACH TO:

Spontaneous Pneumothorax

DEFINITIONS

PNEUMOTHORAX: This is a pathologic condition where air enters the pleural space. With the accumulation of air in the pleural space, the mechanics of lung expansion become compromised due to an increase in the work required for inspiration. In some patients, this causes subjective shortness of breath and increased difficulty with air exchange.

PRIMARY SPONTANEOUS PNEUMOTHORAX: This condition is 4 to 10 times more common in men than women and occurs most commonly in thin, tall men. A primary spontaneous pneumothorax occurs in the absence of underlying lung diseases. Rupture of subpleural bullae is the main cause of the condition. Seventy-six to hundred percent of the patients with primary spontaneous pneumothorax have subpleural bullae in the contralateral lung and are at risk for such an occurrence in the opposite lung. Patients with primary spontaneous pneumothorax tend to have mild symptoms, because they do not have underlying pulmonary diseases.

SECONDARY SPONTANEOUS PNEUMOTHORAX: This refers to spontaneous pneumothorax occuring in an individual with underlying lung disease such as COPD, tuberculosis, necrotizing pneumonia, pneumocystis, sarcoidosis, bronchiectesis, interstitial lung disease, endometriosis, cystic fibrosis, pulmonary fibrosis, Marfan's syndrome, and Ehlers-Danlos syndrome. **COPD is responsible for 70% of secondary spontaneous pneumothoraces.** Patients with secondary spontaneous pneumothorax are usually symptomatic and appear breathless as they tend to have less respiratory reserve.

IATROGENIC PNEUMOTHORAX: The incidence of iatrogenic pneumothorax is increasing due to the increase in invasive diagnostic and therapeutic procedures being performed. The **most common causes** of iatrogenic pneumothorax are **thoracentesis, central venous catheter placement (subclavian vein risk >internal jugular vein risk), CT-guided lung biopsies, positive-pressure mechanical ventilation, transbronchial biopsies, bronchoscopy,** and **pleural biopsy.** An important point to remember about this form of pneumothorax is that delayed presentations are relatively common; therefore, it is important to maintain high vigilance for this complication in order to minimize the morbidity/mortality.

TENSION PNEUMOTHORAX: This clinical condition is caused by a flap-valve effect where air continues to enter the pleural space, but is unable to escape. When this condition persists, air in the pleural space can be so large that it displaces the mediastinal structures to the contralateral side of the thorax. If not treated, kinking of the IVC, diminished venous return, and cardiac arrest may occur.

DEFINITIONS OF CLINICALLY STABLE PATIENT WITH PNEUMOTHORAX: The ACCP definition requires respiratory rate <24/minute, pulse rate of 60 to 120 beats/minute, SpO_2 > 90% on room air, and able to speak in full sentences. The British Thoracic Society defines a patient clinically stable when there is no respiratory disturbance.

OPEN PNEUMOTHORAX ("SUCKING CHEST WOUND"): Injury to the chest causing a full-thickness chest wall defect, allowing air to be sucked directly through the defect into the pleural space, leading to pneumothorax.

FLAIL CHEST: Injury to multiple ribs with the injuries in more than one place resulting in the paradoxical inward movement during inspirations. Other physiologic compromises that these patients have are related to the pulmonary contusions that occurs to the lungs directly adjacent to the flail segment and atelectasis in the uninjured lung secondary to pain and splinting.

TUBE THORACOSTOMY (CHEST TUBE): Placement of catheters of various sizes into the pleural space to evacuate air and/or blood. This often will help the lung to fully re-expand.

PNEUMOTHORAX IN PATIENTS WITH AIDS: Pneumothoraces that occur in patients with AIDS are usually due to the presence of pneumocystis pneumonia (PCP). These patients should be treated with chest tube placement because persistent air leaks occur commonly in these individuals. If the patient is able to withstand surgery, surgical treatment is often required because of failure of resolution of the pneumothorax.

PLEURODESIS: This a treatment approach that utilizes chemical (talc or doxycycline) or mechanical irritant (abrasion) on the pleura and lung surface to cause the visceral pleura to become adherent to the parietal pleura which ultimately obliterates the pleural space.

VIDEO-ASSISTED THORACOSCOPIC SURGERY (VATS): This is a minimally invasive thoracic surgical approach that can be applied for the resection of pulmonary blebs or to perform mechanical pleurodesis.

CLINICAL APPROACH

The five important treatment principles/goals to follow in the treatment of patients with spontaneous pneumothorax are: (1) eliminate air from the pleural space; (2) reduce air leakage; (3) heal the pleural fistula; (4) re-expand the lung; (5) prevent future occurrences. The approach to accomplishing these objectives can vary based on the etiologies/pathogenesis of the pneumothorax, patients' symptoms and physiologic conditions, patient preferences, and the availability of medical resources and expertise.

The physical examination findings associated with pneumothorax include respiratory distress, asymmetrical chest expansion, diminished breath sounds, and hyper-resonance on percussion. Changes in vital signs such as tachycardia, tachypnea, and hypotension may occur in patients with tension physiology. Imaging studies are unnecessary for the diagnosis of severely symptomatic cases, and treatment should not be delayed in these circumstances.

Most cases of spontaneous pneumothorax do not progress to respiratory failure or tension pneumothorax; therefore, treatment of patients with this condition can be approached in a case-by-case fashion. **The American College of Chest Physicians (ACCP) defines small pneumothorax as one where the apex of the lung is less than 3 cm away from the normal position.** The ACCP guidelines suggest that relatively an asymptomatic patient with a small primary pneumothorax can be safely observed. For a patients with a secondary spontaneous pneumothorax, the ACCP guidelines state that observation is appropriate only if the pneumothorax is very small (<1cm rim of air).

Treatment

Without ongoing leakage from the lung parenchyma, gas in the pleural space will diffuse back into the surrounding tissue. Reabsorption of oxygen occurs more rapidly than reabsorption of nitrogen or carbon dioxide. Therefore, placing patients on supplemental oxygen will improve the resolution of pneumothorax. Room air reabsorption from the pleural cavity is estimated at 1.25%/day; based on that estimate, resolution of a pneumothorax occupying 25% of the pleural cavity will require about 20 days. If the patient is receiving supplemental oxygen, pneumothorax resolution is accelerated by a factor of 3 or 4-fold. Affected patients should be placed on high-flow oxygen at 10 L/min to promote pneumothorax resolution. In general, it is safer to observe patients with pneumothorax in the hospital. The ACCP guidelines suggest that under unusual circumstances, a patient can be discharged if he/she remains clinically stable and has a repeat CXR after 4 to 6 hours demonstrating no radiographic progression. If the patient is discharged, follow-up is recommended within 2 days.

Simple aspiration of pneumothorax can be performed by placing a small catheter into the pleural space. The reported success rate of simple aspiration is better for primary spontaneous pneumothorax than for secondary spontaneous pneumothorax (75% vs 35-40% for primary and secondary, respectively). In a small, randomized study that compared simple aspiration versus chest tube placement for patients with the first occurrence of primary spontaneous pneumothorax, no difference in effectiveness was noted. The patients who underwent simple aspiration had a shorter duration of hospitalization than patients treated with chest tube placement. After it is inserted, the chest tube is usually placed on suction to facilitate lung re-expansion. Once the lung is fully re-expanded and there is no on-going air leakage, chest tube removal can be considered. There is no consensus regarding role of water-seal prior to tube removal. See Figure 36–1 for management algorithm.

Persistent Air Leak

There is no standard definition for persistent air leak; however, it generally refers to a situation when the pleural-cutaneous fistula persists beyond the normally expected time of healing. The ACCP recommends that additional interventions be considered when air leak persists for >4 days in cases of primary spontaneous pneumothorax, and >5 days in cases of secondary spontaneous pneumothorax. Additional interventions for persistent air leak include surgery for bulectomy (bleb excision) and mechanical pleurodesis, which can be performed either by open surgery or a thoracoscopic approach.

Interventions to Prevent Recurrences

Surgical interventions described for the treatment of persistent air leaks can also be used to prevent pneumothorax recurrences. The often quoted spontaneous pneumothorax recurrence rates are 30% after one episode, 50% after two episodes, and 80% after three episodes. Smoking cessation and proper breathing exercises are helpful in reducing recurrences. Preventative surgeries generally involve the resection of blebs and mechanical pleurodesis. Surgery is effective but not perfect, with recurrence rates of 1% to 5% are reported following operative interventions. Operations performed by open thoracotomy are associated with lower recurrences than those performed thoracoscopically. However, open thoracotomy is associated with

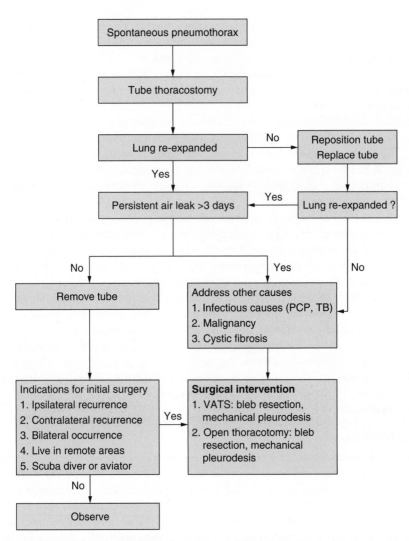

Figure 36–1. Algorithm for the management of spontaneous pneumothorax. PCP, *Pneumocystis jiroveci* pneumonia; TB, tuberculosis; VATS, video-assisted thoracoscopy.

greater postoperative discomfort and prolonged recovery in comparison to thoracoscopic operations.

CASE CORRELATION

- See also Case 6 (Blunt Chest Trauma).

COMPREHENSION QUESTIONS

36.1 A patient is being evaluated by a pulmonologist for recurrent primary spontaneous pneumothorax. Which of the following describes a likely characteristic that this patient exhibits?

   A. Female gender

   B. Age 55 to 70

   C. Tall, thin physique

   D. History of tuberculosis

   E. Recent upper respiratory infection

36.2 The patient described in question 36.1 inquires about the risk of recurrence of his condition. Which of the following factors is most predictive of the recurrence of primary pneumothorax?

   A. Patient's occupation

   B. The location of the blebs

   C. Asthma

   D. Chest tube placement rather than catheter aspiration

   E. The number of prior episodes of pneumothorax

36.3 Following the placement of a left subclavian vein catheter, a 45 year old man develops "air hunger" and chest pain. His breath sounds are diminished on the left, and percussion of the left hemithorax reveals hyper-resonance. His oxygen saturation by pulse-oximetry drops from 97% to 72%. Which of the following is the best treatment?

   A. Oxygen therapy

   B. Placement of a left chest tube

   C. Observation

   D. Left chest tube placement followed by chemical pleurodesis

   E. Intubation and mechanical ventilation

36.4 Which of the following presentations is most consistent with left tension pneumothorax?

   A. Hypotension, distended neck veins, midline trachea, and muffled heart sounds

   B. Hypotension, open 4 cm × 4 cm lateral chest wound

   C. Hypotension, diminished breath sounds on the left, tracheal deviation to the right, and chest x-ray demonstrating opacification of the left hemithorax

   D. Diminished left sided breath sounds, tracheal deviation to right

   E. Diminished left sided breath sounds and deviation of the trachea to the left

36.5 You are assessing a 38-year-old man with respiratory complaints. Your differential diagnosis for the patient is pleural effusion versus pneumothorax. Which of the following physical findings will best help differentiate between these possibilities?

A. Respiratory rate of 33 breaths/minute

B. Agitation due to respiratory distress

C. Somnolence

D. Dullness to percussion over the affected hemithorax

E. Cough

36.6 Which of the following factors has no influence on the recurrence rate of spontaneous pneumothorax?

A. Smoking

B. Concurrent history of pulmonary tuberculosis

C. Gender

D. Surgical treatment

E. Prior history of spontaneous pneumothorax

36.7 Which of the following statements regarding pleurodesis is false?

A. This procedure obliterates the pleural space

B. This can be accomplished with the infusion of a sclerosing agent into the pleural space

C. This can be accomplished by surgical access to the pleural space

D. The effects of pleurodesis can be reversed

E. Pleurodesis increases the risk of recurrent pneumothorax

ANSWERS

36.1 **C.** Primary spontaneous pneumothorax occurs most commonly in young, tall, thin, and otherwise healthy men. This condition is not associated with an underlying pulmonary process such as tuberculosis. Respiratory tract infection is not a known risk factor.

36.2 **E.** The number of prior episodes of primary spontaneous pneumothorax has a prognostic effect on the recurrence of disease. The risk of recurrence after the first episode is 30%, and the risk of recurrence goes up to 50% and 80% respectively after the second and third episodes.

36.3 **B.** The patient described here has an iatrogenic pneumothorax, and the condition has caused the "air hunger," dramatic drop oxygen saturation, and chest pain. For a patient who is symptomatic with these descriptions, observation is not appropriate. Placement of a chest tube or needle aspiration is the treatment that should be initiated at this point.

36.4 **D.** Diminished breath sounds on the left associated with tracheal deviation to the right are findings most compatible with a left tension pneumothorax. The description in choice "A" is compatible with cardiac tamponade.

36.5 **D.** The differentiation between large pleural effusion and pneumothorax in a patient with respiratory distress can be made on the basis of chest percussion findings. The hemithorax affected by a large pleural effusion would likely have dullness on percussion.

36.6 **C.** Smoking, history of tuberculosis, and history of prior episodes of spontaneous pneumothorax all can increase the probability of pneumothorax recurrence. Surgical treatment such as bleb resection and pleurodesis can decrease the probability of recurrences. Gender of the patient has not been shown to influence recurrence patterns.

36.7 **D.** Pleurodesis is the process that obliterates the pleural space, and this is done with the intention of reducing the recurrence of spontaneous pneumothorax in patients. This can be accomplished with the infusion of sclerosing agents into the pleural space. Alternatively, this can be accomplished by mechanical irritation of the visceral and parietal pleura to cause adhesion of these surfaces. Once pleurodesis is performed, this process is generally not reversible.

CLINICAL PEARLS

▶ Most cases of spontaneous pneumothorax can be managed with observation, aspiration, or tube thoracostomy for cases that are high-risk for recurrence (recurrent pneumothorax) or in cases of persistent air leak, surgical treatment should be considered.

▶ The principles of pneumothorax treatment are to eliminate the intrapleural air, reduce the air leakage, promote healing of the pleural fistula, promote re-expansion of the lung, and prevent recurrences.

▶ For primary spontaneous pneumothorax patients, a small randomized study has demonstrated equivocal success rates with aspiration and tube thoracostomy.

▶ Tube thoracostomy is associated with longer length of hospital stay in comparison to simple needle aspiration; however, tube thoracostomy is indicated when the pneumothorax fails to resolve or symptoms do not improve with aspiration.

▶ Spontaneous pneumothorax generally does not progress to tension pneumothorax.

REFERENCES

Choi WI. Pneumothorax. *Tuberc Respir Dis*. 2014;76:99-104.

Huang Y, Huang H, Li Q, et al. Approach to the treatment for pneumothorax. *J Thorac Dis*. 2014;6(S4):S416-S420.

Zarogoulidis P, Kioumis I, Pitsiou G, et al. Pneumothorax: from definition to diagnosis and treatment. *J Thorac Dis*. 2014;6(S4):S372-S376.

A 57-year-old man has a 3-week history of nonproductive cough. He denies weight loss, hemoptysis, or night sweats. His past medical history is significant for hypertension that is controlled with a β-blocker. The patient has had no known history to asbestos and no foreign travels. He has a 25 pack-year history of cigarette smoking. On examination, the patient is afebrile and has no significant abnormal findings. A chest radiograph (CXR) reveals a 2-cm soft tissue density in the perihilar region of the left lung field, which appears to be a new lesion not visualized during a CXR obtained 2 years previously.

▶ What should be your next steps?
▶ What strategies are there for early detection of this disease process?

ANSWERS TO CASE 37:
Solitary Pulmonary Nodule

Summary: A 57-year-old male smoker presents with nonproductive cough and a solitary left lung nodule that is suspicious for a malignancy.

- **Next step:** A contrast-enhanced computed tomography (CT) scan of the chest that includes the liver and adrenal glands should be obtained to better characterize the mass and assess for potential metastatic deposits. Based on the finding of the CT scan, subsequent diagnostic and treatment plans can be implemented. Examples of subsequent management options include bronchoscopy with or without biopsies and brushings, CT guided-biopsies, thoracoscopic or open lung resection.

- **Screening recommendations:** The latest (2013) recommendations by the United States Preventive Services Task Force (USPSTF) is to screen for lung cancer with low-dose CT in adults age 55 to 80 years with a 30 pack-year smoking history who are either current smokers or have quit within the past 15 years.

ANALYSIS

Objectives

1. Be familiar with the strategy for diagnostic evaluation and management of a lung mass in patients with or without known history of malignancy.

2. Be familiar with the staging, treatment, and follow-up of non-small cell and small cell lung cancers.

3. Understand the role of surgery in the management of pulmonary metastasis.

Considerations

This solitary pulmonary nodule most likely represents nonsmall cell lung cancer. The presence of a cough, although nonspecific and common in smokers, should prompt further evaluation when it is new and persistent. With the typical lung cancer doubling time, a 2-cm lung cancer would have been present for nearly 1 year; therefore, visualization of a lung nodule on CXR that was not present 2 years earlier helps to narrow the differential diagnosis to either an infectious or a malignant process. The fact that the patient has no history or physical examination findings that indicate infectious processes further increases the probability that this lesion is a primary lung cancer. A CT scan of the chest and upper abdomen is helpful at this time not only to help characterize the lesion, but may be helpful to look for regional and distant metastases (pulmonary hila, mediastinum, hepatic, and adrenal) and can be helpful for biopsy and surgical planning.

APPROACH TO:
Solitary Pulmonary Nodules

DEFINITIONS

SOLITARY PULMONARY NODULE: This is defined as a round opacity that is at least moderately well marginated and is not more than 3 cm in maximal diameter seen by radiographic imaging. A solitary pulmonary nodule is the initial finding leading to 20% to 30% of the lung cancer diagnosis in the United States.

SMALL SOLITARY PULMONARY NODULE: This describes a nodule less than 1 cm in diameter.

GROUND-GLASS ATTENUATION: This radiographic term describes a less-defined mass lesion that has greater density than background tissue but does not have the same degree of density as a nodule.

SUBSOLID PULMONARY NODULE: This is a radiographic description of a nodule that has solid, partially solid, or ground-glass attenuation. A subsolid nodule is a lesion with less density than a solitary pulmonary nodule. Adenocarcinoma is one of the clinically important differential diagnoses for subsolid nodules. Since primary adenocarcinoma of the lung can occur in younger patients without smoking histories, a history of smoking is not a consideration in the management of subsolid nodules.

CLINICAL APPROACH TO PRIMARY LUNG CANCER

Lung cancer is the leading cause of cancer death worldwide. Globally, the lung cancer incidence and mortality closely parallel each other, which reflect the high case-fatality of the disease. The incidence of lung cancer has been rising, particularly in developed high-income countries. Lung cancer is the third most common cancer in the United States behind breast and prostate cancers. Cigarette smoking is the single most important risk factor for the development of lung cancers, and **radon exposure is the second leading cause of lung cancers** in the United States. Due to the asymptomatic nature of lung cancers during the early stages, many patients with the disease are unfortunately diagnosed at rather advanced incurable stages.

POSITRON EMISSION TOMOGRAPHY (PET) SCAN

This imaging modality is often combined with CT to create PET-CT images. PET scans are obtained after positron-emitting glucose analogue administration, and the images produced are designed to detect tissues with high metabolic rates. Malignant cells generally have higher metabolic rates than normal tissues and can therefore be differentiated from nonmalignant structures.

CLINICAL APPROACH

Lung Cancer Screening

Even though treatment and diagnostic advances have steadily improved 5-year survivals for breast cancer (90%), colon cancer (65%), and prostate cancer (~100%) in the United States, there has been little improvement in United States lung cancer survival that stands currently at 18% at 5 years. The new USPSTF screening recommendation was patterned after the National Lung Screening Trial (NLST) results which were published in 2002. The NLST screened 50,000 asymptomatic adults ages 55 to 74 with ≥30 pack-year smoking history, and their findings suggested that low-dose CT screening contributed to a reduction in all-cause-related mortality and lung cancer-related mortality. Mathematical modeling suggests that the new USPSTF screening guidelines should lead to an overall 14% reduction in lung cancer mortality in the United States.

In an effort to improve lung cancer early detection and survival, the USPSTF in 2013 recommended annual screening with low-dose CT scans for individuals 55 to 80 years old who are current smokers or former smokers with ≥30 pack-year smoking history. These screening recommendations have caused significant controversy within the medical community, as screening for lung cancer is expected to lead to early cancer detection for some individuals. However, large-scale lung cancer screening can be costly and cause potential harm, including unnecessary diagnostic procedures following false-positive findings, radiation-induced malignancies, and psychological stress associated positive screening tests.

The potential harm from radiation exposure from medical imaging is a well-publicized concern among practitioners and the general public. To put this issue in perspective, naturally occurring **background radiation exposure for an average person in the U.S. is about 3 milli Sieverts (mSv) per year,** and for residents of high-altitude environments such as Colorado or New Mexico, the background exposure is 1.5 mSv greater or a total of 4.5 mSv annually. Radiation exposure from common diagnostic chest imaging studies are **0.1 mSv for chest x-ray** (equivalent to 10 days of background radiation dose), **1.5 mSv for low-dose CT** (6 months of background radiation dose), and **7 mSv for regular chest CT** (2 years of background radiation dose).

Diagnosis and Treatment

Most patients with primary lung cancers are symptomatic at diagnosis, with cough, chest pain, and respiratory distress being the most common symptoms. Adenocarcinoma is the most common type of lung cancer responsible for 45% of all cases, with most of the lesions located in the periphery of the lungs. Adenocarcinomas tend to metastasize earlier than squamous cell lung cancers and often metastasize to CNS structures. Squamous cell carcinomas make up approximately 30% of the lung cancers, tend to be more centrally located in the lungs, and are more likely to undergo central necrosis and compressions of the airways. Small cell carcinomas make up 20% of the lung cancers and are most likely centrally located. Regional metastases occur frequently within the lungs and to mediastinal lymph nodes.

Lung cancers can also metastasize systemically, with common metastases to the brain, adrenal glands, and bones.

A new lung nodule presenting in smokers have as high as 70% chance of being cancerous; therefore, **lung lesions in smokers should be approached with a high degree of suspicion.** The evaluation of a new lung nodule can begin with a review of prior CXRs. With serial x-rays, the radiologist can determine the rate of growth that helps differentiate between benign and malignant causes. When the clinical and radiographic pictures are suggestive of pneumonia, a 10 to 14 day course of antibiotics can be prescribed with re-imaging performed following the completion of the treatment course. If the lesion persists, additional evaluations must be carried out.

Lung nodules or masses located centrally are more likely to cause symptoms and are often amenable to bronchoscopic evaluations. For lesions that are located in the periphery of the lungs, CT-guided percutaneous biopsies are often possible for tissue diagnosis. When initial evaluations are nondiagnostic, patients with sufficient pulmonary reserve can undergo either video-assisted thoracoscopic surgical resection (VATS) or open lung biopsies. All patients who are under considerations for lung resection for primary lung cancers should have cardiopulmonary evaluations to determine if he/she can tolerate an anatomic pulmonary resection. Anatomic resections for primary lung cancers have been shown to be associated with greater disease-free survival in comparison to nonanatomic resections (eg, wedge resections). The lung resection can be done either by open surgery or thoracoscopically; resections by thoracoscopic approach have shown to produce more rapid postoperative recoveries and good oncologic outcomes. Recently, the use of focused radiation therapy or stereotactic ablative radiation therapy (Gamma Knife) has been applied for curative intent in patients who do not have sufficient physiologic reserve to withstand surgery. Results of Gamma Knife treatments have been quite favorable, with local disease control rates reported at 30% to 50% and 5-year survival rates reported at 10% to 30%. There are currently on-going clinical trials directed at widening the applications of this technique. See Tables 37–1 and 37–2 for staging.

Patients with stage IB to IIB non-small cell lung cancers generally will benefit from adjuvant chemotherapy or chemoradiation therapy after surgical resections. Adjuvant chemotherapy with cisplatin-based doublet adjuvant regimen is the most often prescribed therapy. Occasionally, patients with stage IIIA locally advanced nonsmall cell lung cancers are treated initially with systemic chemotherapy in the attempt to achieve more complete surgical resections. Adjuvant targeted therapy, such as anti-VEGF and anti-EGF therapies have been found to provide additional survival benefits for some patients with certain gene profiles.

APPROACH TO METASTASES TO THE LUNG

The lung is the second most common site of metastases for many solid tumors (liver is the most common site of metastasis). In some patients, lung metastases represent the only active disease for the individuals; therefore, it is conceivable that these patients may receive benefit from resection of their pulmonary metastases (metastasectomy). This pattern of metastatic disease has been referred to as

Table 37–1 • DEFINITIONS OF T, N, AND M CATEGORIES FOR CARCINOMA OF THE LUNG

Category	Description
T: Primary tumor	
TX	Tumor proven by the presence of malignant cells in bronchopulmonary secretions but not visualized
T0	No evidence of a primary tumor
Tis	Carcinoma in situ
T1	A tumor that is ≤3.0 cm in greatest dimension, surrounded by lung or visceral pleura, and without evidence of invasion proximal to a lobar bronchus on bronchoscopy[a]
T2	A tumor >3.0 cm in greatest dimension, or a tumor of any size that either invades the visceral pleura or has associated atelectasis or obstructive pneumonitis extending to the hilar region. On bronchoscopy, this tumor involves the lobar bronchus or at least 2.0 cm distal to the carina. Any associated atelectasis or obstructive pneumonitis must involve less than the entire lung
T3	A tumor of any size with direct extension into the chest wall (including superior sulcus tumors), diaphragm, or mediastinal pleura or pericardium without involving the heart, great vessels, trachea, esophagus or vertebral body, or a tumor in the main bronchus within 2 cm of the carina without involving the carina, or associated atelectasis or obstructive pneumonitis of the entire lung
T4	A tumor of any size with invasion of the mediastinum or involving the heart, great vessels, trachea, esophagus, vertebral body, or carina, or with the presence of malignant pleural or pericardial effusion[b] or with satellite tumor nodules within the ipsilateral, primary tumor lobe of the lung
N: Nodal involvement	
N0	No demonstrable metastasis to regional lymph nodes
N1	Metastasis to lymph nodes in the peribronchial or the ipsilateral hilar region or both, including direct extension
N2	Metastasis to ipsilateral mediastinal lymph nodes and subcarinal lymph nodes
N3	Metastasis to contralateral mediastinal lymph nodes, contralateral hilar lymph nodes, ipsilateral or contralateral scalene, or supraclavicular lymph nodes
M: Distant metastasis	
M0	No (known) distant metastasis
M1	Distant metastasis present.[c] Specify site(s)

[a]*An uncommon superficial tumor of any size with its invasive component limited to the bronchial wall that may extend proximal to the main bronchus is classified as T1.*
[b]*Most pleural effusions associated with lung cancer are due to tumor. There are, however, a few patients in whom cytopathologic examination of pleural fluid (on more than one specimen) is for tumor; the fluid is nonbloody and is not an exudate. In such cases where these elements and clinical judgment dictate that the effusion is not related to the tumor, the patient should be staged T1, T2, or T3 excluding effusion as a staging element.*
[c]*Separate metastatic tumor nodules in the ipsilateral nonprimary tumor lobe(s) of the lung also classified M1.*

"oligometastatic disease": a pattern that is not always easy to recognize. The selection of patients for metastasectomies is not straightforward, as the majority of patients with metastatic disease do not benefit from metastasectomies. Patients with **oligometastatic disease** generally have fewer than five lesions limited to one

Table 37–2 • AJCC STAGE GROUPING OF TNM SUBSETS			
Stage 0	Carcinoma in situ		
Stage IA	T1 N0 M0		
Stage IB	T2 N0 M0		
Stage IIA	T1 N1 M0		
Stage IIB	T2 N1 M0 T3 N0 M0		
Stage IIIA	T3 N1 M0 T1 N2 M0	T2 N2 M0	T3 N2 M0
Stage IIIB	T4 N0 M0 T1 N3 M0 T4 N3 M0	T4 N1 M0 T2 N3 M0	T4 N2 M0 T3 N3 M0
Stage IV	Any T	Any N	M1

or two organs. Some important considerations for patient selection include primary tumor type, the locations of the lesions, the number of metastatic lesions, and interval between primary disease and metastatic disease presentation. With regards to primary tumor type, it appears that patients with germ cell tumors, melanomas, sarcomas, and epithelial cancers (most commonly colorectal carcinoma) are the most likely to benefit from metastasectomies. Whereas, patients with metastatic cancers from the lung and breast rarely benefit from resections of their metastases. In some cases where the indications for resection are in question, additional observation time can often help answer the question.

Results of metastasectomies from several institutions have suggested that thoracoscopic approach in these patients can result in potentially missing some metastatic

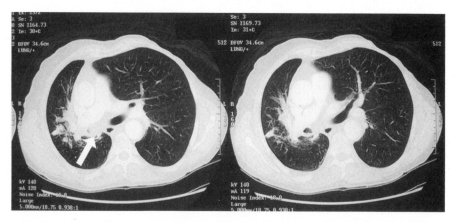

Figure 37–1. Chest CT of an obstructed right main stem lung tumor. Arrow indicates location of right main stem bronchus. *(Reproduced with permission from Brunicardi FC, Andersen DK, Billiar TR, et al, eds. Schwartz's Principles of Surgery. 8th ed. New York, NY: McGraw-Hill;2005:569.)*

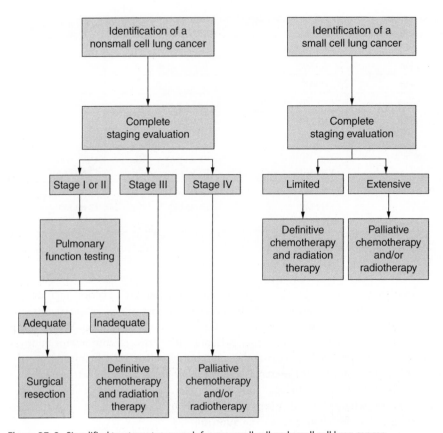

Figure 37–2. Simplified treatment approach for nonsmall cell and small cell lung cancer.

lesions that cannot be easily identified during thorascopy; therefore, a number of groups currently recommend open resections for these patients.

COMPREHENSION QUESTIONS

37.1 A 45-year-old nonsmoker is noted to have a 2-cm soft tissue mass in the left lung field. Which of the following is the most appropriate next step?

A. Perform a CT-guided biopsy of the mass
B. Obtain sputum samples
C. Evaluate all prior CXRs
D. Obtain a repeat CXR in 6 months
E. Perform a video-assisted thoracoscopic resection

37.2 A 45-year-old man with a persistent cough is noted to have a suspicious lesion on CXR. The physician orders a CT scan of the chest. Which of the following describes the main purpose of CT imaging for a patient with a suspicious lung mass?

A. Discern between exudative pleural effusion and transudative effusion

B. Differentiate between malignant and benign lesions

C. Determine if the mass is infectious in origin

D. Differentiate between primary and metastatic disease

E. Determine anatomic location of the mass

37.3 Which of the following patients is the best candidate for pulmonary resection?

A. A 33-year-old female nonsmoker presents with two isolated left lung masses each measuring 3 cm in diameter. Biopsy of the lesions reveals adnenocarcinoma of unknown primary source

B. A 46-year-old man with a history of left thigh soft tissue sarcoma, who underwent complete resection of the primary tumor. He has remained without evidence of disease for 3 years. During the most recent follow-up, he is noted to have a single 2-cm lesion in the left lung with CT-guided biopsy revealing metastatic sarcoma

C. An 86-year-old woman with a history of chronic obstructive pulmonary disease who had undergone resection of rectal cancer 3 years prior. At that time, she did not receive systemic chemotherapy because of her poor physiologic condition. She now has a solitary left middle lobe metastatic lesion measuring 2 cm in diameter

D. A 23-year-old man with a pigmented lesion on the left shoulder with biopsy demonstrating malignant melanoma. Imaging studies demonstrated a suspicious mass in the left frontal portion of his brain and two 1-cm nodules in the left lung

E. A 45-year-old man with a 6-cm left lung mass with biopsy demonstrating small cell lung cancer

37.4 A 53-year-old man with a 20 pack-year smoking history presents with a 2-week history of a productive cough. The chest x-ray reveals a right middle lobe infiltrate. Which of the following is the most appropriate management for this patient?

A. CT scan of the chest, pulmonary function tests, and thoracoscopic wedge resection of the right middle lobe

B. Antibiotic therapy for 2 weeks, followed by repeat CXR. If the infiltrate persists, obtain CT of chest and bronchoscopy

C. CT scan with CT-guided biopsy

D. Right thoracotomy and right middle lobe resection

E. Bronchoscopy with brushings and biopsy

37.5 For which of the following tumor characteristics of a nonsmall cell lung cancer is surgical resection contraindicated?

A. Involvement of the parietal pleura by a 3-cm tumor

B. 2.5-cm tumor with a single peribronchial lymph node on the ipsilateral side

C. 3-cm left lower lobe tumor with left pleural effusion containing malignant cells

D. 5-cm tumor involving the right upper and right middle lobes

E. 4-cm central lesion involving the right mainstem bronchus

37.6 For which of the following patients can the term oligometastatic disease be applied as a description of his/her condition?

A. A 33-year-old man with malignant melanoma of the leg who has two 3-cm metastatic lung lesions involving the left upper lobe and right middle lobe, and three 1-cm lesions in the left lobe of the liver

B. A 44-year-old man with a 8-cm small cell carcinoma of the lung with two brain metastases

C. A 28-year-old man with a history of a 2-mm deep melanoma of the leg who had wide local resection, and sentinel lymph node biopsy that was negative. Four years after resection of the primary tumor, he presents with six 1-cm lung masses in the periphery of the left upper lobe and right lower lobe

D. A 63-year-old woman with left breast T2N1 invasive ductal carcinoma who presents with two left lung nodules, a brain metastasis, and a left adrenal lesion 2 years after her initial resection

E. A 44-year-old man with a 6-cm left calf soft tissue sarcoma resected by wide local resection. Three years after the resection he presents with a single 4-cm metastasis to the right middle lobe of his lung

37.7 Which of the following statements regarding primary lung cancer is true?

A. Nonanatomic resection and anatomic resections of primary lung cancers have similar cancer-related outcomes

B. Contralateral subcarinal node involvement with metastatic disease is a contraindication for pulmonary resection

C. Stereotactic ablative radiation treatment of lung cancer only provides local disease palliation

D. The addition of chemotherapy does not improve survival over pulmonary resection alone for a patient with Stage IIB nonsmall cell lung cancer

E. Adjuvant targeted biologic agents have not been found to improve treatment outcomes in patients with nonsmall cell lung cancers

ANSWERS

37.1 **C.** For this 45-year-old man who is a nonsmoker found with an incidental lung mass, the most appropriate first step is to determine if this is a new lesion. If the mass has been visualized previously by imaging studies and has not changed or grown in size, then the mass is likely noncancerous. In that case, it can be observed with follow-up imaging study in 3 months. If the mass is new or has changed in size or character in comparison to prior imaging studies, then the mass is more likely cancerous and should be resected.

37.2 **E.** The CT scan for this patient can be helpful in determining the exact anatomic location of the "suspicious lesion," and the CT can be helpful in this patient to help evaluate the mediastinal and peribronchial lymph nodes. CT scan in this case not only provides anatomic information for surgical planning, but also provides valuable information for tumor staging.

37.3 **B.** Based on descriptions provided, the patients described in choices "B" and "C" are individuals who may have disease processes that fit the descriptions for oligometastatic diseases. The individual described in "B" has an apparent single pulmonary metastasis from an extremity soft tissue sarcoma that was completely resected 3 years prior. The woman described in "C" has a pulmonary metastasis from rectal adenocarcinoma. Even though her disease state may fit the description of an oligometastatic disease state, she may be a poor surgical candidate based on her medical comorbidities and limited physiologic reserve. She is someone who should be considered for stereotactic radiation ablation therapy rather than surgical resection.

37.4 **B.** A 53-year-old man with a smoking history presents with cough and a pulmonary infiltrate. This appears to be a straightforward case of pneumonia; however, some patients with lung cancers can present this way secondary to airway obstruction by the tumors. A course of antibiotic therapy with follow-up imaging is the most reasonable choice given.

37.5 **C.** Pleural effusion occurs fairly commonly in the setting of a patient with lung cancer. For many patients, this process is secondary to a concurrent infectious process or related to airway obstruction. When there are tumor cells retrieved from the pleural effusion, the pleural effusion is said to be a malignant effusion and suggests disseminated spread of tumor within the pleural space thus making the disease nonresectable.

37.6 **E.** The 44-year-old man with a single lung metastasis in the right middle lobe of his lung 4 years after resection of primary extremity soft tissue sarcoma most likely has a disease state that can benefit from excision of the metastasis.

37.7 **B.** Lung cancer with involvement of the contralateral subcarinal lymph node is staged at IIIB, and is not curable by surgical resection; therefore, this situation should be considered a contraindication for surgical resection. Anatomic resection of primary lung cancers is associated with better cancer-related outcomes than nonanatomic resections. Stereotactic ablative radiation therapy can be applied for curative intent. Stage IIb nonsmall cell lung cancer survival is improved with adjuvant chemotherapy. Adjuvant targeted therapy such as anti-VEGF and anti-EGF treatments have been shown to produce improved survival following lung cancer resections.

CLINICAL PEARLS

▶ Approximately 95% of patients with lung cancer present with symptoms related to the disease, whereas only 5% of patients present with asymptomatic chest findings.

▶ Cough is the initial presenting symptom in 75% of patients with lung cancer, caused by endobronchial tumor growth irritation of the airway.

▶ Approximately 10% to 20% of the lung cancer patients are affected by paraneoplastic syndrome. These syndromes are most commonly associated with small cell carcinoma and squamous cell carcinoma.

▶ The risk for developing lung cancer increases in patients with first-degree relatives with lung cancer.

▶ Small nodules less than 4 mm in diameter have a less than 1% chance of being a primary lung cancer even in patients who are smokers. With nodule size of 8 mm, the risk of malignancy increases to 10% to 20%.

REFERENCES

Eckardt J, Licht PB. Thoracoscopic or open surgery for pulmonary metastasectomy: an observer blinded study. *Ann Thorac Surg.* 2014;98:466-470.

Gould MK, Donington J, Lynch WR, et al. Evaluation of individuals with pulmonary nodules: when is it lung cancer? *Chest.* 2013;143:e93S-e120S.

Treasure T, Milosevic M, Fiorention F, Macbeth F. Pulmonary metastasectomy: what is the practice and where is the evidence for effectiveness? *Thorax.* 2014;69:946-949.

Truong M, Ko JP, Rossi SE, et al. Update in the evaluation of the solitary pulmonary nodule. *Radiographics.* 2014;1658-1679.

A 22-year-old man was walking past a construction site when a brick fell off the scaffold and struck him in the head. Witnesses reported that the patient was unconscious immediately after the incident and did not regain consciousness for approximately 10 minutes. The paramedics placed the patient in cervical spine precautions and brought him to the emergency department. During the primary survey at the emergency department, the patient has apparent normal air exchange, a respiratory rate of 18 breaths/minute, blood pressure of 138/78 mm Hg, and a pulse rate of 80 beats/minute. The patient does not open his eyes in response to voice commands, but has eye opening in response to painful stimuli. He withdraws from painful stimuli, with diminished motor responses in his left upper and lower extremities. His only verbal responses are incomprehensible sounds. The secondary survey demonstrates a 3-cm scalp laceration and soft tissue contusion over the right temporal region. The right pupil is 6 mm and sluggishly reactive to light, and the left pupil is 4 mm in diameter and reacts briskly to light. No blood is visualized behind his tympanic membranes. The examination of his truncal areas and extremities reveal no abnormalities.

▶ What is the most likely diagnosis?
▶ What should be your next steps in management?

ANSWERS TO CASE 38:

Traumatic Brain Injury

Summary: A 22-year-old man has an injury mechanism and findings that are compatible with traumatic brain injury. He has an initial Glasgow Coma Scale (GCS) of 8 (Table 38–1).

- **Most likely diagnosis:** Severe traumatic brain injury (TBI) with possible mass effect.

- **Next steps:** Immediate endotracheal intubation to control and optimize his oxygenation and ventilation. Early CT imaging is important to delineate the brain injury and to determine if the patient would benefit from neurosurgical intervention. The neurosurgeon should be alerted of the findings in this patient even prior to the CT results being available.

ANALYSIS

Objectives

1. Be able to calculate and know the significance of the GCS.

2. Learn the causes and preventive measures for secondary brain injury.

3. Learn the emergent management for patients with intracranial mass lesions and increased intracranial pressures.

4. Learn the assessment and recommendations for sports-related concussions.

Table 38–1 • GLASGOW COMA SCALE*	
Assessment Area	Score
EYE OPENING	
Spontaneous	4
To speech	3
To pain	2
None	1
VERBAL RESPONSE	
Oriented and coherent	5
Confused speech	4
Inappropriate words	3
Incomprehensible sounds	2
None	1
BEST MOTOR RESPONSE	
Obeys commands	6
Localizes pain	5
Withdraws to pain	4
Decorticate posture (abnormal flexion)	3
Decerebrate posture (abnormal extension)	2
No response	1

*The GCS is calculated as the aggregate of all three categories.

Considerations

This patient clearly is at risk for traumatic brain injury (TBI) and likely has severe TBI based on an initial GCS of 8. Because of the injuring mechanism, he is not only at risk for TBI but also at risk for cervical spine injury. Most prehospital personnel are aware of the association of TBI and spinal cord injury, therefore spinal precaution is nearly always applied in the prehospital setting and should be maintained until spinal injuries can be ruled-out. The priorities for this patient are to limit the extent of his brain injury by limiting secondary brain injury, which is best accomplished with the **avoidance of hypoxia, hypercarbia, and hypotension.** Alarming findings in this patient are findings that suggest that there is already significant right-hemispheric intracranial hypertension causing unequal papillary responses and left-side hemiparesis. The **Monroe-Kellie doctrine** is the governing principle for severe TBI management, and this equation states that the volume of brain, intravascular blood, and CSF fluid all influence the intracranial pressure (ICP). Under normal circumstances, the ICP is 5 to 10 mm Hg; however, in the setting of TBI, the cranial vault must accommodate brain, intravascular blood, CSF, blood clot, and cerebral edema. Unfortunately, the only way this additional volume can be accommodated is through the elimination of venous blood and CSF from the intracranial space, and these mechanisms can only accommodate a limited increase in volume prior to herniation.

Once this patient is intubated and ventilated, and has appropriate intravenous access placed, intravenous mannitol should be given at a dose of 0.5 to 1.0 g/kg, which can help provide temporary reduction in cerebral edema and hopefully reduce the ICP. The patient must be sufficiently resuscitated before the administration of mannitol, since this medication can produce hypotension in hypovolemic patients. Optimal ventilation for this patient is controlled hyperventilation with target $PaCO_2$ of 35 to 40 mm Hg. An important point that cannot be overemphasized is clear communication with the neurosurgeon should be made prior implementation of these secondary measures for ICP reduction.

APPROACH TO:
Traumatic Brain Injury

DEFINITIONS

EPIDURAL HEMATOMA: The collection of blood outside of the dura but beneath the skull, most frequently in the temporal region (due to middle meningeal artery laceration). These hematomas are uncommon, occurring in 0.5% of all head trauma cases and 9% of severe TBI. Epidural hematoma patients generally have a better prognosis than other types of cerebral hematomas. The classic appearance is a biconvex or lens-shape opacification on noncontrast CT.

SUBDURAL HEMATOMA: The collection of blood between the brain surface and the dura, commonly produced by tearing of the bridging veins. These lesions are far more common than epidural hematomas and carry a worse prognosis than epidural hematomas because the associated primary brain injury is generally more severe.

CONCUSSION: This describes TBI often associated with transient loss of consciousness, but without CT abnormalities. These types of injuries can cause long-term cognitive and functional deficits.

MILD TBI: GCS of 13 to 15.

MODERATE TBI: GCS of 9 to 12.

SEVERE TBI: GCS <9.

COMA: A vague term that generally describes a patient with GCS <9.

BURR HOLE: A hole drilled through the skull for decompression, usually done on the side of the enlarged pupil. This procedure can be life-saving; however, there is significant risk of causing harm without patient benefits when untrained individuals attempt this procedure.

CLINICAL APPROACH

For TBI patients, **the initial approach is the same as in most trauma patients, where the priorities are assessment and optimization of the airway, breathing, and circulation (ABCs).** The goals in the management of TBI patients is to identify and address immediate life-threatening injuries first before providing definitive treatment of TBI (eg, sources of hemorrhage). In patients with injury mechanisms associated with the potential for multisystem injury, the current approach taken by many experts is the use of the "pan-CT-Scan" for rapid initial survey of injuries. The "pan-scan" entails a CT of the brain, C-spine, chest, abdomen, and pelvis, and its application has been demonstrated to help identify subtle injuries that might otherwise be missed.

TBI patient outcomes are heavily dependent on the age and GCS of the patients. (younger adults generally do better than older adults, and patients with higher GCS do better than those with lower GCS). A comatose patient (those with GCS < 9) with abnormal pupillary responses often signifies an ipsilateral mass lesion. With the mass effect and pressure exertion on the temporal lobe, uncal herniation can occur. Uncal herniation compresses the parasympathetic nerve fibers that travel along the third cranial nerve; this leads to unopposed sympathetic activity to the pupil, which produces ipsilateral pupil dilation and the classic finding of a "blown" pupil. The initial GCS is one of the most important factors driving the management of TBI patients. The initial GCS is important but GCS trend is of importance as deterioration of the GCS of two or more points is often an indication of worsening TBI. (See Table 38–2 for TBI severity and management).

Management of Patients on Anticoagulants and/or Antiplatelet Agents

With the general increasing age of our population, there are more numbers of individuals receiving long-term anticoagulants and/or antiplatelet agents as primary, secondary, or tertiary prevention strategies for cardiovascular and cerebral vascular diseases. A recent prospective observational study has demonstrated that the

Table 38–2 • TBI SEVERITY AND MANAGEMENT

TBI Severity	Treatment Recommendations	Expected Outcomes
Mild (GCS 13-15) ~80% of patients fall into this group	-Inpatient observations with CT if the patient's GCS remains <15 or with high-risk features*; consider repeat CT within 4-6 hours for patients with high-risk features – Consider CT and possible discharge if the patient's examination has returned to normal and patients do not have high-risk features	Most patients have uneventful recovery.~3% of patients may have unexpected deterioration
Moderate (GCS 9-12) ~10% of patients fall into this group	Initial CT should be done in all patients with follow-up CT if the condition worsens; all patients should be observed as in-patients	90% of the patients will improve and can be discharged with outpatient follow-up.~10% of these patients will develop clinical deterioration and may need neurosurgical interventions
Severe (GCS 3-8) ~10% of patients fall into this group	Address the ABCDEs with early intubation. Optimize oxygenation, ventilation, and blood pressure support. Early CT, neurosurgical consultation, and consider pharmacologic therapy if indicated (eg, mannitol and anticonvulsants)	All patients will need ICU monitoring and many will need neurosurgical invasive monitoring or interventions. Most of the patients will need some neurologic rehabilitation

*High-risk features: loss of consciousness >5 minutes, retrograde amnesia >30 minutes, severe headaches, focal neurologic deficits, age >65, alcohol intoxication/illicit drug influence, and patients on **anticoagulants** and/or **antiplatelet agents**.

relative risk of traumatic intracranial hemorrhage development is increased among individuals receiving **clopidogrel (Plavix)** or **aspirin** prior to their injuries, with relative risks ratios of 2.5 and 1.5 reported, respectively. In addition, observational studies suggest that patients who are receiving prehospital aspirin, warfarin, and/or clopidogrel have a higher likelihood of experiencing worsening of CT findings during repeat scans. In summary, patients receiving prehospital anticoagulants and/or antiplatelet therapy are high-risk patients for the development of immediate and/or delayed intracranial hemorrhage and deserve immediate CT evaluation, close observation, and repeat CT scans.

Neurobehavioral Sequelae of Traumatic Brain Injury

Many patients experience neurobehavioral sequelae (NBS) following TBI. It is estimated that 30% to 80% of patients with mild to moderate TBI experience NBS for up to 3 months following the initial injuries. NBS in TBI patients can manifest as cognitive dysfunction, depression, dizziness, lack of concentration, fatigue, memory difficulties, irritability, and insomnia. Persistence of NBS beyond 3 months postinjury is reported in up to 15% of the patients with mild TBI; therefore, to optimize patient outcomes following TBI, it is important to provide the patients and their families with short-term and long-term rehabilitation and counseling support to help the victims and their families cope with potential social and occupational difficulties.

Concussions and Sports-Related Brain Injuries

An estimated 3.8 million concussions occur in the United States each year during competitive sports and recreational activities, and nearly 50% of these concussions go unreported. **Females have been reported to sustain higher rates of concussions when performing similar athletic activities as male athletes.** Overall, concussions in male athletes are more likely to go unreported in comparison to injuries in female athletes. Atheletic acitivies with the highest reported incidences of concussions are football, hockey, soccer, rugby, and basketball. With greater number and severity of concussions and increases in the duration of symptoms following a concussion, the greater the likelihood that the recoveries will be prolonged. An athlete with a history of concussion is also at an increased risk of sustaining another concussion (~2-6-fold increased probability).

The important steps and goals of concussion management are: (1) initial evaluation and diagnosis; (2) postinjury evaluation; (3) symptoms management; (4) safe return to activities participation. The identification of concussions is critical to protect the individual from premature return to potentially injurious activities. **There is evidence to suggest that excessive cognitive or physical activity before complete brain recovery contributes to prolonged brain dysfunction.** Of the many signs and symptoms of a concussion, headache and dizziness are the most and second most common reported symptoms, respectively (see Table 38–3 for the list of signs and symptoms). **In most studies, 80% to 90% of athletes with concussions have symptom resolution by 7 days after the injury; however, it is important to note that based on neuropsychiatric testing, persistent deficits may linger even after symptom resolution.** Because the presence and severity of neuropsychiatric deficits can be difficult to determine, some authorities have recommended liberal testing policies to help identify individuals who may benefit from counseling and treatment.

There are a number of validated assessment systems utilized in the initial assessment of injured athletes, and it has been demonstrated that the sensitivity and specificity of the assessments improves when several are applied in combination. Once the individual is diagnosed with a concussion, the general rule of

Table 38–3 • CONCUSSION SIGNS AND SYMPTOMS
Physical Signs and Symptoms
Headache, nausea, vomiting, dizziness, fatigue, light sensitivity, noise sensitivity, balance difficulties, feeling dazed or stunned, visual disturbances, numbness/tingling
Cognitive Dysfunctions
Feeling mentally "foggy," feeling slow, difficulty with concentration, memory lapses, confusion regarding events, slow to answer questions, repeating questions
Emotional Disturbances
Irritable, sad, overly emotional, nervous
Sleep Disturbances
Drowsiness, sleeps more than usual, sleeps less than usual, insomnia

management is to closely monitor the individual's level of function and behavior during the acute setting (0-12 hours). During this initial observation period, it is important to try to avoid sedatives and medications that may mask patient's symptoms or alter the individual's level of mentation. The patients and their families should be instructed regarding potential sleep, cognitive, and mood disturbances. After initial stabilization of symptoms, the recommendation for most individuals with concussions is to take a graduated return to work, school, or play schedule, with monitoring of progress during each of the steps. For contact-sport athletes, the schedule for their returning to sports activities will progress in a step-wise manner, with initially no activity, followed by progression to light aerobic activities, to sport-specific activity, to non-contact drills, to limited full contact participation, and ultimately to full participation.

Emerging Concepts

At the time of this writing, TBI-specific biomarkers, systemic and head cooling, and nanotechnology were areas being investigated for the treatment of TBI. There is insufficient evidence to support their practical use in an ongoing basis, but there is hope for future use.

CASE CORRELATION

- See also Cases 6 (Blunt Chest Trauma), Case 7 (Multiple Blunt Trauma), and Case 8 (Hemorrhagic Shock [Trauma]).

COMPREHENSION QUESTIONS

38.1 Which of the following is the most accurate statement regarding concussions?

A. Immediate loss of consciousness is necessary for the diagnosis

B. Concussions are not associated with long-term neuropsychiatric disorders

C. Concussions do not contribute to cognitive deficits

D. The reporting rates of concussions are lower for male athletes

E. Early return to activities helps athletes with concussions regain function earlier

38.2 A 46-year-old intoxicated man was driving down the highway in the wrong direction when his vehicle struck a pickup truck head-on. He presented with a pulse rate of 130 beats/minute, blood pressure of 90/62 mm Hg, and respiratory rate of 32 breaths/minute. His pupils are 5 mm and are equally round and reactive to light bilaterally; he does not open his eyes to painful stimuli, moans with painful stimuli, and withdraws from painful stimuli. His oxygen saturation with oxygen by face mask is 86%. In addition to the possibility of traumatic brain injury, what are other important factors that can be contributing to this man's low GCS that we need to identify and address immediately?

A. Hypoxia

B. Polysubstance abuse

C. History of seizure disorder

D. Alcohol intoxication

E. Chronic syphilis infection

38.3 The man described in Question 38.2 underwent endotracheal intubation a short time after arrival to the emergency department. Shortly thereafter, he underwent placement of bilateral chest tubes for pneumothoraces. He also received a bolus of 1000 mL of lactated Ringers solution that improved his blood pressure to 120/80 and reduced his heart rate to 100 beats/minute. With painful stimuli, the patient does not open his eyes and withdraws all extremities. A CT scan of the brain demonstrates bilateral frontal contusions, subarachnoid hemorrhage, and diffuse brain edema bilaterally. Which of the following is the most appropriate next step?

A. Craniectomy for the evacuation of subarachnoid blood

B. Mechanical ventilation, intravenous fluids, and placement of ICP monitor

C. Placement of bilateral burr holes in the ED

D. Administer intravenous corticosteroids and mannitol at 1-g/kg dose

E. Administer mannitol (1 g/kg)

38.4 An 18-year-old man who was skiing without a helmet ran into a tree while going down a hill. He presents with a normal blood pressure, does not open his eyes to painful stimuli, has abnormal flexion of the upper extremities with pain, and moans with painful stimuli. Which of the following is the most appropriate next step?

A. CT scan of the brain

B. 2000 mL of Lactated Ringers bolus

C. Intravenous mannitol

D. Contact the neurosurgeon

E. Endotracheal intubation

38.5 An unhelmeted bicyclist struck a parked car while trying to avoid another oncoming car. He is brought to the emergency center where he is noted to be screaming random words and phrases, localizing to pain, and opening his eyes to his name. Following your initial evaluation, you contact the neurosurgeon for advice and consultation. How would you classify the severity of his TBI?

A. Mild

B. Moderate

C. Severe

D. Unable to evaluate

E. Uncooperative

38.6 Which of the following is a false statement regarding concussions?

A. The degree of disability is related to the number of concussions that the individual has suffered

B. The type of sport and player style strongly influence the risk of concussions

C. 3.8 million concussions occur each year during competitive sports and recreational activities in the United States

D. Roughly half of concussions are unreported

E. Balance disturbance is not a specific indicator of concussion

ANSWERS

38.1 **D.** Male athletes are less likely to report concussions than female athletes. Male athletes are more likely to sustain concussions than female athletes, and this is related to the types of sports that male athletes compete in, and the general difference between player styles of male and female athletes. Overall, the rates of concussions are higher for female athletes competing in the same types of sports activities.

38.2 **A.** This is a patient presenting after polytrauma. His initial GCS is 7 (E1, V2, M4). His oxygen saturation is 86%. His low GCS can be contributed by several factors that are listed, including alcohol intoxication, polysubstance abuse, and hypoxia. Of these contributing factors, the hypoxia is a problem that we need to address immediately, because TBI outcomes are adversely affected by hypoxia. Improving this patient's oxygenation and ventilation are the immediate priorities for this patient.

38.3 **B.** Following intubation and initial interventions, this patient's GCS is now 6T (E1, V1T, M4). His hypoxia and hypotension have improved with the initial interventions. At this time, he is found to have bifrontal cerebral contusions, cerebral swelling, and subarachnoid hemorrhage. Although the brain CT findings are causes for alarm, these findings are not amendable to operative treatments. Midline shifts and focal mass lesions are generally considered injuries that are more amenable to operative interventions. The primary goals for this patient are to optimize his oxygenation, ventilation, and blood pressures with ventilation and intravenous fluids. Intracranial pressure monitoring is also helpful to guide the management of ventilation and direct pharmacologic therapy if needed (eg, mannitol administration). Steroids are not indicated for TBI. It is generally not advisable to administer mannitol prior to CT or physical examination findings indicating mass effects in the brain.

38.4 **E.** This patient presents with a normal blood pressure and an initial GCS of 6 (E1, V2, M3). Based on these findings, he has severe brain injury until proven otherwise. Immediate intubation to optimize oxygenation and ventilation is important.

38.5 **A.** This patient is noted to be screaming random words and phrases (V3), opens eyes to name (E3), and localizes to pain (M5) which gives him a GCS of 11 and places him in the mild TBI category.

38.6 **E.** Balance disturbance is a specific indicator of concussion, although it is not a highly sensitive indicator. Balance testing of athletes on the sidelines can be helpful in identifying individuals with concussions. All of the other statements are true regarding concussions.

CLINICAL PEARLS

► An athlete with history of concussion is at 2-6-fold increased risk of suffering another concussion.

► Balance disturbance is a specific indicator of concussion but not a sensitive indicator (eg, not all concussed individuals have balance problems, but concussion is highly likely if the person has balance difficulties.

► Prevention of secondary brain injury begins with optimizing the patient's oxygenation, ventilation, and brain perfusion by correcting/avoiding hypoxia, hypercapnia, and hypotension.

► The initial GCS determined at the emergency department and the patient's age are the most important indicators of outcome in TBI patients.

► Pupillary reflex and the GCS are the cornerstones of initial neurologic evaluations for TBI patients.

► A dilated pupil usually indicates an ipsilateral mass lesion.

► Neurobehavioral sequelae (NBS) may occur even following mild brain injuries; therefore, it is important to provide follow-up, assessments, and rehabilitation for these patients.

REFERENCES

Harmon KG, Drezner JA, Gammons M, et al. American Medical Society for Sports Medicine position statement: concussion in sport. *Br J Sport Med*. 2013;47:15-26.

Levin HS, Diaz-Arrastia RR. Diagnosis, prognosis, and clinical management of mild traumatic brain injury. *Lancet Neurol*. 2015;14:506-517.

Nishijima DK, Offerman SR, Ballard DW, et al. Risk of traumatic intracranial hemorrhage in patients with head injury and preinjury warfarin or clopidogrel use. *Acad Emerg Med*. 2013;20:140-145.

A 55-year-old man complains of a 4-month history of low back pain that is worsened by walking and sitting, and improved by standing and lying down. He denies back trauma, heavy lifting, or problems voiding or with bowel movements. He states that at times, the pain radiates to the back of his right leg. On physical examination, his blood pressure is 130/78 mm Hg, pulse rate is 80 beats/minute, and he is afebrile. He is slightly overweight. The findings from his heart and lung examinations are normal. The back is without scoliosis. Raising either leg produces the pain, which radiates to the right leg. The results of his neurologic examinations are normal.

► What is the most likely diagnosis?
► What is the best test to confirm the diagnosis?

ANSWERS TO CASE 39:

Low Back Pain: Lumbar Prolapsed Nucleus Pulposus

Summary: A 55-year-old man presents with a 4-month history of chronic low back pain that radiates to his right leg, which is worsened by walking and sitting. It is relieved by standing and lying down. He denies trauma to the back, heavy lifting, or urologic abnormalities. He is slightly overweight. The back is without scoliosis. Raising either leg reproduces the pain, which radiates to the right leg. The neurologic examination is normal.

- **Most likely diagnosis:** Lumbar prolapsed nucleus pulposus.

- **Best diagnostic test:** Magnetic resonance imaging (MRI) or myelography.

ANALYSIS

Objectives

1. Know the differential diagnosis of low back pain.

2. Know the typical clinical presentation of lumbar disc prolapse.

3. Understand that MRI and myelography are the imaging tests that confirm the diagnosis.

Considerations

This 55-year-old man presents with a 4-month history of low back pain with radiation of pain to the posterior aspect of his right leg. The pain is worse when walking and during straight leg raising. His history and findings are typical for chronic back pain (defined as greater than 3 months duration) possibly related to herniated lumbar pulposus, possibly causing compression of the nerve root that are typically at the levels of L4-5 (L4: medial aspect of calf and ankle; L5: lateral ankle and foot). Pain radiation to the lateral or posterior aspect of the leg is a common complaint, as are paresthesias in the affected dermatome distributions. In some patients, motor weaknesses associated with the affected nerve roots can also be detected (L4: anterior tibialis; L5: extensor hallicus longus). MRI is an excellent noninvasive method for patient evaluation, and this imaging modality has largely replaced myelography as the diagnostic test of choice. Importantly, if the patient had significant motor deficits or bladder/bowel dysfunction, a more urgent evaluation and treatment would be paramount to preserve nerve function.

APPROACH TO:

Low Back Pain

DEFINITIONS

ACUTE LOW BACK PAIN: Pain less than 4 weeks.

SUBACUTE LOW BACK PAIN: Pain present between 4 weeks to 3 months.

CHRONIC LOW BACK PAIN: Pain present for more than 3 months.

MECHANICAL LOW BACK PAIN: This refers to the common low back pain experienced by many adults. Roughly two-thirds of adults will experience at least one episode during his/her lifetime. This is the second most common complaint encountered in ambulatory medicine. Most patients with mechanical low back pain will have spontaneous symptoms resolution within 2 to 4 weeks.

LUMBAR DISC HERNIATION: Disc herniation at L_5-S_1 level with S_1 nerve root compression is most common (40%-50%), L_4-L_5 level herniation with L_5 nerve root compression occurs in 40% of the cases, and L_3-L_4 disc herniation with L_4 nerve root compression occurs in 3% to 10% of the herniated discs.

ENTRAPMENT NEUROPATHIES: This involves compression of nerve roots or nerves, such as sciatica produced by a prolapsed disc compressing the nerve root contributing to the lumbosacral plexus.

CAUDA EQUINA SYNDROME: Compression of the sacral nerve bundle, which forms the end of the spinal cord. Common symptoms associated with this syndrome include bladder and bowel dysfunctions, pain and/or weakness in the legs. Identification of the process early during the course of disease is important in avoiding nerve entrapment that ends up producing long-term dysfunctions.

CLINICAL APPROACH

Low back pain is an extremely common compliant and more than 80% of adults will complain of low back pain at least once in their lifetime. It is one of the most common reasons leading to activity limitation and work absence. Lower educational status is associated with increased prevalence of low back pain and associated with worse outcomes associated with the problem. Occupational activities are contributors of low back pain, with higher prevalence reported in manual workers. For majority of individuals, low back pain is self-limiting within a 2 to 4 weeks period; however, one in three individuals reports persistent pain up to 1 year after initial presentation, and one in five reports long-term substantial limitation in activities.

History

The focused history during the work-up should include duration of symptoms, description of symptoms along with exacerbating and alleviating factors, presence of absence of neurologic functions, bowel and bladder functions, and infection-related symptoms such as fevers or night sweats (see Table 39-1). Important information in the past medical history includes history of osteoporosis, prior history of back pain, previous spine surgeries, cancers, and active infections. A number of symptoms and historical items have been identified as indicators of potentially serious conditions (**red-flag symptoms or factors**) which include **age >50, presence of systemic symptoms such as fever, night sweats, weight loss, history of malignancy, night pain, immune suppressed status, history of intravenous drug use, failure to respond to initial treatments, prolonged corticosteroid use, diagnosis of osteoporosis,** and **trauma.**

Table 39–1 • SPINE-RELATED CAUSES OF BACK PAIN	
Cause	Clinical Features
Muscle strain	Associated with ache or muscle spasms in the back and may radiate to the buttock or posterior thigh worsened with activity or bending
Herniated disc	Pain starts in the back with radiation to corresponding dermatomes in the lower extremity; worse with sitting and relieved with standing; may be associated with motor and/or sensory deficits
Lumbar spondylosis	Generalized back pain that is worse immediately after waking up; improves throughout the day; pain fluctuates with activity and is worse with extension of the spine
Spinal stenosis/neurogenic claudication	Back pain with radiculopathy worsened by extension /standing; improvement with flexion, sitting
Spondylolisthesis	Back pain with radiation down one or both legs, exacerbated by flexion/extension
Spondylolysis, stress fractures	Common in children and adolescents
Ankylosing spondylitis	More common in young males; morning stiffness, low back pain radiating to buttock that improves with exercise
Infection with epidural abscess	Severe pain with insidious onset that is unrelenting. Night pain, often with motor and sensory deficits
Malignancy	History of cancer, new onset back pain; often age >50; frequently with radiculopathy and/or motor/sensory deficits
Cauda equina syndrome	Urinary retention or fecal incontinence; decreased rectal tone; saddle anesthesia
Conus medullaris syndrome	Same as cauda equina but also with upper motor neuron signs (eg, hyperreflexia, clonus)
Vertebral compression fracture	History of osteoporosis or corticosteroids use; older patients
Trauma	Variable findings depending on the injury site and extent

Physical Examination

Complete neurologic examination is important in the lower and upper extremities to try to identify upper motor neuron disorders and spinal cord related symptoms. Examination of deep tendon reflexes and sensory examination correlating to various dermatomes, and motor examination related to the various nerve root levels are important to identify the affecting anatomic site (See Table 39-2).

Laboratory Testing

General laboratory testing is not indicated but there are specific laboratory tests that can be helpful to identify certain abnormalities. For example, complete blood count and differentials, C-reactive protein and erythrocyte sedimentation rates may help identify inflammatory or infectious conditions, HLA-B27 testing is specific for ankylosing spondylitis, and serum 1,25-dihydroxyvitamine D_3 level may help verify osteoporosis.

Table 39–2 · LOWER EXTRMITY NERVE ROOTS AND CORRESPONDING NEUROLOGIC EXAMINATIONS			
Nerve Root	Muscle Group (motor strength)	Sensory Dermatome	Deep Tendon Reflex
L_2	Hip flexor	Anterior medial thigh	none
L_3	Quadriceps	Anterior thigh to knee	Knee jerk
L_4	Anterior tibialis	Medial calf and ankle	Knee jerk
L_5	Extensor hallicus longus	Lateral ankle to dorsum of foot	None
S_1	Gatrocnemius/soleus/paroneals	Plantar and lateral foot	Ankle jerk

Imaging

Most clinical studies suggest that the majority of patients with acute back pain do not require imaging, because the majority will get better on their own in 2 to 4 weeks' time; imaging studies such as MRI usually will reveal any findings that would lead different treatments. Imaging studies should be considered in patients with "red flag" symptoms or factors and in patients whose symptoms persist for greater than 4 to 6 weeks of conservative management. The role of imaging in these patients is to rule out fracture, tumor, or infections. The initial radiographic study can be plain radiography of the lumbar region. MRI is indicated in the presence of neurologic complaints or when there is concern for tumor, fracture, or infectious involvements.

Treatment

The majority of patients with low back pain without worrisome neurologic symptoms will improve within a few weeks. Common recommended interventions are activity modification, rest, nonsteroidal anti-inflammatory drugs (NSAIDs), and physical therapy. For some patients, the combination of oral analgesics, antidepressants, and opioids seem to produce better responses. **It is important to closely monitor long-term opioids use for some of the patients to avoid habituation.** Prescription opioid use has become an epidemic in the US, and is one of the leading causes of death in middle aged individuals.

A small percentage of patients with low back pain may have persistence of pain for greater than 6 months, and for these patients, imaging studies such as MRI, and referral for evaluation by a back specialist may be indicated. Patient education is important to help define expectations and a long range goal. For these patients, the realistic goals might be improvement in function and reduction in pain rather than cure. For certain patients with persistent pain, anatomic lesions are identified that may respond to surgical care. The indications for surgical treatment include identifiable anatomic nerve compression, neurologic deficits, and/or intractable pain. Surgical treatment for herniated discs involves laminectomy and removal of the protruding disc(s). If several levels of disc spaces are involved, posterior spinal fusion in addition to the disc extraction is indicated.

COMPREHENSION QUESTIONS

39.1 A 36-year-old man presents with back pain and some lower extremity symptoms that are believed to be related to disc herniation with L_5 and S_1 nerve root impingement on the right. Which of the following physical examination findings most likely correlates with this pathology?

A. Numbness in the anterior thigh down to his right knee

B. Decreased patellar tendon reflex and numbness of the dorsum of right foot and plantar region

C. Decreased strength in the right hip flexors

D. Decreased strength on right foot plantar flexion and right foot numbness

E. Decreased strength on right knee flexion

39.2 Impingement of which of the following nerve roots can cause decreased strength in big toe dorsi-flexion?

A. L5

B. L3

C. L2

D. S1

E. L4

39.3 Which of the following descriptions best fits a patient with cauda equina syndrome?

A. Normal lower extremity motor weakness affecting ankle flexion and extension

B. Urinary retention and fecal incontinence, normal motor and sensory functions in lower extremities

C. Urinary retention, fecal incontinence, hyperreflexia, clonus of the lower extremities

D. Back pain that radiates to the buttock with activity or upon bending forward

E. Severe back pain, with lower extremities motor and sensory deficits, fever, and night sweats

39.4 A 56-year-old mailman is diagnosed with probable lumbar prolapsed nucleus pulposus. Which of the following is most consistent with this diagnosis?

A. Pain in the lower back radiating down the anterior thigh

B. Decreased patellar deep tendon reflex

C. Pain worsens with Valsalva

D. Decreased sensation in the medial thigh and weakness of the adductor muscles of the lower leg

E. Bilateral lower extremity paralysis

39.5 A 47-year-old woman complains of lower back pain with radiation to the right leg, and she is treated with ibuprofen and bed rest. Over the next 3 weeks, the pain worsens, and she complains of difficulty with voiding and some fecal incontinence. Which of the following is the most likely diagnosis?

A. Spinal stenosis

B. Lumbar neoplasm

C. Cauda equina syndrome

D. Tuberculosis of the spine (Pott's disease)

E. Compression fracture

39.6 A 61-year-old man has low back pain of 3 weeks, duration that has not diminished with rest. He is diagnosed with a "herniated disk." Which of the following describes the most common location of disk herniation in the lumbar region?

A. L_1-L_2

B. L_2-L_3

C. L_3-L_4

D. L_4-L_5

E. L_5-S_1

ANSWERS

39.1 **D.** Decreased plantar flexion strength of the foot and foot numbness are consistent with neuropathy corresponding to the S_1 nerve root.

39.2 **A.** Dorsiflexion of the big toe is controlled by extensor hallicus longus contraction, and this reflects motor activity related to the L_5 nerve root.

39.3 **B.** Urinary retention, fecal incontinence, decreased rectal tone, and saddle anesthesia are findings consistent with the cauda equina syndrome. Bowel and bladder dysfunction in addition to hyper-reflexia and clonus are consistent with conus medullaris syndrome (due to compression at L_1, L_2 levels).

39.4 **C.** Pain associated with herniated lumbar disk is exacerbated with Valsalva, straight leg raise, and sitting. The pain typically radiates down the back to the posterior or lateral legs, and the anterior legs are usually uninvolved.

39.5 **C.** The bowel and bladder complaints are typical of cauda equina syndrome. Cauda equina involvement usually constitutes a surgical emergency as permanent nerve damage can occur if the condition is not promptly treated.

39.6 **D.** The L_4-L_5 levels are the most common location for herniated disks, and the second most common level is at the L_5-S_1 level.

CLINICAL PEARLS

▶ The most common locations of herniated lumbar disc disease are at L4-L5, followed by L5-S1.

▶ Bowel and bladder complaints with lower back pain are suggestive of cauda equine syndrome, which must be diagnosed early to avoid permanent nerve damage.

▶ The initial treatment for herniated lumbar pulposus is bed rest and the administration of nonsteroidal anti-inflammatory drugs.

▶ "Red flag" features associated with low back pain include age >50, presence of systemic symptoms such as fever, night sweats, weight loss, history of malignancy, night pain, immune suppressed status, history of intravenous drug use, failure to respond to initial treatments, prolonged corticosteroid use, diagnosis of osteoporosis, and trauma. Diagnosis and management should be approached with some urgency in patients with "red flag" features.

▶ The majority of patients with low back pain get better on their own without specific treatment other than modification of activities, rest, and non-narcotic analgesics.

REFERENCES

Golob AL, Wipf JE. Low back pain. *Med Clin N Am*. 2014;98:405-428.

Patrick N, Emanski E, Knaub MA. Acute and chronic low back pain. *Med Clin N Am*. 2014;98:777-789.

A 44-year-old woman complains of a 6-week history of progressive numbness and pain in her right hand that occasionally wakes her up at night. She states that her thumb and index finger are especially affected. The patient is employed as a computer programmer, and indicates that she recently began to drop objects that she is holding in her right hand, due to decreased hand strength. She denies any history of trauma, exposure to heavy metals, or a family history of multiple sclerosis. She is otherwise healthy and takes no medications.

▶ What is the most likely diagnosis?
▶ What are the cause and risk factors associated with this disorder?
▶ What is your next step?

ANSWERS TO CASE 40:

Carpal Tunnel Syndrome

Summary: A 44-year-old otherwise healthy woman complains of a 6-week history of progressive numbness and pain in her right hand occurring especially at nighttime and affecting her thumb and index finger. She states that she is beginning to drop objects as the result of decreased grip strength in her right hand.

- **Most likely diagnosis:** Carpal tunnel syndrome (CTS)

- **Causes and risk factors:** Median nerve compression is the cause, and reported risk factors include trauma, overuse, inflammatory conditions, diabetes, and hypothyroidism

- **Next step in therapy:** Modification of activities, nighttime splint application, and nonsteroidal anti-inflammatory drugs (NSAIDs)

ANALYSIS

Objectives

1. Learn the clinical presentation, pathophysiology, contributing factors, and diagnostic evaluations for CTS.

2. Learn the medical and surgical options for treating CTS, and learn the indications for surgical therapy.

Considerations

This 44-year-old otherwise healthy woman presents with pain, progressive hand weakness, and numbness involving the median nerve distributions of her right hand. She indicates that her symptoms are worse at night, and that she has recently noticed a decrease in her right hand grip strength that is causing her to drop objects. These symptoms are fairly typical for carpal tunnel syndrome (CTS). **We can make the diagnosis of CTS on the basis of history and physical examination alone because her history and physical examination findings are very straightforward. Electrophysiologic testing is unnecessary in her case.** The physical examination in this patient begins with visual inspection and palpation of the hand, because in severe cases of median nerve entrapment, thenar muscle atrophy can be present. In addition, the hand and wrist area need to be closely inspected for masses such as cysts or ganglia that can also cause nerve compression symptoms. A thorough motor and sensory examination will need to include evaluations of the median, radial, and ulnar nerve motor and sensory functions, with focused evaluation of median nerve functions. There are several findings associated with median nerve entrapment that we should try to verify; which include thumb abduction strength (abducter pollicis brevis muscle strength), **Tinel's sign, modified Phalen's test,** and **Durkan's compression test.** These specific tests are considered to be helpful for the diagnosis when two or more of the signs are present, because the tests applied individually are less sensitive and specific. Although rheumatoid arthritis, diabetes, and hypothyroidism can contribute to CTS, it is generally not advisable or cost-effective to perform diagnostic studies to look for these causes in a patient who has no clinical evidence of these conditions. Her initial management will consist of splinting the affected wrist in a neutral position (0-degree extension). A small, randomized study of 176 patients with CTS assigned patients to initial splinting versus surgery, and splinting improved symptoms in 37% of the patients to an extent that surgeries were avoided. If splinting does not improve the symptoms, corticosteroid injection is an alternative. Unfortunately, the results assessing corticosteroid injection are not very favorable. One trial suggested that symptom improvement was achieved at 10 weeks following injections, but 75% of the patients went on to surgical treatments due to symptom relapse. Operative treatment, which at this time is not indicated in this patient, consists of carpal tunnel release that is effective but can contribute to complications and scarring.

APPROACH TO:
Carpal Tunnel Syndrome

DEFINITIONS

CARPAL TUNNEL SYNDROME: Median nerve compression at the wrist leading to paresthesias of the lateral three digits, pain, and sometimes hand weakness.

TINEL SIGN: The patient is asked to place his/her wrist on a table with the palm up as the examiner gently taps along the median nerve at the wrist. A positive or abnormal response is when this maneuver reproduces the patient's symptoms.

PHALEN'S TEST: The patient is asked to have both hands in front, palms pointing down ward. He/she is then asked to actively and maximally flex his/her wrists. A positive or abnormal test is when this maneuver causes tingling, pain, or altered sensation in the thumb, index finger, middle finger, and radial half of the ring finger.

DURKAN'S COMPRESSION TEST: The patient is asked to place his/her hand flat on a table with the palm up. The examiner places three fingers directly over the carpal tunnel and compresses the area for 30 seconds. A positive or abnormal test is when the patient reports tingling, numbness, or altered sensation in the thumb, index finger, middle finger, or radial half of the ring finger.

ELECTROPHYSIOLOGIC TESTING: This consists of tests such as nerve conduction studies to investigate sensory nerve conduction and motor innervation.

CLINICAL APPROACH

The carpal tunnel serves as a mechanical conduit for the digital flexor tendons. The walls and floor on the dorsal surface of the canal are formed by the carpal bones, and the ventral aspect of the tunnel is confined by the strong, inelastic,

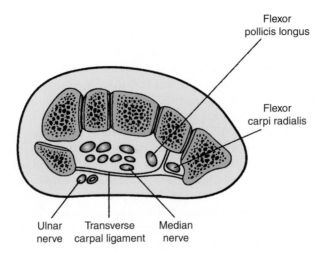

Figure 40–1. The carpal tunnel. The wrist in cross section reveals that the median nerve is susceptible to impingement.

transverse carpal ligament. Significant canal narrowing occurs during extreme flexion and extension of the wrist (Figure 40–1). Exacerbation of symptoms at night is thought to be caused by edema, and in some cases by tenosynovitis. CTS is associated with endocrine disorders such as diabetes and hypothyroidism. Other conditions that are associated with CTS include myxedema, acromegaly, pregnancy, and some autoimmune conditions. Differential diagnoses for CTS include cervical radiculopathy, diabetic neuropathy, osteoarthritis, inflammatory arthritis, other peripheral neuropathies, and Raynaud's phenomenon. Confirmatory physical examination findings include Tinel sign, Durkan's compression test, and Phalen's test.

Conservative management is the initial approach for most patients, including include activity modification, wrist splints, NSAIDS, and corticosteroids injections. If significant improvements are not seen after 4 months of conservative treatments, surgical therapy should be considered. A number of randomized controlled trials comparing nonsurgical treatments to surgical decompression suggest that patients who underwent surgical decompression therapies were two and a half times more likely to have normal nerve conduction studies but also experienced high rates of complications related to surgery. Based on these investigations, it is currently recommended that nonoperative treatments be attempted first, and surgical decompression reserved for individuals who fail an initial course of nonoperative therapy (see Figure 40–2).

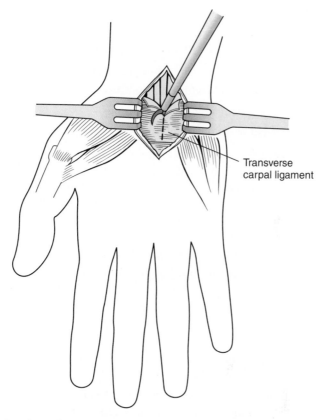

Transverse
carpal ligament

Figure 40–2. Carpal tunnel release. The transverse carpal ligament is incised (palmar view of the wrist).

COMPREHENSION QUESTIONS

40.1 A 24-year-old medical student reports that she has noted numbness and tingling involving the fifth finger. Which of the following nerve is most likely the
site of irritation?

A. Median nerve

B. Radial nerve

C. Ulnar nerve

D. Lateral cutaneous nerve

E. Long thoracic nerve

40.2 Which of the following patients has the greatest likelihood of developing carpal tunnel syndrome?

A. A 45-year-old woman with diabetes insipidus

B. A 45-year-old woman with hypothyroidism

C. A 45-year-old woman with Addison's disease

D. A 45-year-old woman with hypertension

E. A 45-year-old woman with fibromyalgia

40.3 A 30-year-old man complains of numbness and tingling of his thumb and index finger. He also has pain at night on the same hand. The Tinel sign is positive. He is diagnosed with CTS and fitted with nighttime wrist splint. After 4 months, his symptoms appear to have worsened. An electrophysiologic study is done, and the results of the study are equivocal. Which of the following is the best next step for this patient?

A. Refer the patient to a psychiatrist for biofeedback training

B. Inquire regarding drug-seeking type behavior

C. Refer the patient for cervical spine evaluation

D. MRI of the wrist

E. X-ray of the wrist

40.4 Which of the following is a true statement regarding physical examination findings of the wrist for CTS?

A. An abnormal finding when eliciting the Tinel's sign is specific for CTS

B. The Phalen's test is the least sensitive of the tests for CTS

C. Durkan's has the greatest sensitivity for CTS diagnosis

D. Generally, an abnormal finding during the Phalen's test, Tinel sign, or Durkan's compression test is sufficient for CTS diagnosis

E. The combination of the Phalens' test, Tinel sign, and Durkan's compression test improve the sensitivity and specificity of CTS diagnosis

40.5 A 44-year-old woman presents with numbness involving both thumbs and index fingers that occur mostly at night. During the physical examination, her thumb adduction strengths are noted to be slightly diminished bilaterally and her Tinel's signs and Durkan's compression tests are abnormal bilaterally. Which of the following is not indicated in the care of this patient?

A. Thyroid functions test and fasting glucose tests

B. Nighttime bilateral wrist splints

C. Modification of activities

D. Nonsteroidal anti-inflammatory agents

E. Steroid injections

ANSWERS

40.1 **C.** The sensory innervation of the little finger and the ulnar side of the ring finger is through the ulnar nerve. Median nerve sensory distribution involves the thumb, index finger, and middle finger on the palmar aspect.

40.2 **B.** Hypothyroidism (as well as diabetes mellitus, hyperthyroidism, pregnancy, and acromegaly) is associated with CTS. Diabetes insipidus is associated with loss of diluted urine and is not associated with CTS.

40.3 **D.** In this patient whose symptoms appear to be worsening and has equivocal findings during electrophysiologic testing, an MRI can be helpful to evaluate the carpal tunnel and assess for possible nerve compression.

40.4 **E.** The combination of the Phalen's test, Tinel sign, and Durkan's compression test improves the sensitivity and specificity of CTS diagnosis. The tests individually lack sensitivity and specificity for the diagnosis of CTS.

40.5 **A.** Even though hyperthyroidism and hypothyroidism can lead to CTS, it is not cost-effective or indicated to obtain specific testing to rule out the presence of the various endocrinopathies in a patient presenting with CTS and no signs and symptoms to suggest endocrine diseases.

CLINICAL PEARLS

▶ CTS usually presents with pain in the radial three fingers, especially at night.

▶ Electrophysiologic testing is indicated when the diagnosis is not clear based on the patient's history and physical examination.

▶ The initial treatment of CTS includes administration of NSAIDs and the use of wrist splints.

▶ Patients with significant symptoms of CTS who undergo nonoperative treatments for 4 months without improvements are not likely to achieve additional benefits from their treatments, and surgical decompression should be considered in these patients.

▶ Randomized controlled trials have shown that surgical decompression is associated with increased likelihood normalization of nerve conduction findings at the cost of surgery related complications. Based on these observations, it is reasonable to attempt an initial course of nonoperative treatment for most individuals.

REFERENCES

Middleton SD, Anakwe RE. Carpal tunnel syndrome. *BMJ*. 2014;349:g6437-g6443.

Shi Q, MacDermid JC. Is surgical intervention more effective than non-surgical treatment for carpal tunnel syndrome? A systematic review. *J Orthopedic Surg Res*. 2011;6:17-25.

Tang DT, Barbour JR, Davidge KM, Yee A, Mackinnon SE. Nerve entrapment: update. *Plastic Reconst Surg*. 2015;135:199e-215e.

During the routine physical examination of a 33-year-old, fair-complexioned white man, you discover a 1.5-cm pigmented skin lesion on the posterior aspect of his left shoulder. This lesion is flat, nonindurated, has ill-defined borders, and is without surrounding erythema. Examination of the patient's left axilla and neck revealed no abnormalities. No other pigmented lesions are noted during a thorough evaluation of the patient's skin. According to the patient's wife, the lesion has been there for the past several months, and has increased in size and become darker over this time. The patient is otherwise healthy.

► What is your next step?
► What is the most likely diagnosis?
► What is the best treatment for this problem?

ANSWERS TO CASE 41:
Malignant Melanoma

Summary: A 33-year-old man presents with a suspicious pigmented skin lesion on his left shoulder.

- **Next step:** Perform a full-thickness excisional biopsy.

- **Most likely diagnosis:** Malignant melanoma.

- **Best treatment:** Excision of the lesion with the appropriate radial margin based on depth of penetration of the melanoma is the most appropriate initial treatment. Patients with intermediate depth melanomas may benefit from evaluation of the regional lymph node basin by a sentinel lymph node biopsy (SLNB) procedure. Patients with stage III or stage IV disease may benefit from additional systemic therapy.

ANALYSIS

Objectives

1. Learn to recognize clinical presentation of malignant melanoma.

2. Learn the principles involved in the biopsy of suspected melanomas.

3. Learn about the treatment and prognosis associated with melanomas.

Considerations

This man presents with a skin lesion on the left shoulder with several worrisome features: (1) pigmented skin lesion, (2) irregular borders, (3) report of growth and color change. The ABCDE approach is the recommended approach to help one recognize and identify a melanoma. (A) **Asymmetry;** (B) **border irregularity;** (C) **color change;** (D) **diameter over 6 mm;** (E) **enlargement or elevation.**

All skin lesions that are concerning for malignant melanoma should be biopsied. Tissue biopsy helps confirm the diagnosis as well as determine the tumor thickness. **Accurate tumor depth assessment is vital for patients with malignant melanomas because this information provides prognostic information and serves as a guide for treatment.** During the initial biopsy, it is important to take a full-thickness skin biopsy, which provides important microstaging information. It is unnecessary and undesirable to take a wide margin during the initial biopsy, because the size of the margin for definitive treatment is dictated by tumor thickness. Once the biopsy demonstrates melanoma and the depth of penetration is determined, the patient will need a second procedure to excise the surgical bed with an appropriate skin margin. Patients with intermediate depth melanomas (1.0-4.0 mm) should also undergo lymphoscintigraphy and SLNB to assess for regional spread of disease, because selected patients with disease involvement in the regional lymph nodes benefit from therapeutic lymph node dissection.

APPROACH TO:
Pigmented Skin Lesions

DEFINITIONS

MELANOMA MICROSTAGING: This refers to the measurement of melanoma depth. Clark Level and Breslow Measurement are the two most commonly applied microstaging methods. Breslow measurements are more accurate than Clark level measurements for disease prognostication.

CLARK LEVEL: Describes the depth of invasion in relationship to surrounding skin and subcutaneous structures. Level I: intraepidermal; Level II: in papillary dermis; Level III: fills papillary dermis; Level IV: penetrates reticular dermis; Level V: enters subcutaneous tissue.

BRESLOW MEASUREMENT: Measures the primary tumor in millimeters. This measurement is taken from the top of the epidermal granular layer to the base. In cases of ulcerated tumors, the measurement is taken from the base of the ulcer to the bottom of the tumor. Stage I is <0.75 mm; stage II is 0.75 to 1.5 mm; stage III is 1.51 to 2.25 mm; stage IV is 2.25 to 3.0 mm; stage V is >3.0 mm.

PROGNOSIS BASED ON TUMOR DEPTH: (Estimated 5-year survival); <1 mm: 95% to 100%; 1 to 2 mm: 80% to 96%; 2.1 to 4 mm: 60% to 75%; >4 mm: 50%.

IN-TRANSIT DISEASE: These lesions represent tumor deposits in between the primary lesion and the primary lymph node drainage basin(s). The spread of the tumor is by the dermal and subdermal route. The occurrence of in-transit lesions is dictated by the tumor biology of the primary melanoma rather than adequacy of the primary tumor excision.

LYMPHOSCINTIGRAPHY: An imaging technique used to identify the lymphatic drainage basin for an area. This involves injection of special radioactive labeled substance into the skin at the tumor site or prior biopsy site. The pattern and site(s) of drainage can then be visualized or mapped with nuclear medicine imaging. This technique is helpful to decide which lymph node basin(s) to perform the SLNB.

THERAPEUTIC LYMPH NODE DISSECTION: Complete lymph node clearance of the lymph node basin where melanoma has already spread to, as evidenced by (+) SLNB or clinically enlarged lymph nodes. There is evidence to suggest that this treatment produces improved survival in some patients with melanoma metastases isolated to the regional lymph nodes. This operative treatment can produce significant lymphedema. Therefore, it is important to weigh the potential risk-benefit of the procedure in each individual patient.

PROPHYLACTIC LYMPH NODE DISSECTION: The approach of performing complete lymph node dissection without definitive knowledge that there is regional spread of disease to the lymph node basin. This is rarely done today because SLNB can be done to identify occult disease in the lymph node basin before proceeding with complete nodal dissection.

SUBUNGUAL MELANOMA: Melanomas originating in the nail bed follow principles of wide local excisions for other anatomic regions, with margins determined on the basis of the depth of penetration. Excision for subungual melanoma of the distal finger would require amputation of one phalanx proximal to the melanoma.

REGIONAL THERAPIES: These are treatments to be considered for patients with extensive disease isolated to an extremity. The options of regional therapy include isolated limb perfusion and isolated limb infusion, utilizing local infusion of melphalan. These techniques have the advantages of delivering extremely high doses of chemotherapeutic medications to regional diseases. However, these techniques are associated with high locoregional toxicity and often functional losses of the involved extremities.

CLINICAL APPROACH

The incidence of melanoma is increasing worldwide. In 2014, the incidence of melanoma in the United States is estimated at 76,000, with 9700 projected deaths from the disease. Currently, melanoma accounts for 4% of all newly diagnosed cancers in the United States and responsible for 1% of all cancer deaths. Melanoma is the fifth most common cancer in men and the seventh most common cancer in women in the United States. Risk factors for melanoma include family history, sun exposure, dysplastic nevus, a history of blistering sunburns, prior history of melanoma, and fair complexion. Patients with these risk factors should have thorough skin examinations on a regular basis by a trained healthcare professional. Suspicious skin lesions may be recognized based on **ABCDE** (Asymmetry, Borders, Color, large Diameter, and Enlargement or Elevation) characteristics (Table 41–1).

The four types of melanoma are (1) **superficial spreading**, (2) **nodular sclerosing**, (3) **lentigo maligna**, and (4) **acral lentiginous**. By far, the most common form is the *superficial spreading*, which accounts for 70% of all melanoma cases. This type of lesion has a slight female predominance and typically has a prolonged radial growth phase (1-10 years) and a late vertical growth phase. In comparison to the other forms of melanomas, the superficial spreading type has a more favorable prognosis with the exception of the lentigomaligna type. *Nodular sclerosing* is the second most

Table 41–1 • RISK FACTORS FOR MELANOMA		
Genetic[a]	Environmental Factors	Other
Fair skin (2.1)	Sunlight (especially ultraviolet B)	Age
Red hair (3)	Areas near the equator	Gender
White (5-10)	First sunburn at young age	Tanning lamps
>20 nevi on body (3.4)		Ultraviolet A
Blue eyes (4.5)		Higher socioeconomic class
Easily burned and unable to tan (4.5)		Immunosuppression
Familial cases (4-10)		Halogenated compounds
Prior history of melanoma (900)		Alcohol/tobacco
		Coffee/tea

[a]*Relative risk is shown in parentheses.*

common type (~15%), is associated with rapid vertical growth phase, and is most commonly found in the head and neck, and truncal regions. The *lentigo maligna* variant occurs in approximately 4% to 10% of patients and has a prolonged radial growth phase (5-15 years) with a better prognosis. *Acral lentiginous* type represents 35% to 60% of the melanoma cases seen in African Americans, Asians, and Hispanics. These lesions occur primarily on the palms and soles of the hands and feet and in nail beds.

Melanoma incidence is directly related to sun exposure. To minimize sun damage, patients are advised to avoid sun exposure between the hours of 10 AM to 4 PM, seek shade, and apply sunscreen liberally. Additional protective measures include the application of titanium dioxide or zinc oxide for ultraviolet A (UVA) protection.

Once a suspicious lesion is recognized, the next steps are to perform a thorough search for other skin lesions and then perform a biopsy. Biopsy goals are to determine the histological diagnosis, and in the case of melanoma, identify the depth or thickness of the tumor (microstaging). Excisional biopsy can be performed for small lesions. For lesions that are larger or are in a cosmetically sensitive area, a full-thickness punch biopsy of the thickest portion of the lesion should be performed. When performing extremity biopsies, the skin incisions should be oriented in the longitudinal directions. Once the thickness of the primary tumor has been determined by biopsy, a wide-local excision should be performed with margin size based on the tumor depth (see Table 41–2).

The regional lymph node basin is the most common first area of melanoma spread, and the sentinel lymph node(s) is/are the first node(s) where metastatic disease occurs. The probability of nodal involvement increases with increasing thickness of the primary tumor. Surgical lymphadenectomy is the primary therapy for patients with nodal involvement. Prior to the introduction of the SLNB technique in the late 1980s, patients with intermediate thickness (1-4 mm) melanomas often underwent prophylactic lymph node dissections, which often contributed to lymphedema in the affected area/extremity. Following the introduction of SLNB in the late 1980s, patients with intermediate thickness melanoma first undergo SLNB to identify lymph node metastasis, and therapeutic lymph node dissections is only performed if SLNBs reveale positive node(s) (Table 41–3).

Table 41–2 • RECOMMENDED WIDE LOCAL EXCISION MARGINS	
Primary Melanoma Thickness	Margin Size
Melanoma in situ	5 mm
<1 mm	1 cm
1.01-2 mm	1-2 cm
2.01-4 mm	2 cm
>4 mm	>2cm (depending the feasibility of large excision and cosmetic importance of the location)*

*More extensive local excision for melanomas >4 mm in depth is not always associated with improved survival because of the increased rates of regional and distant metastases associated with these thick tumors.

Table 41–3 • 2009 AJCC CANCER STAGING CLASSIFICATIONS FOR MELANOMA			
Stage	T Classification	N Classification	M Classification
	Thickness	**Lymph Node**	**Metastases**
IA	T <1.0 mm no ulcerations or mitosis		
IB	T <1.0 mm with ulceration or mitosis 1-2 mm no ulceration		
IIA	T 1.01-2 mm with ulceration 2.01-4 mm no ulceration		
IIB	T 2.01-4 mm with ulceration T >4.0 mm no ulceration		
IIC	T >4.0 mm with ulceration		
IIIA	Any thickness, no ulceration	Micrometastasis 1-3 lymph nodes	
IIIB	Any thickness, with ulceration Any thickness, no ulceration Any thickness, no ulceration	Micrometastasis 1-3 lymph nodes 1-3 palpable lymph nodes No involved lymph nodes but with in-transit or satellite metastasis	
IIIC	Any thickness, with ulceration Any thickness, with or without ulceration Any thickness, with ulceration	Up to 3 palpable LN 4 or more matted LN or in-transit disease + LN No LN but with in-transit metastasis or satellite metastasis	
VI			Lung metastases or all other sites of metastases or elevated LDH

The Multicenter Sentinel Lymphadenectomy Trial I (MSLT-I) published in 2006 reported the findings of a randomized controlled trial of patients with primary melanomas >1 mm in depth and no clinical nodal disease. The patients were randomized to clinical observation versus SLNB. When SLNB was positive or when clinical nodal recurrences occurred, the patients underwent therapeutic lymph node dissections. Overall, there was no difference in patient survival between the two treatment arms; however, when patients with positive SLNB were compared to patients randomized to initial observation and subsequently developed clinical nodal disease, those patients randomized to initial SLNB were found to have improved overall survival. The observations from this trial verified the accuracy of the SLNB technique for patients with melanoma and suggested that early identification and treatment of microscopic nodal disease offered an advantage over initial observation alone. Subset analysis of the MSLT-I trial suggests that patients with intermediate thickness melanomas (defined as 1.2-3.5 mm) benefited the most from early therapeutic lymph node dissections. The MSLT-II trial is currently ongoing, and is designed to assess the actual benefits of therapeutic lymph node dissection in patient with primary melanoma >1.2 mm and positive SLNBs. Patients fitting these inclusion criteria are being randomized to immediate complete lymph node dissection versus ultrasound surveillance of the lymph node basin. Results of the MSLT-II should provide additional evidence to determine the subsets of patients with microscopic lymph node involvement who would benefit from therapeutic lymph node dissections.

Unfortunately, patients with thick melanomas and melanomas with regional lymph node involvements are at high risk for systemic disease recurrence. For those patients with confirmed lymph node metastasis, the initial evaluation with CT scans or PET scans can be helpful in identifying occult distant metastasis. Adjuvant therapy with interferon-2A (Intron-A) is a therapeutic option for patients with stage III melanoma, but is associated significant side-effects on the patients' physical and emotional well-being. There are several options currently offered for patients presenting with melanoma with distant metastasis. These include surgical excision for isolated distant disease, dacarbazine, interleukin-2 (IL-2), and biologic response modifier such as ipilimumab (an anticytotoxic T-cell antigen 4 monoclonal antibody) and vemurafenib (BRAF inhibitor). The selection of optimal treatment options for patients with advanced diseases is not well-defined and needs to be individualized.

Follow-up

Follow-up of patients after surgical resection of melanomas is important because recurrences commonly occur, especially for patients with thick melanomas or nodal disease involvement. Patients with melanomas have an increased risk of developing a second melanoma, basal cell carcinomas, and squamous cell carcinomas of the skin. The overall risk of developing a second melanoma is in the range of 5% to 10% over the patient's lifetime. Therefore, all melanoma patients require life-long dermatologic surveillance. Recommended laboratory surveillance during routine follow-up include, CBC, liver functions test, and LDH which may indicate metastatic recurrences (Table 41–4).

Table 41–4 • PATIENT PROGNOSIS BY STAGE		
AJCC Stage	5-year Survival	10-year Survival
IA	97%	95%
IB	92%	86%
IIA	81%	67%
IIB	70%	57%
IIC	53%	40%
IIIA	78%	68%
IIIB	59%	43%
IIIC	40%	24%
IV	15-20%	10-15%

Information source: American Cancer Society Web Site. Accessed on September 9, 2014.

COMPREHENSION QUESTIONS

41.1 A 50-year-old man is noted to have a growing, pigmented skin lesion over his left posterior shoulder. Surgical biopsy revealed malignant melanoma. Which of the following type of melanoma is most likely?

A. Superficial spreading

B. Nodular sclerosing

C. Lentigomaligna

D. Acral lentiginous

E. Ulcerative

41.2 The patient in question 41.1 is scheduled for surgery. Which of the following is the most accurate predictor of clinical prognosis in the microstaging of his melanoma?

A. Clark's level

B. Presence of T-cell infiltration

C. Diameter of the primary tumor

D. Patient age

E. Breslow's level

41.3 Based on the current consensus recommendations, which of the following is the most appropriate radial margin measurement for a 2.2-mm-deep superficial spreading melanoma located over the left posterior back?

A. 0.5 cm

B. 1 cm

C. 2 cm

D. 3 cm

E. 5 cm

41.4 A 30-year-old man had an excision of a small nodular pigmented skin lesion from his left forearm. The pathology revealed a melanoma with maximal depth of 1.8 mm with microscopically uninvolved margins. Which of the following is the most appropriate treatment for this man?

A. Thorough dermatologic examination, wide excision of the scar with a 2-cm margin, and interferon alpha treatment

B. Thorough dermatologic examination, wide local excision with a 2-cm margin, and PET scan

C. Thorough dermatologic examination, wide local excision with a 1-cm margin, and left axillary SLNB

D. Thorough dermatologic examination, wide local excision with a 2-cm margin, and left axillary SLNB

E. Thorough dermatologic examination, wide local excision with a 2-cm margin, lymphoscintigraphy, and SLNB

41.5 A 43-year-old woman with a 1.8 mm malignant melanoma over the left thigh underwent wide local excision and left groin SLNB that did not reveal any disease spread 3 years ago. She now presents with a single 2-cm left pulmonary nodule in the peripheral lung field. Her physical examination is otherwise normal. A CT-guided needle aspiration of this lesion revealed malignant melanoma. A PET scan reveals no other hypermetabolic lesions in the body. Which of the following is the most appropriate treatment for this patient?

A. Interferon alpha treatment and serial CT scan surveillance of the lung nodule

B. Thoracotomy and pulmonary wedge excision of the lung nodule

C. Thoracotomy and pulmonary wedge excision followed by whole body radiation treatment

D. Wide local excision of the old left thigh surgical scar, thoracotomy and pulmonary wedge resection

E. Whole body radiation treatment

41.6 Which of the following is the most appropriate management strategy for a 38-year-old man with a 3.2-mm-thick melanoma of the left shoulder?

A. Wide local excision of the melanoma followed by alpha interferon treatment

B. Lymphoscintigraphy, SLNB, wide local excision of the melanoma, and alpha-interferon treatment

C. Wide local excision and axillary SLNB

D. Lymphoscintigraphy, SLNB, wide local excision of the melanoma

E. Wide local excision of the melanoma and radiation therapy to the axilla

41.7 Which of the following statement is TRUE regarding the acral lentiginous form of melanoma?

A. This type of melanoma is rarely found in the nail beds

B. This is the most commonly occurring melanoma subtype

C. This form of melanoma occurs more commonly in the African American patient population

D. This type of melanoma carries the best prognosis

E. This type of melanoma has a very slow vertical growth phase

ANSWERS

41.1 **A.** Superficial spreading melanoma is the most commonly occurring melanoma, representing 70% of the melanomas diagnosed; therefore, statistically
it would be the most likely type of melanoma encountered. In comparison
to the other forms of melanoma, this type of lesion has a better prognosis.
Ulceration is a finding that is not uncommon with melanomas and can occur
with all types of melanomas; this is a simple description of the characteristic
and no a unique subtype per se. Acral lentigious is the second most common
type of melanoma encountered (35%-60%), and this type of lesion tends to
occur more commonly on the soles and hands of African American, Hispanic,
and Asian patients.

41.2 **E.** Breslow and Clark staging classifications are both highly valuable prognosticators for patients with melanomas. However, between these two microstaging classifications, the Breslow depths of invasion have been found to be
a more accurate outcome prognosticator than the Clark levels. The patient's
age, the diameter of melanoma lesions, and the presence of T-cell infiltration
are not valuable independent prognosticators for melanoma patients.

41.3 **C.** The current consensus recommendation is to have a 2-cm margin when
performing a wide local excision for melanoma measuring 2.01 to 4 mm
in depth. The recommendation for margin size in melanoma resection are
developed to minimize local recurrence in the hopes of improving survival.
Increasing the margin size for thicker lesions makes sense up to a point where
local disease control offers no additional benefits; the benefits must also be
weighed against the impact of wide local excision on functionality and cosmesis. For these reasons, once a tumor exceeds 4 mm in depth, the use of a wider
excision is not necessarily better.

41.4 **E.** A thorough dermatologic examination is always indicated for patients
with melanoma, and based on tumor depth, a 2-cm surgical margin is recommended. A 1.8 mm melanoma falls into the intermediate depth category, and
based on findings of the MSLT-1 trial, there is potential benefit in performing a SLNB. The appropriate first lymphatic drainage basin from a melanoma on the forearm can be in the axilla or in the epitrochlear region. The
lymphoscintigraphy is needed prior to the SLNB to identify the lymph node
drainage basin containing the sentinel lymph node(s) for this lesion.

41.5 **B.** This patient presents with an apparent solitary pulmonary metastasis
3 years following resection of her primary melanoma on the thigh. As the
PET scan suggests, this is the only site of metastasis, therefore resection is
indicated. Additional systemic chemotherapy or targeted biologic response
modifier treatment might also be indicated for this patient. Whole body
radiation is not a treatment option for patients with melanoma. Similarly,
without evidence of recurrence on the thigh, re-excision of the surgical scar is
not indicated.

41.6 **D.** This patient has an intermediate depth melanoma (3.3 mm) on the shoulder. Based on the depth, there is increased risk for regional spread of disease, therefore a SLNB is indicated. There are several potential lymph node draining basins for melanoma on the shoulder, therefore lymphoscintigraphy is indicated to identify the most appropriate lymph node basin that the SLNB should be performed. Prophylactic radiation to the axilla is not generally given and can produce lymphedema.

41.7 **C.** Acral lentiginous melanoma is the most common melanoma discovered in African Americans, Hispanics, and Asians. It occurs primarily on the soles of feet, palms, and nail beds. Acral lentignous melanoma has an aggressive vertical growth phase and carries a poor prognosis.

CLINICAL PEARLS

▶ A shave biopsy should never be done for a lesion suspicious of being a melanoma.

▶ **A**symmetry, **B**order irregularity, **C**olor change, **D**iameter over 6 mm, and **E**nlargement or **E**levation associated with skin lesions should raise the suspicion for melanoma.

▶ Excision of the melanoma with appropriate skin margins is the mainstay of treatment for melanomas.

▶ An additional resection margin is taken from the excision scar for patients who have had melanoma excision with insufficient margins.

▶ Minor lymph node drainage basin for melanomas on the lower leg includes the popliteal fossae.

▶ Minor lymph node drainage basin for melanomas on the hands and forearm includes epitrochlear nodes.

▶ Minor lymph node drainage for truncal melanomas may include lymph nodes near the tip of the 12 rib.

▶ Melanoma is responsible for 6 out of 7 deaths associated with skin cancers.

▶ Sentinel lymph node biopsy is potentially beneficial for patients with intermediate thickness (1-4 mm) melanomas.

▶ Selective patients with isolated distant metastasis from melanoma can have improved survival following resection of the metastatic lesion.

REFERENCES

Cole P, Heller L, Bullocks J, Hollier LH, Stal S. The skin and subcutaneous tissue. In: Brunicardi FC, Andersen DK, Billiar TR, Dunn DL, Hunter JG, Mathews JB, Pollock RE, eds. *Schwartz's Principles of Surgery.* 9th ed. New York, NY: McGraw-Hill; 2010:405-422.

Jarkowski III A, Norris L, Trinh VA. Controversies in the management of advanced melanoma: "gray" areas amid the "black and blue". *Ann Pharmacother* 2014. DOI: 10.1177/1060028014544165.

Leung AM, Faries MB, Morton DL. The management of cutaneous melanoma. In: Cameron JL, Cameron AM, eds. *Current Surgical Therapy*. 11th ed. Philadelphia, PA: Elsevier Saunders; 2014: 700-706.

Morton DL, Thompson JF, Cochran AJ, et al. Final trial report of sentinel-node versus nodal observation in melanoma. *N Eng J Med*. 2014;370:599-609.

A 33-year-old man presents for evaluation of swelling in his right thigh. He first noticed this swelling 8 to 10 weeks ago and attributed it to injuries incurred during an informal soccer match with some friends. The patient has no known medical problems and has not had any problems regarding ambulation or physical activities. He is physically fit and runs 3 to 4 miles daily and plays soccer on weekends. On examination, he is found to have a 6 × 5cm, firm nontender mass in the anterior portion of the right thigh. There are no skin or motor/sensory changes in the right lower extremity. There are no evidence of lymphadenopathy in the right groin. A radiograph of the femur reveals no bony abnormalities.

► What is the most likely diagnosis?
► How would you confirm the diagnosis?
► What is the best treatment for this patient?

ANSWERS TO CASE 42:

Sarcomas of the Soft Tissue, Retroperitoneum, and Gastrointestinal (GI) Tract

Summary: A 33-year-old man presents with a large, nontender, soft tissue tumor of the right thigh that is highly suggestive of an extremity soft tissue sarcoma.

- **Most likely diagnosis:** Soft tissue sarcoma (STS) should be highly suspected whenever an individual presents with a firm, non-fatty soft tissue mass, and without any recent history of trauma or infections.

- **Confirmation of diagnosis:** Confirmation of the diagnosis can be established by core needle biopsy, or incisional biopsy of the lesions if core biopsy is non-diagnostic.

- **Best treatment:** Extremity sarcomas are best treated by wide local excision with negative margins. Adjuvant therapy such as pre- or postoperative radiation therapy can be given to improve the local control of disease when the margins are close, or to help decrease the extent of resection in anatomically difficult locations.

ANALYSIS

Objectives

1. Know the presentations of extremity, truncal, and retroperitoneal sarcomas and the importance and principles of tissue biopsies for early diagnosis and treatment.

2. Learn the treatment options and outcomes for patients with sarcomas.

3. Learn the genetic conditions and risk factors associated with sarcoma development.

4. Learn the management of gastrointestinal stromal tumors (GIST).

Considerations

This patient's presentation is very typical for an individual presenting with extremity soft tissue sarcoma (STS). Patients with STSs often are aware of their tumors, but it is not uncommon for patients and medical providers to initially attribute their lesions to traumatic or infectious causes. Several suspicious features described in this patient's presentation are highly suggestive of STS. These include the size of the mass (6 cm × 5 cm), the absence of specific traumatic events that could have caused the formation of a soft tissue hematoma, the firmness of the mass, and the absence of infectious features associated with the mass. As a rule, most patients with STSs do not present with regional lymphadenopathy or with systemic symptoms such as weight loss, night sweats, or cachexia. In some cases, STSs can produce local erythema, pain, and tenderness as the result of tumor necrosis; therefore, it is important to include STSs in the differential diagnosis even in patients presenting with inflammatory changes associated with soft tissue masses.

The initial approach for this patient should include biopsy of the mass for tissue diagnosis. The biopsy can be obtained initially using a core-needle ($\geq$14-16 gauge needle). If the core-needle biopsy is nondiagnostic, an open incisional biopsy should then be performed. **Excisional biopsies of suspected STSs are strongly discouraged because they frequently are associated with positive resection margins**, which necessitate additional surgeries for local disease control. **The failure to achieve an R0 (resection with macroscopic- and microscopic-negative margins) resection at the initial operation is one of the most common causes of local treatment failures.**

Once STS is confirmed by biopsy, we need to stage the patient's disease locally and systemically prior to tumor resection. MRI or CT imaging can provide valuable information regarding the local extent of the lesion, and CT scans of the chest, abdomen, and pelvis are helpful to assess for possible distant metastases. Complete staging evaluation prior to resection is important because the presence of distant metastatic disease would alter our treatment strategy. Surgical resection with microscopically clear margins is the best initial treatment for extremity STS. Patients with small, superficial, and low-grade STSs rarely experience local recurrences or die from the disease. On the other hand, patients with stage II and stage III diseases are at risk for local recurrences as well as distant recurrences; therefore, radiation therapy should be considered if the final staging for this patient is stage II or stage III. There is some evidence to suggest that patients with high-risk STSs may derive some benefits with adjuvant systemic chemotherapy, and the risks/benefits of adjuvant chemotherapy should also be discussed in multidisciplinary forum such as the tumor board at the treatment facility.

APPROACH TO:
Definitions

AJCC SOFT TISSUE SARCOMA STAGING: This STS staging system takes into account of tumor **size** ($\leq$5 cm or >5 cm), **depth** (superficial or deep to fascia), **nodal involvement** (+) or (−), **metastasis** (+) or (−), and **histologic grade** (well-, moderate-, or poorly-differentiated). Based on these criteria, the anatomic stages are assigned as Stage IA, IB, IIA, IIB, III, or IV. AJCC stages correlate closely with prognosis and survival following treatment.

R2 RESECTION: Surgical resection with gross (+) margin involvement. This is rarely done because of the lack of patient benefits.

R1 RESECTION: Surgical resection with gross (−) margin but microscopically (+) margin.

R0 RESECTION: Surgical resection with microscopically (−) margin.

NEOADJUVANT RADIATION THERAPY: Radiation therapy given prior to STS resection. The studies comparing neoadjuvant versus adjuvant (postoperative) radiation therapy have not demonstrated differences in local recurrences, distant recurrences, or progression-free survival. The potential benefits of neoadjuvant radiation therapy include the need for smaller radiation fields and lower radiation doses, tumor shrinkage prior to surgery, and reduced radiation-related morbidities. The drawback of neoadjuvant radiation therapy is increased rate of wound complications following tumor resections.

POSTOPERATIVE DISEASE-SPECIFIC SURVIVAL NOMOGRAMS: Nomograms taking into account various prognostic factors have been introduced to help estimate sarcoma-specific survival for patients with soft tissue sarcomas (12-year survival calculations), retroperitoneal sarcomas (7-year survival calculations), and GISTs (2-year and 5-year survival calculations).

GIST-TUMOR RELATED GENETIC MUTATIONS: A gain-of-function mutation in the tyrosine kinase receptor (KIT) has been identified in 80% to 85% of GISTs. 5% to 7% of GISTs occur as the result of primary platelet-derived growth factor receptor alpha (PDGFRA).

CARNEY'S TRIAD: The original triad included GIST, paraganglioma, and pulmonary chondroma. More recently, esophageal leiomyoma and adrenal adenoma have been added to the group of described abnormalities.

TYROSINE KINASE INHIBITORS (TKIs): Several TKIs have been developed for postoperative adjuvant therapy for high-risk GISTs and for the treatment of patients with metastatic GIST tumors. (Currently available agents: first-line-**imatinib**, second-line-**sunitinib**, and third-line-**regorafenib**.)

CLINICAL APPROACH

Soft tissue sarcomas (STSs) are a heterogeneous group of solid, mesenchymal cell tumors originating from muscle, fat, vascular tissue, fibrous connective tissue, peripheral neural tissue, and visceral tissue. STSs are rare tumors and make up less than 1% of the newly diagnosed cancers in adults and 6% of newly diagnosed cancers in children. A major reason that delays in diagnosis occur is that STSs are uncommon tumors; therefore, many medical providers do not have extensive experiences dealing with patients with these diseases. **It is imperative to consider STS whenever an unexplained soft tissue mass or swelling is identified in an individual of any age.**

The anatomic origins of STSs are important in affecting treatments and outcomes. Several large case series have found that 60% of STSs originate on the extremities, 20% in the truncal region, 15% are intra-abdominal or retroperitoneal, and 5% are located in the head and neck region. Approximately 10% of patients with STSs have distant metastases at presentation, with the lungs being the most common site. It is important to note that myxoid liposarcoma is a variant of liposarcoma, and has the unusual propensity to metastasize to extrapulmonary sites including the abdominal cavity (Table 42–1).

Table 42–1 • CHARACTERISTICS OF EXTREMITY SOFT TISSUE SARCOMAS		
Characteristic	Favorable	Unfavorable
Size	≤5 cm	>5 cm
Grade	Low	High
Depth	Superficial	Deep

Surgical Treatment

The primary goal of surgery is to accomplish an R0 resection (defined as complete resection with macroscopic- and microscopic-negative resection margins). Prior to the early 1980s, standard surgical treatment for extremity STSs consisted of limb amputations. A landmark randomized control study published in 1982 comparing limb-amputation to limb-sparing surgery found no difference in survival between the two treatment groups. Following the publication of this study, limb-sparing operations became the standard of care. The standard surgical resection for extremity STSs between the 1980s and mid-1990s involved removal of the entire muscle compartment from which the tumor originated; however, this approach was found to not be more effective for local and distant disease control than wide local excision. Currently, **the guiding principle in STS surgery is to achieve ≥2.0 cm uninvolved tissue margins or an intact fascia in the resected specimen.** The optimal surgical resection for a patient with STS requires a fine balance between a complete resection of the primary disease and preservation of functionality.

Chemotherapy

The most recent NCCN guidelines suggest that adjuvant chemotherapy should be considered for patients with stage IIB or higher stage disease. Chemotherapy is given either in the neoadjuvant setting or adjuvant setting. There are considerable controversies regarding the benefits of adjuvant chemotherapy, because the current available regimens are not highly effective. Even though most large RCT have not demonstrated a survival advantage for patients who received adjuvant chemotherapy, a recent meta-analysis of published data concluded that patients who received doxorubicin-based chemotherapy had a 6% improvement in local recurrence rate and 10% improvement in relapse-free survival rate in comparison to patients who received no adjuvant chemotherapy. Adjuvant combination chemoradiation is currently under investigation and appears to offer some survival and local disease control benefits.

Genetic and Environmental Predisposition to Sarcomas

There are several known environmental and genetic factors predisposing to STSs development. Known physical factors for sarcoma development include history of radiation, lymphedema, and chemical exposures (including prior chemotherapy). Table 42–2 lists the genetic predisposing factors. Patients with neurofibromatosis are prone to develop sarcomas arising from nerve structures, as well as paragangliomas and pheochromocytomas. Individuals with LFS (Li-Fraumeni syndrome) with mutations in the *p53* gene, and individuals with mutation in the retinoblastoma

Table 42–2 • GENETIC PREDISPOSITION ASSOCIATED WITH SARCOMAS
Neurofibromatosis
Li–Fraumeni syndrome
Retinoblastoma
Familial polyposis coli (Gardner syndrome)

gene (*Rb-1* gene) have autosomal-dominant mutations predisposing to the early development of sarcomas and a variety of other tumors. Patient with LFS have increased risk of developing a variety of cancers, and patients with *Rb-1* mutations are at risk of developing osteosarcomas. Individuals with familial polyposis coli syndromes have increased risk of developing desmoids tumors in addition to the risk of developing adenocarcinomas of the colon and small bowel.

RETROPERITONEAL SARCOMAS

Retroperitoneal sarcomas account for approximately 15% of all sarcomas. Most patients with retroperitoneal sarcomas remain relatively asymptomatic until the lesions have grown to large sizes. Consequently, the median size at diagnosis is 15 to 20 cm. When they occur, symptoms are mostly compressive in nature, with early satiety and lower extremity venous congestion being most common complaints. CT scans of the abdomen and pelvis or MRI are helpful for diagnosis and to define the extent of the lesions. Because retroperitoneal sarcomas often have distinct imaging characteristics, biopsies of the lesions generally unecessary always necessary prior to resection. However, tissue sampling should be considered in cases of diagnostic uncertainty, or when considering neoadjuvant therapies. Most biopsies can be obtained with image-guided core needle placements. Retroperitoneal sarcomas are mostly liposarcomas with or without de-differentiation. Lesions with de-differentiation are associated with up to 80% probability of local recurrence. **Retroperitoneal sarcomas rarely metastasize to distant sites.** Risk factors for post-resection local recurrence include incomplete resection (eg, R1 or R2), patient age, and stage III disease. Because of the high propensity for local recurrence, the resection of these tumors often requires multivisceral resection in order to accomplish an R0 resection. Long-term survival of patients following resection can be determined based on published nomograms. Overall, the 5-year rates of local disease control are 40% to 80% and the 5-year overall survival rates are reported at 50% to 70%. The role of adjuvant radiation and/or chemotherapy remains unclear in this patient population.

GASTROINTESTINAL STROMAL TUMOR (GIST)

GIST is a rare tumor that account for only 0.1% to 3% of all reported GI malignancies. GIST specifically refers to a tumor arising from the GI tract with a *KIT* or *PDGFRA*-activating mutation. The median age at diagnosis is 60. Most patients with GIST tumors have sporadic disease although familial GIST tumors have been reported in individuals with neurofibromatosis and in the setting of Carney syndrome. The stomach is the most common site of origin of GIST

(50%-70%), followed by small bowel (25%-15%), colon and rectum (5%-10%), omentum (7%), and esophagus (<5%). Approximately 70% of the patients with GISTs are symptomatic at diagnosis, while the remainder of patients have them identified incidentally or at autopsies. GISTs originate from the GI tract smooth muscles and symptoms are related to size and location of the tumors. **Bleeding** is the most common symptom related to GISTs, mostly as the result of tumor necrosis. Between 15% and 50% of patients with GISTs have metastatic disease at diagnosis with the most common sites of metastasis being the peritoneum, omentum, and liver. Primary GISTs generally appear as well-circumscribed masses arising from the walls of a hollow viscus. Contrast-enhanced CT scan is the imaging modality most commonly used for diagnosis prior to surgery. MRI is a more useful imaging modality for the assessment of patients with GISTs arising from the rectum or in the pelvis. The typical finding during GI endoscopy is the presence of a submuscosal mass with or without mucosal defect, and associated with tumor necrosis. Forcep biopsies obtained during endoscopy are sometimes nondiagnostic because the tumors are located beneath the mucosa. Endoscopically directed or other image-guided needle biopsies are the most common techniques leading to tissue diagnosis. Tissue biopsies prior to surgery are often unnecessary when patients present typical CT images and with symptoms or complications related to their GISTs.

Surgical Resection and Adjuvant Therapy

Completion resection of the tumor provides the best opportunity for cure. The ideal margin of resection for GISTs remains unknown, but it appears that a resection with either microscopically (R0) or macroscopically clear (R1) margins offers a better chance of disease cure than a macroscopically incomplete resection (R2). Most gastric GISTs can be resected by either a wedge resection of partial gastrectomy. Small bowel and colorectal GISTs are treated by segmental resections. Occasionally, patients with locally advanced GISTs benefit from neoadjuvant TKI treatment, which have been shown to improve the resectability in patients with locally advanced GISTs. Alternatively, surgical debulking procedures followed by adjuvant TKI treatments can be applied for patients with locally advanced GISTs.

Long-term prognosis following the resection of GISTs is determined by the anatomical location of the primary tumor, size of primary tumor, and completeness of resection. In general, gastric GISTs have the best prognosis in comparison to small bowel and colonic involvement. Recurrences following GIST resection is common, especially with high-risk tumors; therefore, adjuvant TKI therapy is indicated for patients who are high-risk for recurrences. A nomogram has been developed at the Memorial Sloan-Kettering Cancer Center to stratify recurrence risks and identify patients who would benefit from adjuvant TKI therapy. The ACOSOG Z9001 trial is a randomized controlled study that examined the benefits of adjuvant imatinib for patients following complete resections of c-kit-positive GIST larger than 3 cm in diameter. This trial showed that adjuvant imatinib (400 mg/qd) × 1 year in patients with high-risk GISTs experienced a significant improvement in one-year disease-free survival in comparison to patients who received placebo treatment.

COMPREHENSION QUESTIONS

42.1 A 35-year-old man notices a firm, nontender, 12-cm mass in his thigh after falling off a ladder. Which of the following is the most appropriate first step after a complete history and physical examination?

A. Observation to see if this mass changes over the next several weeks

B. Core needle biopsy followed by a CT scan of the lower extremities

C. Wide local resection of the mass

D. Ultrasonography of the mass

E. Incisional biopsy of the mass

42.2 A 41-year-old woman underwent excision of a presumed superficial lipoma in the left upper arm. The pathology results revealed a 6-cm high-grade sarcoma with gross positive margins. Which of the following is the most appropriate treatment at this time?

A. Follow-up examination in 3 months to see if local recurrence occurs

B. External beam radiation therapy

C. Systemic chemotherapy

D. Tyrosine kinase inhibitor therapy

E. Re-excision to achieve negative margins

42.3 A 28-year-old man has leiomyosarcoma of the right lower leg. He is found to have metastatic disease by imaging studies. Which of the following is the most likely site of metastasis?

A. Groin lymph nodes

B. Liver

C. Lungs

D. Bones

E. Brain

42.4 A 63-year-old woman is seen in follow-up after resection of a 15-cm retroperitoneal liposarcoma. Which of the following sites is the most likely site of recurrence?

A. Peritoneal cavity or retroperitoneal space

B. Liver

C. Lung

D. Recurrence rarely occurs

E. Brain

42.5 A 53-year-old man had segmental small bowel resection for small bowel GIST, where all gross disease was removed during the operation. The pathology revealed an 8-cm c-kit-positive GIST with 15 mitotic figures per 50 high-power fields. Which of the following is the most appropriate next step?

A. Systemic chemotherapy with doxorubicin-based chemotherapy

B. Imatinib 400 mg daily for 1 year

C. Radiation therapy

D. Doxorubicin + imatinib

E. Tamoxifen + imatinib

42.6 Which of the following conditions has NOT been found to be associated with the increase in lifetime risk of developing soft tissue sarcomas?

A. Li-Fraumeni syndrome

B. Radiation therapy

C. Lymphedema

D. Lipoma excision

E. Cigarette smoking

42.7 Which of the following best indicates a complete local resection of an extremity soft tissue sarcoma?

A. Surgical specimen with macroscopically negative margins

B. Postoperative MRI reveals no evidence of residual tumor

C. PET-CT demonstrates no evidence of residual disease

D. Surgical specimen with microscopic and macroscopic negative margins

E. Absence of local recurrence at 6 months following resection

42.8 Which of the following is the best treatment approach for a 46-year-old man who underwent resection of a 15-cm retroperitoneal sarcoma, whose resection margins were found with microscopic disease involvement?

A. Radiation therapy

B. Doxorubicin-based chemotherapy

C. Combined chemoradiation

D. Re-operation to remove the area of suspected positive margins

E. Observation

42.9 Which of the following is NOT a risk factor for GIST recurrence following resection?

A. c-kit mutation

B. Anatomic site of primary tumor

C. Mitotic index

D. Tumor size

E. R2 resection

ANSWERS

42.1 **B.** A 35-year-old man presents with a 12-cm painless, soft tissue mass in the thigh that he noticed after falling of a ladder. The size and **painlessness** of the mass makes it suspicious for STS. Biopsy of the mass is indicated at this time, and a core needle biopsy will help in most cases. Core needle biopsy followed by CT scan is the best choice available. Observation alone is not appropriate, because the lesion is not explained by the trauma. An ultrasonography will not help avoid tissue biopsy in this patient. Incisional biopsy of the mass is more invasive than core needle biopsy and is appropriate, if the core-needle biopsy is non-diagnostic. Wide local excision of a suspected STS without tissue confirmation can be overly aggressive and can lead to over-treatment in some cases.

42.2 **E.** This patient underwent excision of a superficial soft tissue mass in the upper arm that was presumed to be a lipoma. The pathology evaluation revealed a 6-cm high-grade sarcoma with involved margins. Re-excision to achieve a negative margin is the most appropriate approach given that the tumor is superficial in nature. Resection to negative margins is the preferred treatment in this case to reduce local failure. Radiation therapy is applied when the margins are close and the tumor is in an anatomically difficulty location. Systemic chemotherapy is not generally used for local disease control. TKI is used in the adjuvant treatment of GISTs and is not effective for STS treatment. Simple follow-up without additional local treatment is not appropriate for a patient with incomplete resection of superficial extremity STS.

42.3 **C.** The lungs are the most common site of distant metastasis for patients with extremity STS.

42.4 **A.** Local failure is the most common form of disease recurrence following resection of retroperitoneal sarcomas. In this case, the recurrence would be intraperitoneal and retroperitoneal.

42.5 **B.** This patient has a high-risk GIST (small bowel in origin, >3 cm in size, and >5-10 mitotic figures/50 HPF). Results of the ACOSOG Z9001 trial suggest that adjuvant therapy with imatinib 400 mg PO daily would provide her with additional survival benefits. Standard chemotherapeutic agents such as doxorubicin, radiation therapy, and anti-estrogen therapy have not been shown to be beneficial for patients with GISTs.

42.6 **D.** A history of lipoma excision is not associated with increase in lifetime risk of STS whereas Li-Faumeni syndrome, history of radiation therapy, lymphedema, and cigarette smoking have all been linked to increased lifetime risk of STSs.

42.7 **D.** A surgical specimen that demonstrates no microscopic tumor involvement at the margins is the best indicator of complete resection of STS. This is defined as a R0 resection. Resection with microscopic involvement at the specimen margins is termed an R1 resection. Resection with macroscopic involvement at the specimen margins is termed an R2 resection. Absence of recurrence at 6 months and PET-CT demonstration of no residual disease are not as helpful in reassuring that a complete resection had been undertaken.

42.8 **E.** Retroperitoneal sarcoma recurrence after resection is common because of the lack of clear anatomical boundaries that these tumors occur in. Consequently, positive microscopic margins occur quite commonly. There does not appear to be a defined role for re-excision of microscopically involved margins. Radiation and chemotherapy are not effective against retroperitoneal sarcomas and do not play a role in this setting. Observation for recurrence is most appropriate.

42.9 **A.** Anatomic site of GIST origin is an important prognosticator, with intestinal GISTs having worse prognosis than gastric GISTs. Increase in mitotic index, larger tumor sizes, and incomplete resections (R2 resections) are factors contributing to recurrences of disease. *c-kit* mutation is found in 80% to 85% of all GISTs and does not appear to have any prognostic implications.

CLINICAL PEARLS

▶ Features of an extremity mass suggestive of sarcoma include its size, the absence of specific events to account for a hematoma formation, its firmness, noticeable growth over weeks to months, and the absence of surrounding skin changes suggestive of inflammatory or infectious processes.

▶ The diagnosis of STS begins with a high clinical suspicion based on history and physical examination, followed by diagnostic core needle biopsy or fine-needle biopsy.

▶ Extremity STSs do not have pathognomonic characteristics based on imaging that can establish diagnosis. Tissue sampling is the only way to determine the diagnosis.

▶ The current standard therapy for extremity STS patients is wide local excision with negative microscopic margins, followed by radiation therapy for patients with high-risk tumors. Adjuvant radiation therapy and chemotherapy may provide additional survival benefits for patients following the resections of high-risk STSs. Decisions for adjuvant therapy must be closely weighed against the harm associated with these treatments.

▶ Prior radiation therapy and chemotherapy as well as genetic factors such as neurofibromatosis are risk factors for STS.

▶ Cigarette smoking is associated with an increase in lifetime risk of developing STS.

▶ c-kit mutations are found to be associated with 80% to 85% of GISTs.

▶ One-year of imatinib adjuvant therapy has been found to reduce recurrence following the resection of high-risk GISTs (tumor >3 cm, nongastric origin, and >5-10 mitotic figures/50 HPF).

▶ Imatinib is effective only for patients with GISTs with c-kit mutations.

▶ Neoadjuvant therapy with imatinib should be considered for patients with GIST located in the periampullary duodenum to help limit the extent of surgery.

REFERENCES

Kneisl JS, Coleman MM, Raut CP. Outcomes in the management of adult soft tissue sarcomas. *J Surg Oncol.* 2014;110:527-538.

Raut CP, Gronchi A. The management of soft tissue sarcoma. In: Cameron JL, Cameron AM, eds. *Current Surgical Therapy.* 11th ed. Philadelphia, PA: Elsevier Saunders; 2014:706-717.

Raut CP, Pawlik TM. Gastrointestinal stromal tumors. In: Cameron JL, Cameron AM, eds. *Current Surgical Therapy.* 11th ed. Philadelphia, PA: Elsevier Saunders; 2014:96-103.

Seerrano C, George S. Recent advances in the treatment of gastrointestinal stromal tumors. *Adv Med Oncol.* 2014;6:115-127.

A 48-year-old man with a history of alcoholism and cirrhosis presents to the emergency department for evaluation for severe left leg pain and fever. The patient says that his symptoms began after he scraped the lateral aspect of his knee at home 3 days ago. During the past 2 days, he has had subjective fever and noticed decreased urinary frequency. The patient has self-medicated with aspirin for these symptoms. He consumes approximately 16 oz (473 mL) of whiskey per day and smokes one pack of cigarettes per day. On physical examination, his temperature is 39.2°C (102.6°F), pulse rate is 110 beats/minute, blood pressure is 115/78 mm Hg, and respiratory rate is 28 breaths/minute. His skin is mildly icteric. The findings from his cardiopulmonary examination are unremarkable. The abdomen is soft and without hepatosplenomegaly or ascites. The left leg is edematous from the ankle to the upper thigh. The skin is tense and exquisitely tender; however, it is without erythema, fluctuance, necrosis, or vesicular changes. Examination of the right leg reveals normal findings. Laboratory studies demonstrate a WBC count of 26,000/mm^3 and normal hemoglobin and hematocrit values. Other laboratory studies reveal sodium 128 mEq/L, glucose 180 mg/dL, total bilirubin 3.8 mg/dL, and direct bilirubin 1.5 mg/dL. Radiographs of the left leg reveal no bony injuries and no evidence of air in the soft tissue space.

▶ What is the most likely diagnosis?
▶ What is the best therapy for this condition?

ANSWERS TO CASE 43:
Soft Tissue Infections

Summary: A 48-year-old man with alcoholism and cirrhosis presents with a severe soft tissue infection following a seemingly trivial trauma to his left lower extremity.

- **Most likely diagnosis:** Severe soft tissue infection of the left lower extremity.

- **Best therapy:** Antimicrobial therapy, imaging to determine the nature and extent of the soft tissue infection, and possible surgical drainage and/or debridement if indicated (based on imaging results).

Considerations

This patient with alcoholic cirrhosis presents with severe soft tissue infection of the left lower extremity following a trivial soft tissue injury 3 days ago. His vital signs and laboratory studies (fever, tachycardia, tachypnea, high WBC count, and low sodium) indicate that he is already septic. An individual with alcohol-induced cirrhosis is considered immune compromised, and has increased susceptibility to multiple types of infections and septicemia. Blood cultures should be obtained promptly, followed by the initiation of intravenous fluids and empiric antibiotic therapy to cover potential polymicrobial infections. In this patient's case, vancomycin and piperacillin/tazobactam are an appropriate initial treatment regimen. Next, a CT scan of the affected lower extremity should be obtained to evaluate the possibility of deep tissue space infections and to assess the extent of the soft tissue infection. Although his history is suggestive of a skin-based soft tissue infection, the findings on his affected extremity are not specific for a necrotizing soft tissue infection (NSTI) and may be compatible with a deep-seated abscess with extensive adjacent soft tissue infection. A CT scan is valuable to guide the extent of the wound exploration/debridement and help identify potential hidden abscesses. Surgical debridement and/or wide drainage are very important adjuncts in this patient's treatment, and delays in surgical treatment have been demonstrated to negatively affect the outcomes of patients with NSTIs. It is important to collect tissue and fluid specimens for culture and Gram Stain to optimize the antibiotic treatment. Distant end-organ dysfunction including acute respiratory insufficiency, acute liver dysfunction, and acute kidney injuries can occur in individuals with NSTI, and close monitoring is needed for prompt implementation of supportive care.

The surgical approach should begin with incision and inspection of the soft tissue space and fascia. Easy separation of the subcutaneous tissue from the underlying fascia indicates microvascular thrombosis and necrosis and should be treated with soft tissue debridement. The deep fascia overlying the muscle should be inspected for viability, and if discoloration and necrosis is encountered, debridement of the fascia should be carried out. Muscle fascia is a natural protective layer for the muscles, and infections deep to the fascia occur uncommonly unless a deep puncture wound with bacterial inoculation into the muscle has occurred.

Because of the rich blood supple to the skin, patients with NSTI generally do not develop skin necrosis and bullous changes until late in the disease process. The **absence of skin abnormalities is one of the leading factors contributing to delays in recognition of NSTI.** When the process is recognized, all necrotic tissue should be excised. Infectious involvement of the muscles is uncommon except with deep puncture wounds into the muscles and in cases of infections involving *Clostridium* species. When patients with NSTI fail to improve with supportive care, antibiotic therapy, and surgical debridement, consideration should be given that not all affected soft tissue has been identified and debrided. The lack of improvement in patients is often due to inadequate debridement and/or inappropriate antibiotic selection (source control) (Table 43–1).

APPROACH TO:
Soft Tissue Infections

DEFINITIONS

SIMPLE CELLUTITIS: Milder form of soft tissue infection without microvascular thrombosis and necrosis. Clinically, patients do not exhibit systemic signs and symptoms. Antibiotics therapy are sufficient treatment.

NECROTIZING CELLULITIS: This term refers to skin and superficial subcutaneous fat infection associated with microvascular thrombosis and necrosis. The patient often exhibits systemic signs and symptoms. This process is generally related to infection with group B streptococcus or community-acquired MRSA. Treatment consists of antibiotics, local debridement, and supportive care.

NECROTIZING FASCIITIS: This term refers to infection of the skin, subcutaneous fat, and fascia. This process is frequently associated with microvascular thrombosis and tissue necrosis. Soft tissue debridement is an essential component of treatment.

FINGER TEST FOR NSTI DIAGNOSIS: This is an adjunct method of diagnosing NSTI. A 2- to 3-cm skin incision is made under local anesthesia and carried down to the fascia. This is then followed by insertion of gloved finger to digitally evaluate the fascia. With NSTI, the subcutaneous fat will separate easily without bleeding, and there will often be a presence of murky "dishwater" fluid in the subcutaneous tissue.

IMMUNE-DEFICIENT HOSTS WITH NSTI: Immune-deficient hosts include individuals with who use corticosteroids, with active malignancy, receiving chemotherapy or radiation therapy, with positive HIV status, receiving immunosuppressive medications for bone marrow or solid organ transplantation, with cirrhosis, and with alcoholism. Studies have shown that immunocompromised hosts do not exhibit the usual responses to NSTI, and therefore, are susceptible to delayed treatments and misdiagnoses. Increasing vigilance for this condition in susceptible individuals is important.

Table 43–1 • SKIN AND SOFT TISSUE INFECTIONS			
Infection Type	Clinical Findings	Bacteriology	Treatment
Superficial non-necrotizing soft tissue infection	Cellulitis (erythema and inflammation in the epidermis and dermis); Impetigo (discrete purulent skin lesions), Erysipelas (red, tender, painful, raised plaques)	Gram-positive organisms. Impetigo is associated with β-hemolytic streptococcus and/or S. aureus. Erysipelas is associated with S. pyogenes	Antibiotics and drainage if needed
Abscess	Findings differ depending on location and depth. Abscesses are always painful ± skin changes	Superficial abscesses are most often associated with skin flora. Abscesses related to the aerodigestive tract or genitourinary tract may be Gram- negative or polymicrobial (such as perirectal abscess, diabetic foot abscess)	Adequate drainage is most important and if surrounding cellulitis (>2 cm) and/or sepsis is present or if patient is immune compromised, antibiotic treatment should be added
Necrotizing cellulitis	Skin is inflamed and indurated and often with subcutaneous fat involvement. This process is due to infection with certain toxic strains of bacteria, systemic signs may be present	β-Hemolytic streptococci or community-acquired MRSA	Surgical debridement in addition to antibiotic treatment and supportive care
Necrotizing fasciitis	Skin and subcutaneous fat with "woody" induration, extensive edema, pain, and often without skin discoloration. Patients always exhibit systemic signs of sepsis	Type 1: Polymicrobial. Type 2: Monomicrobial (β-hemolytic streptococcus or community-acquired MRSA). Type 3: Monomicrobial with pathogenic bacilli species	Radical surgical debridement, antibiotic treatment, and supportive care
Fournier's gangrene	Rapidly progressive soft tissue infection of the skin, subcutaneous fat, and fascia in the scrotum, penis, or perineal areas. Skin necrosis and crepitance can be rapidly progressive. Patients always present with systemic signs and symptoms	Polymicrobial infection with aerobic and anaerobic organisms	Radical surgical debridement, antibiotic therapy, and supportive care
Necrotizing myositis	Pain within 24 hours of injury with progressive skin changes to paleness then to a bronze color. Later, bullae and crepitance may develop	Clostridial species. C. perfingens is most common, but other pathogens include C. novyi, C histolyticum, C septicum	Radical surgical debridement, antibiotic treatment, supportive care, and possibly hyperbaric treatment

NSTI ASSOCIATED WITH SURGICAL SITES: Occasionally, this can occur and can be difficult to diagnose and differentiate from simple wound infections. The systemic signs associated with this process are often easily attributed to other conditions, such as pneumonia or atelectasis.

COMMUNITY ACQUIRED-MRSA INFECTION (CA-MRSA): These infections are becoming increasingly more common. CA-MRSAs are genetically and pheno-typically different from hospital-acquired MRSA. CA-MRSA may produce the pathogenic Panton-Valentine leucocidin (PVL) toxin, which destroys white blood cells. Oral antibiotic options for CA-MRSA include clindamycin, trimethoprim-sulfamethoxazole, tigecycline, doxycycline, minocycline, linezolid, or daptomycin.

TETANUS IMMUNIZATION: Tetanus is the clinical sequelae associated with *Clostridium tetani* infections. Individuals residing in the United States are given a set of initial immunization shots during infancy, childhood, and adolescence. Booster shots are recommended every ten years for adults. *Clostridium tetani* is an organism that can be found in soil, dust, and animal feces, and in high-risk wounds include animal bites, human bites, and dirty wounds.

TETANUS IMMUNE GLOBULIN: This is an IgG antibody that neutralizes the toxins that would cause tetanus. Administration provides transient passive immunity for individuals who are not properly immunized (or have unknown tetanus immunization history) and have been exposed to or suspected of having been exposed to the tetanus toxin.

DAPTOMYCIN: This newer antibiotic with good tissue penetration has been found to be effective for soft tissue infections treatment. In direct comparison studies against vancomycin and semi-synthetic penicillins, daptomycin has been shown to be equally efficacious.

CLINICAL APPROACH

Soft tissue infections should be suspected in individuals with pain and edema involving the skin, an extremity, or a body region, which may or may not be associated with inflammatory changes in the skin. It is important to elicit a detailed history from the patient regarding recent trauma to the affected area, including trivial trauma such as skin abrasions and minor lacerations. Severe soft tissue infections should be suspected when individuals described above exhibit systemic signs such as tachycardia, fever, tachypnea, hypotension, or oliguria. Physical examination of the affected soft tissue area can be extremely helpful. **Pain out of proportion to skin changes is a highly suspicious finding, and is often thought to be related to microvascular thrombosis and tissue ischemia associated with NSTI.** It is extremely important to pay attention to the patients' descriptions of symptoms and not disregard their complaints due to absence of specific skin changes. Laboratory studies are helpful in identifying patients with NSTI and may be helpful for disease severity stratification. WBC count over 20,000 mm^3 and hyponatremia (serum sodium < 130 mEq/L) have been reported to prognosticate poor outcomes. For patients with possible NSTI, deep abscesses, and unclear extent of their infectious processes, a CT scan can be very helpful to identify fat stranding, fluid and/or gas collections tracking along fascial planes, which are early signs of NSTI. In addition, CT scans can identify deep soft tissue abscess that clinically may present as a simple soft tissue infection. CT imaging have been reported to be associated with 100% sensitivity and 81% specificity for NSTI diagnosis. Visualization of the subcutaneous tissue and fascia are important during surgical exploration for NSTI. The finger test helps to identify tissue necrosis along the fascia. In addition, the findings of marked subcutaneous tissue edema and "dish-water"-appearing fluid in the subcutaneous space are highly suggestive of NSTI. Close monitoring of patients following the initial wound exploration and/or soft tissue debridement is vital, because if the patients do not show improvements, re-exploration and/or modification of antibiotic treatments should be implemented (Table 43–2).

Group A β-Hemolytic Streptococcus Soft Tissue Infection

This type of infection has been referred to in the lay press as the "flesh-eating bacterial infection". This form of NTSI frequently affects individuals with immune compromised conditions (alcoholic, diabetic, and malnourished patients). Surprisingly, these infections can also affect healthy individuals following trivial soft tissue trauma such as skin abrasions. Approximately, 75% of these infections are community acquired. Bacteremia and toxic shock syndrome are associated with these infections in about 50% of the cases. The local process usually spreads rapidly over hours to days. The combination of clindamycin and penicillin has been touted to

Table 43–2 • CLINICAL MANIFESTATIONS OF NECROTIZING SOFT TISSUE INFECTION			
Clinical Setting	**Organisms**	**Clinical Manifestations**	**Antibiotics**
Acquired after contact with fish or seawater	*Vibrio* species	Rapid progression of soft tissue infection, fever, rigors, and hypotension	Ceftazidime plus quinolone or tetracycline
Mixed synergistic infection; progression of perirectal infection or complications of gastrointestinal surgery	Mixed gram-negative aerobes and anaerobes	Clinical progression over several days; may involve perineum and abdominal wall	Multiple regimens developed to cover gram-negative bacilli, and anaerobes
Gas gangrene may complicate trauma or ischemia	Clostridial species	Swollen, tense skin, crepitation, and skin vesicles; frequently present with systemic toxic therapy	Penicillin (questionable benefit with hyperbaric therapy)
Necrotizing soft tissue infection related to injectional drug abuse (IDA) or "skin popping"	Clostridial species and other gram-positive anaerobic organisms	Swelling and systemic toxicity due to the release of exotoxins. Because injections pass through the fascia and into the muscles during "skin popping," the area of infection is in muscles and below the fascia. These infections have very high mortality due to sepsis and organ failure	Penicillin, clindamycin, and vancomycin

produce superior results compared to penicillins alone. There is limited evidence suggesting that adjunctive treatment with intravenous immunoglobulins (IVIG) will help neutralize the bacteria-produced superantigens and improve outcomes.

Toxic Shock Syndrome (TSS)

TSS is a clinical syndrome caused by pyrogenic toxin superantigens produced by certain community-acquired *MRSA* species and *Group A β-Hemolytic Streptococcus* species. The binding of the superantigens to major histocompatibility complex class III molecules lead to T-cell clonal expansion and massive release of proinflammatory cytokines by macrophages and T cells. Patients with TSS frequently develop mental obtundation, hyperdynamic shock, and multiple-organ dysfunction syndrome (MODS). The systemic findings of TSS frequently do not correlate with the local extent of the soft tissue or pelvic (vaginal) infections and thus can cause delays in diagnosis and treatment.

Fournier's Gangrene

This is a **rapidly progressive soft tissue infection of the perineal, scrotal, and penis area in males,** but the process can occur less commonly in the perineal region in females. The infection can lead to skin necrosis, sepsis, and death within hours to days if unrecognized and untreated. Fournier's gangrene was originally described in 1883 as scrotal soft tissue infections in a group of healthy young men. The infection is commonly a polymicrobial synergistic type of infection leading to sepsis and MODS. Treatment consists of broad-spectrum antibiotics directed at aerobic and anaerobic organisms and radical debridement of the affected soft tissue.

COMPREHENSION QUESTIONS

43.1 Which of the following statements is true regarding NSTI treatment in immune-compromised hosts?

A. Antibiotic therapy is not effective treatment for these individuals

B. The outcome of NSTI treatments in immune-compromised hosts is the same as in healthy normal hosts

C. NSTI in immune-compromised hosts usually is caused by different bacterial organisms from the usual population

D. Clinical presentations of NSTI is the same for immune compromised individuals and immune competent individuals

E. Treatment is often delayed in immune compromised hosts because of variability in clinical presentation

43.2 Which of the following is most accurate for the diagnosis of NSTI?

A. CT scan

B. History and physical examination

C. Blood and skin swab culture

D. Serology

E. Clinical experience

43.3 Which of the following soft tissue infection processes can be treated with antibiotics alone?

A. Superficial abscess

B. Necrotizing cellulitis

C. Deep muscle infection following hip prosthesis implantation

D. Necrotizing myositis

E. Impetigo

43.4 A 38-year-old man with a history of injection heroin abuse presents to the emergency center with tenderness and swelling that extends circumferentially around his left upper arm. The entire area is minimally erythematous, but it is tense and swollen. The patient indicates that he had injected some "black tar heroin" into the area 6 days ago. His temperature is 39.5°C (103°F), heart rate is 125 beats/minute, and WBC is 46,000 mm³. CT scan of the arm reveals no evidence of abscess or venous thrombosis, but there is extensive tissue stranding along the muscle fascia and in the muscles. Which of the following is the most appropriate treatment?

A. Admit to the hospital for IV antibiotics, and if he does not improve then repeat the CT to look for an abscess

B. Perform radical debridement of the affected area followed by intravenous antibiotics therapy

C. Perform a transesophageal echocardiography to look for endocarditis and treat patient with IV antibiotics

D. Admit the patient for antibiotics treatment and hyperbaric oxygen treatment

E. Perform radical debridement of the affected area

43.5 A 33-year-old house painter sustained an abrasion and superficial laceration of the left shoulder 2 days ago. He presents to the outpatient clinic with an area of erythema extending 3 cm along the area of skin abrasion and superficial laceration. There is an area of fluctuance underneath the skin, and the tenderness does not appear to extend beyond the area. His temperature and vital signs are normal. Which of the following is the most appropriate treatment?

A. Oral antibiotics for 3 days followed by reassurance. Perform incision and drainage if it does not improve

B. Topical antibiotic ointment application and dressing changes

C. Oral antibiotics for 1 week

D. Incision and debridement of the area

E. Incision and drainage of the area, followed by 1-week course of oral antibiotics

43.6 A 62-year-old man with diabetes returns to the emergency department 3 days after undergoing incision and drainage of a perirectal abscess. The patient complains of fever and malaise. Evaluation of the perirectal area reveals an open draining wound with a 20-cm area of surrounding induration and erythema, with some localized blistering of the skin. The infection appears to have extended to involve his entire perineum, scrotum, and the anterior abdomen. Which of the following is most likely the process that is occurring?

A. Toxic shock syndrome

B. Clostridial gas gangrene

C. NSTI caused by group A β-hemolytic streptococcus

D. Polymicrobial synergistic NSTI

E. Community-acquired MRSA

43.7 A 55-year-old man with diabetes presents with a swollen, painful right hand that developed 1 day after sustaining a puncture wound to the hand while fishing in the Gulf of Mexico. His temperature is 39.5°C (103.1°F), pulse rate is 120 beats/minute, and blood pressure is 96/60 mm Hg. His right hand and forearm are swollen, and a puncture wound with surrounding ecchymosis is present on the hand. There is drainage of brown fluid from the wound. Which of the following therapies is the most appropriate?

A. Supportive care, penicillin G, and hyperbaric treatment

B. Supportive care, penicillin G, tetracycline, ceftazidime, and surgical debridement

C. Supportive care, penicillin G, tetracycline, ceftazidime, surgical debridement, and hyperbaric treatment

D. Supportive care, penicillin G, clindamycin, and Intravenous Ig

E. Supportive care and penicillin G

ANSWERS

43.1 **E.** Observational studies suggest that immunocompromised patients with NSTI had delays in diagnosis and surgical treatment, because many of the patients failed to exhibit the usual clinical signs and did not have the usual WBC responses associated with NSTIs. Clinicians need to maintain a higher level of vigilance, consider additional imaging studies, and earlier surgical evaluations.

43.2 **A.** CT scan is highly sensitive and specific for the diagnosis of NSTI. The reported sensitivity is 100%, specificity of 85%, positive predictive value of 76%, and negative predictive value of 100%; therefore, the CT scan is an excellent tool to rule-out NSTI.

43.3 **E.** Impetigo is a common skin infection with small pustules that develop along with soft tissue inflammation. This process is nearly always caused by β-hemolytic streptococcus infections or *Staphylococcus aureus*. Treatment is antimicrobial therapy and skin care. The superficial abscess requires drainage, necrotizing cellulitis requires debridement, deep muscle infection following hip prosthesis placement will require surgical drainage and possibly removal of hardware. Necrotizing myositis will require debridement.

43.4 **B.** This patient has findings consistent with NSTI associated with injectional drug abuse. Based on the history of black-tar heroin injection, the infection is likely a polymicrobial synergistic infection. Early, aggressive surgical debridement and broad-spectrum antimicrobial therapy are the keys to reduce mortality associated with this process. The role of hyperbaric treatment in this population is unclear.

43.5 **E.** The descriptions given are consistent with a soft tissue abscess with a 3-cm rim of surrounding cellulitis. Incision and drainage of the abscess with antibiotics treatment are the most appropriate for this patient.

43.6 **D.** The origin of the infection in this patient is the perirectal area. Abscesses that originate in that location are most likely polymicrobial in nature, and if left untreated, they can progress to develop polymicrobial synergistic NSTI. Hyperbaric treatment for NSTI has not been shown to reduce mortality; in fact, there is a general lack of strong clinical evidence to apply hyperbaric treatments for NSTI, and increase in hospital costs.

43.7 **B.** This man developed a severe infection of the hand and forearm following a puncture wound to the hand that he sustained during a fishing trip in the Gulf of Mexico. Because the infectious organisms might be water-borne bacteria, antimicrobial therapy needs to include coverage for *Vibrio* species (Ceftazidime, tetracycline), and at the same time penicillin G should be included to cover for Gram positive organisms. Incision and drainage are also very important components of his treatment.

CLINICAL PEARLS

▶ The most common findings in a patient with NSTI are local edema and pain in the presence of systemic signs such as high fever (hypothermia in some patients), tachycardia, and often mental confusion.

▶ NSTI should be suspected when pain and tenderness extend beyond the area of skin erythema.

▶ When NSTI is strongly suspected, exploration of the wound through a limited incision may help to establish the diagnosis. Drainage of "dish water" fluid and easy separation of the subcutaneous tissue from the affected fascia is seen during digital exploration.

▶ Rapid, aggressive surgical debridement is the most important treatment for NSTI.

▶ Lack of improvement after initial treatment of NSTI may be related to inadequate debridement and/or inappropriate antibiotic selection (lack of source control).

REFERENCE

Sartelli M, Malangoni MA, May AK, et al. World Society of Emergency Surgery (WSES) guidelines for management of skin and soft tissue infections. *World J Emerg Surg.* 2014;9:57-75.

Stevens DL, Bisno AL, Chambers HF, et al. Practice guidelines for the diagnosis and management of skin and soft tissue infections: 2014 update by the Infectious Disease Society of America. *Clin Infect Dis.* 2014;59:e10-e52.

An otherwise healthy 23-year-old female medical student presents with an asymptomatic neck mass that was found during a practice head and neck examination performed by a fellow medical student. Physical exam reveals a 3-cm nontender, firm mass in the inferior pole of the right thyroid lobe. The remaining physical exam is normal. She denies symptoms of hyper- or hypothyroidism and has no exposure to ionizing radiation. There is no family history of thyroid disease nor other endocrinopathies. Serum TSH and T_4 levels are normal.

► What is your next step in management?
► What is the most likely diagnosis?
► What are the treatment options based on pathology?

ANSWERS TO CASE 44:

Thyroid Nodule

Summary: A 23-year-old woman presents with an asymptomatic thyroid mass who is clinically euthyroid without concerning personal or family history.

- **Next step:** Ultrasound of the thyroid with fine needle aspiration biopsy of the nodule for cytologic assessment

- **Most likely diagnosis:** Despite the absence of risk factors, the non-tender firm mass is consistent with thyroid carcinoma.

- **Treatment options:** Treatment of thyroid carcinoma generally consists of thyroidectomy with lymph node dissection when cervical lymph nodes are involved. Adjunct therapies are based on the type of carcinoma and extent of disease.

ANALYSIS

Objectives

1. Understand the basic approach to evaluation of a solitary thyroid nodule.

2. Review the diagnostic evaluation and surgical indications for patients with thyroid nodules.

3. Identify the treatment plan for thyroid nodules based on FNA cytology.

Considerations

This is a 23-year-old healthy and asymptomatic woman with a 3-cm nontender mass of the thyroid. The patient should be questioned carefully about symptoms such as possible compression on the trachea or esophagus, or possible symptoms of hyperthyroidism or pheochromocytoma. A prior history of head or neck radiation is very important since the risk of thyroid cancer is much higher with this history. A careful family history should be obtained about thyroid disease but also other cancers, especially those within MEN II A and B. On physical exam, the mass should be palpated for location, tenderness, texture, and movement with the thyroid gland during swallowing. Lymph nodes should be palpated. An ultrasound exam of the mass and an FNA biopsy are reasonable to assess for the possibility of thyroid carcinoma.

APPROACH TO:

Thyroid Nodules

DEFINITIONS

PAPILLARY THYROID CARCINOMA: The most common type of thyroid carcinoma, usually well-differentiated and with a favorable prognosis.

FOLLICULAR ADENOMA: Benign thyroid nodules, which are fairly common in adults. They cannot be differentiated from follicular carcinoma by fine-needle aspiration (FNA) due to lack of architecture and inability to confirm invasion.

MEDULLARY THYROID CARCINOMA (MTC): A more aggressive type of thyroid cancer which arises from parafollicular c-cells. It may occur sporadically or in associated familial clusters such as MEN2.

ANAPLASTIC THYROID CARCINOMA: An extremely aggressive type of dedifferentiated thyroid cancer which has a preponderance for local invasion. Prognosis is dismal and treatment of is palliative and multimodal.

CENTRAL NECK DISSECTION: A functional lymph node dissection of the anterior neck that is bordered laterally by the carotid arteries, superiorly by the hyoid bone, and inferiorly by the suprasternal notch. The benefits of routine prophylactic central lymph node dissection in patients with papillary and follicular thyroid cancers are controversial.

MULTIPLE ENDOCRINE NEOPLASIA 2A (MEN 2A): An autosomal dominant genetic syndrome that includes medullary thyroid carcinoma, pheochromocytoma, and parathyroid hyperplasia.

MULTIPLE ENDOCRINE NEOPLASIA 2B (MEN 2B): An autosomal dominant genetic syndrome that includes medullary thyroid carcinoma, pheochromocytoma, marfanoid habitus, and mucosal neuromas.

CLINICAL APPROACH

The prevalence of thyroid nodules and thyroid carcinoma is on the rise due to increased diagnoses, mainly because of advancements in imaging technology. Thyroid nodules larger than 1 cm are considered clinically significant and require further evaluation. A patient with a thyroid nodule should be questioned about symptoms of hyper- or hypothyroidism, compressive symptoms such as dyspnea, coughing, or choking spells, dysphagia or hoarseness, and a prior history of head or neck irradiation. Patients should also be asked about a family history of thyroid cancer, hyperparathyroidism, or pheochromocytoma.

Symptoms of hyper- or hypothyroidism may be present in patients with thyroiditis. Symptoms of hyperthyroidism are also seen in patients with benign functioning follicular adenomas. TSH is the single most useful test in the workup for thyroid function, and thyroid uptake scans now have limited utility except in the hyperthyroid patient. Compressive symptoms, which occur from thyroid enlargement and impingement on adjacent structures (trachea, esophagus, and recurrent laryngeal nerve) are indications for surgery. **A patient with a solitary thyroid nodule and a prior history of low-dose head or neck irradiation has a 40% risk of carcinoma.** A family history of thyroid cancer should increase the physician's suspicion of carcinoma in a patient with a thyroid nodule. An estimated 20% to 30% of medullary thyroid cancers occur as part of a familial syndrome, most notably MEN 2A and MEN 2B (Table 44–1). Twenty-five percent of medullary thyroid cancers are familial cancers with the remainder being sporadic.

Table 44–1 • MULTIPLE ENDOCRINE NEOPLASIA
Multiple endocrine neoplasia 2A
• Medullary thyroid cancer
• Pheochromocytoma
• Hyperparathyroidism
• Lichen planus amyloidosis
• Hirschsprung disease
Multiple endocrine neoplasia 2B
• Medullary thyroid cancer
• Pheochromocytoma
• Marfanoid habitus
• Mucosal neuromas
• Ganglioneuromatosis of the gastrointestinal tract

On physical examination, the size and character of the thyroid nodule should be noted. The thyroid gland should be examined for other nodules, and the neck evaluated for associated cervical lymphadenopathy. The presence of associated adenopathy should increase suspicion of malignancy.

The primary challenge in the management of a thyroid nodule is selecting patients with a high risk of cancer for surgery while avoiding operations in patients with benign disease who would not benefit from surgery. Ultrasound is an important adjunct in the workup and management of thyroid nodules.

Nodule characteristics seen by thyroid ultrasound are useful in determining risk of carcinoma and to guide the use of fine needle aspiration biopsy (FNAB). Historically, nuclear scintigraphy (thyroid uptake scan) was a standard part of the workup of thyroid nodules looking for "cold" versus "hot" nodules to assess malignancy risk. With the increased access and improved resolution of thyroid ultrasound, thyroid uptake scans are reserved for patients with thyroid nodules and hyperthyroidism to differentiate a hyperfunctioning nodule from diffuse toxic goiter. **Currently, FNAB is the initial and most important step in the diagnostic evaluation of a dominant thyroid nodule.** Management of nodular thyroid disease is guided by results from the FNAB (Figure 44–1). Thyroidectomy is reserved for patients with progressive nodule enlargement, compressive symptoms, or a malignant FNAB. A cytologic diagnosis of malignancy is very reliable with only a 1% to 2% incidence of false-positive results. Patients with benign FNAB results are followed with a yearly physical examination of the neck and a serum TSH-level test. The incidence of false-negative FNAB results is approximately 2% to 5%.

A cellular FNAB result refers to a specimen with cytologic features consistent with either a follicular or a Hürthle cell neoplasm. A follicular or Hürthle cell carcinoma cannot be distinguished from a follicular or Hürthle cell adenoma using cytologic criteria alone. Diagnosis of carcinoma is based on the presence of capsular or vascular invasion as observed in a tissue sample. Diagnostic thyroid lobectomy is recommended for patients with a cellular FNAB because of the 20% to 30% incidence of carcinoma. If pathology returns as invasive carcinoma, completion thyroidectomy should be performed.

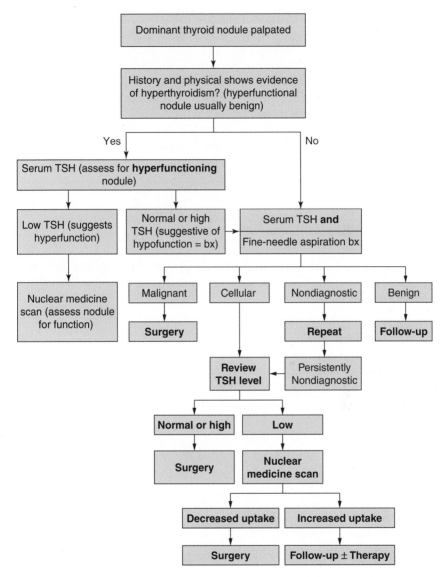

Figure 44–1. Algorithm for the evaluation of patients with a dominant thyroid nodule. Reproduced, from McHenry CR, Sgusarczyk SJ, Askari AT, et al. Refined use of scintigraphy in the evaluation of nodular thyroid disease. *Surgery.* 1998;124:660, with permission from Elsevier.

In patients with nondiagnostic FNAB results, the biopsy should be repeated because an adequate specimen is obtained with a repeated biopsy in more than 50% of patients. Surgery is recommended for patients with a second nondiagnostic FNAB. A 9% incidence of carcinoma has been reported in the subset of patients with a persistently nondiagnostic FNAB results and a hypofunctioning nodule.

Patients with FNA proven thyroid cancers are ideally treated by surgery consisting of total thyroidectomy. The benefits of prophylactic central lymph node dissection remains controversial in papillary and follicular carcinomas because of the marginal benefits and the high-rate of temporary and permanent hypoparathyoidism associated with the procedure. Postoperative radioactive iodine ablation (RAI) is recommended for patients with large primary cancers, metastatic disease, and cancer extension outside of the thyroid gland. Patients with medullary thyroid carcinoma should be screened for MEN2 prior to thyroid surgery, and if a pheochromocytoma is present, it should be treated before the thyroid procedure. A central lymph node dissection is indicated at the time of surgery due to the more aggressive medullary thyroid carcinoma and ineffectiveness of RAI. The prognosis of anaplastic thyroid carcinoma is dismal and involves multimodality palliative treatment with a mean survival of less than 6 months.

COMPREHENSION QUESTIONS

44.1 A 38-year-old woman is noted to have a 1.2 cm thyroid nodule. In which of the following situations would the results of thyroid scintigraphy most likely impact treatment?

A. Fine-needle aspiration biopsy (FNAB) results consistent with a malignant neoplasm

B. FNAB results consistent with a benign neoplasm

C. FNAB results consistent with a follicular neoplasm

D. Prior history of head or neck irradiation

E. FNAB demonstrating nondiagnostic result

44.2 A 40-year-old woman presents with a single thyroid nodule. Which of the following situations would be associated with the highest risk of malignancy?

A. A prior history of head or neck irradiation

B. Hyperfunction of the nodule seen on thyroid scintigraphy

C. Hypofunctioning of the nodule seen on scintigraphy (cold nodule)

D. History of Graves disease

E. The presence of a dominant nodule within a goiter

44.3 A 55-year-old man is noted to have a 1.4-cm nodule in the right thyroid lobe. For which of the following situations is thyroidectomy the best treatment option?

A. Initial nondiagnostic FNAB results

B. Hypothyroidism

C. A mother who had papillary carcinoma

D. FNAB results consistent with a benign neoplasm when compressive symptoms are present

E. Patient has underlying hyperplastic thyroid disease (goiter)

44.4 Which of the following procedures should be performed routinely in a patient with a thyroid nodule who is clinically euthyroid?

A. FNAB and determination of a screening serum TSH level

B. Measurement of radioiodine uptake and thyroid scintiscanning

C. Measure of serum T_4, triiodothyronine (T_3), and TSH levels

D. Ultrasound examination of the thyroid gland to distinguish a solid from a cystic nodule

E. Thyroid scintigraphy

44.5 A 60-year-old man is noted to have a 2-cm nodule in the right lobe of the thyroid. He is asymptomatic, and FNAB has been attempted on three separate occasions demonstrating nondiagnostic findings. Ultrasound has shown a solid thyroid nodule without other abnormalities, and iodine-123 scintigraphy has revealed a nonfunctioning nodule. Which of the following management approaches is most appropriate?

A. Place patient on suppressive dose of levothyroxine and repeat FNA in 3 months

B. Right thyroidectomy

C. Place patient on suppressive dose of levothyroxine and repeat ultrasound in 3 months

D. Total thyroidectomy with central neck dissection

E. Ethanol injection of the nodule under ultrasound guidance

44.6 A 52-year-old woman with a history of asymptomatic carotid stenosis undergoes follow-up ultrasound of the neck that revealed stable stenosis of the carotid and an incidental finding of several solid and fluid-filled nodules seen in both lobes of the thyroid gland. The largest of these nodules measure 0.3 cm in diameter. Her serum TSH is within the normal range. Which of the following is the most appropriate management for this patient?

A. Total thyroidectomy

B. I^{131}-radioablation of the thyroid

C. Observation

D. Placement on suppressive dose of levothyroxine

E. Aspiration of the fluid-filled nodules

ANSWERS

44.1 **C.** Radionuclide scanning can determine the function of the nodule. With a fine-needle aspirate showing a follicular pattern, a "cold" hypofunctioning pattern is associated with a significant risk of cancer (20%-35%), whereas a "warm or hot" functioning pattern is associated with a low (1%) risk of cancer.

44.2 **A.** A history of head and neck irradiation greatly increases the risk of a thyroid nodule being malignant. A cold nonfunctioning nodule increases the risk of cancer, but not as significantly as the history of irradiation. Dominant nodules arising from a goiter do not have an increased risk of being cancerous; however, a clinical diagnosis based on the physical examination can be difficult because of the background abnormality.

44.3 **D.** Compressive symptoms can become life threatening; therefore, urgent surgical intervention is considered the best therapy.

44.4 **A.** FNAB and a TSH level test for the assessment of thyroid function and determination of the histology of the lesion are the two most important initial tests for evaluating a thyroid nodule.

44.5 **B.** Right thyroidectomy is an appropriate option for this patient because an overall cancer rate of 9% has been reported for this population. Thyroxine suppression would not change the fact that this is a nonfunctioning nodule. Total thyroidectomy is not indicated since a diagnosis is not yet ascertained. Ethanol injection is a reasonable option for the ablation of recurrent, benign thyroid cysts. However, this is not an appropriate treatment for a nodule of unknown significance.

44.6 **C.** Thyroid nodules less than 1 cm in diameter are common findings in women, and most of these are of no clinical consequences, do not progress, and have low probability of being malignant. The probability of cancer in this patient is further reduced because there are multiple nodules seen. Observation with repeat ultrasound is generally appropriate for these patients.

CLINICAL PEARLS

▶ FNAB is the initial and most important step in the diagnostic evaluation of a dominant thyroid nodule and guides subsequent management

▶ The role of thyroid uptake scans has been replaced by ultrasound but may be useful in the setting of thyroid nodules in the hyperthyroid patient.

▶ A patient with a prior history of neck irradiation or a family history consistent with MEN syndromes has a high risk of thyroid cancer.

▶ Indications for surgical removal are compressive symptoms, functioning nodules, or suspicion of malignancy (history, size, growth, ultrasound characteristics, FNA findings)

▶ Papillary and follicular thyroid carcinomas are treated with total thyroidectomy with postoperative RAI in high-risk patients. Prophylactic central neck dissection is controversial.

▶ Initial treatment of a follicular neoplasm is a diagnostic thyroid lobectomy to look for invasive carcinoma which cannot be determined by FNA biopsy.

▶ Medullary thyroid carcinoma is associated with familial genetic syndromes in 25% of cases. MEN2 or pheochromocytoma should be assessed prior to thyroidectomy in patients with MTC.

REFERENCES

Cooper DS, Doherty GM, Haugen Br, et al. Revised American Thyroid Association management guidelines for patients with thyroid nodules and differentiated thyroid cancer. *Thyroid.* 2009;19: 1167-1214.

Lal G, Clark OH. Thyroid, parathyroid, and adrenal. In: Brunicardi FC, Andersen DK, Billiar TR, Dunn DL, Hunter JG, Mathews JB, Pollock RE, eds. *Schwartz's Principles of Surgery.* 9th ed. New York, NY: McGraw-Hill; 2010:1343-1407.

Mittendorf EA, McHenry CR. Management of thyroid nodules. In: Cameron JL, ed. *Current Surgical Therapy.* 9th ed. Philadelphia, PA: Mosby Elsevier; 2008:602-608.

A 43-year-old woman was found to have an elevated serum calcium during a cardiac workup for fatigue. The results of her physical examination were unremarkable, and no cardiac abnormalities were identified. On routine blood work during the evaluation, she was noted to have a serum calcium level of 11.8 mg/dL (8.4-10.4 mg/dL), a phosphate level of 1.9 mg/dL (2.5-4.8 mg/dL), and a chloride level of 104 mmol/L (95-109 mmol/L).

▶ What is the most likely cause of this patient's hypercalcemia?
▶ How would you confirm the diagnosis?
▶ What is the most appropriate therapy?

ANSWERS TO CASE 45:

Hyperparathyroidism

Summary: A 43-year-old woman is found to have incidental hypercalcemia and hypophosphatemia.

- **Cause of hypercalcemia:** Primary hyperparathyroidism.

- **Confirmation of diagnosis:** An elevated serum parathyroid hormone (PTH) level and the absence of a familial pattern of hypocalciuric hypercalcemia.

- **Treatment:** The treatment for primary hyperparathyroidism is surgical removal of the offending gland(s) assuming that the patient is an acceptable surgical candidate.

ANALYSIS

Objectives

1. Formulate a differential diagnosis for hypercalcemia.

2. Describe the diagnosis and treatment of primary hyperparathyroidism.

3. Appreciate the natural history and long-term consequences of untreated primary hyperparathyroidism.

Considerations

In the ambulatory setting, primary hyperparathyroidism is by far the most common cause of hypercalcemia, while malignancy is the most common cause in hospitalized patients. In this patient, the chloride/phosphate ratio is greater than 33:1, suggestive of hyperparathyroidism. The diagnosis can be confirmed by an elevated serum PTH and 24-hour urinary calcium measurement demonstrating normal or increased calcium excretion. For this 43-year-old woman, localization and surgical exploration are warranted if the serum PTH and urinary calcium levels confirm primary hyperparathyroidism, then localization and surgical exploration are warranted.

APPROACH TO:

Hypercalcemia and Hyperparathyroidism

DEFINITIONS

PRIMARY HYPERPARATHYROIDISM: A disorder of elevated parathyroid function caused by the hyperfunctioning of one or more parathyroid glands. The most common cause is a sporadic single parathyroid adenoma, followed by parathyroid hyperplasia, and rarely parathyroid carcinoma.

FAMILIAL HYPOCALCIURIC HYPERCALCEMIA: A condition of mild elevations of serum calcium. Most cases are associated with mutations in the Calcium Sensing Receptor gene. Diagnosis is confirmed with low 24-hour urine calcium levels. FHH is benign and does not require treatment.

PARATHYROID ADENOMA: A benign tumor of the parathyroid gland. It is the most common cause of primary hyperparathyroidism which is usually a sporadic, single hyperfunctioning gland that has resulted from a clonal mutation. Treatment is operative removal.

PARATHYROID HYPERPLASIA: A condition of diffuse enlargement of all 4 parathyroid glands. The result is elevated parathyroid hormone and serum calcium levels. It may occur sporadically or as part of a familial syndrome.

PARATHYROID CARCINOMA: A rare neuroendocrine tumor of the parathyroid gland. The usual presentation is that of primary hyperparathyroidism with higher serum calcium levels or an associated neck mass. Treatment is en bloc removal with the ipsilateral thyroid lobe and adjacent tissue.

CLINICAL APPROACH

The differential diagnosis for hypercalcemia is extensive (Table 45–1). Primary hyperparathyroidism and malignancies account for 90% of all causes of hypercalcemia. In the ambulatory setting, 50% to 60% of all cases of hypercalcemia are caused by primary hyperparathyroidism. Hypercalcemia is the hallmark of primary hyperparathyroidism. Patients may also have a low or low-normal serum phosphorus level, a high or high-normal serum chloride level, and mild metabolic acidosis. This is a result of the inhibitory effects of PTH on the reabsorption of phosphorus

---

Table 45–1 • DIFFERENTIAL DIAGNOSIS FOR HYPERCALCEMIA

Hyperparathyroidism
• Primary, tertiary (result of autonomous parathyroid function that develops in patients with long-standing secondary hyperparathyroidism, usually after improvement of chronic renal failure after renal transplantation)

Malignancy
• Pseudo-hyperparathyroidism (secretion of parathyroid hormone-related peptide by renal cell carcinoma, squamous cell carcinoma of the lung, carcinoma of the urinary bladder), hematologic malignancies (multiple myeloma, lymphoma, leukemia)

Other endocrine disorders
• Hyperthyroidism, hypothyroidism, adrenal insufficiency, pheochromocytoma, VIPoma

Granulomatous diseases
• Tuberculosis, sarcoidosis, fungal infection, leprosy

Exogenous agents
• Calcium, vitamin D, vitamin A, thiazide diuretics, lithium, milk alkali

Other etiologies
• Immobilization
• Paget disease
• Familial hypocalciuric hypercalcemia (an autosomal dominant disorder characterized by hypercalcemia, hypocalciuria, none of the complications of hypercalcemia, and a urinary calcium clearance of <0.010 mmol/24 h)

and bicarbonate in the renal tubule. Because of the increased excretion of bicarbonate, additional chloride is reabsorbed with sodium to maintain electroneutrality. A **chloride-to-phosphorus ratio of greater than 33:1 is consistent with a diagnosis of primary hyperparathyroidism.** In malignancy related hypercalcemia, phosphate may also be low or normal, but chloride is generally normal. Other causes of hypercalcemia are usually associated with normal to elevated phosphate levels.

The definitive diagnosis of hyperparathyroidism is made by documenting an elevated serum intact PTH levels. With the exception of familial hypocalciuric hypercalcemia which may be associated with a mild increase in serum PTH levels, all other causes of hypercalcemia are associated with suppressed PTH levels. Primary hyperparathyroidism is differentiated from familial hypocalciuric hypercalcemia by 24-hour urine calcium measurements.

Most patients with primary hyperparathyroidism are diagnosed after incidental hypercalcemia is detected on routine blood testing. The clinical manifestations of primary hyperparathyroidism are variable (Table 45–2). Most patients admit to nonspecific symptoms such as weakness, fatigue, irritability, or constipation. Kidney stones are the most common metabolic complication, occurring in 15% to 20% of patients with primary hyperparathyroidism. The potential development of skeletal manifestations such as generalized demineralization, osteoporosis, and pathologic fractures are of particular concern for postmenopausal women. Gastrointestinal manifestations include peptic ulcer disease and pancreatitis. Patients may experience joint manifestations related to gout or pseudogout, as well as a wide variety of psychiatric symptoms. Hyperparathyroidism is also associated with well-described cardiovascular effects including an increased prevalence of hypertension, left ventricular hypertrophy, and calcification of the myocardium and the mitral and aortic valves.

A **hypercalcemic crisis** may occur in 1.6% to 3.2% of patients with primary hyperparathyroidism. It manifests with marked hypercalcemia, with serum calcium levels usually >15 mg/dL and an altered mental status. Patients may present with nausea, vomiting, dehydration, lethargy, and confusion or frank coma. **Treatment of hypercalcemic crises consists of hydration and forced diuresis with normal saline infusion and furosemide administration.** Saline reduces serum calcium by blocking the proximal tubule calcium absorption while furosemide blocks distal tubule calcium absorption.

Long-Term Effects

Untreated hyperparathyroidism reduces patient survival by approximately 10% when compared to age- and gender-matched control subjects without hyperparathyroidism. This increased risk for premature death is primarily related to cardiovascular disease, for which surgical parathyroidectomy can alter the progression.

Indications and Preparation for Parathyroidectomy

The definitive treatment for primary hyperparathyroidism is parathyroidectomy. Patients with symptoms should be referred for parathyroidectomy. The guidelines from the Fourth International Workshop on asymptomatic primary hyperparathyroidism identified any of the following criteria as an indication for surgery: age less than 50 years old, serum calcium levels greater than 1.0 mg/dL above the normal limit, 24-hour urine calcium >400mg/d, creatinine clearance <60 ml/min,

Table 45-2 • CLINICAL MANIFESTATIONS OF PRIMARY HYPERPARATHYROIDISM	
Symptoms	**Metabolic Conditions**

Skeletal
  Bone pain
  Pathologic fractures
  Joint pain
  Joint swelling
	Osteitis fibrosacystica
	Osteopenia
	Osteoporosis
	Gout
	Pseudogout
	Hyperuricemia

Renal
  Colic
  Hematuria
  Polyuria
  Polydipsia
  Nocturia
	Nephrolithiasis
	Nephrocalcinosis
	Hypercalciuria
	Reduced creatinine clearance

Gastrointestinal
  Constipation
  Abdominal pain
  Nausea
  Vomiting
	Peptic ulcer disease
	Pancreatitis

Psychiatric
  Lethargy
  Memory loss
  Confusion
  Hallucinations
  Delusions
	Depression
	Psychosis
	Coma

Neuromuscular
  Fatigue
  Muscle weakness
  Malaise	

Cardiovascular	Hypertension Left ventricular hypertrophy Heart block Cardiac calcifications

Dermatologic
  Brittle nails
  Pruritus	

nephrolithiasis, or osteoporosis (DXA T-score < -2.5 at lumbar spine, total hip, femoral neck, or distal 1/3 radius), or vertebral fracture. (see Table 45–3). Because parathyroidectomy may improve the vague nonspecific symptoms and render survival benefits in patients with primary hyperparathyroidism, many experts advise that in the absence of prohibitive operative risk, all patients with primary hyperparathyroidism be treated with parathyroidectomy.

Surgical Treatment

The etiology of primary hyperparathyroidism is most commonly parathyroid adenoma (85%-96%), followed by hyperplasia (4%-15%) and carcinoma (1%). Surgical

Table 45-3 • FOURTH INTERNATIONAL WORKSHOP GUIDELINES FOR THE MANAGEMENT OF ASYMPTOMATIC PRIMARY HYPERPARATHYROIDISM
• Age < 50   • Markedly elevated serum calcium (>1.0 mg/dL above upper limit of normal)   • Creatinine clearance <60 ml/min   • 24-hour urine calcium >400 mg/d   • Presence of nephrolithiasis or nephrocalcinosis detected by imaging   • Osteoporosis as determined by direct measurement (dual energy x-ray absorptiometry *T*-score   <-2.5)   • Vertebral fracture

management addresses removal of offending glands and is based on the location and number of abnormal parathyroids. The 2002 NIH Consensus Workshop recommended that all patients under consideration for parathyroidectomy undergo preoperative localization studies to assist in operative planning and to determine the feasibility of minimally invasive parathyroidectomy or unilateral explorations. The preferred localization modality varies based on local expertise and technological availability. The most commonly utilized localization modalities are ultrasonography, nuclear imaging (sestamibi), CT, and MRI. When patients have biochemically documented primary hyperparathyroidism and nonlocalized pathology by preoperative imaging, there is a higher probability parathyroid hyperplasia exists. These individuals may require more extensive parathyroid explorations, subtotal parathyroidectomy, and have a lower chance of cure. It is important to have more extensive discussions of risks and benefits prior to the planning surgery in these patients.

With unilateral parathyroid exploration or the minimally invasive approach, intraoperative parathyroid hormone assay is generally used to verify removal of the parathyroid gland responsible for hyperparathyroidism. Published results show that a greater than 95% cure rate can be expected for primary hyperparathyroidism when parathyroid exploration is performed by an experienced surgeon after obtaining appropriate preoperative evaluations and localization studies.

COMPREHENSION QUESTIONS

45.1 A 60-year-old postmenopausal woman with osteoporosis has a serum calcium level of 11.4 mg/dL, a serum phosphorus level of 2.0 mg/dL, and a 24-hour urine calcium excretion of 425 mg. Which of the following serum tests is most likely to establish the cause of her hypercalcemia?

A. Chloride/phosphorus ratio

B. PTH-related polypeptide

C. Urine calcium clearance

D. Intact PTH level

E. A sestimibi scan

45.2 You are asked to evaluate a patient in the hospital with hypercalcemia. A diagnosis of hyperparathyroidism has been excluded. Which of the following is the most likely cause?

A. Familial hypocalciuric hypercalcemia

B. Sarcoidosis

C. Induced by medication

D. Nephrogenic diabetes insipidus

E. Malignancy

45.3 Which of the following is the most common metabolic complication of primary hyperparathyroidism?

A. Kidney stones

B. Osteoporosis

C. Pancreatitis

D. Gout

E. Hyperthyroidism

45.4 Which of the following abnormalities is most likely to be caused by hyperparathyroidism?

A. Hypocalciuria

B. Hyperphosphatemia

C. Hyperchloremia

D. Elevated serum bicarbonate

E. Elevated serum creatinine

45.5 A 49-year-old woman with primary hyperparathyroidism has severe symptoms. Preoperative imaging fails to localize an abnormal gland. What is the best treatment for this patient?

A. No intervention

B. Medical management with cinacalcet

C. Unilateral parathyroid exploration

D. Total parathyroidectomy

E. Total parathyroidectomy with partial parathyroid reimplantation

45.6 During parathyroid exploration for a 36-year-old woman with primary hyperparathyroidism, you see an enlarged inferior parathyroid gland which appears to be adhered to the thyroid gland and surrounding soft tissue. What is your next step in management?

A. Left inferior parathyroidectomy

B. En-bloc left parathyroidectomy and thyroid lobectomy with removal of adjacent soft tissue

C. Total parathyroidectomy

D. Modified radical neck dissection

E. Radical neck dissection

ANSWERS

45.1 **D.** An intact PTH level is highly specific for hyperparathyroidism. A chloride/phosphorus ratio greater than 33:1 is only suggestive of hyperparathyroidism, while an elevated PTH is confirmatory. A sestimibi scan is a localization study most useful to localize the parathyroid adenoma prior to operative resection.

45.2 **E.** Malignancy is the most common cause of hypercalcemia encountered in patients in the in-patient setting, particularly when hyperparathyroidism is ruled out. Familial hypocalciuric hypercalcemia, medications, and sarcoidosis are all less common causes of hypercalcemia. Nephrogenic diabetes insipidus is not a cause of hypercalcemia but can be seen in patients with hyperparathyroidism, as increased serum calcium inhibits the kidneys' response to antidiuretic hormone.

45.3 **A.** Kidney stones are the most common metabolic complication associated with hyperparathyroidism, occurring in 15% to 20% of patients with the disease.

45.4 **C.** Hyperparathyroidism is associated with a high secretion of calcium in urine (hypercalcinuria), low serum phosphate, high serum chloride, and low serum bicarbonate levels. Increased serum creatinine is generally not seen in patients with primary hyperparathyroidism unless there is damage to the kidneys from long-standing nephrocalcinosis. Elevated creatinine or chronic renal insufficiency causes increased serum phosphorous and lead to the increase in PTH levels (secondary hyperparathyroidism).

45.5 **E.** This patient with nonlocalized primary hyperparathyroidism likely has parathyroid hyperplasia. The procedures of choice are subtotal parathyroidectomy (3½ gland removal) or total parathyroidectomy with forearm reimplantation of ½ of a gland to prevent postoperative hypoparathyroidism.

45.6 **B.** A locally infiltrating parathyroid gland represents parathyroid carcinoma. Surgical treatment involves unilateral parathyroidectomy, and thyroid lobectomy with en-bloc resection of adjacent lymph nodes and soft tissue to prevent recurrence.

CLINICAL PEARLS

▶ Hypercalcemia with hypophosphatemia is suggestive of hyperparathyroidism. The diagnosis is confirmed by an elevated PTH level.

▶ The two most common causes of hypercalcemia are hyperparathyroidism and malignancy in the outpatient and inpatient settings, respectively.

▶ Surgical indications for primary hyperparathyroidism include presence of symptoms, age less than 50, markedly elevated serum calcium or a hypercalcemic crisis, kidney stones, or osteoporosis. The best treatment for primary hyperparathyroidism is surgical parathyroidectomy.

▶ Support for parathyroidectomy in an asymptomatic patient is based on the increase in cardiovascular complications and 10% survival reduction associated with patients with untreated primary hyperparathyroidism. This survival advantage is most notable in younger patients (age < 50).

▶ Preoperative localization is recommended to limit the extent of the operating and to determine the likelihood of cure prior to surgery

▶ Causes of primary hyperparathyroidism include adenoma, hyperplasia, and carcinoma which are surgically treated by parathyroidectomy, 3½ gland removal, or en-bloc ipsilateral removal with thyroid lobectomy, respectively.

▶ Intraoperative parathyroid hormone management can be used to confirm removal of hyperfunctioning parathyroid glands and to determine the extent of exploration

REFERENCES

Ambrogini E, Cetani F, Cianferotti L, et al. Surgery or surveillance for mild asymptomatic primary hyperparathyroidism: a prospective, randomized clinical trial. *J Clin Endocrinol Metab.* 2007;92:3114-21.

Biliezikian JP, Brandi ML, Eastel R, et al. Guidelines for the management of asymptomatic primary hyperparathyroidism: statement from the fourth international workshop. *J Clin Endocrinol Metab.* 2014;99:3561-3569.

Caron NR, Pasieka JL. What symptom improvements can be expected after operation for primary hyperparathyroidism? *World J Surg.* 2009;33:2244-2255.

Chen H. Primary hyperparathyroidism. In: Cameron JL, Cameron AM, eds. *Current Surgical Therapy.* 10th ed. Philadelphia, PA: Mosby Elsevier; 2011:610-613.

A 37-year-old nurse complains of a 3-year history of intermittent palpitations, irritability, shakiness, nausea, and diaphoresis, which have worsened in the past 6 months. Her symptoms are worse in the morning and at the end of her work shifts, but seem to improve after eating. She has no significant past medical history. The results of her physical examination are unremarkable, but she has an isolated serum glucose of 44 mg/dL.

▶ What is the most likely diagnosis?
▶ How would you confirm the diagnosis?
▶ What are the main considerations in the treatment of this condition?

ANSWERS TO CASE 46:

Insulinoma and Pancreatic Endocrine Neoplasm

Summary: A 37-year-old healthcare worker has symptoms consistent with hypoglycemia that resolve with ingestion of food in the absence of physical exam abnormalities.

- **Most likely diagnosis:** Insulinoma is very likely with this constellation of symptoms that worsens with fasting and improves with ingestion of glucose.

- **Confirmation of diagnosis:** 72-hour fasting glucose levels demonstrate low blood sugars with onset of symptoms. C-peptide levels are elevated suggesting endogenous overproduction of insulin.

ANALYSIS

Objectives

1. Recognize the constellation of clinical signs and symptoms of functional pancreatic endocrine neoplasms.

2. Understand the diagnosis and management principles of pancreatic endocrine neoplasms.

Considerations

This 37-year-old nurse has symptoms of hypoglycemia, which is confirmed with a markedly low serum glucose level. Because of the numerous nonspecific symptoms caused by low blood sugar, many patients are incorrectly clinically diagnosed with hypoglycemia. The signs and symptoms include shakiness, nervousness, irritability, hunger, diaphoresis, clumsiness, lightheadedness, weakness, and confusion. Sequelae of hypoglycemia can be severe and may result in seizures, coma, and death.

Whipple's triad endorses a hyperinsulinemic cause of hypoglycemia. Once hypoglycemia has been confirmed, etiologies should be determined to facilitate immediate therapy. The most common cause is the use of oral diabetes mellitus medications such as sulfonylureas. Among the many causes of low blood sugar, exogenous administration of insulin must be ruled out in the workup of a low-serum glucose.

The diagnosis of an insulinoma is confirmed through biochemical workup which may require a 72-hour fast. Results reveal a blood glucose below 50 mg/dL in the setting of elevated insulin and C-peptide levels. Elevated insulin with normal C-peptide levels indicate exogenous use of insulin, and patients should be checked for use of oral hypoglycemic agents which can result in high insulin levels and low serum glucose. Following confirmation of the diagnosis of an insulinoma, localization and staging are performed to determine the multidisciplinary treatment plan. Treatment may be multimodal and is based on the extent and location of disease.

APPROACH TO:
Pancreatic Endocrine Neoplasm

DEFINITIONS

PANCREATIC ENDOCRINE NEOPLASM (PEN): This describes a rare tumor of multipotent endocrine pancreatic stem cells that are classified by size, mitotic rate, or the presence or absence of a syndrome due to hormone production.

INSULINOMA: The most common functional neoplasm of the endocrine pancreas. It associated with Whipple's triad. Insulinomas arise equally in all parts of the pancreas. They have a low malignant potential but may be multifocal.

GASTRINOMA: PEN linked to elevated serum gastrin levels, peptic ulcer disease, and diarrhea. The majority are located in the gastrinoma triangle (junction of the cystic duct and common bile duct, 2nd to 3rd portion of the duodenum, junction of head and neck of pancreas).

GLUCAGONOMA: PEN most commonly associated with severe migratory dermatitis, diabetes mellitus, stomatitis, and anemia.

SOMATOSTATINOMA: This is the least common of the five generally accepted functional pancreatic endocrine neoplasm syndromes. Clinical manifestations include diabetes, cholelithiasis, steatorrhea, hypochlorhydria, and obstructive jaundice.

VIPOMA: This is PEN associated with episodic WDHA syndrome (watery diarrhea hypokalemia achlorhydria).

NON-FUNCTIONING PEN: The majority of pancreatic endocrine neoplasms are not associated with a defined clinical syndrome or hormonal elevations.

MULTIPLE ENDOCRINE NEOPLASIA 1 (MEN 1): This is an autosomal dominant genetic syndrome that includes pancreatic endocrine neoplasia, parathyroid hyperplasia, and pituitary adenoma.

WHIPPLE'S TRIAD: This describes three criteria that confirm a hyperinsulinemic cause of hypoglycemic symptoms. In this triad, a patient must demonstrate (1) symptoms consistent with hypoglycemia, (2) low plasma glucose measured at the time of symptoms, and (3) resolution of symptoms when glucose levels are corrected.

CLINICAL APPROACH

Pathogenesis and Clinical Presentation

Pancreatic endocrine neoplasms (PEN) account for 1% of pancreatic neoplasms. The etiology has not been fully elucidated but the former use of the term islet cell tumor has been replaced by PEN or PNET.

The best classification of PENs is under debate, but more recent systems such as the that proposed by the World Health Organization in 2010 are based on mitotic rate or size of the tumor. They can be further classified as functional or nonfunctional based on whether an associated clinical syndrome of hormonal secretion is present. Functional PENs are named after the hormone of interest while nonfunctional PENs now account for the majority of cases.

Although most often sporadic, PENs may be associated with familial genetic syndromes such as Multiple Endocrine Neoplasia 1, von Hippel-Lindau syndrome, neurofibromatosis 1, and tuberous sclerosis. Inherited familial syndromes in the setting of PENs may affect disease, prognosis, and treatment patterns.

Diagnosis

Pancreatic endocrine neoplasms present primarily as incidental findings on imaging, as an obstructive pancreatic mass, or by a constellation of symptoms associated with the pancreatic endocrine overproduction. The five generally recognized syndromes with PENs are insulinoma, gastrinoma, glucagonoma, VIPoma, and somatostatinoma. Diagnoses are generally obtained by combination of characteristic clinical syndromes and detection of hormone elevations.

Workup

Preoperative imaging has become an integral component of the workup and management of pancreatic endocrine neoplasms. Although there is no single best modality for the various types of lesions, the preferred initial imaging technique is a high-resolution computed tomography scan. Multiphase CT is accurate in detecting primary pancreatic endocrine neoplasms and in assessing the size, anatomy, and presence or absence of hepatic metastases. Alternative techniques include magnetic resonance imaging, somatostatin receptor scintigraphy, endoscopic and intraoperative ultrasound, or venous sampling.

Treatment

Therapeutics for PENs depend on the type of neoplasm, malignant potential, and staging, but is often surgical. Patients with localized tumors are candidates for resection for cure. For patient with even unresectable disease, surgery may be performed to limit symptoms, and PENs are one of the few tumors for which a survival advantage can be obtained through surgical debulking. Multimodality treatment includes the use of surgery, ablative procedures, chemotherapy, and biotherapeutics.

CASE CORRELATION

- See also Case 47 (Thymoma and Myasthenia Gravis).

COMPREHENSION QUESTIONS

46.1 A 28-year-old nurse is found in the nursing break room and is confused and shaky. Her fasting blood glucose is 42 mg/dL, C-peptide and urine sulfonylureas are normal. What is your next step in management of this patient?

A. CT scan of the abdomen

B. Cessation of diabetes mellitus medications

C. Endoscopic ultrasound

D. Psychiatric evaluation

E. 72-hour fast

46.2 The CT scan of a 59-year-old man with a metastatic pancreatic endocrine neoplasm reveals nonresectable large hepatic masses in the right and left lobes. Which of the following therapies is most useful in his treatment?

A. Total hepatectomy

B. Liver transplant

C. Radiofrequency ablation of liver lesions

D. Platinum-based chemotherapy

E. No effective treatments are available

46.3 A 63-year-old man has a long history of peptic ulcer disease despite maximal doses of gastric acid suppression medications and a surgical acid-reduction surgery. How do you obtain the diagnosis?

A. Secretin stimulation test

B. Urinary pancreatic polypeptide

C. Octreotide scan

D. Venous sampling

E. MRI

46.4 A 43-year-old woman with a known pancreatic mass returns to the office with high blood sugars, foul smelling stools, and gallstone related pain. What is the most likely diagnosis?

A. Insulinoma

B. Gastrinoma

C. Glucagonoma

D. VIPoma

E. Somatostatinoma

46.5 A 72-year-old woman has been seen by numerous specialists for an erythematous rash that has migrated from the groin to the buttocks and abdomen. She is noted to also have recent onset hyperglycemia. What is the most likely diagnosis?

    A. Insulinoma

    B. Gastrinoma

    C. Glucagonoma

    D. VIPoma

    E. Somatostatinoma

46.6 A 49-year-old woman with a history of previous pancreatic surgery has a return of intermittent voluminous diarrhea. Her stool sample is negative for ova and parasites, but her chemistry reveals a low potassium. What is the most likely diagnosis?

    A. Insulinoma

    B. Gastrinoma

    C. Glucagonoma

    D. VIPoma

    E. Somatostatinoma

ANSWERS

46.1 **D.** This healthcare worker has a factitious disorder, and she has been injecting insulin. The normal C-peptide indicates an exogenous source of insulin rather than an insulinoma. Normal sulfonylureas rule out diabetes medications as a cause. Workup includes workup to determine the reasons behind the use of insulin.

46.2 **C.** Up to 75% of endocrine neoplasms develop metastases to the liver depending on type. Surgical resection is the treatment of choice when feasible but is not indicated with extensive bilobar disease. Radiofrequency ablation of liver lesions provides symptomatic relief in a large percentage of patients with adequate survival.

46.3 **A.** Gastrinoma or Zollinger-Ellison syndrome frequently presents with diarrhea and refractory peptic ulcer disease. Failure to improve despite surgical antiulcer surgery should prompt workup. Gastrin levels greater than 1000 pg/mL or a rise of over 200 pg/mL above the basal level on secretin stimulation test support a diagnosis of gastrinoma.

46.4 **D.** The steatorrhea, diabetes, and cholelithiasis suggest a somatostatinoma and the overall slowing of gastrointestinal function.

46.5 **C.** Necrolytic migratory erythema, diabetes, anemia, stomatitis, and weight loss are the classic presentation of a glucagonoma.

46.6 **D.** The constellation of watery diarrhea, hypokalemia, achlorhydria, acidosis (WDHA) is suggestive of a VIPoma (Verner-Morrison syndrome).

CLINICAL PEARLS

▶ Pancreatic endocrine neoplasms are a group of tumors that have functional capacity and malignant and metastatic potential.

▶ Initial localization with CT helps assess anatomy and extent of PENs.

▶ Insulinomas present with Whipple's triad with high C-peptide and normal levels of sulfonylurea.

▶ Gastrinoma should be in the differential for patients with refractory peptic ulcer disease.

▶ Common glucagonoma findings are a characteristic migratory erythematous rash, diabetes, stomatitis, and anemia.

▶ VIPoma presents with a classic syndrome of watery diarrhea, hypokalemia, and achlorhydria.

▶ The clinical syndrome of steatorrhea, cholelithiasis, and diabetes may represent the rare somatostatinoma.

REFERENCES

Kennedy E, Brody J, Yeo C. Neoplasms of the endocrine pancreas. In: Mulholland et al., eds. *Greenfield's Surgery: Scientific Principles & Practice.* 5th ed. Lippincott Williams & Wilkins. 2011.

Klimstra DS, Modlin IR, Coppola D, et al. The pathologic classification of neuroendocrine tumors: a review of nomenclature, grading, and staging systems. *Pancreas.* 2010;39(6):707-712.

Mathur A, Gorden P, Libutti S. Insulinoma. *Surg Clin North Am.* 2009;89:1105-1121.

Niederle B, Happel B, Kurtaran A, O'Toole D, Schima W. Pancreatic imaging: the value for surgery of neuroendocrine pancreatic tumors. In: Hubbard, Inabnet, Lo, eds. *Endocrine Surgery: Principles and Practice.* Philadelphia: Springer; 2009.

Oberg K. Pancreatic endocrine tumors. *Semin Oncol.* 2010;37:594-618.

A 44-year-old woman is found to have an incidental anterior mediastinal mass as revealed by a pre-employment chest radiograph. The patient has no known medical problems, and she denies respiratory or gastrointestinal symptoms. On examination, she is found to have mild bilateral ptosis and no neck masses. The results of the cardiopulmonary examination are unremarkable, and there is no generalized lymphadenopathy. The neurologic examination reveals normal sensation and diminished muscle strength in all of her extremities with repetitive motion against resistance. A CT scan of the chest shows the presence of a 4.5-cm well-circumscribed solid mass in the anterior mediastinum.

▶ What is the most likely diagnosis?
▶ What is the best therapy?

ANSWERS TO CASE 47:

Anterior Mediastinal Mass and Myasthenia Gravis

Summary: A 44-year-old woman has a 4.5-cm well-circumscribed anterior mediastinal mass and symptoms suggestive of myasthenia gravis (MG).

- **Most likely diagnosis:** An incidentally identified thymoma in a patient with class IIA MG.

- **Best therapy:** The best treatment for thymoma is complete excision.

ANALYSIS

1. Know the pathogenesis and medical management of MG.

2. Learn the role of thymectomy in the treatment of MG, with and without the presence of thymoma.

3. Learn the strategies for diagnosing anterior mediastinal masses.

Considerations

This patient presents with an incidentally discovered anterior mediastinal mass. She is noted on physical examination to exhibit muscle fatigue with repetitive movements, which is consistent with the diagnosis of MG. MG is a disorder of the neuromuscular junction associated with the loss of nicotinic receptors due to autoimmune damage of the receptors. Symptoms of MG include weakness that worsens after exercise and improves after rest. Other symptoms may include ptosis, diplopia, dysarthria, dysphagia, and respiratory fatigue. The diagnoses can be tentatively made on the basis of history and physical examination, and the diagnosis can be confirmed by provocative testing (Edrophonium-Tensilon test). The Myasthenia Gravis Foundation of America (MGFA) Clinical classification is a commonly used system to characterize the neurologic dysfunction in patients with MG (Table 47–1). The medical management for this patient will depend on her responses to treatment from the various pharmacologic options that include anticholinesterase drugs, glucocorticoids (prednisone), intravenous immune globlin G (IVIG), immunosuppressive drugs (azathioprine, cylcophosphamide, and tacrolimus), and plasmapheresis. Thymomas are present in about 50% of the patients with MG, and thymectomy improves symptoms of MG in up to 60% of the patients with MG, with symptom improvements occurring over extended periods of time (months). Some of the potential benefits of thymectomy in MG patients include reduction in episodes of symptoms exacerbation, reduction in maintenance medications usage, and improved possibility of long-term remissions.

Because of the multiple options available for the treatment of MG, it is important that these patients be managed in a multidisciplinary fashion, where management decisions take into consideration the severity of the baseline illness, severity of the flare-ups (crisis), benefits of thymectomy, and the medical management of the patient in the perioperative period.

Table 47–1 • MG FOUNDATION OF AMERICA (MGFA) CLASSIFICATION FOR MYASTHENIA GRAVIS SEVERITY

Class	Symptoms
I	Any *ocular muscle weakness* with all other muscle strengths being normal
IIa	*Mild muscle weakness* predominantly affects limb and/or axial muscles. May have lesser involvement of oropharyngeal muscles
IIb	*Mild muscle weakness* predominantly affecting oropharyngeal and/or respiratory muscles. May have lesser involvement of limb and/or axial muscles
IIIa	*Moderate muscle weakness* predominantly affecting limb and/or axial muscles and may have lesser involvement of oropharyngeal muscles
IIIb	*Moderate muscle weakness* predominantly affecting oropharyngeal and/or respiratory muscles. May also have lesser involvement of limb and/or axial muscles
IVa	Severe weakness involving predominantly limbs, axial muscles, or both. May have lesser oropharyngeal involvement.
IVb	Severe weakness predominantly affecting oropharyngeal and/or respiratory muscles. May have lesser or equal limb and/or axial involvement, or needing feeding tube but without need for intubation.
V	Requiring intubation with/without mechanical ventilation, except when requiring support in the postoperative setting only.

APPROACH TO:
Anterior Mediastinal Mass and Myasthenia Gravis

DEFINITIONS

MYASTHENIA GRAVIS: An uncommon autoimmune disorder of the peripheral nerves in which antibodies form against the acetylcholine (Ach) nicotinic post-synaptic receptors at the myoneural junction. A reduction in the number of Ach receptors results in progressive reduction in muscle strength with repeat usage of the muscles. In addition, the recovery following muscle usage is delayed. The eye muscles tend to be affected early on to produce ptosis and diplopia. A subset of patients with MG harbor antibodies against muscle-specific receptor tyrosine kinase (MuSK).

THYMOMA: This is the most common anterior mediastinal tumor in patients over the age of 40.

WHO CLASSIFICATIONS FOR THYMIC EPITHELIAL NEOPLASMS: (listed in order from best-to-worst prognosis) Type A is medullary thymoma; Type AB (mixed thymoma); Type B1 is predominantly cortical thymoma; Type B2 is cortical thymoma; Type B3 is a well-differentiated thymic carcinoma; Type C is thymic carcinoma.

ANTERIOR MEDIASTINAL TUMORS IN PATIENTS UNDER 40 YEARS OF AGE: Hodgkin lymphoma and non-Hodgkin's lymphoma are the most common anterior mediastinal tumors in women under age of 40. Among men under the age of 40, the most common anterior mediastinal tumors are nonseminomatous germ cell tumors, followed by non-Hodgkin's lymphoma/Hodgkin's disease.

MASAOKA STAGING SYSTEM OF THYMOMA: Stage I: no evidence of capsular invasion; Stage II: microscopic capsular invasion of gross involvement of surrounding fat or pleura; Stage III: gross involvement of adjacent organs; Stage IVa: pleural or pericardial metastases; Stage IVb: hematogenous or lymphangenous metastases.

GERM CELL TUMORS: The most common extragonadal site of germ cell tumor spread is the anterior mediastinum, with tumor sub-types including seminomas and nonseminomatous tumors (with primary mediastinal seminomas being more common). With nonseminomatous germ cell tumors, tumors markers such as alpha fetal protein (AFP) and beta-HCG are often elevated in patient with nonseminomatous germ cell tumors, while patients with seminoma often have normal or only minimally-elevated tumor markers.

LYMPHOMAS: Lymphomas represent about 20% of the tumors in the mediastinum, and these can occur in the anterior or middle mediastinum. Hodgkin's lymphomas are much more common than NHLs presenting as mediastinal tumors.

SUBSTERNAL GOITERS: Substernal thyroid goiters most commonly present as extensions of cervical goiters, but can rarely be primary thyroid goiters originating from the mediastinum. Goiters that develop de novo in the mediastinum have arterial inflow directly from the aortic arch and need to be differentiated from substernal goiters that extend down from the neck that have arterial inflow from cervical vessels. Resections of primary mediastinal goiters require direct approaches to the mediastinum to control the arterial inflow.

CLINICAL APPROACH TO MEDIASTINAL TUMORS AND THYMOMAS

Evaluation and Treatment of an Anterior Mediastinal Mass

The mediastinum is generally divided into three separate compartments: anterior (superior), middle, and posterior. Posterior mediastinal tumors are relatively unusual and make up about 15% of the mediastinal tumors in adults and 50% of the mediastinal tumors in children. Neurogenic tumors are usually located in the posterior mediastinum. **Masses in the middle mediastinum are often associated with lymphoproliferative disorders such as lymphomas and Castle's disease.** Anterior mediastinal tumor differential diagnoses can be variable based on patient ages (greater or less than 40 years) and differ slightly between males and females. Serum tumor markers for male patients can be useful in identifying men with nonseminomatous germ cell tumors. Tissue biopsies are important to help differentiate the various tumors and direct treatments.

Indications for Mediastinal Mass Biopsies

Patients with mediastinal masses are often referred for surgical biopsy to help establish tissue diagnoses. Fine-needle aspirations (FNAs) are low-risk procedures that can be obtained under image-guidance, but unfortunately are often nondiagnostic. It remains controversial whether localized thymoma biopsies are indicated prior to resections. Open biopsies can be accomplished for most anterior mediastinal tumors, especially if the lesion is suspected to be a lymphoma, germ cell tumor, or Masaoka stage III or stage IV thymoma.

Outcomes of Patients with MG Following Thymoma Resections

At 5-years postresection, 25% to 30% of patients show complete remission of MG; 35% to 60% of the patients have improvement in symptoms with decrease in medications requirement; 20% have no change in status; 10% to 15% of the patients have disease progression.

Thymectomy in Myasthenia Gravis Patients without Thymomas

The utility of thymectomy for patients with MG and no thymoma is a little less well understood. The reason for thymectomy in patients with non-thymomatous MG is based on the observations that some of these patients have thymic hyperplasia and may derive benefits from thymectomy. Unfortunately, there is no high-quality randomized controlled trial evidence available to guide therapy in these patients. A recent literature review published in 2014 suggests that overall remission rates reported in this patient population are remission rates of 38% to 72% at 10 years. **The patients reported to have the most benefits were female patients under the age 45 years with lower preoperative MG severity classes.** Based on these observations, thymectomies may improve the chance of remission for some younger patients with non-thymomatous MGs (Table 47–2).

Table 47–2 • EVALUATION AND TREATMENT OF ANTERIOR MEDIASTINAL MASSES

Tumor	Diagnosis	Treatment
Thymoma	Surgical resection	Surgical resection, possible XRT, chemotherapy
Lymphoma	Open mediastinotomy, video-assisted thoracoscopy if fine-needle aspiration biopsy is equivocal	Chemotherapy or XRT, depending on cell type
Germ cell tumor		
Teratoma	Surgical resection	Surgical resection
Seminoma	PE	XRT
Nonseminoma	PE, positive β-human chorionic gonadotropin, and α-fetoprotein tests	Chemotherapy
Parathyroid adenoma	Hyperparathyroidism, CT scan, sestamibi scan	Surgical resection
Aberrant thyroid	CT scan	Surgical resection if symptomatic
Lipoma, hemangioma, thymic cyst	CT scan, MRI	Surgical resection if symptomatic or to rule out malignancy

Abbreviations: CT, computed tomography; MRI, magnetic resonance imaging; PE, physical examination; XRT, radiotherapy.

> **CASE CORRELATION**
>
> - See also Case 46 (Insulinoma and Pancreatic Endocrine Neoplasia).

COMPREHENSION QUESTIONS

47.1 In which of the following patients is CT-guided biopsy of the mediastinal mass indicated?

   A. A 35-year-old man with HIV who develops a large, ill-defined anterior mediastinal mass that appears to closely involve the mediastinal vessels

   B. A 47-year-old man with enlarged cervical lymph nodes, axillary lymph nodes, and mediastinal lymph nodes

   C. A 28-year-old man with left testicular mass, markedly elevated serum alpha-fetal-protein level, and a large ill-defined mass in the anterior mediastinum

   D. A 55-year-old woman with a thyroid mass that has been growing over the past 15 years complaining of compressive symptoms whenever she lies flat. There is also evidence of tracheal deviation in the upper mediastinum secondary to the mass

   E. A 23-year-old woman with biopsy-proven papillary thyroid cancer with lymphadenopathy involving the right lateral neck and central neck

47.2 A 25-year-old medical student is reading a chapter on myasthenia gravis and recalls that his grandmother had this disorder. She had a thymectomy for her condition. Which of the following statements is most accurate regarding thymectomy and MG treatment?

   A. Thymectomy is indicated for all patients with MG

   B. Anticholinesterase medications are used in the treatment of MG

   C. Thymectomy is most effective for the treatment of MG when performed during an acute crisis

   D. The indication for thymectomy for a patient with a 3-cm well circumscribed thymoma is to prevent the occurrence of MG

   E. MG is always associated with the presence of thymoma

47.3 Which of the following patients has the best potential for MG remission following thymectomy?

   A. A 32-year-old woman with no evidence of anterior mediastinal tumor and class IVa MG

   B. A 50-year-old man with no evidence of anterior mediastinal tumor and class IVa MG

   C. A 32-year-old man with no mediastinal tumor and class IVa MG

   D. A 32-year-old woman with no mediastinal tumor and class IIa MG

   E. A 32-year-old man with no mediastinal tumor and class IIa MG

Questions 47.4 to 47.6 For questions 47.4 to 47.6, match the following mediastinal locations (A, B, C) to the most appropriate diagnosis.

   A. Anterior

   B. Middle

   C. Posterior

47.4 Neurogenic tumor

47.5 Thymoma

47.6 Castleman's disease

47.7 By which of the following modalities is the staging of thymomas primarily determined?

   A. Surgical resection

   B. Immunohistochemistry assay

   C. MRI evaluation

   D. CT scan evaluation

   E. Mediastinoscopy

ANSWERS

47.1 **A.** The 35-year-old man with HIV who develops a large, ill-defined anterior mediastinal mass could have lymphoma or a seminomatous germ cell tumor. In either case, biopsy is helpful for tissue diagnosis to help direct chemotherapy or radiation therapy. For the man descried in choice "B," biopsy of the cervical lymph nodes may be less invasive. For the patient described in choice "C," orchiectomy should be performed to help establish the diagnosis. For the patient described in choice "D", biopsy of the substernal goiter is not likely to help change treatment. Since the patient is highly symptomatic, thyroidectomy with resection of the mediastinal goiter can be performed without prior biopsy.

47.2 **B.** MG is an autoimmune disorder causing injury to the nicotinic cholinergic receptors, and anticholinesterase is a form of treatment. Thymectomy is indicated for a subset of patients with MG who have a thymoma; thymectomy in these patients can help improve remission of MG but is also indicated because thymomas have the potential to undergo malignant transformation. Thymectomies for MG patients should not be performed during acute myasthenia crisis, as the postoperative complications are dramatically increased under those circumstances. MG is diagnosed in 30% to 50% of the patients with thymomas.

47.3 **D.** The benefits of thymectomy for patients with nonthymomatous MG has not been evaluated by randomized controlled trials; however, literature review of nonrandomized thymectomy outcomes suggest that young (<45 years) females with lower clinical stages of MG tend to have the best long-term response to thymectomy.

47.4 **C.** Neurogenic tumors are most likely found in the posterior mediastinum.

47.5 **A.** Thymomas are most likely found in the anterior mediastinum.

47.6 **B.** Middle mediastinal masses are often associated with lymphoproliferative disorders such Castleman's disease.

47.7 **A.** The Masaoka staging system for thymoma is based on microscopic evaluation of the surgical specimen and visual inspection of the thymoma and its relationship to surrounding structures; therefore, surgical resection is the best staging method for thymoma staging.

CLINICAL PEARLS

▶ Anterior mediastinal masses often require surgical resection for diagnosis and treatment.

▶ Staging of thymoma takes place at the time of surgical resection and during microscopic evaluation during pathologic evaluation.

▶ Proper staging and complete resection determine the prognosis for thymoma.

▶ With regards to nonthymomatous MG, woman younger <45 years of age, with lower clinical stages of MG tend to have the best clinical responses in their MG following thymectomy.

▶ Given the list of differential diagnoses, FNAs of mediastinal masses are often low-yield in providing a definitive diagnosis.

▶ Thymomas can be associated with paraneoplastic syndromes causing red cell dysplasia, immunodeficiencies, and collagen vascular diseases, but these conditions are not often resolved with thymectomy.

REFERENCES

Carter BW, Marom EM, Detterbeck FC. Approaching the patient with an anterior mediastinal mass: a guide for clinicians. *J Thorac Oncol.* 2014;9:S102-S109.

Diaz A, Black E, Dunning J. Is thymectomy in non-thymomatous myasthenia gravis of any benefit? *Interact Cardiovasc Thorac Surg.* 2014;18:381-389.

Hubka M, Wood DE. Primary tumors of the thymus. In: Cameron JL, Cameron AM, eds. *Current Surgical Therapy.* 11th ed. Philadelphia, PA: Elsevier Saunders; 2014:761-764.

Muniappan A, Mathisen D. Mediastinal masses. In: Cameron JL, Cameron AM, eds. *Current Surgical Therapy.* 11th ed. Philadelphia, PA: Elsevier Saunders; 2014:755-761.

A 59-year-old woman was brought to the emergency department as a trauma activation after a high-speed motor vehicle collision. Pan-computed tomographic (CT) scan revealed an incidental 3.5-cm solid mass in the left adrenal gland. After discharge from the trauma service, she was instructed to follow up for outpatient evaluation of her left adrenal mass. During the office visit, she feels well and is asymptomatic. Her heart rate is 70 beats/minute and blood pressure is 138/86 mm Hg. Her physical examination is normal.

▶ What is the differential diagnosis for an incidental adrenal mass?
▶ What are the important elements of the history and physical examination in a patient with an adrenal mass?
▶ What is the most likely diagnosis?

ANSWERS TO CASE 48:

Adrenal Incidentaloma and Pheochromocytoma

Summary: A 59-year-old woman is found to have an incidental 3.5-cm solid adrenal mass.

- **Differential diagnosis:** Includes benign functioning and nonfunctioning adrenal adenomas, adrenocortical carcinoma, and metastatic tumors.

- **History and physical examination:** The history should include symptoms of hypertension, previous malignancies, endocrinopathies, and family medical problems. The physical examination should include the patient's general appearance, an abdominal examination, and blood pressure readings.

- **Most likely diagnosis:** Nonfunctioning adrenal adenoma.

ANALYSIS

Objectives

1. Learn the significance of clinically unapparent adrenal masses otherwise referred to as adrenal incidentalomas.

2. Become familiar with functioning and nonfunctioning adrenal tumors as well as other clinical entities that may manifest as an incidentaloma.

3. Understand the diagnostic evaluation and management of an adrenal incidentaloma.

4. Recognize the clinical presentation of a patient with pheochromocytoma.

5. Outline a diagnostic and treatment plan for a patient with a pheochromocytoma.

Considerations

This is a 59-year-old woman who had pan-CT imaging due to a motor vehicle accident, which revealed a 3.5-cm incidental adrenal mass. The patient has no apparent medical issues that would indicate a functional tumor such as pheochromocytoma, and also no findings that would indicate a metastatic lesion. Even though the history and physical do not point to a functional or metastatic lesion, baseline biochemical studies and further imaging is helpful to confirm this suspicion. If this evaluation is reassuring, then re-imaging is recommended in 3-4 months. The adrenal mass is most likely a benign finding.

APPROACH TO:
Adrenal Incidentalomas

CLINICAL APPROACH

The term "adrenal incidentaloma" refers to a clinically unapparent adrenal mass that is discovered inadvertently in the course of diagnostic testing for other conditions. They are found in 0.7% to 4.3% of patients undergoing abdominal CT scans and in 1.4% to 8.7% of patients at autopsy. Most adrenal incidentalomas are nonfunctioning adenomas, accounting for 55% to 94% of all cases. Functioning tumors, which include pheochromocytoma, aldosterone-producing adenoma, and cortisol-producing adenoma, are less common. Other adrenal lesions that can appear as incidentalomas are ganglioneuromas, adrenocortical carcinoma, and metastases. The differential diagnosis also includes myelolipoma, cysts, and hemorrhage which can be diagnosed on the basis of imaging criteria alone. An adrenal hematoma is not an infrequent finding in a patient who sustains abdominal trauma, and the diagnosis is confirmed with resolution of the mass on follow-up imaging.

The evaluation of a patient with an adrenal incidentaloma commences with history and physical examination, and making functional and anatomic assessment of the adrenal mass (see Table 48–1). **Signs and symptoms of excess catecholamines, aldosterone, cortisol, and androgens should be actively sought in the history and on physical examination.** Patients should be asked about a history of hypertension, headaches, palpitations, profuse sweating, abdominal pain, anxiety, and prior history of malignancy. When present, adrenal masses are metastases in up to 75% of patients. In addition to obtaining a resting heart rate and a blood pressure reading, patients should be examined for features suggestive of Cushing syndrome such as truncal obesity, moon facies, thin extremities, prominent fat deposition in the supraclavicular areas and the nape of the neck, hirsutism, bruising, abdominal striae, and facial plethora.

The functional assessment consists of three main diseases. Measurement of metanephrine and catecholamine levels is performed to look for pheochromocytoma. Plasma aldosterone and renin activity can be measured to evaluate for an aldosterone-producing adenoma (Conn syndrome) where an aldosterone-renin ratio greater than 30 is suggestive of hyperaldosteronism. An overnight 1-mg

Table 48–1 • BIOCHEMICAL EVALUATION OF PATIENTS WITH ADRENAL INCIDENTALOMA

Functional Adrenal Lesion	Screening Study	Confirmatory Study
Subclinical Cushing syndrome	1-mg dexamethasone suppression test (DST)	Low adrenocorticotrophic hormone (ACTH) and dehydroepiandrosterone sulfate (DHEAS)
Pheochromocytoma	Plasma metanephrines	24-hour urine metanephrine
Primary aldosteronism	Plasma aldosterone-renin ratio >30	Saline salt loading test or captopril challenge

dexamethasone suppression test (DST) is useful during the initial evaluation for hypercortisolism. Aldosterone and cortisol-producing lesions require hormone lateralization to determine the utility of surgical resection.

After determining whether an adrenal mass is functioning or nonfunctioning, anatomic assessment is performed, preferably with CT or magnetic resonance imaging (MRI). Positron emission tomography (PET) scanning is used for the evaluation of an adrenal mass in a patient with a known extra-adrenal cancer because of its ability to separate benign from metastatic lesions. It is also important in excluding the presence of other metastases. Myelolipomas, cysts, and hemorrhage of the adrenal gland can be identified on the basis of CT criteria alone. Imaging characteristics suggestive of adrenocortical carcinoma include irregular margins, inhomogeneous density, scattered areas of decreased attenuation, and local invasion. Other CT criteria that increase the probability of malignancy include large size and enlargement over time. Primary adrenocortical carcinomas are rare, and the majority of them are 6 cm or greater. The CT characteristics that are highly specific for adrenal adenomas are Hounsfield units less than 10 during noncontrast CT and early contrast washout during a CT with intravenous contrast (defined as >60% contrast clearance at 10-15 minutes after contrast injection). One or both of these CT features has extremely high negative predictive value for malignancy, and incidentalomas with these findings can be managed with observation only.

Surgery is recommended for all functioning tumors, nonfunctioning tumors 4 cm or greater, tumors that enlarge (growth of >0.8-1.0 cm during a 3- to 12-month period), tumors with imaging characteristics suspicious for carcinoma, or solitary adrenal metastases.

Treatment in Patients with Other Malignancies

The adrenal gland is a frequent site of metastasis which include breast, kidney, colon, stomach, melanoma, and most commonly lung cancer. Patients with an adrenal incidentaloma and a prior history of malignancy should undergo biochemical assessment to exclude a functioning tumor. PET scanning may exclude the presence of metastatic disease. Fine-needle aspiration (FNA) biopsy should be rarely performed and is reserved for a solitary nonfunctioning lesion where the result will alter therapy. Patients with negative results from an FNA biopsy are treated nonoperatively. Finally, nonsurgical treatment is recommended for patients with diffuse metastases (Figure 48–1).

Follow-up

Patients with nonfunctioning adrenal incidentalomas smaller than 4 cm usually undergo follow-up imaging at 3 and 15 months. A change in size greater than 1 cm may prompt adrenalectomy. In the absence of change, the patient is followed annually with history and physical examination with repeated biochemical testing is reserved for abnormal history or physical findings.

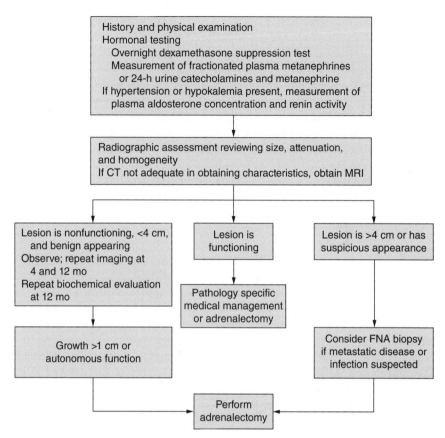

Figure 48–1. Algorithm for the evaluation of patients with an adrenal incidentaloma. CT, computed tomography; DST, dexamethasone suppression test; FNA, fine-needle aspiration; MRI, magnetic resonance imaging.

APPROACH TO:

Pheochromocytoma

Pheochromocytoma is a tumor that arises from the chromaffin cells of the adrenal medulla and secretes catecholamines. It is historically known as the **"10% tumor"** because 10% are bilateral, extra-adrenal, multiple, malignant, and over 10% familial. The hallmark clinical manifestation of pheochromocytoma is paroxysmal hypertension and episodic headaches, palpitations, anxiety, and sweating. Because of the increasing application of CT imaging, up to half of the patients with pheochromocytoma are identified during biochemical testing for clinically silent incidentaloma.

The diagnosis of pheochromocytoma requires demonstration of excess catecholamine production by one of two methods: a 24-hour urine collection to test for metanephrine, normetanephrine, and VMA and/or measurement of plasma-free metanephrine levels. Plasma measurements are more sensitive but less specific with a sensitivity of 99% and a specificity of 89%.

Imaging and Localization

Once a pheochromocytoma has been diagnosed, localization is performed to exclude multiple, bilateral, or extra-adrenal pheochromocytomas (paragangliomas). Abdominal CT imaging and MRI have at least 95% sensitivity in detecting an adrenal pheochromocytoma. A pheochromocytoma usually appears bright on a T2-weighted MRI. Both CT imaging and MRI have a specificity of as low as 50% in some studies related to the high frequency of adrenal masses that are not pheochromocytomas. An iodine-131 metaiodobenzylguanidine (MIBG) scan may be obtained for confirmation or evaluation of nonlocalized pheochromocytoma because of its superior specificity of 90% to 100%. PET imaging can be used when conventional imaging studies cannot localize the tumor.

Patient Preoperative Preparation

A preoperative chest radiograph should be obtained for all patients because the lung is one of the most common sites for metastasis. Electrocardiography and echocardiography are frequently useful because **chronic catecholamine excess may cause cardiomyopathy.** Preoperative blood pressure management is essential to minimize the risk of hypertensive crises. The preferred method is administration of an α-adrenergic–blocking agent 1 to 2 weeks before surgery. This allows for relaxation of the constricted vascular tree and correction of the reduced plasma volume which prevents hypotension that often occurs following tumor removal. A β-adrenergic–blocking agent may be added to oppose the reflex tachycardia associated with α-blockade. Administration of a β-blocking agent should not be started without prior α-blockade due to the potential precipitation of a hypertensive crisis related to unopposed α-receptor stimulation.

Traditionally, phenoxybenzamine has been the preferred α-adrenergic antagonist. α-Methyl-p-tyrosine, which is often used in combination with phenoxybenzamine, competitively inhibits tyrosine hydroxylase, the rate-limiting enzyme in catecholamine synthesis. Newer, selective α_1-blocking agents and calcium-channel blockers have also been used with good results.

Surgical Concerns

Intraoperative medical management is critical because of the danger of large fluctuations in blood pressure, heart rate, and fluids. Continuous blood pressure monitoring is accomplished with an arterial line, and central venous and Foley catheters are inserted for volume assessment and intravenous fluid replacement. An intravenous nitroprusside continuous infusion can be administered for the control of hypertension, and a short-acting β-blocker such as esmolol is used to control tachycardia. Adrenalectomy can be accomplished either laparoscopically or through an open technique. Acute hypotension may occur following excision of a pheochromocytoma related to sudden diffuse vasodilatation. Continuous intravenous norepinephrine is used when blood pressure fails to respond to fluid administration. Postoperatively, a normotensive state is achieved in approximately 90% of patients following tumor excision.

Follow-up

Because malignant potential is not always identified on initial histopathology, all patients are followed for the rest of their life. Plasma-free metanephrine levels should be measured 1 month after surgery and at yearly intervals thereafter.

> ## CASE CORRELATION
>
> • See also Case 46 (Insulinoma and Pancreatic Endocrine Neoplasia).

COMPREHENSION QUESTIONS

48.1 A 44-year-old otherwise healthy man has a 3-cm left adrenal mass found during CT evaluation for acute appendicitis. Following his appendectomy, a serum metanephrine level during his hospitalization revealed mild elevation in value. Which of the following is the most appropriate next step?

A. A 24-hour urine collection for VMA, metanephrine, and normetanephrine

B. MIBG scan

C. CT-guided needle biopsy of the adrenal gland

D. Alpha blockage for 1 week followed by laparoscopic adrenalectomy

E. Monitor the lesion with CT scans annually

48.2 A 3.5-cm right adrenal mass was discovered incidentally on an abdominal CT scan obtained for a 62-year-old man who was a victim of motor vehicular trauma. His medical history was notable for a right upper lobe lung resection 3 years previously for a stage I carcinoma. He is asymptomatic. Which of the following is the next most appropriate step in the evaluation?

A. FNA biopsy of the adrenal mass

B. Repeated CT scanning in 3 months

C. A functional assessment of the adrenal mass

D. MRI of the adrenal gland

E. Perform a PET scan to look for other sites of possible metastatic disease

48.3 For which of the following patients is observation alone appropriate?

A. A 53-year-old healthy man with a 8-cm nonfunctioning left adrenal mass

B. A 46-year-old man with a history of hypertension and unexplained hypokalemia

C. A 32-year-old woman with elevated serum metanephrines and urinary VMA, metanephrines, and an asymptomatic 2-cm right adrenal mass

D. A 66-year-old man with a history of malignant melanoma on the leg at age 50, who presents with a newly diagnosed 4-cm right adrenal mass

E. A 44-year-old woman with a 8-cm left adrenal mass that appears to be a myolipoma based on CT

48.4 Which of the following is the most appropriate management for an 85-year-old nursing home resident, with severe dementia and congestive heart failure (CHF), and a 6-cm left adrenal mass?

    A. Evaluate the tumor for functionality and treat with laparoscopic adrenalectomy

    B. Evaluate the tumor for functionality and perform CT-guided biopsy

    C. Expectant management

    D. Medically optimize the patient and perform laparoscopic adrenalectomy

    E. Monitor the lesion with repeat CT scan every 6 months

48.5 Which of the following statements regarding adrenalectomy for a pheochromocytoma is most accurate?

    A. It results in blood pressure improvement, but blood pressure rarely normalizes

    B. It corrects hypertension only in patients with benign disease

    C. It may lead to profound intraoperative hypotension

    D. It should be reserved for patients with hypertension refractory to drug therapy

    E. Preoperative management is not needed if laparoscopic surgery is planned

48.6 Which of the following imaging studies has the *highest specificity* when used to confirm the presence of a pheochromocytoma?

    A. MIBG imaging

    B. CT imaging

    C. MRI

    D. PET

    E. Ultrasonography

ANSWERS

48.1 **A.** A 24-hour urinary collection for VMA, metanephrines, and normetanephrine is needed in this patient to confirm the diagnosis of pheochromocytoma. While a normal serum metanephrine level has a high negative predictive value for the absence of pheochromocytoma, elevated serum values do not always indicate the presence of a pheochromocytoma, and the possibility of a pheochromocytoma needs to be further explored with the more specific urinary catecholamine analyses. If the biochemical analysis confirms pheochromocytoma, the lesion should be removed rather than observed.

48.2 **C.** The initial step in evaluating an adrenal mass is performing functional studies. The presence of an adrenal mass in a patient with a prior history of early-stage lung cancer cannot be assumed to be metastatic disease.

48.3 **E.** CT is accurate for the diagnosis of myolipoma of the adrenal gland. To be more complete, it is not unreasonable to obtain biochemical studies to rule out a functional adrenal adenoma and pheochromocytoma in this patient. The patient with a prior history of melanoma may have an adrenal metastasis and needs biochemical evaluations first to rule out the usual causes, followed by biopsy of the mass. The patient with hypertension and unexplained hypokalemia needs biochemical analysis to rule out aldosterone-producing adrenal adenoma.

48.4 **C.** Expectant management is acceptable for this patient with severe comorbidities and an asymptomatic adrenal mass. While the possibility of an adrenocortical carcinoma exists in this patient, the risks of treatment would exceed the potential benefits associated with further diagnostic studies and/or treatment.

48.5 **C.** Excision of a pheochromocytoma may result in immediate intraoperative hypotension. Preoperative treatment of the patients with α-blockers is critical prior to laparoscopic and open adrenalectomy.

48.6 **A.** An MIBG scan is highly specific in confirming pheochromocytoma.

CLINICAL PEARLS

▶ Initial evaluation of a patient with an adrenal mass involves assessment of functional status and risk for carcinoma

▶ Functional assessment consists of evaluation for pheochromocytoma, aldosterone-producing adenoma, and a cortisol-producing tumor.

▶ Cancer is considered in adrenal lesions larger than 4 cm in diameter, growth over time, imaging characteristics, or a history of previous malignancy.

▶ Lung cancer is the most common metastatic tumor to the adrenal gland. Other tumors include carcinoma of the breast, kidney, colon, stomach, and melanoma.

▶ Biopsy of an adrenal mass is rarely indicated and should be performed only when diagnosis would change surgical management.

▶ Adrenalectomy should be performed for functioning adenomas, suspicion of cancer, or metastatic disease.

▶ Patients with aldosterone or cortisol producing tumors should obtain functional localization to determine laterality and whether surgical therapy is indicated.

▶ Pheochromocytomais classically known as the 10% tumor because 10% are bilateral, extra-adrenal, multiple, malignant, or familial.

▶ Preoperative management of pheochromocytoma includes volume resuscitation with α-blockade followed by β-blockade.

REFERENCES

Mazzaglia PJ, Miner TJ. Adrenal incidentaloma. In: Cameron JL, Cameron AM, eds. *Current Surgical Therapy*. 10th ed. Philadelphia, PA: Elsevier Saunders; 2011:565-570.

Silberfein E, Perrier ND. Management of pheochromocytoma. In: Cameron JL, Cameron AM, eds. *Current Surgical Therapy*. 10th ed. Philadelphia, PA: Elsevier Saunders; 2011:579-584.

Young WF. The incidentally discovered adrenal mass. *N Engl J Med*. 2007;356:601-610.

A 62-year-old woman presents to the emergency department with an open wound on her left foot. This patient has a history of non-insulin-dependent diabetes mellitus, which is treated with an oral agent. She states that she has not had any prior foot infections or foot problems, and denies any recent trauma to her foot. Her wound has not been particularly painful, and she only noticed the wound when yellow drainage appeared on her socks over the past several days. Her temperature is 37.9°C (100.2°F), and her vital signs are normal. Her peripheral vascular examination reveals palpable pulses in both femoral regions and normal pulses in both feet. The left foot is swollen over the plantar region and has a 1.5-cm open wound over the plantar surface of the foot overlying the second and third metatarsal heads. There is minimal amount of yellow drainage from the area, and the surrounding skin is erythematous and warm. There is no exposed bone appreciated at the base of the ulcer. Her white blood cell count is 14,000 cell/m³ and the serum glucose is 280 mEq/dL.

▶ What is the diagnosis?
▶ What are the next steps in this patient's management?
▶ What are the complications associated with this process?

ANSWERS TO CASE 49:
Diabetic Foot Complications

Summary: A 62-year-old woman with type II diabetes presents with a plantar ulcer on the foot that is associated with surrounding inflammation, low-grade fever, and leukocytosis.

- **Diagnosis:** Diabetic foot infection associated with a plantar surface area ulcer. Charcot neuroarthropathy cannot be ruled out at this time.

- **Next Steps:** Assess the wound and patient for signs of infections. Biopsy the wound for culture and send blood cultures. Obtain x-ray of the foot to look for Charcot neuroarthropahy and/or osteomyelitis. This patient should be placed on bed rest, intravenous antibiotics, and strict glycemic control.

- **Complications:** Non-healing wounds and progression of infections may lead to limb loss and quality of life compromises in diabetic patients.

ANALYSIS
Objective

1. Learn to recognize and monitor diabetic foot complications.

2. Learn the terminologies applied for foot diseases in diabetic patients.

3. Learn the principles and strategies applied for the treatment of diabetic foot complications.

Considerations

A 62-year-old diabetic female presents with fever and a new plantar ulcer associated with a swollen and erythematous foot. Her clinical presentation is highly suspicious for a neuropathic ulcer causing a diabetic foot infection. The presence of palpable pulses in the foot and the location of the ulcer suggest that macro-arterial disease is unlikely a contributing factor for this non-healing wound. The **PEDIS** classification can be applied during the evaluation of her foot ulcer, which requires us to consider **P**erfusion, **E**xtent (area size), **D**epth, **I**nfection, and **S**ensation. Because all open wounds are colonized by microbes but not necessarily infected, the diagnosis of active infection should be based on the combination of culture results and clinical assessment rather than wound cultures alone. In this patient's case, she has local signs of infection (redness, drainage, and swelling), systemic signs of infection including leukocytosis (WBC count of 14,000) and hyperglycemia. Documentation of tissue infection and identification of the infectious organisms should be based on tissue biopsy and not a tissue swab. It is important to begin empiric antimicrobial treatment even before microbiology culture results become available. Given that the most common pathogens involved in diabetic foot infections are *Staphylcoccus aureus* and β-hemolytic Streptococcus, the initial empiric treatment can be amoxicillin-clavulanic acid, ciprofloxacin, cephazolin, or vancomycin. The possibility of polymicrobial infection with aerobic Gram-positive cocci, Gram-negative bacilli, and anaerobic organisms is less likely for this patient because she has not previously received antimicrobial therapy and does not have arterial insufficiency. The optimal duration of antibiotics treatment for diabetic foot infections has not been determined on the basis of randomized controlled trials. Most practitioners will give 7 to 14 days of antibiotics for individuals without osteomyelitis. With osteomyelitis involvement, a 4- to 6-week course of antibiotics is usually prescribed. Glycemic control in patients with diabetic foot infections is an essential component of the treatment, as hyperglycemia contributes to leukocyte dysfunction and compromises the host's response to infections. If bony destruction is seen during radiographic evaluation in this patient, it could difficult to differentiate osteomyelitis from Charcot neuroarthropathy; long-term antibiotics (4-6 weeks) course may be necessary. For a patient a with diabetic foot infection, local wound care is very important in promoting healing, and local care may include sharp debridement, larval therapy with medicinal maggots, topical agents, and in some cases surgical drainage and minor amputations. For many patients without active infections, contact casting can be helpful to offload pressure from the wound site. Once healing of the ulcer occurs, it is important to carry out a thorough evaluation to identify any modifiable factors (eg, limited joint mobility of the foot and ankle, calluses, bunions, hammer toes, clawed toes, etc.) that may have contributed to her infection, and address these issues to prevent additional neuropathic ulcer formation.

APPROACH TO:
Diabetic Foot Complications

DEFINITIONS

DIABETIC NEUROPATHIES: Up to 60% of diabetic patients may have neuropathies affecting the lower extremities. Nerve dysfunction may include sensory neuropathies that disrupt pain and temperature sensations and increases susceptibility to trauma. Motor neuropathies to the intrinsic muscle of the foot can cause imbalance between the flexor and extensor mechanism contributing to foot deformities and increased vulnerability to injuries. Autonomic neuropathies can contribute to the loss of sweat gland functions, skin cracking, soft tissue edema, and osteopenia.

BIOFILM: A slimy matrix of extracellular polymeric substance that is produced by bacteria when they aggregate together. Biofilms are common in chronic wounds, and the presence of biofilm impedes antibiotic penetrance into the tissue. Treatment of biofilm containing wounds generally requires debridement of tissue.

BUNION: A bunion (hallux valgus) is an enlargement of the bony tissue and surrounding soft tissue at the base of the big toe that can develop in diabetic and nondiabetic individuals. This is generally associated with angulation of the first-toe toward the other toes. The process occurs mostly in women and is often related to wearing tight, pointed, and confining shoes. Bunion predisposes to injuries in the overlying skin and soft tissue.

HAMMERTOES: Hammertoes are contracture of the toes (often sparing the big toe) that can occur in diabetic and nondiabetic individuals. The typical appearance is upward bend to the second to fifth toes at the metatarsal-proximal phalangeal joint and downward bend of the distal portion of the toes producing the typical "clawed toes." This deformity occurs nearly uniformly in women and is believed to be due to muscle-tendon imbalance produced by tight shoes with heels.

CHARCOT FOOT: This is a type of neuropathic osteoarthropathy that occur most commonly in diabetic patients. Charcot foot occurs in approximately 16% of patients with diabetes and neuropathic ulcers, and can be difficult to differentiate clinically from diabetic foot infection with osteomyelitis. The pathogenesis is believed to be multifactorial and begins as a neurally mediated vascular reflex causing inflammation, increased blood flow, and metabolic changes in the bones in the foot/ankle. With these changes, the foot is at risk for fractures and soft tissue trauma in the mid-foot that produces a "rocker-bottom" deformity in the foot during the later stages of disease progression.

OFFLOADING: This is an important treatment strategy for patients with Charcot foot early during the disease process. The affected foot is immobilized in a total contact cast to rest the injuries and prevent the injury from progressing to permanent deformity.

FOOT ULCER CLASSIFICATIONS: Neuropathic foot ulcers are located over weight-bearing portions of the foot and are associated with normal arterial examination. Vasculogenic ulcers are generally located at the tips of the toes where perfusion is most susceptible. Ulcers can also develop initially as neuropathic ulcers and then persists as the result of decreased blood flow and poor tissue perfusion.

DIABETIC MICROVASCULAR DISEASE: This is tissue level hypoperfusion that develops as the result of long-standing diabetes mellitus. The process is believed to begin with increased micro-arterial pressure and flow leading to endothelial injury and sclerosis of the microvasculature. This process causes a reduction in capillary flow and loss of vasoconstriction at the tissues level. In addition, there is often increased arterio-venous shunting secondary to the autonomic neuropathy.

CLINICAL APPROACH

Disease of the foot is common and one of the most feared complications associated with diabetes. The "diabetic foot" refers to a number of common pathologic conditions encountered in the diabetic population, and these include diabetic neuropathy, ischemic vascular disease, Charcot neuroarthropathy, skin ulcerations, soft tissue infections, and osteomyelitis. **The lifetime risk of foot ulcer development in a diabetic individual is reported as high as 25%, and infections related to diabetic foot is responsible for 80% of the nontraumatic amputations performed.** The prevention of diabetic foot complications is possible through patient education and close patient surveillance so that conditions predisposing to pressure ulceration and trauma could be avoided, identified early, and treated. The National Institute for Clinical Excellence (NICE) has made the following recommendations for diabetic foot surveillance based on patient risk stratification. *Low-risk patients* with intact sensation and normal pulses are recommended to have examination and maintenance care annually. *Moderate-risk individuals* with neuropathy or absence of pulses are recommended to have examinations and maintenance care every 3 to 6 months. *High-risk patients* are individuals with neuropathies, skin changes, foot deformities, prior history of ulcers, and absence of pulses, and these patients are recommended to undergo evaluations and maintenance care every 1 to 3 months. During the scheduled maintenance evaluations, all patients undergo thorough evaluations for **neuropathies, structural abnormalities** (calluses, bunions, hammer toes, etc.), and **vascular abnormalities** (ankle-brachial index and ischemic skin changes). Patients found to have active foot ulcerations are then recommended to undergo aggressive treatments by a multidisciplinary foot care team.

Challenges in the evaluation of diabetic foot disease are the asymptomatic nature of the disease and the absence of traumatic events producing the injuries. As the result of microvascular disease, superficial cellulitis can progress to more extensive soft tissue infection and osteomyelitis if not carefully monitored and aggressively treated. Hence, attention must be directed at (1) identifying and intervening for deep space infections or osteomyelitis, (2) preventing superficial infections from progressing to more extensive processes, (3) educating the patient and family in preventive care and early recognition of problems. Diabetic ulcers (Figure 49–1) may develop on pressure points or areas of vascular insufficiency (tips of toes). **Pain, swelling, and wound drainage are often signs of deep space infections, and when present, imaging studies and/or wound explorations should be strongly considered to address the problems early.** Most deep space infections will require wound debridement and/or drainage in addition to antibiotics therapy. Osteomyelitis should be considered in the differential diagnosis, whenever patients present with deep ulcers, elevated WBC count, swelling, and pain. Due to their relative immune suppressive conditions, fever is not always present in diabetic patients with deep space infections; therefore clinical vigilance is important for early recognition of the condition. Plain radiographs are often inadequate for the detection of osteomyelitis, therefore radionuclear imaging such as a **gallium scan should be considered for early diagnosis of osteomyelitis.**

Since atherosclerotic vascular disease occurs commonly in diabetic individuals, the contribution of arterial insufficiency in diabetic foot complications should never be overlooked. When macrovascular occlusive disease is present, the arterial stenoses in diabetic patients tend to occur in more distal locations than in nondiabetic individuals, where stenoses occur at the tibial-peroneal level rather than the femoral-popliteal level. Based on the level of arterial disease, diabetic patients are expected to report foot claudication with ambulation; however, foot claudication symptoms often can be masked by the patients' diabetic neuropathy. During their medical visits, all patients with diabetic foot complications need to have ABI measurements or measurement of toe-brachial indices. It is also important to keep in mind that the ABIs in diabetic patients can be falsely elevated due to arterial calcifications. Due to the distal nature of disease and the occurrence of multilevel

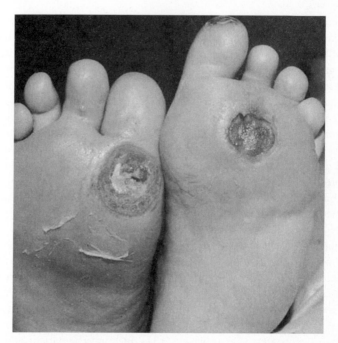

Figure 49–1. Diabetic, neuropathic ulcers on the soles of the feet due to significant long-standing diabetes-associated neuropathy. *(Reproduced, with permission, from Wolff K, Johnson RA, Suurmond D. Fitzpatrick's Color Atlas & Synopsis of Clinical Dermatology. 5th ed. New York, NY: McGraw-Hill; 2005:436.)*

disease, the occlusive processes in diabetic patients are generally less amendable to endoluminal interventions, and revascularization often entails open bypasses. The healing of chronic ulcers in patients with ABI less than 0.5 is highly unlikely without revascularization, and if revascularization is not an option then there is a high likelihood that an amputation will be required.

CASE CORRELATION
- See also Case 50 (Claudication Syndrome).

COMPREHENSION QUESTIONS

49.1 A 53-year-old man with type 2 diabetes presents with ulcers over the tips of the first and second left toes. His pulses are normal in the left femoral artery and popliteal artery, and no palpable pulses are found in the left foot. The ABI in his left leg is 0.4. Which of the following is the best treatment?

   A. Local debridement, wound care, and systemic antibiotics

   B. Local debridement, wound care, systemic antibiotics, and hyperbaric oxygen therapy

   C. Local debridement, wound care, antibiotics, angiography and revascularization

   D. Local debridement, wound care, and if no improvement left below the knee amputation

   E. Local debridement, wound care, and systemic vasodilator therapy

49.2 Which of the following options is not a part of the PEDIS evaluation process for foot ulcers?

   A. Wound depth

   B. Sensation

   C. Size of ulcer

   D. Duration of ulcer

   E. Perfusion

49.3 Which of the following factors contributes to polymicrobial diabetic foot infections?

   A. Hyperglycemia

   B. Patient age

   C. Age of ulcer

   D. Prior antibiotics treatment

   E. Neuropathic ulcers

49.4 Which of the following statements regarding Charcot neuroarthropathy is true?

   A. This is strongly associated with osteomyelitis

   B. Bone fracture in the foot rules out the diagnosis

   C. Charcot neuroarthropathy always occurs with foot ischemia

   D. Bony destruction is a key radiographic feature

   E. Open wounds are always found in this condition

49.5 A 46-year-old diabetic male is being seen in the office for an ulcer of the right foot and ankle that appeared approximately 10 days ago. There is some tenderness over the lateral malleolus. An x-ray of the ankle does not show any abnormalities. Which of the following is most likely to help in the detection of osteomyelitis?

A. Needle aspiration of the region in question

B. MRI of the ankle

C. Bone biopsy

D. Serum erythrocyte sedimentation rate

E. Radionucleotide scan of the ankle

49.6 A 55-year-old man with type 2 diabetes presents with complaint of "foot infection." He is noted to have foul-smelling and purulent drainage from a 10-cm left plantar ulcer with exposed bone. His temperature is 39.4°C (102.9°F) and blood pressure is 90/50 mm Hg. The WBC count is 35,000 cells/m³, and an x-ray indicates extensive osteomyelitis involving several metatarsal bones and gas within the soft tissue space in the lower leg. Which of the following is the most appropriate treatment?

A. Below the knee amputation

B. Piperacillin-tazobactam + clindamycin

C. Piperacillin-tazobactam + vancomycin and wound care

D. Below the knee amputation, piperacillin-tazobactam + metronidazole

E. Transmetatarsal amputation and piperacillin-tazobactam + metronidazole

49.7 A 51-year-old man presents for an appointment to your office for a recurrent foul-smelling diabetic foot infection. There does not seem to be ischemia in the soft tissue in the area. You noted that the infected area initially had improved after a 2-week course of vancomycin therapy. Which of the following is the best antimicrobial therapy for this patient at this time?

A. Metronidazole

B. Fluconazole

C. Clindamycin

D. High dose vancomycin

E. Piperacillin-tazobactam

ANSWERS

49.1 **C.** For this patient with a nonhealing ulcer in the toes and ABI of 0.4, healing of the ulcer is unlikely to occur without revascularization. In principle, chronic wounds that do not heal should trigger us to investigate for possible ischemia, infection, and poor nutritional state.

49.2 **D.** The PEDIS classification of ulcer evaluation assesses for **P**erfusion, **E**xtent of wound (wound size), **D**epth, **I**nfection, and **S**ensation. Duration of ulcer occurrence is not part of the evaluation process.

49.3 **D.** Most new diabetic foot ulcers do not have polymicrobial involvement unless the patient has received prior antimicrobial therapies.

49.4 **D.** Charcot neuroarthropathy is associated with increased tissue blood flow and bony destruction. Ischemia is not a contributing factor and the process may occur without osteomyelitis. Open wounds may or may not be an associated finding.

49.5 **E.** A gallium scan can be useful to help identify osteomyelitis in this patient with open wounds of the foot and ankle.

49.6 **D.** This diabetic patient is presenting with late stage diabetic foot infection that is associated with septic shock. For patients with diabetic foot infections that are less severe, it is often helpful to try to preserve the foot; however, at this time the patient is exhibiting severe systemic signs that are suggestive of an ongoing life-threatening process. Amputation and systemic broad-spectrum antibiotics therapy are the best treatment for this patient.

49.7 **E.** For this 56-year-old man with prior history of antibiotics treatment targeting Gram-positive organisms and now has recurrence of foul-smelling drainage associated with the wound; this presentation following the sequence of prior treatment is highly suggestive of a polymicrobial infection at this time. Piperacillin-tazobactam is a good initial empiric antibiotic choice at this time. Anaerobic organisms are less likely to develop in diabetic foot infections unless also with arterial insufficiency and tissue ischemia. Fungal infection is uncommon in diabetic foot infection. Increasing the dosage of vancomycin is not likely to improve the infection unless the peak and trough levels of the drug are low.

CLINICAL PEARLS

▶ Neuropathic and vasculopathic ulcers may be differentiated based on ulcer locations, where neuropathic ulcers occur at pressure and weight-bearing areas of the foot and vasculopathic ulcers occur at the tips of toes.

▶ Acute Charcot foot is associated with acute pain, soft tissue swelling, erythema, and increased warmth in the foot, and these features can be easily confused with cellulitis, deep venous thrombosis, and osteomyelitis.

▶ Hammertoes are contracture of the toes (often sparing the big toe) that can occur in diabetic and nondiabetic individuals. The typical appearance is an upward bend to the second to fifth toes at the meta-tarsal-proximal phalangeal joint and a downward bend of the distal portion of the toes producing the typical "clawed toes. These occur mostly in women.

▶ A bunion (hallux valgus) is an enlargement of the bony and surrounding soft tissue at the base of the big toe that can develop in diabetic and nondiabetic individuals. This is associated with angulation of the first-toe toward the other toes. The process occurs mostly in women and is contributed by wearing tight, pointed, and confining shoes. Bunion predisposes to injuries in the overlying skin and soft tissue.

REFERENCES

Boulton AJM. The diabetic foot. *Medicine*. 2014;43:33-37.

Noor S, Zubair M, Ahmad J. Diabetic foot ulcer-review on pathophysiology, classification and microbial etiology. Diabetes Metabol Syndrome. *Clin Res Rev*. 2015, http://dx.doi.org/10.1016/j.dsx.2015.04.007.

Rogers LC, Frykberg Rg, Armstrong DG, et al. The charcot foot in diabetes. *Diab Care*. 2011;34: 2123-2129.

CASE 50

A 64 year-old-man with a history of hypertension presents with pain in his legs upon exertion. The patient relates that these symptoms have been present over the past 12 months and have worsened slightly. He currently has pain and tightness in both calves that develop after walking more than one block, but the symptoms always resolve after several minutes of rest. He denies pain without exertion. His past medical history is significant for hypertension and dyslipidemia. He smokes approximately half a pack of cigarettes each day. On examination, his feet are warm and without lesions. The femoral pulses are normal bilaterally; however, his popliteal, dorsalis pedis, and posterior tibial pulses are absent bilaterally. Doppler examination of the lower extremities reveals the presence of Doppler signals in both feet with ankle-brachial indices (ABIs) demonstrating moderately severe occlusive disease: ABI on the left is 0.58, and the ABI on the right is 0.56.

▶ What is the most likely diagnosis?
▶ What are the risk factors for this condition?
▶ What is the most appropriate next step?
▶ What is the best initial treatment for this patient?

ANSWERS TO CASE 50:
Lower Extremity Arterial Occlusive Disease

Summary: A 64-year-old-man presents with bilateral leg claudication. Based on the history and pulse examination, the patient's symptoms are likely due to arterial insufficiency with occlusive lesions in the superficial femoral arteries (SFA).

- **Most likely diagnosis:** Peripheral artery disease (PAD) with bilateral SFA occlusive disease.

- **Risk factors for the condition:** Non-modifiable risk factors include age, sex, and ethnicity. Modifiable risk factors include smoking, diabetes mellitus, hypertension, renal insufficiency, and dyslipidemia.

- **Next step:** Assessment of disability, patient counseling to discuss natural history of the disease process, treatment options, and risks/benefits of invasive interventions.

- **Best initial treatment:** Lifestyle modification with smoking cessation, exercise program, and pharmacological treatment at reducing cardiovascular risks.

ANALYSIS

Objectives

1. Learn to differentiate vascular and nonvascular causes of claudication.

2. Be able to recognize the indications for lower extremity revascularization and benefits and limitations of open surgical and endovascular treatment approaches.

3. Learn the noninvasive modalities available for the evaluation and follow-up of patients with claudication.

Considerations

This patient's presentation is very typical for individuals with lower extremity arterial occlusive disease: a history of pain in the lower extremity muscles that develops with exertion and improves with rest. Pain in the legs with exertion can occur as the result of a number of different disease processes other than arterial insufficiency, with differential diagnoses that include bones and join abnormalities, and central and peripheral neurologic causes. To help differentiate arterial insufficiency from the other causes, it is important to obtain additional details regarding his symptoms (Table 50–1). Since arterial insufficiency pain is produced by inadequate blood flow to meet the metabolic demands associated with exercise, a patient with arterial insufficiency usually reports symptoms that are reproduced each and every time that he exerts the same work load. For example, if a patient says that his symptoms are variable in that he occasionally has "good days" when he can walk much

	Location of Pain	Association with Exercise	Relieving Factors	Additional History/ Conditions
Table 50–1 • DIFFERENTIAL DIAGNOSIS OF LEG PAIN				
Condition	**Location of Pain**	**Association with Exercise**	**Relieving Factors**	**Additional History/ Conditions**
Intermittent Claudication	Buttock, thigh, or calf	Always and reproducible	Stopping	Pain lasting only minutes
Osteoarthritis	Hips, knees, ankles	Variable, not always reproducible	Variable, relieved with NSAIDs	Pain duration variable. Patient may have history of arthritis, older age, and obesity
Lumbar Stenosis	Buttock, thighs, hips, calf	Yes and can be associated with standing	Back flexion	History of chronic back pain is common
Herniated Disc	Radiation down the leg	Variable	Variable, relieved with NSAIDs	History of back pain or back injuries

further without symptoms, then most likely he has symptoms that are not caused by arterial insufficiency. As for the location of the pain, symptoms produced by insufficient blood flow should consistently manifest in the muscle groups below the location of the arterial obstruction or the flow-disturbing lesion(s). In this patient with bilateral calf claudication, the locations of the arterial occlusions are most likely in the superficial femoral arteries.

One of the important initial considerations in the management of a patient with peripheral arterial disease (PAD) is to determine whether the disease falls into the category of intermittent claudication (IC) or critical limb ischemia (CLI). Based on the patient's symptoms, pulse examination, and his ABIs, this man's PAD falls into the category of IC.

The diagnosis of CLI is characterized by ischemic rest pain lasting greater than 2 weeks in duration, and with the patient often becoming dependent on opiate analgesia for relief. In order to confirm that the symptoms are due to poor blood flow and not another cause such as peripheral neuropathy, the pulse examination, ankle/brachial index, and noninvasive imaging studies are helpful for confirmation of arterial insufficiency. Critical limb ischemia (CLI) represents an advanced form of lower extremity arterial insufficiency. A patient with CLI generally has claudication symptoms producible by minimal exertion and often reports pain in the foot and toes at rest (rest pain). Patients with CLI have ankle-brachial index (ABI) of less than 0.40, and in patients with heavily calcified blood vessels, CLI diagnosis requires symptoms and a toe pressure of less than 30 mm Hg. It is important to quantify the disease severity in all patients with PAD, because it allows us to monitor the patients for symptoms and disease progression. PAD severity can be classified using either the Fontaine Classification System or the Rutherford Classification system (Tables 50–2 and 50–3). The severity of arterial obstruction in patients with PAD should be serially monitored using the ankle-brachial index measurements.

Table 50–2 • FONTAINE CLASSIFICATION SYSTEM FOR PERIPHERAL VASCULAR DISEASE	
Stage	History
I	Asymptomatic
IIa	Mild claudication (symptoms onset >200 m)
IIb	Moderate-severe claudication (symptoms onset <200 m)
III	Ischemic rest pain
IV	Tissue loss or ulceration

After establishing the diagnosis of IC, the initial management for this patient should include life style modifications (smoking cessation, dietary modifications, and weight loss) and pharmacological treatment to reduce his cardiovascular disease risk. Some important points to discuss with this patient are that the risk of limb-loss for patients with IC is generally quite low (<5% over 5 years); however, as an individual with IC, his combined risk of mortality from cardiovascular and cerebral vascular events are high (42% and 65% at 5 and 10 years, respectively). Our priorities in managing this patient are: (1) to identify, treat, and prevent progression of the systemic manifestations of atherosclerotic disease; (2) to improve functional status of the patient. For this man with suspected femoral-popliteal occlusive disease and claudication, invasive treatments such as angioplasty/stenting and bypass procedures are generally not indicated because the majority of these patients will not progress to a limb-threatening situation. With invasive interventions, patients' symptoms may improve, but there is an associated risk of failure, that may contribute to limb loss.

Table 50–3 • RUTHERFORD CLASSIFICATION OF PERIPHERAL VASCULAR DISEASE		
Category/ Stage	Comparable Fontaine Classification	History
0	I	Asymptomatic
1	IIa	Mild claudication*
2	IIb	Moderate claudication*
3	IIb	Severe claudication*
4	III	Rest pain
5	IV	Ischemic ulceration not exceeding the digits of the foot
6	IV	Severe ischemic ulcers or frank gangrene

*Mild, moderate, and severe claudication under the Rutherford Classification are not clearly quantified.

APPROACH TO:
Lower Extremity Vascular Disease

DEFINITIONS

DYSLIPIDEMIA: Conditions associated with decreased high density lipoproteins (HDL), elevation of total cholesterol, elevation of low density lipoproteins (LDL), and/or elevation of triglyceride. This type of metabolic disorder is known to accelerate PAD. Statin therapy targeting the reduction of LDL levels to <100 mg/dL in average-risk individuals and to <70 mg/dL in high-risk patients with multiple other cardiovascular co-morbidities have been shown to reduce the occurrence of cardiovascular disease-related morbidities.

HYPERTENSION CONTROL: Blood pressure control to targets of 140/90 mm Hg in nondiabetics and 130/80 in diabetics and chronic renal disease patients have been demonstrated to reduce the risk of MI and strokes. Beta-blockers and ACE inhibitors have been shown to reduce the risk of MI and strokes in patients with PAD.

DIABETIC CARE: Patients with PAD and diabetes should have close monitoring of glycemic control targeting HbA1c <7%. In addition, diabetic patient need to be instructed on proper foot care and should be closely monitored and aggressively treated for skin conditions and ulcers on their feet. A common problem associated with PAD in diabetic patients is that the disease is often multilevel with common involvement of femoral-popliteal and tibial level arteries. Because of these factors, diabetic patients with PAD have much higher risk of limb loss in comparison to the nondiabetic patients with PAD.

SMOKING EFFECTS ON PAD: The mechanisms by which cigarette smoking accelerate the progression of atherosclerosis is not well determined. However, epidemiologically, smoking is associated with the acceleration of atherosclerosis, increased failure associated with revascularization, and increased amputation rates in patients with PAD.

ANKLE BRACHIAL INDEX (ABI): Ratio of the ankle systolic pressure by Doppler to the brachial systolic pressure by Doppler. ABI >0.9 is normal; ABI <0.9 signifies PAD, and ABI <0.4 is usually associated with rest pain or tissue loss (CLI).

PHYSIOLOGIC/FUNCTIONAL ASSESSMENT OF PAD: Segmental pressure measurement and Doppler waveform analysis can be obtained simultaneously in the noninvasive vascular laboratories and can help identify the locations of flow disturbing lesions within the vascular system. The drawback of segmental pressure measurement is falsely high pressures are seen in diabetic patients secondary to calcified arteries. Exercise testing is useful when the history, physical examination, and pressure readings are ambiguous.

ANATOMIC ASSESSMENT OF PATIENTS WITH PAD: Anatomic assessment of patients with PAD should be reserved only for individuals for whom invasive interventions are being considered. The available imaging studies include color flow duplex scan, spiral computed tomography (CT), magnetic resonance imaging (MRI), and arteriography. Arteriography is the most invasive of the imaging modalities used, but it is considered the "gold standard." The drawback associated with CT, MRI, and color flow duplex scans is limited resolution thus limiting the visualizing of subtle abnormalities in small vessels, such as arteries below the popliteal level.

CLINICAL APPROACH

Pain in the lower extremities with exercise, pain at rest, and ulcers or tissue necrosis in the feet or legs are common reasons leading to evaluations by vascular specialists. The patient evaluation should always begin with history focusing on his/her atherosclerotic disease risk factors and comorbidities, the patients' activity levels, symptomatology, inciting factors, duration of pain, location of pain, and alleviating factors. Claudication associated with insufficient arterial flow is generally manifested in the largest muscle groups just below the level of the flow disturbing lesion(s). For example, patients with aorto-iliac occlusive disease may complain of pain in the upper thighs and buttock regions with walking. In male patients with this problem, impotence may result from occlusive disease in the internal iliac arteries. The combination of **buttock and thigh claudication, impotence**, and **diminished femoral pulses** is referred to as **Leriche syndrome**. Patients with superficial femoral artery occlusive disease most often manifest with calf claudication.

Patients with critical limb ischemia (CLI) often have claudication with minimal exertion. In addition, these patients often have rest pain, which is described as pain located predominately in the foot and toes at rest, and rest pain is improved or relieved with dependent positioning of the extremity. On physical examination, patients with rest pain have chronic ischemic changes of the feet and lower legs including atrophic and shiny skin and loss of leg hairs. In addition, patients with CLI often have marked erythema of the feet in dependent positions (dependent rubor) and paleness of the feet with elevation (elevation pallor). The diagnosis of CLI ischemia can be established based on the history and physical examination findings just described, in addition to an ABI <0.4.

Once the patient's symptoms are determined to be due to PAD, the important next steps are to educate the patient regarding systemic cardiovascular disease risks, initiate appropriate medical management to reduce atherosclerotic risks, and to determine disease severity and whether imaging studies and invasive interventions should be pursued. When considering interventions for PAD at the femoral-popliteal artery segment, it is important to determine the anatomic locations, the degree of stenosis, and lengths of the occlusive lesions using the TASC Classification. Arterial occlusive disease can often be considered as inflow disease (above the inguinal ligament) or outflow disease (below the inguinal ligament). It is helpful to make the distinction between "inflow" and "outflow" diseases because operative interventions and percutaneous interventions are much more successful and durable for the treatment of inflow diseases. The durability and success of treatments for outflow diseases is further reduced for interventions performed to treat occlusive disease in the below-the-knee arteries such as the distal popliteal and tibial arteries.

Differential Diagnosis

Not all patients presenting with effort-related lower extremity pain have vasculogenic claudication. In some cases, neurogenic causes need to be differentiated from vasculogenic claudication (see Table 50–1). Neurogenic claudication can occur in association with spinal stenosis, which can also produce excruciating lower extremities pain during exertion or with positional changes; however, there are subtle differences that should be appreciated. The onset of neurogenic claudication tends to occur inconsistently with positional changes; whereas, claudication from PAD is related to insufficient blood flow to the major lower extremity muscles during exertion. Because this is a function of work load and blood supply, the symptoms are reproducible with the same amount of work load each and every time. Physical findings such as skin temperature, capillary refill, and peripheral pulses are critical to help differentiate patients with neurogenic causes from those from vascular causes.

Treatment

All patients with PAD should be counseled regarding risk of systemic cardiovascular disease complications; and all patients should be placed on appropriate risk-reduction strategies. In addition, patients need to be counseled regarding the importance of life style modifications. Diabetic teaching is particularly important for patients with PAD, because diabetes is an independent risk factor for ischemia-related limb loss. Some of the difficulties in the care of diabetic patients with PAD include the presence of neuropathy that makes patients more susceptible to tissue trauma in the feet and the increased susceptibility to infectious complications associated with even trivial trauma to the foot.

Invasive Interventions

Interventions are indicated predominantly in patients with CLI or severe claudication that severely compromises the patient's life style. It is important to convey to the patients, the reason to withhold operative or endovascular interventions is that the procedures can be associated with failures, and the failure of interventions can lead to worsening ischemia. Overall, the interventions for occlusive diseases in the aorta and iliac arteries are associated with greater long-term patency than procedures performed in smaller vessels at the below-the-knee level.

An understanding of the arterial anatomy is important to help clinicians localize the pathology in patients with PAD symptoms. Increasing levels of arterial involvement usually affect blood flow more significantly and usually are associated with greater need for open or endovascular interventions. The Trans-Atlantic Inter-society Consensus (TASC) has determined grading of PAD lesions based on location and characteristics. The classifications of anatomic lesions are helpful to determine whether open surgical approaches or endovascular approaches are best for each of the identified artery lesions (see Table 50–4 for patency outcomes after procedures).

Table 50–4 • GENERALLY REPORTED PATENCY RATES ASSOCIATED WITH REVASCULARIZATION FOR PAD*			
Procedure	3-year % patency	5-year % patency	10-year % patency
Aortobifemoral Bypass		~90%	~80%-86%
Axillo-bifemoral Bypass		~75%	
Iliac Artery Angioplasty	~82%	~71%	
Percutaneous Transluminal Angioplasty and Stent Placement for Femoral-popliteal Disease	~64%	~55%	
Femoral-popliteal Bypass (Above Knee)		~50%-75%	
Femoral-popliteal Bypass (Blow Knee)		~50%-60%	

*The patency rates of nearly all interventions are related to the indications for the procedure, such that the patency rates are generally lower for procedures performed in the setting of CLI when compared to claudication. Patency of surgical bypass procedures below the inguinal ligament levels is dependent on the quality and availability of conduits (vein conduits are associated with improved patency in comparison to PTFE conduits).

TASC CLASSIFICATION OF AORTO-ILIAC OCCLUSIVE DISEASE: This classification system was developed by the TASC.

Type A lesions

- Unilateral or bilateral common iliac artery
- Unilateral or bilateral single short stenosis (≤3 cm) of external iliac artery

Type B lesions

- Short (<3 cm) stenosis of infrarenal aorta
- Unilateral common iliac artery occlusion
- Single or multiple stenosis totaling 3 to 10 cm in the external iliac and not extending into the common femoral artery
- Unilateral external iliac artery occlusion not involving the origins of the internal iliac or common femoral artery

Type C lesions

- Bilateral common iliac artery occlusions
- Bilateral external iliac artery stenoses (3-10 cm long) not extending into the common femoral artery
- Unilateral external iliac artery stenosis extending into the common femoral artery
- Heavily calcified unilateral external iliac artery occlusion with or without involvement of the origin or the internal iliac and/or common femoral artery

Type D lesions

- Infrarenal aortoiliac occlusion

- Diffuse disease involving the aorta and both iliac arteries

- Diffuse multiple stenoses involving the unilateral common iliac artery, external iliac artery, and common femoral artery

- Unilateral occlusions of both common iliac artery and external iliac artery

- Bilateral occlusion of the external iliac artery

- Iliac artery stenoses in patient with abdominal aortic aneurysm requiring treatment and not amendable to endograft placement or other lesions requiring open aortic or iliac surgery

TASC CLASSIFICATION OF FEMORAL POPLITEAL ARTERY OCCLUSIVE DISEASE:

Type A lesions

- Single stenosis ≤10 cm in length

- Single occlusion ≤5 cm in length

Type B lesions

- Multiple lesions (stenoses or occlusions), each ≤5 cm

- Single stenosis or occlusion ≤15 cm not involving the infra-geniculate popliteal artery

- Single or multiple lesions in the absence of continuous tibial vessels to improve inflow for a distal bypass

- Heavily calcified occlusion ≤5 cm in length

- Single popliteal stenosis

Type C lesions

- Multiple stenoses or occlusions totaling >15 cm with or without heavy calcification

- Recurrent stenoses or occlusions that need treatment after two endovascular interventions

Type D lesions

- Chronic total occlusions of common femoral artery or superficial femoral artery (>20 cm involving the popliteal artery)

- Chronic total occlusion of common femoral artery or superficial femoral artery (>20 cm involving the popliteal artery)

- Chronic total occlusion of the popliteal artery and proximal trifurcation vessels

TREATMENT APPROACHES AND OUTCOMES BY TASC CLASSIFICATIONS:

Type A lesion: Type A lesions ("simple lesions") in the aorta, iliac, and femoral-popliteal have good results with endovascular treatment techniques (angioplasty and stenting).

Type B lesions: Type B lesions have good results using the endovascular approaches. The endovascular approaches are preferred unless open revascularization is needed for another lesion in the same anatomic region.

Type C lesions: Type C lesions have better long-term results with open revascularization techniques so endovascular approaches should be used only if the patient is at high risk for open surgery.

Type D lesions: Type D lesions have poor results with endovascular treatment, therefore open surgery is the primary treatment.

Adjuvant antiplatelet therapy has been shown to improve the long-term patency of infrainguinal bypass grafts; therefore, acetylsalicylic acid (ASA) is commonly prescribed for patients after revascularization procedures.

CASE CORRELATION

- See also Case 52 (Abdominal Aortic Aneurysm).

COMPREHENSION QUESTIONS

50.1 A 57-year-old man who works as a delivery man has left calf and thigh pain when he walks, and he is only able to walk 120 feet before stopping. He is worried that he may lose his job. The patient is a diabetic and takes an oral hypoglycemic agent, a long-acting β-blocker, and a statin. He smokes a pack of cigarettes each day. On examination, he has normal pulses in the right leg but no pulse in the left groin and leg. Which of the following is the most likely site of arterial occlusion?

A. His left iliac artery

B. His left superficial femoral artery

C. His descending thoracic aorta

D. His infra-renal aorta

E. His inominate artery

50.2 The patient described in Question 50.1 is managed medically. He returns 8 months later with worsening calf pain with minimal exertion and a non-healing ulcer at the tip of his left fourth toe. His pulse examination remains unchanged. His ABI on the left side is 0.37. Which of the following sites is now likely also involved with occlusive disease?

A. Left internal iliac artery

B. Left superficial femoral artery

C. Infra-renal aorta

D. Left profunda femoris artery

E. Thoracic aorta

50.3 The patient described in question 50.2 is found on CT-angiography to have three areas of narrowing and a 5-cm length of complete occlusion of the left common iliac artery; in addition, he has occlusion of an 18 cm portion of the left superficial femoral artery, with reconstitution of the popliteal artery and tibial vessels being patent and intact. What is the recommended management?

A. Continue life style management and risk-factor control

B. Aorto-bifemoral bypass

C. Left iliac artery angioplasty and stent placement followed by left femoral popliteal artery bypass

D. Left iliac artery angioplasty and left superficial femoral artery angioplasty and stent placement

E. Right femoral artery to left femoral artery bypass

50.4 An 82-year-old woman with history of severe dementia and left cerebral vascular accident leaving her with a dense right hemiparesis is noted to have a gangrenous toe and erythema of the foot and lower leg. This woman is severely debilitated by her dementia and stroke to the point where she is now confined to her bed in a long-term care facility. Her physical examination reveals diminished femoral pulses bilaterally, diminished popliteal pulse on the right and absent popliteal pulse on the left, and no palpable pedal pulses bilaterally. Her left first and second toes are gangrenous and she has extensive cellulitis involving her left foot and distal third of her lower leg. Her ABI on the left is 0.25. What is the best treatment option for this patient?

A. Obtain aortography with run-off of the left lower extremity to identify obstructive sites and treat those with angioplasty and stent placement, followed by toe amputations and antibiotic treatment

B. Perform left below the knee amputation

C. Obtain aortography with run-off of the left lower extremity to identify the obstructive sites then perform open bypass to revascularize the left lower leg, followed by toe amputations and antibiotic treatment

D. Toe amputations and antibiotics treatment

E. Hyperbaric oxygen treatment with antibiotics

50.5 A 57-year-old man presents with acute onset of right foot pain. He states that he was in his usual state of good health until 4 hours ago when he develop sudden onset of right foot and leg pain. Following the onset of pain, he has noted numbness in his right toes. His physical examination reveals irregularly irregular heart beat 120 beats/minute, blood pressure 130/78 mm Hg, and respiratory rate 24 breaths/minute. The cardiac monitor shows irregularly, irregular rhythm with the absence of p-waves. His right lower extremity is cool to the touch and has a bluish discoloration below the mid-thigh. The patient is unable to feel his toes and has difficulties moving them. His aortic pulse is normal, the femoral pulses are normal bilaterally, the left popliteal and pedal pulses are normal, and the right popliteal and pedal pulses are absent. Which of the following is the most appropriate treatment option?

A. Systemic heparinization, right femoral artery embolectomy

B. Systemic heparinization, angiography, and placement of right superficial femoral artery stent

C. Systemic heparinization

D. Catheter-directed thrombolytic therapy

E. Right femoral-popliteal bypass

ANSWERS

50.1 **A.** Occlusion of his left iliac artery would most likely be the cause of his symptoms and absence of pulse in his femoral artery and distally.

50.2 **B.** This patient's nonhealing ulcer, worsening claudication symptoms, and ABI of 0.37 are compatible with the diagnosis of critical limb ischemia. It is likely that there has been progression of the arterial occlusive process in his left lower extremity. Occlusion of the left superficial femoral artery (SFA) is most likely the problem. Although occlusion of the left profunda femoris artery is also possible, the SFA is a much more common site of involvement of PAD than the profunda femoris artery.

50.3 **C.** For this patient with critical limb ischemia, short segment left iliac artery occlusion (type B) and 18-cm segment of left SFA occlusion (type C), iliac artery angioplasty and stent placement with open femoral-popliteal bypass grafting is the most appropriate option listed here.

50.4 **B.** This patient has ischemic, gangrenous changes in the left, first and second toes. Her vascular examination suggests that she had occlusive disease at multiple levels above and below the inguinal ligament. Options A and C are appropriate if our goal of care is to establish blood flow to her left lower extremity to allow the local amputations to heal in her toes. The most important details regarding this patient's case are that she has severe dementia, neurologic deficits from a prior stroke, and she is nonambulatory and bed bound. Revascularization of the ischemic extremity is not justifiable and not beneficial for a patient who is bed bound and nonambulatory; therefore, below the knee amputation is the best option for her.

50.5 **A.** Systemic heparinization and femoral artery embolectomy is the most appropriate choice for this patient without history of chronic arterial occlusive disease symptoms presenting with new onset atrial fibrillation, and acute right femoral artery occlusion. Most likely, this patient has suffered from an acute embolization to that artery. Heparinization is important to minimize extension of the thrombus. The patient has ischemic symptoms with some findings of advanced ischemia (bluish discoloration with motor and sensory neuropathy). Surgical embolectomy and catheter-directed thrombolytic therapy are all options that would help revascularize the right leg. The surgical approach is more likely to re-establish perfusion faster than thrombolytic therapy and is a preferable option for him. Stent placement and femoral-popliteal artery bypass procedures are revascularization strategies for patients with chronic obstructions and are not necessary for this patient who likely does not have structural narrowing of the SFA.

CLINICAL PEARLS

▶ Medical management is critical in the treatment of patients with PAD, with a strong emphasis on smoking cessation, life style modification, and pharmacological therapy.

▶ Medical management targeting atherosclerotic risk reduction will diminish patient mortality and improve amputation-free survival.

▶ When considering invasive interventions, endovascular interventions should be first-line therapy for patients with TASC A, B, and C type lesions in the aortoiliac vessels or TASC A and B lesions in the femoral-popliteal vessels.

▶ Vasculogenic claudication is characterized by pain in the lower extremity muscles that occur with exertion and is relieved with rest.

▶ Neurogenic claudication is inconsistent and can be brought on or relieved with positional changes.

▶ Rest pain is pain located in the toes and feet that is relieved with dependent positioning.

▶ Critical limb ischemia (CLI) is associated with an ABI <0.4.

REFERENCES

Friedell ML, Stark KR, Kujath SW, Carter RR. Current status of lower-extremity revascularization. *Curr Probl Surg*. 2014;51:254-290.

Norgren L, Hiatt WR, Dormandy JA, et al. Inter-society consensus for the management of peripheral artery disease (TASCII). *Eur J Vasc Surg*. 2007;33(Suppl 1):S1-S75.

Silva Jr MB, Choi L, Cheng CC. Peripheral artery occlusive disease. In: Townsend Jr CM, Beauchamp RD, Evers BM, Mattox KL, eds. *Sabiston Textbook of Surgery: The Biological Basis of Modern Surgical Practice*. 19th ed. Philadelphia, PA: Elsevier Saunders; 2012:1725-1784.

A 58-year-old woman complains of the sudden onset of right chest pain and shortness of breath 4 days following an uncomplicated laparoscopic left hemi-colectomy for adenocarcinoma of the descending colon. Prior to this time, the patient has had an uncomplicated course, and was in the process of receiving her instructions for discharge from the hospital. During your assessment, she appears anxious and complains that she is unable to "catch her breath." Her temperature is 37.9°C (100.3°F), pulse rate is 105 bpm, blood pressure is 138/80 mm Hg, and respiratory rate is 32 breaths/minute. She is receiving O_2 by nasal cannula with an O_2 saturation of 96% by pulse oximetry. Despite her O_2 saturation, the patient is complaining that she is having difficulties with her breathing. There is no jugular venous distension. Her lungs are clear with slightly diminished breath sounds at both bases. Her legs are mildly edematous bilaterally and her left calf is mildly tender to palpation. Laboratory studies reveal a white blood cell (WBC) count of 10,000/mm^3 with normal differential, normal hemoglobin, hematocrit, and plate-let count. The serum electrolytes are normal. An arterial blood gas reveals pH 7.45, PO$_2$ 73 mm Hg, PCO$_2$ 34 mm Hg, and HCO$_3$ 24 mEq/L. A 12-lead electrocar-diogram (ECG) reveals sinus tachycardia. Serum creatinine kinase and troponin levels are within normal limits. A portable chest radiograph (CXR) demonstrates no infiltrates, no effusion, and minimal atelectasis in both lower lung fields.

▶ What is the most likely diagnosis?
▶ What should be your next steps?

ANSWERS TO CASE 51:

Venous Thromboembolism (VTE)

Summary: A 58-year-old woman develops sudden onset of chest pain and shortness of breath 4 days following laparoscopic colectomy for adenocarcinoma of the colon. Her physical examination does not identify any significant abnormalities other than calf tenderness. Her laboratory studies are non-contributory. Arterial blood gas reveals hypoxemia and respiratory alkalosis. The CXR and ECG do not demonstrate obvious pathology.

- **Most likely diagnosis:** Pulmonary embolism (PE) is likely given the sudden onset of chest pain and shortness of breath in a patient without prior history of pulmonary pathology, who has just undergone laparoscopic colectomy for adenocarcinoma of the colon.

- **Next steps:** Initiate systemic anticoagulation therapy for presumptive diagnosis of PE, transfer the patient to the intensive care unit, and obtain confirmatory imaging studies.

ANALYSIS

Objectives

1. Learn to risk-stratify patients and determine pretest probability for VTE.

2. Learn the applications of prophylaxis for VTE for surgical patients.

3. Learn the diagnostic and therapeutic approaches for patients with VTE.

Considerations

The differential diagnosis for a 58-year-old woman who develops the sudden onset of chest pain and shortness of breath during the postoperative period, which includes acute coronary syndrome, acute lung injury, respiratory infection, pneumothorax, and PE. Since all of these possible diagnoses are potentially lethal if not identified and treated in a timely fashion, the clinician must be prepared to investigate and address the patient's symptoms immediately. Her physical examination is essentially normal with the exception of calf tenderness and nonspecific diminished breath sounds at both lung bases. The laboratory data such as CBC, cardiac enzymes, and ABG are useful during the initial evaluation to point us toward or away from certain diagnoses. The ECG and CXR are equally important to help establish or rule out certain cardiac and pulmonary processes. We know that at this time, the patient has a history of colon cancer and a postoperative course that had been unremarkable up until this time. Her physical examination does not reveal pulmonary edema or pneumonia. The fact that she has had an unremarkable recovery from her colectomy reduces our suspicion for acute lung injury; this complication is commonly caused by an intra-abdominal infectious process in patients following intestinal surgery. The cause of her calf tenderness is currently unknown but may represent deep venous thrombosis (DVT) in that location. Her ABG results suggest respiratory alkalosis and hypoxemia. For all the reasons mentioned above, this patient has a high pretest probability for VTE, and based on our initial assessment, it is acceptable to initiate systemic anticoagulation therapy for the presumptive diagnosis of PE. Once this is initiated with appropriate supportive care, we can obtain the necessary confirmatory studies.

APPROACH TO:
Deep Venous Thrombosis and Pulmonary Embolism

DEFINITIONS

VENOUS DUPLEX IMAGING: An accurate, non-invasive imaging modality combining ultrasonography and Doppler technology to assess the patency of veins. This modality is very useful for evaluations of the upper and the lower extremities.

VENTILATION/PERFUSION (V/Q) SCAN: A radioisotope scan applied to identify V/Q mismatches, which can indicate PE when there is no other pathology (such as pneumonia and atelectasis) in the areas of mismatches. This diagnostic technique is less commonly performed since the introduction of the CT-angiography for PE diagnosis.

COMPUTED TOMOGRAPHY ANGIOGRAPHY (CTA): This vascular contrast study using CT technology has diagnostic sensitivities for PE reported from 64% to 93%. CTAs are highly sensitive for PEs involving the larger central pulmonary arteries and less sensitive for subsegmental PEs. There is evidence to suggest that when CTAs are obtained with concurrent CT venography of the pelvis, the diagnostic sensitivity is improved.

PULMONARY ANGIOGRAPHY: Considered the "gold standard" for PE diagnosis. Its accuracy is reported at 96%, and more importantly, pulmonary angiography has a low false-negative rate (0.6%). The advantage of pulmonary angiography is that, catheter directed treatments can be delivered to dissolve the clots in the pulmonary arteries. The draw-backs of this technique include delays in preparation for this study and procedure-related major complications in 1.3% of patients and reported mortality rate of 0.5%.

THROMBOLYTIC THERAPY FOR PE: Thrombolysis for PE are beneficial, especially for patients with large PEs causing persistent systemic hypotension. Tissue plasminogen activator (TPA) is the most commonly used agent, and it can be delivered systemically or by catheter-directed delivery to the pulmonary arteries. Recent major surgery (within 10 days) and/or recent traumatic brain injuries are considered contraindications to systemic thrombolytic therapy.

CATHETER-DIRECTED OR SURGICAL PULMONARY THROMBECTOMY: These treatment approaches require greater expertise and time to set up for the procedures. These procedures should be considered for patients with PEs with hemodynamic instability who failed initial thrombolytic therapy.

PROVOKED v. UNPROVOKED VTE: Characterization of VTE is an important part of the assessment and treatment process, prior to initiating treatments for first VTE events in patients. The assessment takes into account risk factors and recent events (eg, trauma, surgery, long plane rides, and cancer). Patients who are suspected to have unprovoked VTE often need life-long anticoagulation to prevent recurrences; whereas, patients with provoked VTE may by treated with shorter, defined courses.

D-**DIMER ASSAY:** Fibrin D-dimer is released into the circulation following degradation of cross-linked fibrin by plasmin. D-dimer can be measured using a number of commercially available assays. Elevation of D-dimers suggests that there is thrombus formation and degradation that is ongoing. The problem is that D-dimer elevations are not specific and also occur with sepsis, recent myocardial infarction, strokes, trauma, and surgery. Because of the multiple causes of D-dimer elevations in the hospitalized, surgical patients, this assay is of limited value to the assessment of patients with suspected VTE. **The combination of low-suspicion Wells score and nonelevated D-dimer is helpful to rule out VTE for patients in the outpatient settings.**

CLINICAL APPROACH

VTE is a major cause of morbidity and mortality in hospitalized patients and the leading cause of preventable hospital deaths. Approximately two-thirds of the patients with VTE present with DVT, with the remaining one-third of patients present with PE alone. The 30-day mortality of patients suffering a thrombotic event is 25%, and of those patients who survive their initial event, 30% will develop recurrent VTE within 10 years. A number of **genetic risk factors** for VTE has been identified, which include Factor V Leiden, protein C deficiency, protein S deficiency, and anti-thrombin deficiency. Similarly, there are a number of **acquired risk factors** (aging, cancer, obesity, congestive heart failure, stroke, and anti-phospholipid antibodies) and **transiently acquired risk factors** (immobility, trauma, hospitalization, pregnancy, central venous catheters, oral contraceptives, and hormonal therapy). Certain hospitalized patient populations are recognized to have higher risks of developing VTE, and this list of patients include hip or knee surgery patients, spinal cord injury patients, major trauma patients, cancer patients, neurosurgery patients, and patients undergoing major general surgery or gynecological surgery procedures. Patient populations with relatively lower VTE risks have also been identified (medical patients, gynecological, and general surgical patients undergoing minor surgery). **Risk stratification of VTE risk is important during any patient encounter, because without proper VTE risk-stratification and prophylaxis, the DVT incidences in some high-risk patients are reported to be as high as 80%.**

VTE Prophylaxis

VTE prophylaxis protocol is a well-recognized and effective approach to reducing VTE in hospitalized patients. The most effective way of implementing VTE prophylaxis protocols is to incorporate them into standardized orders such as admission, postoperative, and transfer orders. For most patients, prophylaxis consists of mechanical and/or pharmacologic measures. Hospitalized surgical patients are at

Table 51-1 • APPROXIMATE DEEP VENOUS THROMBOSIS PREVALENCE WITH AND WITHOUT PROPHYLAXIS			
Treatment	General Surgery (%)	Total Hip Replacement (%)	Trauma (%)
No therapy	25	51	50-58
Low-dose heparin	8	31	44
Low-molecular-weight heparin	7	15	30; proximal deep vein thrombosis reduced to 6
Elastic stockings	9 (data include only low-risk patients)	22	No evidence available
Intermittent pneumatic compression device	10 (only low- to moderate-risk patients)	38	No evidence available

significantly increased risk of VTE development secondary to stasis, hypercoagulability, and venous endothelial injury that are produced by local and systemic effects of trauma, operations, aging, and pre-existing conditions. The incidence of DVT in general surgical patients without appropriate prophylaxis is roughly 20% to 30%, with most of the patients being relatively asymptomatic. Patients with major traumatic injuries, spinal cord injuries, as well as orthopedic surgery patients undergoing joint replacements are among the highest risk populations for VTE. The application of appropriate VTE prophylaxis cannot be overemphasized in these high-risk populations. See Table 51–1.

Diagnosis

The Wells criteria are a set of validated assessment criteria to determine the pretest probability of PE during the evaluation of patients with suspected PE. Patient with score less than 2 are classified as low suspicion; patients with scores of 2 to 6 are moderate risk, and patients with scores >6 are high risk (see Table 51–2). Determination of VTE pretest probability helps to identify patients in whom empiric therapy should be initiated prior to obtaining confirmatory studies. In addition, risk stratification can also help eliminate unnecessary imaging studies in some patients. See Figure 51–1 for suggested diagnostic and management decisions.

Table 51-2 • WELLS CRITERIA	
Clinical characteristics	Score
Signs of DVT (Leg swelling, pain, tenderness with palpation of deep veins)	3
Immobilization or surgery in previous 4 weeks	1.5
Previous DVT/PE	1.5
Hemoptysis	1
Malignancy	1
An alternative diagnosis is less likely than PE	3

Total Wells score:	Mean probability of PE
Low suspicion <2	4%
Moderate suspicion 2-6	21%
High suspicion >6	67%

Treatment

Systemic anticoagulation therapy is the primary treatment modality for patients with VTE. This therapy is helpful in preventing PE or PE recurrences and in reducing clot propagation. Early initiation of therapy and early attainment of therapeutic levels of anticoagulation are two factors that have been demonstrated to reduce VTE recurrences (See Table 51-3). Anticoagulation is usually delivered by intravenous unfractionated heparin or with weight-based dosing of low-molecular weight heparin (LMWH). Unfractionated heparin dosing is typically titrated to maintain an activated partial thromboplastin time (aPTT) of 2 to 2.5 times normal. LMWH administration has the advantage of not needing monitoring and can be administered by subcutaneous dosing. Once initial anticoagulation is established, most patients are then transitioned to oral warfarin therapy. **The overlapping of heparin or LMWH with warfarin is important because initiation of warfarin without prior**

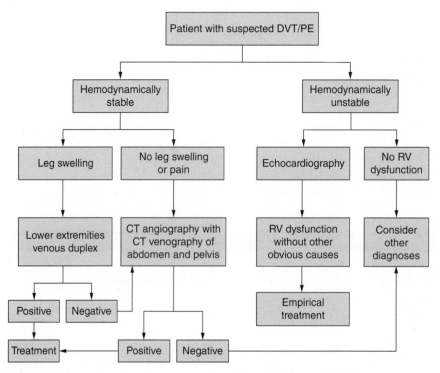

Figure 51-1. Diagnostic and treatment strategy for patients with suspected DVT/PE.

Table 51–3 • DEEP VEIN THROMBOSIS TREATMENT AND EFFICACY	
Unfractionated heparin	6% recurrence; 3% major bleeding; 1%-3% risk of heparin-induced thrombocytopenia
Low-molecular-weight heparin	3% recurrence; 1% major bleeding; associated with a lower risk of heparin-induced thrombocytopenia
Thrombolysis therapy	Indicated for iliofemoral deep vein thrombosis; contraindicated in recently postoperative patients or after recent head trauma

anticoagulation with heparin or LMWH can cause a transient hypercoagulable state secondary to the inhibition of proteins C and S. Some patients with long-term anticoagulation needs are being maintained on newer oral agents that include direct thrombin inhibitor (dibigatran), and factor Xa inhibitors (rivaroxaban, apixaban). Several clinical trials have verified that these newer agents are not inferior in comparison to warfarin.

The duration of anticoagulation can be highly variable depending on the patient and the VTE event. In general, a patient with femoral–popliteal DVT without persistent risk factors would only require 3 months of systemic anticoagulation therapy. Patients with PE and no genetically determined hypercoagulable conditions should receive 6 months of anticoagulation therapy. Patients with unprovoked VTE often require 12 months or longer periods of systemic anticoagulation. Patients with genetic causes of VTE should be managed with life-long anticoagulation therapy.

Vena Caval Filters

Inferior vena caval filters are indicated for the following conditions: (1) VTE recurrence or propagation in the face of therapeutic anticoagulation; (2) VTE and contraindication to systemic anticoagulation. The protection rate of patients with IVC filters from PE is reported to be similar to the rate (~95%) reported for patients undergoing systemic anticoagulation therapy. IVC filters are associated with increased local complications including IVC thrombosis and erosion. Retrievable filtered are being applied increasingly to reduce the rate of filter-related complications.

CASE CORRELATION

- See also Case 2 (Perioperative Management of Antithrombotic and Antiplatelet Therapies).

COMPREHENSION QUESTIONS

51.1 A 49-year-old man with diabetes underwent laparoscopic colectomy 5 days ago. He now complains of right calf and thigh swelling and pain. His vital signs are normal. Which of the following is the most appropriate next step for this patient?

A. Begin systemic thrombolytic therapy

B. Perform CTA of the chest and CTV of the pelvis

C. Perform a pulmonary angiography

D. Determine D-dimer level, and obtain a pulmonary angiogram if this value is elevated

E. Perform lower extremity venous duplex scan

51.2 In which of the patients with confirmed femoral vein thrombosis is unfractionated heparin contraindicated?

A. A hemodynamically stable 80-year-old man with symptomatic left femoral DVT

B. A 20-year-old man who sustained a concussion (TBI with no CT abnormalities) during a car crash 8 days ago

C. A 23-year-old woman in her third-trimester of pregnancy

D. 44-year-old woman with heparin-induced thrombocytopenia

E. 28-year-old man with grade 3 liver laceration sustained following a gunshot wound to the abdomen

51.3 A 35-year-old man is hospitalized for right femur fracture suffered after a car crash. He develops dyspnea and pain in the left thigh on postinjury day 5. He subsequently underwent a V/Q scan that is interpreted as "low probability" for PE. Which of the following statements is most accurate?

A. The probability of PE is less than 1%

B. The probability of PE is as high as 40%

C. A D-dimer assay should be obtained for confirmation

D. Pulmonary angiography should be obtained to definitively rule out PE

E. Systemic heparinization should not be initiated unless PE is confirmed

51.4 Which of the following choices is the most appropriate VTE prophylaxis for a 33-year-old man who just underwent an exploratory laparotomy, distal pancreatectomy, splenectomy, and repair of gastric perforation for injuries suffered from a gunshot wound to the abdomen? He had approximately 3000 mL of blood loss during the operation. Following the operation, he has been stable in the ICU with hematocrit measurement of 28% and international normalized ratio (INR) of 1.5. He does not have any signs of active blood loss currently.

A. LMW heparin

B. 5000 unit of unfractionated heparin TID

C. 5000 unit of unfractionated heparin BID

D. Pneumatic compression devices

E. Withhold DVT prophylaxis until the INR normalizes

51.5 A 72-year-old man who had right hip replacement surgery 4 days ago is diagnosed with a small subsegmental PE. Which of the following studies is probably the most helpful for the diagnosis?

A. Chest x-ray

B. Troponin levels

C. Venous duplex scan of the lower extremities

D. CT-angiography

E. 12-lead ECG

51.6 Which of the following patients has the lowest pretest probability of having PE?

A. A 65-year-old man with history of CHF who is hospitalized after undergoing right hip replacement

B. A 47-year-old woman with stage 3 ovarian cancer undergoing chemotherapy

C. A 26 year-old 38-week pregnant woman whose pregnancy is complicated by HELLP syndrome

D. A 21-year-old man who had an uncomplicated laparoscopic appendectomy 3 days ago

E. A 38-year-old man with a history of right femoral DVT 3 years ago after a 6-hour plane ride

51.7 A 57-year-old man who had an indwelling central venous catheter placed 1 day ago for chemotherapy administration for his recently diagnosed non-Hodgkin lymphoma develops sudden onset of pleuritic chest pain and dyspnea. His vital signs are normal. His lungs are clear and the remainder of his physical examination is noncontributory. Which of the following studies is least helpful in this patient?

A. D-dimer assay

B. CT-angiography of the chest

C. VQ scan

D. Chest x-ray

E. 12-lead ECG

ANSWERS

51.1 **E.** This man's presentation is suspicious for right femoral–popliteal DVT. Lower extremity venous duplex study is the most appropriate diagnostic study for this patient. Systemic thrombolytic therapy is usually given only to a patient with proven proximal DVT. CTA of the chest and CTV of the pelvis would be appropriate if the patient had symptoms suggestive of PE. Pulmonary angiography is not indicated in this patient with suspected DVT and no symptoms of PE. The D-dimer is most likely elevated in this patient who had recent surgery, and this assay result would not be helpful to direct further testing.

51.2 **D.** The woman with a history of heparin-induced thrombocytopenia, which is an IgG-induced reaction, has a contraindication to unfractionated heparin therapy. A man with mild TBI without CT abnormality 8 days ago does not have a contraindication for systemic heparinization. The man with liver injury following gunshot wound to the liver has increased risk of bleeding with anticoagulation, but treatment is not contraindicated. Unfractionated heparin does not cross the placenta and is not contraindicated during pregnancy.

51.3 **B.** In this patient with high pretest probability of having VTE, PE probability can be as high as 40% even with a "low probability" VQ scan. If the patient has low clinical suspicion and a "low probability" VQ scan, the probability of PE is only about 4%. The D-dimer assay is not helpful because in this setting it will be abnormally elevated for a variety of reasons that may not be related to VTE. Systemic heparinization should be administered for high-risk patients with high clinical suspicion for PE even prior to ordering confirmatory studies having been obtained, because delays in treatment can contribute to recurrences.

51.4   **A.** LMW heparin is more effective than unfractionated heparin in the chemoprevention of VTE in high-risk patients. Trauma patients with a history of large amount of blood losses are considered extremely high risk for VTE. For these trauma patients with massive blood losses, once the bleeding sources have been controlled, VTE prophylaxis can be initiated within 36 hours. Pneumatic compression devices are not very effective in the prevention of VTE in the high-risk population. The elevation of INR after massive blood losses generally reflects a coagulopathy, and this INR elevation does not appear to confer any protective benefits against VTE development.

51.5   **D.** This 72-year-old man is diagnosed with a small subsegmental PE following hip replacement surgery. The CT-angiography is the most useful diagnostic study listed that would help make the diagnosis. CXR and 12-lead ECG are often nonspecific in a patient with small subsegmental PE. Venous duplex of the lower extremities would identify DVTs if the PE originated in the lower extremities. Troponin elevation is not frequently observed in patients with PEs.

51.6   **D.** An otherwise healthy man who underwent laparoscopic appendectomy does not have a significant risk of VTE, unless the procedure is prolonged or complicated by sepsis of blood loss. A 65 year-old man with history of CHF and recent hip replacement has a significant risk of VTE. The woman with ovarian carcinoma has increased risk of VTE. The pregnant woman with HELLP syndrome has increased VTE risk from pregnancy and critical illness. The woman with a prior history of DVT has a higher pretest probability of VTE than someone without this prior history.

51.7   **A.** This 57-year-old man develops pleuritic chest pain and dyspnea. He had a central line placed 1 day ago. The two leading possible causes for his current condition are PE and delayed presentation of pneumothorax following his central line placement. Acute coronary syndrome can also be a possibility given his age, but this would be lower on our differential diagnosis. All of the studies listed with the exception of the D-dimer assay are likely helpful to help identify the cause of his symptoms.

CLINICAL PEARLS

▶ Up to 95% of patients with VTE have recognizable risk factors and therefore would benefit from prophylactic measures.

▶ The benefits of prophylactic measure against VTE are additive and should be applied together to reduce risks maximally in the very high-risk patients.

▶ Liberal application venous duplex studies should be considered in the very high-risk patients even with prophylactic measures in place.

▶ Heparin-induced thrombocytopenia is a contraindication to heparin administration.

▶ Upper extremity DVT (such as sublavian vein DVT) carries much higher risk of PE than lower extremity DVT.

▶ Retrievable inferior vena caval filters are indicated for patients who develop PE or DVT propagation in the setting of appropriate anticoagulation therapy for DVT.

▶ Retrievable filter are indicated for patient with lower extremity DVT and with contraindication to systemic anticoagulation.

▶ The Wells score is a scoring system to stratify a patient's clinical risk of having VTE.

▶ The combination of low Wells score (<2) and normal D-dimer helps to rule out the diagnosis of VTE.

REFERENCES

Gould MK, Garcia DA, et al. Prevention of VTE in nonorthopedic surgical patients. *Antithrombotic Therapy and Prevention of Thrombosis*. 9th ed. American College of Chest Physicians evidence-based clinical practice guidelines. *Chest*. 2012;141(s):e227S-e277S.

Pollak AW, McBane II RD. Succint review of the new VTE prevention and management guidelines. *Mayo Clin Proc*. 2014;89:394-408.

Turney EJ, Lyden SP. The Prevention of venous thromboembolism. In: Cameron JL, Cameron AM, eds. *Current Surgical Therapy*. 11th ed. Philadelphia, PA: Elsevier Saunders; 2014:972-976.

During a routine physical examination, a primary care physician identifies an asymptomatic pulsatile mass in the abdomen of a 62-year-old man. An ultrasound evaluation revealed a 4.8-cm aneurysm in the infrarenal aorta. This patient is subsequently referred to the vascular surgeon for evaluation and management. The patient's past medical history is significant for hypertension and stable angina. He has a 40-pack-year smoking history. His current medications include aspirin, a beta-blocker, and nitrates. The patient describes himself as an active man who just retired and plays 18-holes of golf two times a week. On examination, the carotid pulses and upper extremity pulses are normal. The abdomen is nontender with a prominent aortic pulse. Pulses in the femoral and popliteal regions are readily palpable and appear more prominent than usual.

▶ What are the complications associated with this disease process?
▶ What is the best treatment?

ANSWERS TO CASE 52:
Abdominal Aortic Aneurysm

Summary: A 62-year-old man presents with an asymptomatic abdominal aortic aneurysm (AAA) measuring 4.8 cm in diameter.

- **Complications:** Rupture, thrombosis, distal embolization, and increased risk for arterial aneurysms at other sites.

- **Best treatment:** The best treatment for this patient is to continue surveillance. Given the AAA size, the risk of repair outweighs the benefits at this time.

ANALYSIS

Objectives

1. Learn the presentations, evaluations, treatment, and follow-up of patients with abdominal aortic aneurysms.

2. Learn the risks and outcomes associated with elective open aneurysm repairs.

3. Describe the role of elective endovascular aneurysm repairs (EVAR) and the repair of ruptured aneurysms.

Considerations

A 62-year-old man with hypertension and stable angina presents with a 4.8 cm asymptomatic infrarenal AAA. The patient's physical examination is suggestive of aneursymal disease in the femoral and popliteal arteries. Based on the current size of his AAA, it is best to just follow the AAA with repeat physical examinations and follow-up ultrasound examinations every 6 months. In addition, it is important to obtain ultrasound, CT-angiography, or MR-arteriography to assess the femoral and popliteal arteries since the physical examination findings are suspicious for the presence of aneurysmal changes in those areas. The reason for continuing surveillance rather than repairing the AAA at this time is that randomized controlled trials comparing observation vs. elective repairs of small asymptomatic AAA (4.0-5.0 cm) showed that elective repairs were associated with increased 30-day mortality and did not improve patient survival over a mean follow-up period of 20 months. The current recommendations for open or endovascular interventions for AAA are based on **size, growth rate,** and **symptoms**; criteria are specifically: (1) **Diameter >5.5 cm in men** or **diameter >5.0 cm in women**; (2) **Rapid growth of >0.5 cm/6 months**; (3) **Symptomatic AAA (pain or distal embolism)**.

Even though intervention for his aneurysm is not currently indicated based on the size and the asymptomatic nature, it is important to educate the patient regarding risk reduction strategies to minimize AAA expansion and rupture. The control of hypertension, hypercholesterolemia, and coronary artery disease seem to be beneficial in reducing the risk of AAA expansion.

APPROACH TO:
Abdominal Aortic Aneurysm

DEFINITIONS

ANEURYSM: By definition, an aneurysm exists when a segment of an artery increases in size to more than 50% of the normal diameter (ie, >150% size of native artery). Aneurysm formation is caused by conditions that cause weakening of the arterial walls, including collagen defects, inflammatory conditions, immune responses, and atherosclerotic changes.

INHERITED CONDITIONS ASSOCIATED WITH ANEURYSMS: Marfan syndrome, Ehlers-Danlos syndrome, and familial thoracic aneurysm and dissection (TAAD) syndrome are known hereditary conditions associated with AAA.

ABDOMINAL AORTIC ANEURYSM RISK FACTORS

Nonmodifiable risk factors	Modifiable risk factors
Older age (age >50 for men and age >60 for women) Male sex (4× increased risk vs. female) Family history Race (more common in Whites) Height	Smoking Hypertension Elevated cholesterol levels Obesity

AAA SCREENING RECOMMENDATIONS: The U.S. Preventive Service Task Force recommends one-time ultrasound screening in men age 65 to 75 who have ever smoked, and selective screening for men age 65 to 75 who have never smoked.

AAA SURVEILLANCE: Small aneurysms (3.0-5.4 cm) in men when identified should be monitored for size changes by ultrasonography. Recommended surveillance ultrasonography with these recommended intervals: 2.6 to 2.9 cm re-examine in 5 years; 3.0 to 3.4 cm every 3 years; 3.5 to 4.4 cm every year; 4.5 to 5.4 cm every 6 months.

ESTIMATED RUPTURE RISK BASED ON SIZE: <4 cm (0%/year); 4 to 5 cm (0.5%/year); <5.5 cm (<1%/year); 5–6 cm (3%-15%/year); 6–7 cm (10%-20%/year); 7 to 8 cm (20%-40%/year); >8 cm (30%-50%/year).

ENDOLEAKS FOLLOWING EVAR: Endoleaks are persistence of blood flow outside of the endograft following EVAR, and endoleaks are the most common reasons for secondary interventions following EVAR.

Type I endoleak: Caused by inadequate sealing at either the proximal or distal endograft attachment sites.

Type II endoleak: Caused by blood flow into the aneurysm sac from patent branch vessels such as inferior mesenteric artery and lumbar arteries.

Type III endoleak: Caused by a defect in the fabric of the endograft or leakage between separate graft components deployed.

Type IV endoleak: Leaking between the interstices of the graft fabric.

Type V endoleak or endotension: Aneurysm sac that remains pressurized without visible endoleaks.

CLINICAL APPROACH

Arterial aneurysms develop as the result of a degenerative processes involving the arterial wall. The process is associated with infiltration of the arterial wall by lymphocytes and macrophages, destruction of the elastin and collagen in the media and adventitia of the artery, and loss of smooth-muscle cells resulting in thinning of the arterial wall. Age and family history are two of the most important risk factors associated with AAA formation. The prevalence of AAA increases after the age of 50 in men and after 60-70 in women. The risk of AAA formation is greater in men than women (men: women ratio of 4:1). The majority of individuals with AAA do not have symptoms until rupture occurs; therefore, screening can be valuable in identifying the disease in high-risk populations, such as older men and individuals with family history of AAA. **A number of risk-reduction strategies has been identified to decrease aneurysm ruptures including smoking cessation, control of hypertension and hypercholesterolemia.**

In terms of location, approximately 85% of the AAAs are located in the infrarenal aorta. **Aneurysm size and symptoms are the best predictors of rupture.** When AAA ruptures occur, the overall mortality rate is 85% to 90%. For individuals who are fortunate enough to reach the hospital with ruptured AAA, the reported mortality is 50% to 70%. Given the lethal nature of ruptured AAA, it is most important to identify the patients with high-risk AAAs for elective repairs to prevent ruptures.

Aneurysm Repairs

Most experts recommend elective AAA repairs when the aneurysm reaches 5.5 cm in men and 5.0 cm in women. AAA repair options include open aneurysmectomy and endovascular aneurysm repair (EVAR). The open approach can be performed either by a trans-abdominal approach or a retroperitoneal approach. The open approaches are associated with extensive dissections and significant perioperative fluid shifts. The average reported 30-day mortality for open AAA repair is 4% to 5%, with average hospital stay of 9 days. EVAR on the other hand is a percutaneous approach generally gained through a puncture in the femoral artery. Under image-guidance, covered stent grafts are placed into the aorta and anchored to the normal aorta above the aneurysm and to the iliac arteries below the aneurysm. **EVAR approach is now done for more than 75% of all AAA repairs in the United States.** Based on arterial anatomy and technical limitations, some patients are not candidates for EVAR. The reported 30-day mortality after EVAR is 1% with an average hospital stay of 3 days. Procedure-related cardiovascular, pulmonary, and infectious complications rates are significantly lower following EVAR in comparison to open repairs. Patients require close follow-up after both open AAA repairs and EVAR.

In general, 20% to 30% of patients require secondary interventions within 6 years following EVAR. The monitoring recommendations for patients following EVAR are CT scans at 1 month and 12 months following the procedures, as most endoleaks following repairs tend to present early. The majorities of the reinterventions following EVAR are percutaneous, with only 2% to 4% of the patients requiring open secondary interventions. A reintervention rate of approximately 20% is seen following open AAA repairs; therefore, CT monitoring is recommended at 5-year intervals following open AAA repairs.

CASE CORRELATION

- See also Case 50 (Claudication Syndrome).

COMPREHENSION QUESTIONS

52.1 A 61-year-old man is found on physical examination to have an asymptomatic AAA. Ultrasound evaluation reveals that the AAA measures 4 cm in diameter. Which of the following is the best surveillance strategy for his AAA?

A. Observation with ultrasound evaluation every 3 years

B. Ultrasound evaluation only when the AAA becomes symptomatic

C. Ultrasound evaluation every 6 months

D. Ultrasound evaluation every year

E. CT angiography every 6 months

52.2 For the patient described in question 52.1, when is continued nonoperative treatment most reasonable?

A. The patient complains of back pain without other identifiable causes. His AAA is now measuring 5.2 cm in diameter

B. The patient's aneurysm has increased to 4.8 cm over 2 years; however, he presents with painful ischemic changes in several toes in both feet

C. The aneurysm measures 5.3 cm in diameter at follow-up 3 years after surveillance began

D. The patient's aneurysm grew from 4.6 cm to 5.5 cm over a 6-month interval

E. The patient presents with sudden onset of back pain with CT demonstrating retroperitoneal fluid around the AAA

52.3 Which of the following is a known complication associated with AAA?

A. Early satiety

B. Small bowel obstruction

C. Painful discoloration of the great toe

D. Hematuria

E. Hematochezia

52.4 Which of the following statements is true regarding EVAR?

A. EVAR is associated with higher peri-procedural complication rates in comparison to open repairs

B. EVAR can be applied to 100% of the patients with AAA

C. Most EVAR complications do not require open interventions

D. EVAR is an inferior approach for patients with prior abdominal operations

E. EVAR is no longer recommended due to its peri-procedural complications

52.5 For which of the following patients is nonoperative management most appropriate?

A. A 65-year-old otherwise healthy woman with a 5.2 cm AAA

B. A 96-year-old man with severe dementia and a 6-cm AAA. The patient has been a long-term resident of a chronic care facility due to inability to care for himself secondary to his dementia

C. A 60-year-old man with a 5.3 cm AAA who presents with unexplained back pain over the past 24 hours. No other causes of back pain can be identified

D. A 63-year-old man with 5.4 cm AAA and new onset of painful ecchymoses in the tips of several toes in both feet

E. A 63-year-old man with a known AAA that is under surveillance. His aneurysm has grown from 4.5 to 5.4 cm over the past 6 months

52.6 Which of the following statements is true regarding EVAR?

A. With introduction of EVAR, the minimal size for recommending repairs have changed

B. EVAR is contraindicated in individuals with aneurysms >10 cm

C. EVAR repair is associated with higher rates of leakage within the first year in comparison to open repairs

D. EVAR is contraindicated in individuals with aneurysms involving the iliac arteries

E. EVAR should not be performed in individuals who can tolerate open repairs

ANSWERS

52.1 **D.** The current recommendations for ultrasound surveillance of AAA are: 2.6 to 2.9 cm re-examine in 5 years; 3 to 3.4 cm re-examine every 3 years; 3.5 to 4.4 cm re-examine yearly; 4.5 to 5.4 cm re-examine every 6 months.

52.2 **C.** AAAs measuring less than 5.5 cm and that are asymptomatic in men can be monitored. Symptomatic AAA often represents impending rupture and is an indication for repair. Similarly AAA that has rapid growth defined as >0.5 cm growth over a 6 month period should also be repaired. Patients presenting with "blue toe syndrome" related to their AAA should undergo AAA repair, as this syndrome is related to distal embolization from the aneurysm. Patient described in choice "E" has a leaking AAA that should undergo emergency repair.

52.3 **C.** Painful discoloration of the toes can occur as the result of embolization of aneurysm contents to the distal arteries. This is referred to as the "blue toes syndrome" or "trashed feet."

52.4 **C.** Most EVAR complications are amendable to percutaneous treatments, with only 2% to 4% of patients requiring open interventions for complications. EVAR is associated with lower postoperative complications and shorter hospitalization when compared to open repairs. EVAR is a better approach than open repairs for patients with extensive history of prior abdominal operations. Currently, EVAR outnumbers open AAA repairs in the United States.

52.5 **B.** AAA repair for a man with a 6-cm AAA may be medically indicated; however, given his limited level of function and poor quality of life, AAA repair is not likely to improve his quality of life. It is difficult to justify AAA repair for this individual given that the indications for repair are better in the other individuals described.

52.6 **C.** The endoleaks associated with EVAR are generally present within the first year after the procedures; whereas, complications related to open aneurysm repairs tend to occur later. There is no size limitation to EVAR. The introduction of EVAR has not changed the size criteria for recommending aneurysm repairs.

CLINICAL PEARLS

▶ Patients diagnosed with AAA should have thorough pulse examination to look for aneurysmal disease in other anatomic locations.

▶ AAAs are palpable in the epigastrium, whereas iliac aneurysms can be palpable in the infraumbilical locations

▶ AAA is more common in men than women, but the risk of rupture is higher in women.

▶ AAA greater than 5.5 cm in men and 5.0 cm in women should be considered for repair due to the risk of rupture.

▶ A patient with suspected ruptured AAA associated with hemodynamic instability should undergo exploration and attempted repair rather delaying the repair for confirmatory CT scan.

▶ Rapid growth of AAA, defined as >0.5 cm growth in 6 months is an indication for repair.

REFERENCES

Kent KC. Abdominal aortic aneurysms. *N Engl J Med*. 2014;371:2101-2108.

Orandi BJ, Black III JH. Open repair of abdominal aortic aneurysms. In: Cameron JL, Cameron AM, eds. *Current Surgical Therapy*. 11th ed. Philadelphia, PA: Elsevier Saunders; 2014:777-783.

Shuja F, Kwolek CJ. *Endovascular treatment of abdominal aortic aneurysm*. In: Cameron JL, Cameron AM, eds. *Current Surgical Therapy*. 11th ed. Philadelphia, PA: Elsevier Saunders; 2014:783-787.

Thomas DM, Hulten EA, Ellis ST, et al. Open versus endovascular repair of abdominal aortic aneurysm in the elective and emergent setting in a pooled population of 37,781 patients: a systematic review and meta-analysis. *ISRN Cardiol*. 2014;10:1155. http://dx.doi.org/10.1155/2014/149243.

A 77-year-old woman is seen in the outpatient clinic for the evaluation of weight loss. The patient is a reliable historian and indicates that 6 months ago she weighed 138 pounds (62.7 kg) but over the past several months her weight has steadily declined to 94 pounds (42.7 kg). The patient attributes her weight loss to an inability to eat. She relates that whenever she tries to eat a meal, she develops intense abdominal pain that is severe and diffuse throughout her entire abdomen. To avoid the pain, she has limited herself to small meals and soups. She denies any fever, malaise, nausea, vomiting, or constipation. Her past medical history is significant for hypertension for which she takes an angiotensin-converting enzyme inhibitor. She smokes approximately one pack of cigarettes per day and consumes a glass of wine each day. The physical examination reveals a thin woman in no acute distress. Her skin and sclera are nonicteric, and bilateral carotid bruits are present. The results of her cardiopulmonary examination are unremarkable. The abdomen is scaphoid, nontender, and without masses. Her stool is hemoccult negative. Her femoral pulses are diminished with audible bruits bilaterally. There is audible bruit over her epigastric region. Her pulses are diminished in both lower extremities. Laboratory evaluations are obtained revealing a normal complete blood count and normal electrolyte values. The serum urea nitrogen, creatinine, and glucose values are within the normal ranges, as are the results of a urinalysis. The 12-lead ECG reveals normal sinus rhythm. Her PA and lateral chest x-rays reveal no infiltrates, masses, or other pathology.

- ▶ What is the most likely diagnosis?
- ▶ What is the most likely mechanism causing her problem?
- ▶ What is the best treatment?

ANSWERS TO CASE 53:
Mesenteric Ischemia

Summary: A 77-year-old woman with carotid, abdominal, and femoral bruits presents with signs and symptoms consistent with mesenteric angina, leading to food aversion or "food fear" and significant unintentional weight loss.

- **Most likely diagnosis:** Postprandial abdominal pain, massive weight loss, and signs of advanced systemic atherosclerotic changes suggest chronic mesenteric ischemia.

- **Most likely mechanism causing the problem:** Occlusion of the mesenteric arteries causes mesenteric angina with food ingestion.

- **Best treatment:** Revascularization by either surgical or endovascular approach.

ANALYSIS

Objectives

1. Learn the causes, presentations, diagnosis, and treatment of acute and chronic mesenteric ischemia.

2. Learn the diagnosis and treatment of patients with mesenteric angina related to mesenteric arterial occlusion.

Considerations

This patient presents with the classic symptom complex of food fear with postprandial pain and significant unintentional weight loss, which are the hallmarks of chronic mesenteric ischemia. The typical symptoms that a patient with intestinal angina reports are postprandial cramping and dull abdominal pain that begins shortly after eating and lasting 1 to 2 hours. In some patients, the pain is associated with nausea, vomiting, and diarrhea. Because chronic mesenteric ischemia is an uncommon clinical entity, it is important that we conduct a thorough evaluation for all possible causes of chronic abdominal pain prior to proceeding with mesenteric revascularization. Once the more common causes of upper and lower GI sources of abdominal pain are ruled out by clinical evaluations, endoscopies, and abdominal imaging, the mesenteric arteries can be studied. Duplex ultrasound is a noninvasive study that can be used to evaluate blood flow in the splanchnic circulation. Waveform analyses can be utilized to gauge the severity of narrowing within the mesenteric arteries. Alternatively, computed tomographic angiography (CTA) or magnetic resonance angiography (MRA) can be obtained to help identify narrowing within the mesenteric arteries. A major advantage of CTA is that it is helpful to rule-out occult GI malignancies such as pancreatic cancers or retroperitoneal processes such as lymphomas.

The treatment for chronic mesenteric ischemia is revascularization by either an open surgical or endovascular approach. The decision to proceed with surgical approach or an endovascular approach to revascularization depends on the patient's anatomy and the available technical expertise. Both revascularization approaches can contribute to morbidity and mortality in the peri-procedural period. Surgical revascularization is reported to have better long-term patency in comparison to revascularization by endovascular approaches.

APPROACH TO:
Mesenteric Ischemia

Mesenteric ischemia-related conditions are broadly categorized as acute or chronic. Patients with *acute mesenteric ischemia* present to the hospital with acute abdominal pain that is often sudden in onset, diffuse, persistent, and severe. The anatomical distribution of the arterial blood supply can explain the symptoms (see Table 53–1). The "classic" presentation of **pain out of proportion to the physical examination findings often holds true for these patients until intestinal necrosis with peritonitis sets in.** The patient's histories can provide helpful clues for clinicians to make the diagnosis, because the majority of acute mesenteric ischemia patients have predisposing conditions, such as a history of atrial fibrillation, recent myocardial infarction, hypercoagulable conditions, connective tissue disorder, portal hypertension, or digoxin or vasopressor use.

Arterial occlusive disease is responsible for 40% to 50% of the acute mesenteric ischemia cases, and these cases typically occur in patients with atrial fibrillation or acute myocardial infarction. In these patients, the thrombi typically form in the heart and then dislodge and embolize to arterial strictures anywhere in the body including the SMA (see Figure 53–1). Ischemic injuries to the intestines from this process typically involve the distal small bowel and proximal colon. It is important to keep in mind that embolic events to other organs can occur in patients with SMA embolism; therefore, systemic anticoagulation is important for the management of these patients. Patient with SMA embolism can be managed with operative thrombectomy, catheter-directed thrombolytics treatment, or expectant management, depending on the severity of the embolic event and viability of the intestines.

Table 53–1 · VISCERAL BLOOD SUPPLY		
Arterial trunk	Arterial branches	GI organs perfused
Celiac artery	Hepatic artery, splenic artery, gastric arteries	Liver, stomach, and duodenum
Superior mesenteric artery	Branches to the small bowel, ileocolic artery, right colic artery, middle colic artery	Small bowel, right colon, and transverse colon
Inferior mesenteric artery	Sigmoid artery, superior and middle hemorrhoidal arteries	Descending colon, sigmoid colon, and upper rectum

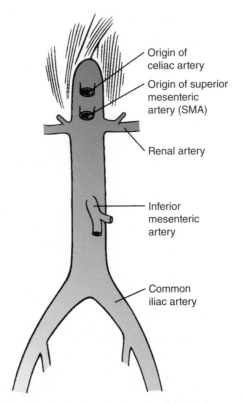

Origin of
celiac artery

Origin of superior
mesenteric
artery (SMA)

Renal artery

Inferior
mesenteric
artery

Common
iliac artery

Figure 53–1. Origins of the visceral arteries arising from the abdominal aorta.

Approximately 25% of acute mesenteric ischemia can result from the formation of thrombi within the mesenteric arteries; in most cases the patients have some underlying atherosclerotic changes within the mesenteric vasculature prior to clot formation. In less than 5% of cases, the acute mesenteric ischemia is related to aortic dissection and the direct shearing of the mesenteric vessels. Unfortunately, when intestinal ischemia occurs as the result of acute SMA thrombosis, ischemic changes generally will involve the entire small bowel distal to the ligament of Treitz and the right colon. **SMA thrombosis generally leads to more devastating losses of intestinal length and function than SMA embolism.** Patients with SMA occlusive disease generally benefit from systemic anticoagulation, resection of the nonviable segments of intestines, and in some cases, catheter-directed thrombolytic administration or catheter-embolectomy.

Nonocclusive mesenteric ischemia is a rarer form of damage responsible for 20% to 30% of cases of acute mesenteric ischemia. This process typically occurs in hospitalized patients with prolonged hypotension in association with the administration of vasopressors or other vasoconstrictive medications such as digoxin or dopamine. The **ischemia patterns produced under these conditions are generally in non-anatomic distributions where patchy areas of necrosis** are identified adjacent to normally perfused and viable intestines. The mainstay of treatment for patients with this condition is to support the cardiac output and blood flow to the intestines and resection of the nonviable portions of the intestines. Systemic anticoagulation may be helpful to minimize extension of the mesenteric thrombosis. Second-look operations are often helpful to allow time for clear demarcation of intestinal viability.

Mesenteric venous thrombosis is a rare cause of acute mesenteric ischemia responsible for only 5% of all cases of acute mesenteric ischemia. Treatment includes systemic anticoagulation, catheter-directed thrombolytic therapy, and resection of clearly non-viable segments of the intestines. Due to the high rate of rethrombosis, second look laparotomies are often recommended in the management of these patients.

Chronic mesenteric ischemic diseases in most situations occur as the results of diffuse atherosclerotic occlusive disease involving multiple mesenteric arteries. The intestinal blood supply normally arises from the celiac artery, superior mesenteric artery, and the inferior mesenteric artery. With excellent collateral blood flow between these arteries, most patients do not develop mesenteric ischemia symptoms until occlusion of at least two of the mesenteric arteries occur. When this occurs, the intestines develop a chronic low perfusion state that is worsened by food ingestion. The typical history includes unintentional weight loss secondary to food avoidance in an individual with other manifestations of generalized atherosclerotic diseases. When unrecognized or untreated, these individuals may present with acute mesenteric thrombosis that often is associated with the loss of most of the small intestines and large intestines. The treatment for mesenteric thrombosis involves resection of the non-viable intestines and revascularization of the mesenteric vessels either by open bypass grafting or stent placement. In some cases catheter-directed thrombolytic infusion can be helpful to temporarily re-establish blood flow in patients prior to the revascularization procedures.

The median arcuate ligament syndrome is an uncommon form of chronic mesenteric ischemia produced by extrinsic compression of the celiac artery by the median arcuate ligament. When occurs, this problem can be treated by decompression procedures that involves division of the arcuate ligament in conjunction with endovascular stenting or surgical reconstruction of the celiac artery.

CASE CORRELATION

- See also Case 18 (Small Bowel Obstruction) and Case 24 (Abdominal Pain [Right Lower Quadrant]).

COMPREHENSION QUESTIONS

53.1 Which of the following is the best treatment strategy for a 44-year-old man presenting with acute abdominal pain, tachycardia, and diffuse abdominal rebound tenderness following cocaine intoxication?

   A. Hydration, observation, and broad-spectrum antibiotics

   B. Hydration, systemic vasodilator (nitroprusside) infusion, and broad-spectrum antibiotics

   C. Hydration, angiography and catheter-directed thrombolytics infusion

   D. Hydration, surgical exploration, broad-spectrum antibiotics

   E. Hydration, surgical exploration, systemic vasodilator (nitroprusside) infusion

53.2 A 58-year-old man presents with atrial fibrillation and sudden onset of severe abdominal pain. Which portions of the intestines are most likely involved with this process causing his abdominal pain?

   A. Jejunum, distal duodenum, and stomach

   B. Distal jejunum, ileum, and right colon

   C. Right colon, transverse colon, and descending colon

   D. Upper rectum and splenic flexure of the colon

   E. Distal jejunum, ileum, and right colon

53.3 In which segment of the intestine is ligation of the inferior mesenteric artery during aortic aneurysm repair most likely to produce ischemia?

   A. Transverse colon

   B. Low rectum

   C. Splenic flexure of the colon

   D. Right colon

   E. Distal small bowel

53.4 A 66-year-old man is admitted to the coronary care unit because of new-onset atrial fibrillation. After 24 hours, he develops acute abdominal pain, distension, and on examination is found to have diffuse peritonitis. The patient is taken to the operating room for abdominal exploration and resection of necrotic intestinal segment. Which of the following is the most important postoperative treatment for this patient?

   A. Intra-arterial thrombolytic infusion with tissue plasminogen activating factor (TPA)

   B. Cardioversion

   C. Systemic heparinization

   D. Early oral feeding to stimulate intestinal growth

   E. Revascularization of the SMA and celiac artery

53.5 A 73-year-old woman with cardiogenic shock following an anterior wall myocardial infarction develops diffuse abdominal pain. On examination, her blood pressure is 85/50 mm Hg and pulse rate is 90 beats/minute. Her abdomen is nontender. Her extremities are cool with skin mottling in the distal lower extremities. Which of the following is the best management approach at this time?

A. Exploratory laparotomy

B. Dobutamine drip

C. Mesenteric angiography

D. Systemic thrombolytic therapy

E. Mesenteric revascularization

53.6 Which of the following clinical presentations is most consistent with mesenteric angina?

A. Diarrhea that occurs after fatty meals, steatorrhea, and chronic epigastric and back pain

B. Daily postprandial abdominal pain and 40-lb (18.2 kg) weight loss

C. Intermittent epigastric pain that occurs approximately one hour after meals

D. Chronic persistent abdominal pain and back pain of 1-month duration, jaundice, and 10-pound (4.5 kg) weight loss

E. Recurrent postprandial abdominal pain, bloating, and vomiting

53.7 Which of the following clinical descriptions best fits food aversion or "food fear" related to chronic mesenteric ischemia?

A. 73-year-old woman with postprandial upper abdominal pain, nausea, and vomiting after ingestion of fatty foods

B. 73-year-old woman with diffuse, nonfocal abdominal pain that occurs following food ingestion

C. 73-year-old woman with epigastric and substernal pain, shortness of breath, and diaphoresis brought on by food ingestion

D. 73-year-old woman with vomiting, abdominal bloating and distension brought on by food ingestion

E. 73-year-old woman with vague abdominal and back discomfort and pulsatile mass in the upper abdomen

53.8 Which of the following statements best describes features of superior mesenteric artery embolism and superior mesenteric artery thrombosis?

   A. SMA embolism-atrial fibrillation, chronic weight loss; SMA thrombosis nonanatomic intestinal ischemia

   B. SMA embolism-atrial fibrillation, sudden onset, distal small bowel inschemia; SMA thrombosis-nonanatomic intestinal ischemia pattern

   C. SMA embolism-atrial fibrillation, sudden onset, distal small bowel ischemia; SMA thrombosis-chronic weight loss, extensive small bowel and proximal colon ischemia

   D. SMA embolism-atrial fibrillation, chronic weight loss, distal small bowel ischemia; SMA thrombosis-extensive small bowel and proximal colon ischemia

   E. SMA embolism-hypercoagulable state, extensive small bowel and proximal colon ischemia; SMA-thrombosis-atrial fibrillation and hypercoagulable state

ANSWERS

53.1 **D.** Presumably this patient has nonocclusive mesenteric ischemia secondary to cocaine (a potent vasoconstrictor). At this point, the patient has peritonitis suggesting that ischemic necrosis with perforation has occurred. Hydration, surgical exploration, and broad-spectrum antibiotics are the most appropriate treatments at this time. At the time of surgery, all necrotic intestines will need to be removed; if there is questionably viable bowel identified, it can be left in place with a planned second-look operation arranged.

53.2 **E.** The patient described here most likely has an SMA embolus. Embolic events involving the SMA usually involves a clot traveling from the heart to the SMA, and this generally produces obstruction of the distal SMA that supplies blood flow to the distal small bowel and right colon.

53.3 **C.** The splenic flexure region of the colon is a classic "water-shed" region of the colon, because the SMA blood supply delivers blood flow to the jejunum, ileum, right colon, and proximal transverse colon. The IMA delivers blood flow the descending colon, sigmoid colon and upper rectum. The splenic flexure of the colon generally relies on collateral blood flow from both the SMA and IMA, and ligation of the IMA puts this region at risk for ischemia. Another "water shed" area within the colon is the mid- to low-rectum, where ligation of the IMA may cause ischemic changes.

53.4 **C.** The patient described has suffered from SMA embolism with subsequent bowel necrosis. The source of the embolus is the heart; in this setting, the patient likely has developed either cardiomyopathy or possibly a ventricular aneurysm following his myocardial infarction. Patients with SMA embolism are susceptible to subsequent embolic events and would benefit from systemic anticoagulation.

53.5 **B.** This patient had a myocardial infarction and appears to have cardiogenic shock based on the description of her physical examination (low blood pressure and cool distal extremities). She does not have any clinical evidence to suggest that a thrombotic/embolic event has occurred, nor does she have any signs of bowel necrosis at this time. Treatment should be directed at correcting her cardiogenic shock. Dobutamine is an agent with inotropic effects as well as after-load reducing effects and may be helpful in improving cardiac performance at this time.

53.6 **B.** Choice "A" is most consistent with a description of chronic pancreatitis with exocrine pancreatic insufficiency. Choice "C" is compatible with symptoms of biliary colic. Choice "D" can be compatible with several possible diagnoses, including pancreatic cancer, abdominal lymphoma, and retroperitoneal sarcoma. Choice "E" is a nice description of a patient with chronic intestinal obstruction.

53.7 **B.** Nonfocal pain that only occurs with food ingestion fits the best description for a patient with mesenteric angina and "food fear." Most individuals with the condition learn over time that food causes pain and learn to avoid food.

53.8 **C.** SMA embolism is usually associated with a clot traveling from the heart to the SMA, and most commonly the clot lodges in the distal SMA past the take-offs of arterial branches that deliver blood to the proximal jejunum thus giving a "proximal-sparing" ischemia pattern. SMA thrombosis usually occur secondary to diffuse atherosclerotic changes in the aorta involving the take-off of the SMA; therefore, thrombosis most commonly occur at the SMA-aorta junction producing ischemic necrosis of nearly all small bowel, right colon, and proximal transverse colon.

CLINICAL PEARLS

▶ A patient with chronic mesenteric ischemia almost always has significant weight loss. If there is no weight loss, then the diagnosis should be questioned.

▶ An abdominal bruit is a very nonspecific finding.

▶ Chronic mesenteric ischemia usually occurs in a patient with diffuse atherosclerotic occlusive disease; therefore, most patients will have lower extremity arterial insufficiency symptoms also.

▶ Chronic mesenteric ischemia is much more frequently encountered in women than men, and it is believed to be related to the difference in SMA-aorta angulations.

▶ A lateral projection of aortagram or MRA provides the most important information regarding occlusive disease within the mesenteric vessels.

▶ Acute mesenteric ischemia is a surgical emergency.

▶ Exposure of the SMA for embolectomy is accomplished by locating the base of the transverse mesocolon and the proximal middle colic artery.

REFERENCES

Stone JR, Wilkins LR. Acute mesenteric ischemia. *Tech Vasc Interventional Rad.* 2015;18:24-30.

Saedon M, Saratzis A, Karim A, Goodyear S. Endovscular versus surgical revascularization for management of chronic mesenteric ischemia. *Vasc Endovasc Surg.* 2015. DOI: 10.1177/153874415585127.

Tracci MC. Median arcuate ligament compression of the mesenteric vasculature. *Techn Vasc Interventional Rad.* 2015;18:43–50.

Cheng CC, Choi L, Cheema Z, Siva Jr MB. Acute mesenteric ischemia. In: Cameron JL, Cameron AM, eds. *Current Surgical Therapy.* 11th ed. Philadelphia, PA: Elsevier Saunders; 2014:939-946.

Wilkins LR, Stone JR. Chronic mesenteric ischemia. *Tech Vasc Interventional Rad.* 2015;18:31-37.

During an office visit, a 66-year-old man tells you that approximately 3 days ago, he experienced weakness in his right hand at work that resulted in a temporary inability to write or hold a pen. These symptoms persisted for 45 minutes and resolved without recurrence. The patient's past medical history is significant for hypertension and coronary artery disease with stable angina. He has a 45-pack-year smoking history and currently smokes 5 cigarettes a day. His medications include aspirin, nitrates, and a beta-blocker. On examination, bruits can be auscultated over both carotid arteries. The remainder of his physical examination is unremarkable. A duplex study of the carotid arteries reveals 80% narrowing of the left internal carotid artery and a 95% narrowing of the right carotid artery.

▶ What is the most likely diagnosis?
▶ What is the best therapy?
▶ What is the optimal timing for intervention?

ANSWERS TO CASE 54:

Carotid Artery Stenosis

Summary: A 66-year-old man presents with signs and symptoms suggestive of a recent transient ischemic attack (TIA) involving the left cerebral hemisphere. His physical examination demonstrates bilateral carotid bruits, and the carotid duplex study confirms bilateral carotid artery stenosis.

- **Most likely diagnosis:** Bilateral carotid artery stenosis with a history of left hemispheric TIA.

- **Best therapy:** The patient should be immediately placed on "best medical management," which includes smoking cessation, blood pressure control, statin therapy to reduce LDL below 70 to 100 mg/dL, initiation of clopidogrel (Plavix) for combination antiplatelet therapy, and staged bilateral carotid artery endarterectomies (CEAs), addressing the left carotid artery (symptomatic side) first.

- **Optimal timing of treatment:** Optimization of medical management should begin immediately. Carotid endarterectomy for symptomatic disease should be performed soon after the symptomatic event (preferably with 2 weeks), as his stroke risk is the highest immediately after the event and remains high for the first few months after a TIA.

ANALYSIS

Objectives

1. Understand the natural history of asymptomatic and symptomatic carotid artery stenosis.

2. Be familiar with the medical and surgical treatments of patients with asymptomatic carotid artery stenosis and symptomatic carotid artery stenosis.

3. Understand the current roles and controversies regarding medical therapy, open-operative treatment, and endovascular treatment of carotid artery stenosis.

Considerations

This patient presents with a history that is highly suggestive of a left cerebral hemispheric TIA; however, TIA symptoms are not always easy for patients or physicians to recognize. Most TIA symptoms are minor and short-lived; therefore, it is easy for patients to attribute TIA symptoms to fatigue or other unrelated events. Neurologic events attributable to carotid disease are unilateral and involve the contralateral extremities or ipsilateral side of the face, with the exception of speech-related difficulties. A careful review of the patient's history, thorough physical examination, and non-invasive imaging of the patient's peripheral arteries and coronary circulation are important, since atherosclerotic disease distribution in is often generalized. In this case, his carotid duplex study has identified high-grade stenosis in both the right and left carotid arteries. Because the patient's TIA symptoms are highly suggestive of a left carotid artery distribution event, the left carotid artery stenosis should be considered as being symptomatic, while the right carotid artery with the higher grade stenosis is the asymptomatic side. The administration of dual platelet therapy (ASA + clopidogrel) in patients with carotid artery stenosis in the perioperative period has been shown to reduce the rate of perioperative neurological events without significant increase in the rate of perioperative bleeding. Statin therapy has been shown to decrease the 30-day risk of stroke and cardiac events among patients undergoing carotid endarterectomy (CEA). Both the clopidogrel and statin should be initiated and continued indefinitely in this patient.

The North American Symptomatic Carotid Endarterectomy Trial (NASCET) was a randomized multicenter study comparing medical management to endarectomy in symptomatic patients with high-grade carotid stenosis. In patients with high grade stenosis (>70%), the 2-year ipsilateral stroke rates for CEA and medical therapy were 9% and 26%, respectively. For patients with a moderate stenosis of (50%-69%), a smaller but significant benefit in 5-year ipsilateral stroke rate reduction was also found with CEA. During the 1990s, randomized trials also compared best medical management to CEA for patients with a symptomatic carotid stenosis, and the results suggest that patients with high-grade asymptomatic carotid artery stenosis benefited from CEA, as long as the perioperative stroke and death rates were kept low. Based on results of these randomized controlled trials, the current recommendation from the Society of Vascular Surgery is to perform CEA and best medical management for patients with symptomatic disease and >50% stenosis, as long as the combined perioperative stroke and death rates can be kept below 6%. Because the risk of stroke from asymptomatic disease is lower, the Society of Vascular Surgery recommendation is to consider best medical management and CEA in asymptomatic patients with carotid artery stenosis greater than 60%, as long as the perioperative combined stroke and death rates can be kept below 3%. With improvements in medical management, indications for CEA depend upon the individual patient and surgeon.

APPROACH TO:
Carotid Artery Disease

DEFINITIONS

ABCD SCORING SYSTEM FOR STROKE RISK: This is five-factor scoring system to help stratify stroke risks in symptomatic patients.

Age > 60 = 1 point. Blood pressure > 140/90 mm Hg = 1 point. Clinical feature: unilateral weakness = 2 points and speech impairment without weakness = 1 point. Diabetes mellitus = 1 point.

Stroke risk based on scores: 0 to 3 points is associated with 1.2% stroke risk in 7 days; scores of 4 to 5 points are associated with 5.4% stroke risk in 7 days; scores of 5 to 6 points are associated with 11.7% stroke risk in 7 days.

TRANSIENT ISCHEMIC ATTACK (TIA): Defined as a reversible neurologic deficit lasting less than 24 hours.

AMAUROSIS FUGAX: This is derived from the Greek phrase meaning "fleeting darkness." This is temporary monocular blindness generally caused by an embolic event originating from the ipsilateral carotid distribution. This is a form of TIA.

CAROTID DUPLEX SCAN: This is an ultrasound and Doppler noninvasive imaging modality that provides anatomic information (B-mode analysis) and flow-velocity patterns (duplex mode) to determine the degree of carotid artery narrowing and identify suspicious plaque patterns (such as ulcerated plaque).

CAROTID ENDARTERECTOMY (CEA): Open surgical procedure that involves opening, controlling, and occluding the common carotid artery, the internal and external carotid arteries and then opening the vessel longitudinally to remove the diseased intima and plaque. The artery can be closed primarily or closed with a patch closure to widen the diameter of the area.

CAROTID ARTERY SHUNTING DURING CEA: Some surgeons perform CEA with an intraluminal shunt in place to minimize ischemia time. Necessity of routine shunting is controversial. Shunting most likely benefits individuals with low cerebral perfusion from the other arteries (contralateral carotid and vertebral arteries). Some surgeons perform CEA with selective shunting, and these groups generally will clamp the common carotid artery and measure the back pressure in the internal carotid and place a shunt when the back-pressures are low (<25-50 mm Hg)

CAROTID ARTERY STENTING (CAS): This is a percutaneous technique through intraluminal access to the carotid artery, followed by balloon dilation and stent placement. The procedure can predispose to distal embolization; therefore, the whole process is usually performed with a cerebral protection device in the carotid artery above where dilation and stenting are being performed.

NORTH AMERICAN SYMPTOMATIC CAROTID ENDARTERECTOMY TRIAL (NASCET): Randomized controlled trial of symptomatic patients managed either by medical management or CEA. For patients with 70% to 99% stenosis, the 2-year stroke rate following CEA was 9% following CEA v. 26% with medical management. For the moderate stenosis group (50%-69% stenosis), the 5-year stroke rates were 15.7% following CEA and 22.2% with medical management. Surgery was found to be beneficial for both the symptomatic patients with high-grade stenosis and moderate stenosis.

ASYMPTOMATIC CAROTID ATHEROSCLEROSIS TRIAL (ACAS): This trial conducted in the early 1990s randomized asymptomatic patients with stenosis >60% to CEA v. medical management. During a 5-year follow-up period, the stroke rate was 11.0% for medically treated patients and 5.1% for CEA-treated patients. Based on these results, treatment recommendations for asymptomatic patients were established.

CLINICAL APPROACH

Stroke is the third leading cause of death in the United States and a leading cause of disability for adults. In a typical Western community, roughly 15% of strokes are hemorrhagic and 85% are ischemic. Of the ischemic strokes, 20% will be in the vertebral-basilar system and 80% will be in the carotid territory. Of the strokes attributable to the carotid territory, 50% will be related to thromboembolic processes, while 25% will be related to small vessel intracranial disease (lacunar stroke), 20% will be cardioembolic, and 5% will be other. Based on this estimate, roughly 34% of all strokes are attributable to thromboembolic processes within the carotid circulation, and some of the patients with strokes arising from the carotid circulation will not have clinically significant stenosis (>50%) that warrant surgical interventions. **The overall estimate is that based on current screening, surveillance, and treatment recommendations, CEA is effective in preventing 20% to 30% of all strokes that present in the general population.** As medical practitioners, we must keep these figures in mind as we counsel patients regarding the risks and benefits of carotid endarterectomy as a stroke prevention strategy. **The bottom line is that CEA will diminish stroke risks in patients with high-risk profiles; however, it is only effective in reducing some thromboembolic stroke risks in the carotid artery distribution. The more important information to convey to the patients is that effective implementation of life-style modifications and pharmacologic interventions directed at reducing cardiovascular disease risk factors are crucial in future stroke and cardiovascular diseases-related mortality prevention for the individual.**

Since the introduction of CEA in 1954 as a stroke prevention strategy, there have been a number of large randomized control trials that have been conducted to help identify patient populations that would benefit from this intervention. The conundrum of CEA as a stroke prevention measure is that CEA prevents strokes but can also cause strokes. Ideally, the best scenario would be to select out patients with the highest risk of future strokes and perform CEA on these patients with the lowest complication rates possible.

Diagnosis

The diagnosis of carotid artery disease is mostly based on history and physical examinations. The older individuals with cardiovascular disease risk factors, history of TIAs, coronary artery diseases, or peripheral vascular diseases constitute the at-risk patient population. Audible bruits can often be identified during auscultation. Presence of bruit often triggers further workups such as carotid duplex scans, however, is not always associated with significant carotid stenosis. In fact, only 50% of patients with carotid bruits have carotid stenosis >30%, and only 25% of patient with bruits have stenosis >75%. Duplex ultrasonography is a very accurate noninvasive imaging modality for the carotid arteries and can be used to measure the severity of stenosis and visualize high-risk plaque features such as ulcers in the plaque. Once high-grade stenosis are identified and surgery is contemplated, CT angiography with reconstruction or magnetic resonance angiography is often obtained for surgical planning. Catheter-based angiography is helpful for surgical planning or for planning of percutaneous interventions; however, angiography is invasive and carries approximately 1% to 2% risk of stroke.

Angiography should not be obtained for sole diagnostic reasons; instead, the study should only be ordered by the operative surgeons or practioners performing the vascular interventions.

Treatment

The treatment of carotid stenosis is one of the best studied areas in medicine with many large randomized controlled trials having been conducted to help identify best managment for symptomatic and asymptomatic patients. At this point, there is still strong evidence to indicate that symptomatic patients with significant carotid stenosis can receive benefits from CEA.

The management of the asymptomatic patients has now become more controversial. One of the reasons causing disagreements between practitioners is that "best medical management" has changed since the publication of some of the important trials from the 1990s. At this point, best medical therapy includes life style and dietary modifications, smoking cessation, combination anti-platelet therapy, blood pressure control, diabetes control, and statins. The introduction of statins and clopidogrel to the medical management regimen has dramatically reduced the stroke risks for patients. Consequently, some practitioners believe that these advances in medical management have overcome the small margin of benefits that CEA conferred for the asymptomatic patients.

Sapphire and Crest Findings

Another area of controversy that has emerged in the management of carotid stenosis is the safety and efficacy of CAS. The Stenting and Angioplasty with Protection in Patients at High Risk for Endarterectomy (SAPPHIRE) trial results were initially published in 2002, in which patients with >80% asymptomatic stenosis and more than 50% symptomatic stenosis and high-risk operative profile were randomized to CAS or CEA. This trial reported 30-day death and major complications rates that favored CAS, and in a 3-year follow-up, there were no long-term survival or stroke rate differences between the groups. Based on the SAPPHIRE findings, CAS was introduced as the preferred treatment procedure for older patients. The Carotid Revascularization Endarterectomy Stenting Trial (CREST) was a North America multicenter trial published in 2010 that randomized symptomatic and asymptomatic patients to CEA v. CAS. The study observed a higher rate of perioperative strokes in CAS patients and a higher rate of perioperative cardiac complications in the CEA patients. Interestingly, the combined rates of stroke and cardiac complications were found to be significantly higher in older patients (6.1% at <64 years, 6.3% at 65-74 years, 7.4% at >75 years). **The findings of CREST seem to have refuted the notion that CAS is the procedure that should be applied in older and more fragile patients.**

CASE CORRELATION

- See also Case 50 (Claudication Syndrome) and Case 52 (Abdominal Aortic Aneurysm).

COMPREHENSION QUESTIONS

54.1 A 63-year-old man has a 4-minute period of documented expressive aphasia that completely resolved. A workup reveals 70% left internal carotid stenosis and a 50% right internal carotid stenosis. In addition to best medical management, which of the following is the most appropriate treatment?

A. Right CEA

B. Left CEA

C. Bilateral CEA

D. Coumadin

E. Continued observation

54.2 An 84-year-old woman has diabetes and congestive heart failure that is refractory to medical treatment. A right carotid bruit is detected on physical examination. A duplex study suggests a 50% to 75% right carotid stenosis. Which of the following is the most appropriate treatment?

A. Right CEA

B. Right CAS

C. Medical management

D. Optimize medical condition then perform right CEA

E. Right CAS

54.3 A 71-year-old man suffers a moderately dense cerebral vascular accident (CVA) affecting movements in his right arm and leg. However, over the past 3 weeks, he has recovered 80% of the strength in his right leg and right arm. It has been 8 weeks since his stroke. A workup reveals 90% left carotid stenosis with complete occlusion of the right internal carotid artery. Which of the following is the most appropriate treatment?

A. Continue best medical management

B. Right CEA

C. Bilateral CEA

D. Left CEA with intraluminal shunt

E. Left CEA

54.4 A 66-year-old woman underwent right CEA for right hemispheric TIA symptoms. The patient suffered complications related to the CEA and expires on postoperative day 2. Which of the following events likely contributed to her death?

A. Myocardial infarction

B. Bleeding

C. Pulmonary embolism

D. Electrolyte imbalance

E. Infection

54.5 Which of the following statements regarding CAS is most accurate?

A. SAPPHIRE study suggests that CAS is associated with higher short term complications than CEA

B. CREST study suggests that older patients have increased combined stroke and death rates in comparison to younger patients

C. CAS is the procedure of choice for all patients with symptomatic carotid disease

D. CAS is a safe procedure that can be used to revascularize completely occluded carotid arteries

E. CREST and SAPPHIRE studies both demonstrate CAS as the preferred procedure for older patients

54.6 Which of the following does not need to be instituted for a patient following carotid endarterectomy?

A. Aspirin

B. Glycemic control in diabetics

C. Coumadin to target an INR of 2 to 3

D. Statin

E. Smoking cessation

54.7 For which of the following patients is a left carotid endarterectomy most indicated?

A. A 74-year-old man with complaints of memory loss who has 55% stenosis in the left internal carotid artery

B. A 83-year-old woman with dizziness and unsteady gait with 100% occlusion of the left carotid artery

C. A 60-year-old man with a left middle cerebral artery distribution CVA with left hemiplegia and expressive aphasia. His carotid duplex demonstrates 80% stenosis

D. A 70-year-old man with transient loss of vision in the left eye that recovered after 20 minutes, and he has 75% left carotid stenosis

E. A 70-year-old man with transient loss of vision in the right eye that recovered after 20 minutes, and he has 60% stenosis in the left carotid and 70% stenosis in the right carotid artery

ANSWERS

54.1 **B.** This patient's history is consistent with him having had a left hemispheric TIA and 70% stenosis of the left ICA. As this man has symptomatic high grade stenosis of the left carotid artery, a left CEA is indicated.

54.2 **C.** This 84-year-old woman with poorly compensated CHF has asymptomatic stenosis shown on duplex to correspond to 50% to75% stenosis of the right carotid artery. The margin of benefit in an asymptomatic patient is smaller than the margin for a symptomatic patient. Given the fact that her CHF has been refractory to medical management, further medical therapy may not improve her operative risks for CEA. Continued optimal medical management may be the best recommendation for this patient. CAS is not a good option as the CREST trial has shown that older patients have higher peri-procedural stroke and death rates.

54.3 **D.** Left CEA with intraluminal shunt is the best choice here for this patient with a right hemispheric CVA 8 weeks ago, who has now recovered significant function. He has 90% left carotid artery stenosis with complete occlusion of the contralateral carotid artery. Because of the contralateral carotid occlusion, a temporary shunt during the operation may be the best choice given.

54.4 **A.** Cardiac complications and strokes are the leading complications affecting patients following CEA.

54.5 **B.** The CREST study showed that patients randomized to CAS had higher peri-procedural stroke rates and lower cardiac complication rates in comparison to patients who underwent CEA; however, the trial demonstrated that complications and stroke rates increased with patient age.

54.6 **C.** Aspirin, glycemic control in diabetics, statin therapy, and smoking cessation are all components of "best medical management" for patients with carotid diseases, and these measures should be continued after CEA.

54.7 **D.** The 70-year-old man with amaurosis fugax involving the left eye and 75% carotid artery stenosis would benefit from left CEA. The patient described in "A" is asymptomatic with 55% stenosis of the left carotid artery. The degree of stenosis is below the 60% studied in the ACAS trial. The patient in "B" has complete occlusion of the left carotid and cannot benefit from revascularization.

CLINICAL PEARLS

▶ The success and complication rates associated with CEA and CAS are highly operator-dependent; therefore, it is important to consider these factors prior to recommending therapy.

▶ Embolization is the most common cause of ischemic event related to carotid stenosis.

▶ Carotid endarterectomy will only prevent 20% to 30% of the potential cases of stroke in a general population.

▶ Optimal medical management is indicated for every patient with carotid artery stenosis; and this should be provided to patients prior to and after CEA or CAS.

▶ Cervical bruit corresponds to turbulent flow in the carotid distribution; only 50% of patients with cervical bruits have carotid stenosis >30%.

REFERENCES

Beaulieu RJ, Abularrage CJ. Carotid endarterectomy. In: Cameron JL, Cameron AM, eds. *Current Surgical Therapy*. 11th ed. Philadelphia, PA: Elsevier Saunders; 2014:811-818.

Gokaldas R, Singh M, LAl S, Benenstein RJ, Sahni R. Carotid stenosis: from diagnosis to management, where do we stand? *Curr Atheroscler Rep.* 2015;17:1-8.

Naylor AR. Why is the management of asymptomatic carotid disease so controversial? *The Surgeon.* 2015;13:34-43.

Yoshida K, Miyamoto S. Evidence for management of carotid artery stenosis. *Neurol Med Chir (Tokyo).* 2015;55:230-240.

A 4-year-old boy informed his mother that he had just passed some blood in his urine. The mother confirmed the hematuria and brings him in today for evaluaton. The child denied any significant recent trauma, and he had been in good health. His medical history is unremarkable. He is in the 56th percentile in height and the 43rd percentile in weight. On physical examination, the patient appears healthy and has normal vital signs. Findings from the cardiopulmonary examinations are within normal limits. A 10-cm mass is palpable in the left upper quadrant of the abdomen. This mass is firm and nontender. No abnormalities are noted in the extremities. The laboratory studies reveal a normal complete blood count (CBC) and electrolytes. The urinalysis reveals 50 to 100 red blood cells per high-power field.

▶ What is the most likely diagnosis?
▶ What is the best treatment?

ANSWERS TO CASE 55:
Wilms Tumor and Pediatric Abdominal Mass

Summary: A 4-year-old boy presents with hematuria and a left-sided abdominal mass.

- **Most likely diagnosis:** Wilms tumor (nephroblastoma) involving the left kidney.

- **Best treatment:** The best treatment will ultimately depend on the staging and local extent of the disease. Operative treatments include nephrectomies and nephron-sparing operations such as partial nephrectomies. In general, treatments are multimodality and include surgical resection, chemotherapy, and/or radiation therapy. Some minor treatment controversies exist because of different recommendations by the different international pediatric oncology groups.

ANALYSIS

Objectives

1. Become familiar with common presentation, differential diagnosis, and the initial evaluation of an abdominal mass in a newborn or pediatric patient.

2. Understand the management and outcome of Wilms tumor and neuroblastoma.

Considerations

Nephroblastomas (also known as Wilms tumor) are renal embryonal neoplasms that occur with peak incidence in young children between the ages of 1 to 5 years and peak age 3 to 4 years of age. Wilms tumors often manifest as asymptomatic abdominal or flank masses. Ten percent of the patients' tumors are incidentally identified after trauma, 25% of the patients have microscopic hematuria, and 25% of the patients have gross hematuria. Hypertension is a finding that occurs in some patients, as the result of excess renin production by the tumors.

Optimal treatment of most patients with Wilms tumors consist of surgical resection, radiation therapy, and chemotherapy. The exception to the multimodality treatment approach is a patient <2 years of age with stage I disease with favorable histology; for this type of patient, surgical resection with close surveillance may be sufficient treatment. Treatment for patients with Wilms tumor follows a protocol at most institutions, with treatments outlined by the various clinical trials (see Tables 55–1 and 55–2 for staging and stratification). Modern multimodality treatment outcomes are excellent for patients with Wilms tumors: Stage I: 88% to 95% 5-year disease-free survival and 99% overall survival. Stage II: 84% 5-year disease-free survival and 94% overall survival. Stage III: 89% 8-year relapse-free survival and 93% overall survival. Stage IV: 81% 2-year relapse-free survival and 90% 2-year overall survival. With modern treatment and long-term survival for patients with Wilms tumors, second malignancies are beginning to be recognized in some of the survivors. The risks of second malignancies can be seen

Table 55-1 • WILMS TUMOR STAGING BY NWTS AND SIOP CRITERIA

	NWTS/COG	SIOP
Stage I	Tumor confined to kidney with complete resection; intact renal capsule; no extension to renal sinus	Same as NWTSG/COG stage I but also with no involvement of the renal pelvis
Stage II	Tumor extends beyond capsule but with complete resection; extension to renal sinus; tumor presence in extrarenal vessels	Same as NWTSG/COG stage II but also includes no infiltration of adjacent organs or IVC
Stage III	Incomplete tumor resection; lymph node involvement; positive surgical margin; tumor spillage; peritoneal implants; non-hematogenous tumor within abdomen	Same as NWTSG/COG stage III but also include tumor thrombi at margin of vessels of ureter; surgical biopsy prior to chemotherapy or surgery
Stage IV	Hematogenous metastasis to lung, liver, brain, or bone	Same as NWTSG/COG stage IV but also include lymph node metastasis outside of abdomen/pelvis
Stage V	Bilateral tumors	Bilateral tumors

NWTS: National Wilms Tumor Study; COG: Children's Oncology Group; SIOP: Societe Internationaled' Oncologie Pediatrique.

up to 20 years after treatment. In the analysis of international cohorts of over 13,000 patients treated for Wilms tumor, the risk of a second solid tumor occurrence was 6.7%. Patients also had increased risk of leukemia development within 5 years of diagnosis and treatment for Wilms tumors. The overall risk of Wilms tumor patients going on to develop end stage renal disease (ESRD) is uncommon (<1%); however, patients with bilateral Wilms tumors and patients with associated genitourinary tract anomalies are at increased risk of developing (ESRD). At 20 years following treatment, ESRD is reported in up to 9% of the treated population when other genitourinary tract anomalies are present.

Neuroblastoma

Neuroblastoma (NBL) is the most common solid extracranial tumor in childhood. These tumors originate from primordial neural crest cells that form the sympathetic nervous system; therefore, the common tumor locations are adrenal glands,

Table 55-2 • RISK STRATIFICATION OF WILMS TUMOR

	NWTS/COG	SIOP
Low risk	Mesoblastic	Mesoblasticnephroma; cystic partially differentiated
Intermediate risk	Favorable histology	Nonanaplastic; focally anaplastic
High risk	Anaplastic; clear cell sarcoma; rhabdoid	Diffuse anaplastic; clear cell sarcoma; rhabdoid

NWTS: National Wilms Tumor Study; COG: Children's Oncology Group; SIOP: Societe Internationaled' Oncologie Pediatrique.

posterior mediastinum, retroperitoneal, pelvis, or neck. NBL is a disease of early childhood with 90% of the patients having disease diagnosis prior to the age of 6. The biological behaviors of NBLs are highly variable, with some tumors being highly aggressive locally and metastasizing early. Other tumors may maintain an indolent course and spontaneously regress. In general, patient with NBLs diagnosed in early infancy have a more favorable prognosis.

When identified in the abdomen, these lesions can grow to large sizes before they produce obstructive symptoms. NBLs in the neck can produce airway compressions. NBLs originating in the chest may also cause airway symptoms, however thoracic NBLs tend to be less aggressive in behavior than abdominal NBLs. Opsomyoclonus is a paraneoplastic syndrome associated with NBL and is seen in 2% to 4% of infants/children at presentation. NBLs can also be associated with excess production of vasoactive intestinal peptide (VIP), which produces watery diarrhea leading to failure to thrive in infants and children. MRI has become the imaging modality of choice for the evaluation of patients with NBL. MRI has the advantage of not only providing detailed anatomic location and extent of the tumors but is superior to CT scans for the identification of bone marrow involvement and spinal canal invasion. CT scans are helpful for some patients for preoperative planning, especially for the evaluation of vascular involvement. The INSS staging system (International Neuroblastoma Staging System) is the most common staging system used in the staging of patients (Table 55–3). For most patients with NBLs, treatment includes a combination of surgery, chemotherapy, and radiation therapy. For patients with high-risk NBLS, the treatment may also include the addition of myeloablative therapy and bone marrow transplantation. The determinations for surgery or chemotherapy as the initial treatment are sometimes dictated by the location and local extent of the tumors, and available surgical expertise.

Table 55–3 • INSS Staging System for Neuroblastomas*	
Tumor stage	**Description**
Stage 1	Localized tumor excision with gross negative margins; negative ipsilateral lymph nodes; nodes attached and removed with tumors may be positive
Stage 2A	Localized tumor with incomplete gross excision; ipsilateral nonadherent lymph nodes negative for tumor
Stage 2B	Localized tumor with or without complete gross excision; ipsilateral nonadherent lymph nodes positive; enlarged contralateral lymph nodes negative for tumor
Stage 3	Unresectable unilateral tumor infiltrating across midline; with or without regional lymph node involvement
Stage 4	Any tumor with distant spread to lymph nodes, bone, bone marrow, liver, skin, and/or other organs (except as defined in $S)
Stage 4S	Localized tumor with disseminated disease limited to skin, liver, and/or bone marrow. (marrow involvement <10% on biopsy and MIBG scan negative for marrow)

*The INSS staging system is a postsurgical staging system, therefore staging can be affected by local surgical expertise.

APPROACH TO:
Abdominal Mass in the Pediatric Patient

DEFINITIONS

PARANEOPLASTIC SYNDROMES ASSOCIATED WITH NBL: Patients with NBL are susceptible to develop paraneoplastic syndrome secondary to substances that are produced by the tumors. **Opsomyoclonus** occurs in 2% to 4% of the patients with NBL and is characterized by a variety of neurologic symptoms. Another common paraneoplastic syndrome is profuse watery diarrhea due to excess production of vasoactive intestinal peptide (VIP).

NEPHROBLASTOMATOSIS: This is considered as immature metanephric tissue or nephrogenic rests. When identified, it is considered a precursor to Wilms tumor formation. When a kidney containing Wilms tumor is removed and contains nephroblastomatosis, the risk of Wilms tumor development in the contralateral kidney is 20%. Other syndromes associated with nephroblastomatosis include Beckwith-Weidemann and Drash syndromes.

IMAGE-DEFINED RISK FACTORS (IDRFs): These are characteristics assigned to NBLs based on CT imaging. In general, they describe the presence, absence, and degree of major vascular involvement, airway involvement, and CNS involvement. Tumors with absence of IDRFs are associated with more complete resections and better prognosis; whereas, tumors with IDRFs are associated with increase difficulties in resection and increased complications.

The etiology of an abdominal mass in a pediatric patient depends to a large extent on the age of the patient at presentation. Knowledge of the patient's age and relevant details from a focused history and physical examination can allow the examiner to formulate a list of differential diagnoses. With this list generated, imaging studies and selective laboratory evaluations can be obtained for definitive diagnosis of the abdominal masses. Table 55–4 lists the likely diagnosis for abdominal masses in neonates (<1 month of age), and Table 55–5 lists the likely diagnosis for abdominal masses in older infants and children.

CLINICAL APPROACH

With the awareness of the possible differential diagnoses listed in Tables 55–4 and 55–5, the causes of the majority of abdominal masses can be determined with a high degree of certainty. During the history and physical examination, it is important to find out from the patient and the family how long the mass has been present or noticed. It is also helpful to illicit other associated symptoms including changes in eating habits, changes in bowel or bladder functions, signs of fatigue, night sweats, abnormal bleeding or bruising, or any other changes in behavior or activities. An important consideration for neonates is the maternal prenatal history, especially data from prenatal ultrasound and information regarding the presence or absence of polyhydramnios. Maternal polyhydramnios may be the

Table 55–4 • ABDOMINAL MASSES IN NEONATES (BIRTH TO 1 MONTH)[a]

Renal:
- Hydronephrosis, eg, from obstruction (ureteropelvic junction, obstruction, posterior urethral valves, other)
- Multicystic dysplastic kidney
- Polycystic kidney disease
- Mesoblastic nephroma
- Wilms tumor

Genital:
- Hydrometrocolpos
- Ovarian mass, simple cyst, teratoma, torsion

Gastrointestinal:
- Duplication cyst
- Complicated meconium ileus
- Mesenteric or omental cyst

Retroperitoneal:
- Adrenal hemorrhage
- Neuroblastoma
- Teratoma
- Rhabdomyosarcoma
- Lymphangioma
- Hemangioma

Hepatobiliary:
- Hemangioendothelioma
- Hepatic mesenchymal hamartoma
- Choledochal cyst
- Hepatoblastoma

[a]The most common etiologies of an abdominal mass in a neonate can be categorized as shown here (from most common to least common).

first sign of neonatal intestinal obstruction, which may present as abdominal masses in newborns.

Radiographic Evaluations and Preoperative Planning

Plain abdominal radiography can be helpful during the initial evaluation of an abdominal mass, because this imaging modality can help identify solid masses occupying the abdomen and identify intestinal obstructive patterns. Calcifications distributed along the intestines within the abdomen of neonates may indicate meconium ileus; whereas, calcifications within a mass in the abdomen may help suggest neuroblastomas in older infants. However, these findings are not diagnostic in themselves. When findings from plain radiography are not helpful, abdominal ultrasound can be the next imaging modality of choice. Ultrasonography can generally help identify the organs of origin of abdominal masses. Furthermore, ultrasonography can characterize the mass as cystic or solid, and blood

Table 55–5 • ABDOMINAL MASSES IN INFANTS AND CHILDREN (1 MONTH TO 18 YEARS)[a]

Renal:
- Wilms tumor
- Hydronephrosis, eg, from obstruction (ureteropelvic junction, obstruction, posterior urethral valves, other)
- Rhabdoid tumor
- Clear cell sarcoma
- Polycystic kidney disease

Retroperitoneal:
- Neuroblastoma
- Rhabdomyosarcoma
- Teratoma
- Lymphoma
- Lymphangioma
- Hemangioma

Gastrointestinal:
- Appendiceal abscess
- Intussusception
- Duplication cyst
- Functional constipation
- Hirschsprung disease
- Mesenteric or omental cyst
- Lymphoma

Hepatobiliary:
- Hepatoblastoma
- Hepatocellular carcinoma
- Benign liver tumors
- Choledochal cyst

Genital:
- Ovarian mass (eg, simple cyst, teratoma, torsion)
- Hydrometrocolpos
- Undescended testicle, neoplasm, or torsion

[a]*Note that although many of the specific etiologies of an abdominal mass are the same as listed for neonates, the most likely causes change with older children.*

flow within the mass can be assessed with the aid of Doppler mode, which can provide additional information regarding the nature of the mass. It is important to recognize that the sensitivity and specificity of ultrasonography is always highly operator dependent.

CT scans are typically obtained if the ultrasound is either nondiagnostic or shows a solid tumor. CT imaging can provide anatomic details and are especially helpful for operative planning. The disadvantage of CT imaging in infants and young children is that sedation often is required to obtain these images, and the long-term carcinogenic effects of ionizing radiation associated with CT imaging are uncertain. It is important to bear in mind that in an infant or child with a neuroblastoma, urinary studies for catecholamines should be obtained to identify and address potential excess catecholamine state related to the tumor. In a patient with an abdominal mass that is suspected to be hepatoblastoma, the serum alpha-fetal-protein level should be assessed prior to tumor resection.

> ## CASE CORRELATION
>
> - See also Case 56 (Neonatal Jaundice [Persistent] as a pediatric condition).

COMPREHENSION QUESTIONS

55.1 Which of the following statement is true of Wilms tumor?
   A. The treatment consists of surgical resection, except for those patients with stage IV disease with unfavorable histology
   B. The risk of end stage renal disease (ESRD) exceeds 50% for patients with Wilms tumor and other genitourinary tract anomalies
   C. Stage V disease indicates bilateral tumors
   D. Stage IV and stage V patients rarely survive 5 years
   E. Patients with stage I disease and favorable histology should be treated with surgery and chemotherapy

55.2 Which of the following is a true statement?
   A. Neuroblastoma is the third most common extracranial solid tumor in children
   B. Wilms tumors occur frequently in association with trisomy 21 genetic defect
   C. Plain film of the abdomen can be specific for the diagnosis of neuroblastomas of the abdomen
   D. Plain film of the abdomen is not indicated for the evaluation of newborn intestinal obstruction
   E. Neuroblastoma has been found to be associated with conditions such as Hirschsprung's disease

55.3 Which of the statements is true regarding opsomyoclonus?
   A. This is a paraneoplastic syndrome associated with nephroblastomas
   B. Manifestations are nonspecific and can include sensory, motor, and gait dysfunctions
   C. This condition is correctable with plasmapheresis
   D. This is a condition that complicates 50% of patients with neuroblastomas
   E. Electromyography (EMG) generally will demonstrate characteristic findings and is highly diagnostic

55.4 A 12-year-old girl presents with left lower quadrant pain and pelvic pain, and she is found to have a vague fullness in her lower abdomen. She is otherwise healthy without other associated symptoms. Which of the following imaging studies will most likely identify the etiology of the mass?

A. Plain radiography of the abdomen

B. Upper gastrointestinal tract contrast study

C. Magnetic resonance imaging of the abdomen and pelvis

D. Ultrasound of the abdomen and pelvis

E. Positron emission tomography (PET) scan

55.5 A 15-year-old boy presents to the emergency department with a fever of 38.9°C (102°F), a firm, fixed mass in the right lower quadrant of the abdomen, and chief complaint of abdominal pain. The patient has been ill for the past 2 weeks but has not sought medical care until now. Which of the following is a CT scan of the abdomen most likely to demonstrate?

A. Neoplasm in an undescended testicle

B. Right hydronephrosis

C. Abscess from a perforated appendix

D. Lymphoma

E. Gastrointestinal stromal tumor

55.6 A 5-year-old girl presents with a 7-cm, vague, left-sided abdominal mass. The patient has also experienced recent weight loss and failure to thrive. The mass is hard and fixed. A plain film reveals fine calcifications in the regions of the mass, and a CT scan shows an irregular, solid mass arising from the left adrenal gland. Which of the following conditions is this most likely?

A. Adrenal hemorrhage

B. Adrenal adenoma

C. Neuroblastoma

D. Wilms tumor

E. Duodenal duplication cyst

55.7 A previously healthy 9-month-old boy is brought to the emergency department with severe, intermittent abdominal pain. During the attacks, which are episodic and occur every 10 to 15 minutes, the child draws up his legs to the abdomen. He has vomited several times and is noted to have hemoccult positive stools. On physical examination, a tender mobile, sausage-shaped mass is found in the mid-abdomen. Which of the following is the most likely diagnosis?

A. Intestinal intussusception

B. Intestinal atresia

C. Neuroblastoma

D. Intestinal duplication cyst

E. Perforated appendicitis

ANSWERS

55.1 **C.** Stage V Wilms tumor indicates bilateral renal involvement; however, it is important during treatment to individually stage each kidney and direct the treatment based on individual staging for each kidney. With treatment, the 2-year survival of patients with stage IV and stage V Wilms approach 90%. Patients less than 2 years of age with stage I favorable histology may be treated with surgery and surveillance. In general, most patients except for some stage I disease should receive surgery, radiation, and chemotherapy.

55.2 **E.** Neuroblastoma has been reported to be associated with Hirschsprung's disease in addition to a number of other conditions, including neurofibromatosis type I, Beckwith–Wiedemann syndrome, and DiGeorge syndrome. Wilms tumor has not been found to be associated with trisomy 21. Neuroblastoma is the most commonly identified extracranial pediatric solid tumor. Plain films are helpful for the initial evaluation of newborn intestinal obstructions, for example the absence of air in the intestine is diagnostic for esophageal atresia. The "double bubble" sign is highly suggestive of duodenal atresia. Plain radiography of the abdomen is often insufficient for the diagnosis of abdominal neuroblastomas.

55.3 **B.** Opsomyoclonus is a paraneoplastic syndrome seen in 2% of the patients with NBLs. This is a nonspecific neurologic disorder with motor, sensory, and gait defects. The EMG findings are nonspecific for this condition. There is no specific treatment for this condition.

55.4 **D.** The ultrasound of the abdomen and pelvis will likely identify an ovarian neoplastic process that is causing this girl's lower abdominal and pelvic symptoms.

55.5 **C.** This patient's history and presentation are most consistent with perforated appendicitis with a walled-off, localized right lower quadrant abscess.

55.6 **C.** This 5-year-old girl has a left-sided abdominal mass with fine calcifications that is arising from the left adrenal gland. With this type of presentation, this mass most likely represents a neuroblastoma arising from the left adrenal gland. A Wilms tumor originates from the kidneys and is not associated with calcifications.

55.7 **A.** This patient's clinical history and presentation are classic for a patient with intestinal intussusception. The intussuscepted segment is most frequently the ileum and will produce a mass that is often found on the mid to right side of the abdomen. Crying and drawing up of the legs during cramping attacks is common. Bloody, mucous containing stool passage is a late finding often associated with some partial-thickness ischemic changes in the affected intestines.

CLINICAL PEARLS

▶ The most common cause of an enlarged renal mass in a neonate is hydronephrosis.

▶ The most common presentation (60%) of Wilms tumor is an asymptomatic upper abdominal or flank mass in a child 1 to 4 years of age.

▶ Bilateral Wilms tumors are staged as stage V, but treatment is based on individual staging of each kidney/tumor.

▶ A neonatal evaluation should include a review of the prenatal and delivery records.

▶ Neuroblastoma is the most common type of retroperitoneal mass in a child older than 1 year.

▶ Neuroblastoma is the common solid extracranial malignancy in childhood and the most common malignancy in children under the age of 1.

REFERENCES

Chung EM, Biko DM, Arzamendi AM, Meldrum FT, Stocker FT. Solid tumors of the peritoneaum, omentum, and mesentery in children: radiologic–pathologic correlation. *Radiographics.* 2015;35:521-546.

Chung DH. Pediatric surgery. In: Townsend CM Jr, Beauchamp RD, Evers BM, Mattox KL, eds. *Sabiston Textbook of Surgery: The Biological Basis of Modern Surgical Practice.* 19th ed. Philadelphia, PA: Elsevier Saunders; 2012:1829-1871.

Dumba M, Jawad N, McHugh K. Neuroblastoma and nephroblastoma: a radiological review. *Cancer Imaging.* 2015;15:5-19.

A six-week-old girl is evaluated for persistent jaundice. The infant was born at 39 weeks, gestation to a 27-year-old woman with no personal or family history of medical problems. The delivery was by Caesarean section after premature rupture of membranes. The infant's birth weight was 3200 g and her Apgar scores were 9 and 9 at 1 and 5 minutes, respectively. She had passage of meconium on the first day of life, and she was mildly jaundiced at the time of discharge from the hospital on day 2 of life. Over the past 2 weeks, she has been having light-colored stools and darkly stained urine. On examination, the patient is deeply jaundiced with an unremarkable cardiopulmonary examination. The liver and spleen are not palpable. No other abdominal masses are identified. The laboratory evaluations reveal a normal CBC. The serum total bilirubin and direct bilirubin levels are 28 and 24 mg/dL, respectively. Her serum γ-glutamyltransferase (GGT), aspartate aminotransferase/alanine aminotransferase (AST/ALT), and alkaline phosphatase are 840, 176/190, and 975 IU/L, respectively.

► What are your differential diagnoses?
► What is your next step(s)?
► Should this be urgently evaluated or electively and definitively diagnosed?

ANSWERS TO CASE 56:

Neonatal Jaundice (Persistent)

Summary: A six-week-old, full-term, female infant with no identifiable prenatal problems has persistent jaundice and abnormalities in her liver function tests.

- **Differential diagnoses:** Neonatal hepatitis, TORCH (toxoplasmosis, other agents, rubella, cytomegalovirus, herpes simplex) infections; metabolic diseases (α-1-antitrypsin deficiency, cystic fibrosis, and others); biliary atresia, and choledochal cyst.

- **Next step(s):** After initial laboratory studies are performed, the evaluation should simultaneously include TORCH and other metabolic studies (as listed in Table 56–1), abdominal ultrasonography, and magnetic resonance cholangiopancreatography (MRCP).

- **Timing:** Hyperbilirubinemia in the neonate that persists beyond 2 weeks of age is rarely physiologic, particularly when it is predominantly conjugated

Table 56–1 • CLINICAL MANAGEMENT OF PERSISTENT JAUNDICE IN CHILDREN			
Disease	Clinical Findings	Studies	Treatment
Unconjugated Hyperbilirubinemia			
Hemolytic diseases	Early, severe jaundice	Coombs positive	Phototherapy; exchange transfusion
Metabolic diseases	Disease specific	Disease specific	Disease specific
Physiologic jaundice	Nonspecific	Fractionated bilirubin	Phototherapy
Conjugated Hyperbilirubinemia			
Biliary atresia	Nonspecific	US; HIDA; liver biopsy; IOC	Portoenterostomy
Choledochal cyst	Abdominal mass; rarely cholangitis	US; HIDA	Cyst excision and hepaticojejunostomy
Biliary hypoplasia (Alagille syndrome)	Cardiovascular, spinal, eye abnormalities and jaundice common	US; HIDA; liver biopsy; IOC; investigate other organ systems	Choleretics
Total parenteral nutrition	Short bowel syndrome (anatomic or functional)	US; HIDA/liver biopsy of diagnosis in question	Enteral feeding
Inspissated bile syndrome	Hemolytic diseases or cystic fibrosis	US	IOC may be diagnostic and therapeutic
Sepsis/infection	Clinically ill	TORCH screen, blood culture	Supportive/specific to disease

Abbreviations: HIDA, hepatoiminodiacetic acid; IOC, intraoperative cholangiogram; TORCH, toxoplasmosis, other agents, rubella, cytomegalovirus, herpes simplex; US, ultrasound.

hyperbilirubinemia. Because surgical correction of biliary atresia is optimally performed before 8 weeks of age (12 weeks maximal), expeditious evaluation and potential preoperative preparations should be undertaken over next several days.

ANALYSIS

Considerations

Jaundice during the first week of life is a common phenomenon that affects approximately two-thirds of newborns. For the majority of newborns, hyperbilirubinemia is self-limiting and represents only transient physiologic jaundice (to be discussed later). **It is important to note that all term infants who remain jaundiced after 14 days of life or preterm infants who remain jaundiced after 21 days should be investigated for liver diseases.** The initial investigation can be with a measurement of conjugated and unconjugated serum bilirubin values. **Physiologic jaundice is associated with increased serum concentrations of unconjugated (indirect) bilirubin, whereas most forms of liver diseases are associated with elevations of conjugated (direct) bilirubin.** Common mechanisms that are responsible for pathologic jaundice in neonates include **biliary obstruction, increased hemoglobin load,** and **liver dysfunction.**

The presentation of this patient is fairly typical of newborns with hyperbilirubinemia referred for surgical evaluations. In most cases, the infant has no specific symptoms. With the clinical suspicion of liver and/or biliary disorder as the cause of jaundice, additional laboratory studies and imaging studies such liver/biliary ultrasonography and MRCP will be helpful. Useful studies to further differentiate the causes of hyperbilirubinemia for this patient include alkaline phosphatase, γ-glutamyl transferase (GGT), AST, and ALT. At presentation, most patients with biliary atresia have GGT values >100 IU/L, alkaline phosphatase values >600 IU/L, and AST/ALT of 80 to 200 U/L, which are consistent with her laboratory findings. The ultrasound of the gallbladder and liver will be important to determine the steps to take for this patient. If the ultrasound shows dilated intrahepatic and/or extrahepatic ductal dilatation, the next step in the investigation is to determine the level and cause of biliary obstruction. Common obstructive processes encountered in newborns include cystic malformations (choledochal cysts), other extrahepatic biliary obstructive processes such as a predominant extrahepatic form of biliary atresia (Type 2).

APPROACH TO:
Neonatal Jaundice

DEFINITIONS

PHYSIOLOGIC NEONATAL HYPERBILIRUBINEMIA: The newborn is susceptible to hyperbilirubinemia because of breakdown of red cell and decreased ability to excrete the bilirubin. For the majority of newborns this process is self-limiting and harmless. Bilirubin production is especially increased in preterm infants because of increased RBC turnover due to shorter life span of RBCs. Another contributing factor to jaundice is the limited ability of newborn liver to conjugate and secrete bilirubin. The average full-term newborn has a peak serum bilirubin of 5 to 6 mg/dL. **Serum bilirubin >17 mg/dL is regarded as pathologic.**

GENERAL CELLULAR TOXICITY DUE TO EXCESS BILIRUBIN: Bilirubin inhibits mitochondrial enzymes and interferes with DNA synthesis, induces DNA-strand breaks, and inhibits protein synthesis and phosphorylation.

KERNICTERUS: This refers to chronic bilirubin encephalopathy. Persistent elevation in serum bilirubin in newborns is associated with bilirubin crossing the blood-brain barrier leading to injuries to neurons by mechanisms that are unclear. Kernicterus is a relatively rare condition that should be preventable with monitoring of newborn serum bilirubin levels. Reported rates of kernicterus in Western Europe and United States are 0.5 to 1.0 per 100,000 live births.

PHOTOTHERAPY: Phototherapy or "bili lights" is the mainstay of therapy for newborns with hyperbilirubinemia. This therapy works by photoconversion of bilirubin molecules to water soluble isomers that can be excreted in the urine and stool.

EXCHANGE TRANSFUSIONS TO TREAT HYPERBILIRUBINEMIA: This is a more invasive therapy for infants with hyperbilirubinemia, which entails simultaneous removal of patient blood and replacement with donated blood. The threshold level suggested is serum bilirubin of >20 mg/dL.

CLINICAL APPROACH

The precise cause of biliary atresia is unknown. Various speculations have been proposed, and these include viral infection and autoimmune processes. Histologically, the biliary tracts contain inflammatory cells surrounding obliterated ductules. The liver shows signs of cholestasis and in later stages, fibrosis. Grossly, the most common finding is fibrosis of the entire extrahepatic biliary tree, followed by proximal duct fibrosis with distal duct patency.

Similarly to biliary atresia, the exact etiology of *choledochal cysts* is unknown. A widely held opinion is that the sharing of a common channel between the common bile duct and pancreatic duct leads to retrograde reflux of pancreatic juices in the biliary tree to produce subsequent biliary dilations. There are five types of choledochal cysts, but the fusiform, or type 1, comprises 90% of all lesions. Infants with choledochal cysts often present with clinical jaundice.

Patient Evaluation

The diagnosis of biliary atresia is based on timing of jaundice presentation and imaging findings that rule out other mechanical causes. Biliary atresia represents a common phenotype and can be grouped into one of four categories: *Isolated biliary atresia* is the most common type, where biliary atresia is the only anomaly; *cystic obliteration* of the biliary tree (cyst + biliary atresia) is when the atresia is associated with cystic changes; *perinatal cytomegalovirus (CMV) infections* can also cause biliary atresia and are categorized as CMV-biliary atresia; in some cases the patients

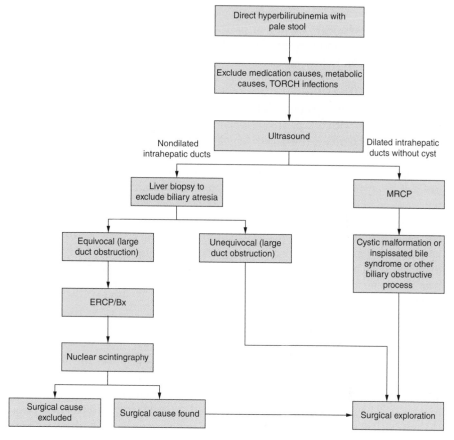

Figure 56–1. Management algorithm for new born jaundice.

may have *syndromic biliary atresia* where patients present with other congenital malformations. Identifying a cause for hyperbilirubinemia is important and the process should be performed in an expeditious manner so that if a portoenterostomy is to be performed, it can be done prior to the onset of irreversible injuries to the liver. See Figure 56–1 for management algorithm.

Biliary Atresia Screening

In some countries, there are widely implemented biliary atresia screening systems, which attempt to identify the disease at the early stages. In Taiwan, the screening protocol involves giving mothers color-coded cards to help them identify pale stools. This screening program has been reported to shorten the time to portoenterostomy to a median infant age of <50 days.

Preoperative Preparation of Patients with Biliary Atresia

Prior to surgical treatment, the patients need to be evaluated for coagulation abnormalities, anemia, and hypoproteinemia. Correction of coagulopathy usually requires both vitamin K and fresh frozen plasma. Anemia may need to be addressed with blood transfusions. Parents of patients with biliary atresia should be made aware of the long-term prognosis of the disease and understand the role of portoenenterostomy.

Treatment of Biliary Atresia

The Kasai portoenterostomy (KPE) is the operation of choice for the treatment of young infants with biliary atresia when synthetic functions of the liver are preserved. The operation involves excision of the entire extrahepatic biliary tree and exploration of the porta hepatis at the liver hilum to expose the ductules within the liver. A Roux-limb (defunctionalized limb) of jejunum is then anastomosed to the cut surface of the liver. This procedure is optimal for patients with preserved liver functions and no cirrhosis; therefore, the timing of diagnosis and referral for surgical treatment is critical for these patients. Some groups believe that best outcomes are achieved with the operations being performed before 8 weeks of age. Unfortunately, there is no clear evidence available to indicate the optimal time when biliary decompression procedures should be accomplished. In some centers, the approach is to forego portoenterostomy and proceed directly to liver transplantation if the patient is older than 100 days of age.

Postoperative Care and Outcomes

Important postsurgical care for these patients includes prevention, detection, and treatment of cholangitis, as infections cause additional liver damage. Important nutritional goals in postoperatively include the preventing malnutrition and addressing the malabsorption caused by liver dysfunction. High-energy and high protein formulas are generally recommended. It is important to treat the steatorrhea and malabsorption of fat soluble vitamins that are common in these patients. Some groups believe that corticosteroid treatment is important based on their anti-inflammatory and immunomodulatory properties; however, postoperative steroids benefits are not substantiated by strong clinical evidence.

Postoperative success following portoenterostomy is defined by a normal serum bilirubin concentration at 6 months following the operation. Following Kasai portoenterostomy, 70% of the patients will develop progressive biliary obstruction. A review of operative outcomes suggests that >80% of the patients will go on to survive more than 10 years following a successful operation. For many individuals with biliary atresia, liver transplantation is the treatment that ultimately gives them the opportunity for prolonged survival. The timing of liver transplantation is largely based on the success of the initial Kasai portoenterostomy. Currently, 90% of the transplant patients receive liver transplantation as a secondary treatment following Kasai portoenterostomies, and only a very small percentage of patients undergo liver transplantation as their primary treatments. Liver transplantations for this population can be either a liver-related partial liver transplantation or orthotopic graft placement. The overall 10-year graft and patient survival are 73% and 86%, respectively for liver transplantation performed in children with biliary atresia.

> **CASE CORRELATION**
>
> • See also Case 55: Wilms Tumor (Pediatric Abdominal Mass), which is another pediatric condition.

COMPREHENSION QUESTIONS

56.1 You are providing preoperative counseling for the parents of a 6-week-old infant with biliary atresia. Which of the following statements is true regarding the portoenterostomy procedure?

A. A successful operation provides the opportunity for 95% of the patients to live a normal life span

B. The operation is associated with better outcomes when it is delayed to let the infant grow larger

C. It is difficult to differentiate patients with biliary atresia from those with choledochal cysts prior to surgical explorations

D. Portoenterostomy rarely improves the hyperbilirubinemia in the majority of patients

E. Liver transplantation may be the better initial surgical option for infants older than 120 days

56.2 A 6-week-old infant develops jaundice. Which of the following diagnostic studies will help differentiate choledochal cyst from biliary atresia as the condition causing his jaundice?

A. The direct bilirubin fraction

B. Ultrasonography

C. The prenatal history

D. Ethnicity

E. TORCH screen

56.3 Which of the following statements is false regarding neonatal jaundice?

A. The average peak serum bilirubin for a term newborn is 5 to 6 mg/dL

B. Pathologic hyperbilirubinemia in newborns is defined as level >17 mg/dL

C. The negative effects of hyperbilirubinemia in the newborn occur only in the neurons

D. Phototherapy is the mainstay of treatment, and it helps to convert bilirubin to its water-soluble isomers

E. Neonatal jaundice is most common in post-term newborns

56.4 A 2-month-old baby is noted to be jaundiced by his pediatrician. Which of the following diagnostic studies will provide a definitive diagnosis of biliary atresia?

A. Abdominal ultrasound

B. HIDA scan (nuclear medicine imaging)

C. Intraoperative cholangiography

D. Magnetic resonance imaging

E. Percutaneous CT-guided cholangiography

56.5 A 7-week-old girl underwent a successful Kasai Portoenterostomy procedure, and she returns one-month postoperatively with fever, leukocytosis, and return of hyperbilirubinemia. Which of the following is the best treatment?

A. Revision of the portoenterostomy

B. Corticosteroids and antibiotics

C. Corticosteroids

D. Percutaneous drainage of the biliary tree

E. Liver transplantation

56.6 A 5-month-old infant presenting with mixed hyperbilirubinemia undergoes percutaneous liver biopsy, MRCP, and abdominal ultrasonography that ultimately revealed the diagnosis of biliary atresia. Which of the following is the best treatment for this patient?

A. Kasai Portoenterostomy

B. Liver transplantation

C. Open biopsy and cholangiography

D. Cholecystostomy tube

E. CT-guided percutaneous drainage of the biliary tree

ANSWERS

56.1 **E.** Portoenterostomy when done early before the onset of irreversible liver damage works best for the patients. In most cases, if the infant is older than 100 days, the long-term success of the procedure is limited and the patient may benefit from liver transplantation as the primary treatment.

56.2 **B.** The ultrasound should demonstrate dilatation of the intrahepatic and/ or extrahepatic biliary tree in patients with choledochal cysts, whereas, bile ducts will be nonvisualizable in cases of biliary atresia. The other choices provided will not be able to help differentiate these two diagonoses.

56.3 **E.** All of the statements are true except for the statement "neonatal jaundice is most common in post-term newborns." Neonatal jaundice is actually more common in premature newborns due to shortened RBC lifespan and less ability in the premature liver to process the bilirubin.

56.4 **C.** The ultrasound, HIDA scans, and MRI will provide helpful information for the diagnosis of biliary atresia; however, the definitive diagnosis is best established with direct visual inspection of the biliary tract and with intraoperative cholangiography.

56.5 **B.** The infant described has a classic presentation of postportoenterostomy cholangitis. This is a frequent complication following portoenterostomy. Revision of the operation is rarely indicated. Occasionally, it is done for procedure that fails primarily immediately postoperatively. Standard treatment for this patient includes supportive care, blood cultures, antibiotics, and steroids (for the choleretic and anti-inflammatory effects).

56.6 **B.** Liver transplantation may be best initial treatment in this 150-day-old infant with biliary atresia, as observations suggest that outcomes are best when portoenterostomies are performed prior to 8 weeks (56 days).

CLINICAL PEARLS

▶ Jaundice in the neonate beyond 2 weeks is rarely physiologic, especially when involving mainly conjugated bilirubin.

▶ The most common complication after portoenterostomy is cholangitis.

▶ Neonates with biliary atresia or choledochal cysts should be assessed for coagulopathy prior to surgery.

▶ Biliary atresia can occur in isolation, as part of a syndrome, or following CMV infections.

▶ BASM Syndrome: biliary atresia splenic malformation syndrome is one of the syndromic presentations of biliary atresia.

▶ Biliary atresia screening in neonates has led to earlier diagnosis of the disease.

REFERENCES

Davenport M. Biliary atresia: clinical aspects. *Seminars Peditr Surg.* 2012;21:175-184.

Hartley JL, Davenport M, Kelley DA. Biliary atresia. *Lancet.* 2009;374:1704-1713.

Maisels MJ. Managing the jaundiced newborn: a persistent challenge. *CMAJ.* 2015;17:335-343.

A 63-year-old man complains of a 6-month history of difficulty voiding and feeling as though he cannot empty his bladder completely. Shortly after voiding, he often has the urge to urinate again. He reports waking up from sleep at least three to four times each night to urinate. He denies urethral discharge or history of sexually transmitted diseases. He has mild hypertension and takes hydrochlorothiazide. The patient reports that he has had two bouts of urinary tract infections during the past year, and these infections have been treated with outpatient antibiotics. His vital signs are normal, and his cardiopulmonary and abdominal examination is unremarkable.

▶ What is the most likely diagnosis?
▶ What is the best initial therapy for this patient?

ANSWERS TO CASE 57:

Benign Prostatic Hyperplasia/Lower Urinary Tract Symptoms

Summary: A 63-year-old man with 6 months history of difficulty voiding, incomplete emptying of this bladder, and frequent nocturia. He has two recent bouts of cystitis.

- **Most likely diagnosis:** Lower urinary tract symptoms (LUTS), which in men occurs most commonly as the result of benign prostatic hyperplasia (BPH).

- **Best initial therapy:** Initial treatment includes life style modification and pharmacologic treatment with either an α-1-blocker or a 5-α reductase inhibitor if the patient is bothered significantly by his symptoms.

ANALYSIS

Objectives

1. Learn the clinical presentation of LUTS/BPH.

2. Learn to determine the severity of BPH and treatment strategies based on clinical severity.

3. Learn the treatments for BPH.

Consideration

BPH is the most commonly occurring internal benign neoplasm found in men. Nearly all older males have some degree of BPH with symptoms that vary in severity and frequency. In general, the BPH Symptoms Score outlined in Table 57–1 can be used to determine whether the symptoms are mild, moderate, or severe.

The BPH score is based on patient responses from the following questions:

1. How often do you have the sensation of not completely emptying you bladder after you finished urinating?

2. How often do you to urinate again less than 2 hours after finishing urinating?

3. How often do you stop and start again several times when urinating?

Table 57–1 • INTERNATIONAL PROSTATE SYMPTOMS OR BPH SYMPTOMS SCORES	
Score	BPH Severity
0-7	Mild
8-19	Moderate
20-35	Severe

4. How often do you find it difficult to postpone urinating?

5. How often do you have a weak urinary stream?

6. How often do you have to push or strain to begin urinating?

7. How often do you have to get up to urinate from the time you go to bed until the time you get up in the morning? (0 = none; 1 = 1 time; 2 = 2 times; 3 = 3 times; 4 = 4 times; 5 = 5 or more times)

Scores for answers to questions 1-6 above
0 = not at all
1 = less than once in 5 times
2 = less than half the time
3 = about half the time
4 = more than half the time
5 = almost always

There are a number of other conditions that can produce LUTS. These include prostate cancer, urethral stricture, bladder and or ureteral stones, bladder tumors, prostatitis, cystitis, and neurogenic bladder. This patient's initial assessment should include a detailed review of systems, detailed history of current symptoms, physical examination to rule out neurologic abnormalities, and laboratory evaluation including CBC, chemistry panel, urinalysis, and a prostate-specific antigen (PSA) test. The digital rectal examination is an important component of the workup because it gives us information regarding the size, contour, and consistency of the prostate.

Treatment

Men with BPH and LUTS who are not bothered by their symptoms do not need specific treatments. Instead these men can be managed by a *watchful waiting approach*. Included in the watchful waiting strategy are serial monitoring of symptoms and serum creatinine, and education regarding life style modifications which include: (1) reducing fluid intake at specific times to reduce urinary frequency at inconvenient times, (2) using relaxed and double-voiding technique, (3) eliminating or limiting caffeine, alcohol, and/or other foods that have diuretic and/or irritating effects on the bladder, (4) urethral milking may help reduce or prevent post-void dribble, (5) bladder retraining by encouraging men to delay urination when having the urge may help gradually increase their bladder capacity, (6) treatment of constipation, (7) adjusting medications to replace or eliminate diuretics and other medications that may produce bladder symptoms. After addressing other potential causes of LUTS, and if the patient's symptoms are bothersome, either an α-1-antagonist or a 5-α-reductase inhibitor can be started concurrently with the instructions for life style modifications to help address the symptoms related to his BPH.

APPROACH TO:

Male Lower Urinary Tract Symptoms and BPH

DEFINITIONS

MICTURITION: The physiologic act of voiding. This involves contraction of the detrusor (bladder muscle) followed by relaxation of the bladder neck and other urinary sphincters to allow for unrestricted and complete emptying of the bladder in a single setting.

LOWER URINARY TRACT SYMPTOMS (LUTS): These symptoms include complaints regarding bladder storage, voiding, and postmicturition symptoms. LUTS can be produced or aggravated by BPH, over-reactive bladder detrusor muscle, and polyuria. It is best to identify the actual cause(s) of LUTS before initiating treatment.

DIGITAL RECTAL EXAMINATION: The prostate is palpated with gloved examination finger inserted into the rectum. The normal prostate has the "feel" of the thenar eminence of the thumb (see Figure 57–1).

URODYNAMICS TESTING: This is a testing procedure that is performed in men and women to help determine how well the bladder stores and empties urine on demand. This testing generally involves the placement of a manometry catheter into the bladder and sometimes a second manometer in the rectum. The bladder is then slowly filled with warm water and patient is asked about sensation and asked to indicate when there is an urge to urinate. Urinary flow measurements are then

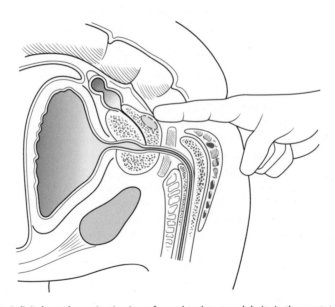

Figure 57–1. A digital rectal examination is performed to detect nodularity in the prostate gland.

taken as the patient is asked to empty his/her bladder. Results of this study may be helpful to further identify the cause(s) of LUTS in a man.

PROSTATE-SPECIFIC-ANTIGEN (PSA): A serum protein that is produced by the prostate. PSA elevation most often reflects pathology and processes specific to the prostate. PSA elevation can occur as the result of increased patient age, prostate cancer, prostatitis, and benign prostatic hyperplasia.

CLINICAL APPROACH

Patients with LUTS may present with bladder storage, voiding, and/or post-micturition symptoms. Specifically, the complaints may include urinary urgency, urinary frequency, nocturia, feelings related to incomplete bladder emptying, difficulty/pain with urination, bladder infections, or decreased urinary stream. The history and physical examination is helpful to sort out the symptoms and possible causes. The digital rectal examination helps characterize prostate size, consistency, and identify abnormal nodularities or tenderness. Abnormal findings during digital rectal examination may be further evaluated by transrectal ultrasonography. Patients with moderate or severe LUTS may benefit from lifestyle management and medication(s), or surgical treatment. Medications for LUTS often can produce side-effects, therefore patients need to be appropriately counseled and followed.

Medications for LUTS

Alpha-blockers: Prostate contraction causes narrowing of the bladder neck and decreasing urine flow; prostate contraction is nearly exclusively mediated by alpha1a-receptor stimulation. α-Blockers cause prostate relaxation and increase in bladder neck and prostatic urethra diameter increase and increase in urine flow. This type of medication generally will produce symptoms improvement within days after treatment initiation. Medications in this class include alfuzosin, doxazosin, tamsulosin, terazosin, and silodosin. Most common side-effects associated with α-blockers are weakness, abnormal ejaculation, and orthostatic hypotension.

5-α-Reductase inhibitors (5-ARIs): These agents block the conversion of testosterone to dihydrotestosterone in the prostatic stroma resulting in the reduction in prostate size. **Patients' clinical responses to this class of medications generally are delayed by several months.** Major side-effects are reduction in libido, erectile dysfunction, and abnormal ejaculation.

Muscarinic-receptor antagonists: Muscarinic receptors are highly expressed in bladder smooth muscle cells, prostate, and bladder urothelial cells. Muscarinic-receptor blockade reduces bladder contraction and bladder sensory threshold (reduces urinary urgency). These drugs are mainly used for the treatment of over-active bladder in men and women. Side-effects include dry mouth, constipation, micturition difficulties, and dizziness.

Vasopressin analogue (desmopressin): This drug controls urine production by binding to the V2 receptor in the renal collecting ducts. The medication causes water reabsorption and decreases in water excretion. This medication is helpful for the management of patients with bothersome nocturia. The medication for these patients would be taken once at bedtime.

Combination therapy: α-1-Blockers and 5-α-reductase inhibitors are often combined to treat patients with LUTS from BPH. Combination therapy may be indicated for patients with moderate to severe LUTS associated with high prostate volume, higher PSA, and advanced age, as these are risk factors for disease progression and future need for surgical treatment.

SURGICAL TREATMENT OF BPH-RELATED LUTS

Transurethral resection of prostate (TURP): This procedure involves resection of the transition zone of the prostate. TURP is indicated for patients with severe bladder outlet obstruction secondary to a large prostate. Alternatively, transurethral incision of the bladder (TUIP) is an option for some patients. The size of the prostate is often the basis determining selection of TURP versus TUIP. Long-term complications associated with these procedures include urinary incontinence, bladder neck strictures, retrograde ejaculation, and erectile dysfunction.

Transurethral needle ablation (TUNA): This treatment involves the delivery of low-level radiofrequency energy through a needle inserted into the prostate. The procedure produces controlled destruction of the prostate and relief of bladder outlet obstruction. This treatment option results in higher retreatment rate than TURP.

Open prostatectomy: This is the most invasive surgical option but is also more effective and more durable than the other surgical options. Patient selection is a key to balance complications and long-term benefits.

Transurethral laser vaporization of the prostate: Several laser energy delivery devices can be introduced by the transurethral route with the delivery of energy to the prostate. The short-term results are good; however, because these are newer treatments, long-term outcomes are not yet available.

COMPREHENSION QUESTIONS

57.1 A 57-year-old asymptomatic patient is noted to have a normal prostate shape and size on digital rectal examination. His laboratory study revealed a PSA of 38 ng/mL (normal ≤2.5 ng/mL). Which of the following choices is the best next step for this patient?

A. Continued observation and monitoring for symptoms

B. Repeat the PSA in 6 months

C. CT scan of the abdomen and pelvis

D. Transurectal ultrasound with prostate biopsy

E. Prescribe a low-dose doxazosin (α-blocker) treatment

57.2 A 72-year-old man without prior history of renal disease has a mildly tender firm lower abdominal mass and constant urinary dribble. His serum creatinine is 2.0 mg/dL (nL for adult male 0.8-1.2 mg/dL). Which of the following is the best next step?

A. CT of the pelvis

B. Enema

C. Placement of a urinary (Foley) catheter

D. Referral to a general surgeon for the abdominal mass and a neurologist for the urinary incontinence

E. Trans-rectal ultrasonography

57.3 A 58-year-old man who is employed as a commercial airline pilot has a confirmed diagnosis of BPH. He is currently taking an α-1 blocker for this problem and has recently presented to the emergency department for dizziness that is affecting his ability to continue as a commercial pilot. Which of the following is the most likely problem?

A. Parkinson's disease causing neurologic symptoms and neurogenic bladder

B. Metastatic prostate cancer

C. Chronic renal insufficiency

D. Medication side-effect

E. Urosepsis from untreated urinary tract infection

57.4 A 49-year-old man presents with moderately severe LUTS and physical examination finding of minimally enlarged prostate size and normal PSA. After detailed discussions with the patient, it appears that his main complaint is noctural urinary frequency (2-3 times/night). He has already reduced his nighttime fluid intake with only minor improvement in symptoms. Which of the following is the most appropriate next step in management?

A. Serial monitoring of PSA and prostate size by digital rectal examination

B. Prescribe nighttime desmopressin therapy

C. Bladder catheterization prior to bed

D. Initiate diuretic therapy with morning medication administration

E. Recommend a TURP

57.5 A 44-year-old man requests a laboratory prostate "test" because his father was recently found to have prostate cancer. This patient's digital rectal examination reveals a normal-sized, smooth, prostate gland. A serum PSA is drawn approximately 10 minutes following his office visit because the patient is anxious and insists that he wants the results as soon as possible. The PSA result returned 5 days later at 3.2 ng/dL (normal < 2.5 ng/dL). Which of the following is the best next step?

A. CT scan of the abdomen and pelvis to identify and stage his prostate cancer

B. Transrectal ultrasonography and biopsy of the prostate

C. Repeat the PSA

D. Radical prostatectomy with pelvic lymph node dissection

E. Reassure that mild elevation can occur and schedule a follow-up in one year

ANSWERS

57.1 **D.** A PSA of 38 is much higher than would be expected with the PSA abnormalities related to other non cancer causes. At this point, a transrectal ultrasound to evaluate the prostate and obtain biopsies of abnormal areas is indicated. Repeating the PSA in 6 month is an option for patients with benign prostate examination and mild PSA elevations. CT of the abdomen and pelvis is helpful for staging once cancer has been diagnosed but tissue biopsy is needed before that. α-Blocker treatment is only appropriate for patient with LUTS due to benign BPH.

57.2 **C.** This patient's clinical presentation is compatible with overflow incontinence and bladder outlet obstruction. Overflow incontinence occurs when the bladder's filling capacity is exceeded. Therefore, when the person coughs, stands, or increases the abdominal pressure, urine leaks outs in a dribbling fashion. The history and physical examination are sufficient to make the diagnosis, and placement of a urinary catheter is the best initial treatment.

57.3 **D.** Alpha-1 Blockers cause smooth muscle relaxation but are associated with side effects of dizziness and orthostatic hypotension.

57.4 **B.** Desmopressin at bedtime may be helpful for this patient with a primary complaint of nocturia and physical examination demonstrating minimal prostate enlargement. It is likely that his symptoms are the result of an overactive bladder rather than bladder outlet obstruction.

57.5 **C.** Transient mild elevation in the PSA can occur following digital prostate examination, therefore a mild PSA elevation found in a patient who just had a prostate examination does not necessarily indicate cancer. The PSA is best used to follow patients who have undergone treatment for prostate cancer. PSA screening per se has not been shown to be beneficial in reducing prostate cancer related mortality.

CLINICAL PEARLS

▶ Men above the age of 50 with LUTS should undergo renal function test (BUN/creatinine), a PSA, urinalysis, and a digital rectal examination.

▶ The International Prostatic Symptoms Score (IPSS) provides objective and quantifiable measurement of LUTS that categorizes patients' disease into mild, moderate, or severe categories.

▶ There is no physiologic relationship between BPH and prostate cancer, however it is important to keep in mind that the age of onset of both problems overlap.

▶ BPH and prostate cancer can occur together in the same patient, therefore one must always rule out cancer as a possible source before attributing LUTS to BPH.

▶ Distinguishing characteristics of prostate cancer include a firm, hard or nodular prostate on digital rectal examination and/or elevations of PSA.

▶ Diagnosis of prostate cancer can be made on imaging abnormalities and transrectal biopsy of the prostate.

▶ α Blockers will produce symptoms improvement within days of treatment initiation; whereas, it may take months after the initiation of 5-ARI treatment before symptom improvements occur.

▶ The combination of α-blocker and 5-ARI is more effective for the treatment of BPH than single agent therapy.

REFERENCES

Coburn M. Urologic surgery. In: Townsend Jr CM, Beauchamp RD, Evers BM, Mattox KL, eds. *Sabiston Textbook of Surgery: The Biological Basis of Modern Surgical Practice.* 19th ed. Philadelphia, PA: Elsevier Saunders; 2012:2046-2078.

Oelke M, Bachmann A, Descazeaud A, et al. EAU guidelines on the treatment and follow-up of nonneurogenic male lower urinary tract symptoms including benign prostatic obstruction. *Eur Urol.* 2013;64:118-140.

A 20-year-old man reports that he has had a nontender, heavy sensation in his scrotal area for 2 months. He jogs several miles every day, but denies lifting heavy objects. He does not recall trauma to the area and has no urinary complaints. On examination, his blood pressure is 110/70 mm Hg, his heart rate is 80 beats/minute, and he is afebrile. His cardiopulmonary examination findings are normal. His abdominal examination is within normal limits. The external genitalia examination reveals a 2-cm nontender mass in the right testis. Transillumination reveals no light penetration. The findings of his rectal examination are normal.

▶ What is the most likely diagnosis?
▶ What is the best therapy for this patient's condition?

ANSWERS TO CASE 58:
Testicular Cancer

Summary: A 20-year-old man has a 2-month history of having a "heavy" sensation in the scrotal area. He is found to have a 2-cm mass in the right testis. The remainder of his history and physical examinations are unremarkable.

- **Most likely diagnosis:** Testicular cancer.

- **Best therapy:** Surgery (radical orchiectomy) with possible chemotherapy.

ANALYSIS

Objectives

1. Know that a non-tender, non-transilluminating testicular mass in a man under the age of 40 should be considered a testicular cancer until proven otherwise.

2. Understand that knowledge of the correct pathological diagnosis or cell type(s) is crucial in directing treatment of testicular cancers.

3. Know that a testicular carcinoma can be cured; however, patient compliance with treatment and surveillance protocols is important.

Considerations

Testicular cancer is the most common malignancy in men between the age of 15 and 35, with the incidence of 3-5/100,000 men. It is more common in white males than black males. Painless scrotal mass is the most common presentation, although patients often will make reference to some trivial trauma that brought their attention to the area. Misdiagnoses of testicular cancers are not uncommon as these tumors can be mistaken as varicocele, spermatocele, hydrocele, epididymitis, or testicular torsion. Regular scrotal self-examination is advocated but rarely performed. In addition, the patients sometimes delay seeking treatments because of embarrassment. For this patient, the initial step is to perform a complete history and physical examination to determine the extent of the disease. Tumor markers including β-HCG and alpha fetal protein (AFP) should be obtained prior to treatment. In addition, lactase dehydrogenase (LDH) levels should be assessed to help determine extent of the disease. Ultrasound imaging of the testicle can be performed to better characterize the testicular mass, and in a case of testicular cancer, the mass will be solid and hypoechoic. Biopsy of the testicular mass is contraindicated because of the risk of tumor contamination of the scrotum and alterations in lymphatic flow from the region. In patients who present with back pain, which may represent extensive retroperitoneal tumor spread, or patients who present with respiratory symptoms secondary to pulmonary metastases, CT scan of the chest, abdomen, and pelvis can be helpful prior to surgery. Once the imaging and laboratory studies have been completed, the next step is to perform a radical orchiectomy, which utilizes an inguinal incision to approach the testicle and the ipsilateral spermatic cord. The orchiectomy will provide much information to help direct the subsequent care, and these data include histological type and local extent of disease. The surgical pathology information, CT imaging, and serum markers are important to help determine the type and stage of testicular cancers.

Once the diagnosis of testicular cancer is confirmed by orchiectomy, further staging should include CT scans of the chest, abdomen, and pelvis. Adjuvant treatments are determined based on the tumor types. Often, there is more than one cell type identified in the tumors which are referred to as "mixed germ cell tumors."

APPROACH TO:
Testicular Cancer

DEFINITIONS

RADICAL ORCHIECTOMY: This is a diagnostic as well as therapeutic procedure for the initial treatment of testicular cancers. The incision is made in the groin over the ipsilateral spermatic cord which then leads to the testicle. This procedure removes the testis, epididymis, and spermatic cord all the way up to the internal inguinal ring. The skin over the scrotum is not violated during this procedure.

RETROPERITONEAL LYMPHADENECTOMY: A surgical procedure to remove the lymph nodes in the lymphatic drainage basin from the testicle. Testicular cancers often progress in an orderly fashion up the lymphatic chain. These nodes often go alone the iliac vessels and proceed along the aorta and vena cava.

GERM CELL TUMORS: Ninety percent of testicular cancers are derived from the germinal epithelium (sperm-containing elements) of the testis. Subtypes of germ cell tumors include choriocarcinoma, embryonal carcinoma, seminoma, teratoma, and yolk sac tumors. The remaining 10% of the testicular tumors are gonadal stromal tumors, secondary tumors of the testis including lymphoma and metastatic disease to the testicle.

CLINICAL APPROACH

When a male patient presents with a chief complaint of a testicular mass, a detailed examination of the genitalia should be performed, delineating the character of the mass, painful versus painless, hard versus soft, and transilluminating versus non-transilluminating. Palpation of the groin lymph nodes, examination of the male breasts, and general survey of signs and symptoms related to not only the genitourinary system but also to the endocrine and neurologic systems are important. See Table 58–1 for staging, and Table 58–2 for risk stratification.

The initial treatment is a radical orchiectomy when the testicular mass is confirmed to be solid. Testicular ultrasound is often useful to help characterize masses within the scrotum. Prior to performing the radical orchiectomy, serum laboratory studies including beta-HCG, AFP, and LDH should be obtained. Serum LDH is helpful for determining tumor burden and helps in disease staging. Following orchiectomy, staging CT scans of the chest, abdomen, and pelvis may be helpful.

Table 58–1 • TESTICULAR CANCER STAGING

Stage	Primary Tumor (T)	Lymph Nodes (N)	Metastasis (M)	Serum Tumor Markers
IA	Involvement of testis, w/wo tunical albulginea involvement; no tunical vaginalis involvement	No nodal involvement or lymphovascular invasion	No metastases	Normal after orchiectomy
IB	Involvement of testis and tunical vaginalis, spermatic cord, and/or scrotum	No nodal involvement but with lymphovascular invasion	No metastases	Normal after orchiectomy
IS	Involvement of the testis with/without tunical albuginea, tunica vaginalis, spermatic cord, or scrotum	No nodal involved and no lymphovascular invasion	No metastases	Remains elevated after orchiectomy
IIA	Involvement of testis with or without involvement of tunica albuginea, tunica vaginalis, spermatic cord, or scrotum	Fewer than 5 retroperitoneal LN involve and each LN <2 cm	No metastases	β-HCG < 5000 mIU/mL, AFP < 1000 ng/ml, LDH < 1.5 times upper limits of normal
IIB	Same as in IIA	>5 retroperitoneal LN involved or at least one LN > 2 m but <5 cm	No metastases	Same as in IIA
IIC	Same as IIA and IIB	Retroperitoneal LN > 5 cm	No metastases	Same as in IIA
IIIA	Same as in stage II	Any retroperitoneal LN status	Distant LN or lungs	Same as in IIA
IIIB	Same as in stage II	Any retroperitoneal LN status	Distant LN or lungs	Beta HCG 5000-50,000 mIU/ml; AFP 1000-10,000 ng/mL; LDH 1.5-10 times normal
IIIC	Same as in stage II	Any retroperitoneal LN status	Nonpulmonary visceral metastases	β-HCG > 50,000 mIU/mL; AFP > 10,000 ng/mL; LDH > 10× normal

Most forms of testicular cancers are highly curable. Patients need to be reassured about the overall prognosis, but at the same time, they need to be educated regarding compliance with adjuvant treatments such as radiation and/or chemotherapy and with follow-up surveillance visits. Pure seminoma is treated differently from the other types of germ cell tumors, as seminomas are exquisitely sensitive

Table 58–2 • TESTICULAR CANCERS RISK-STRATIFICATION

Seminoma				
Low risk	Any primary site	+LN	No nonpulmonary metastasis	Normal tumor markers, any LDH
Intermediate risk	Any primary site	+LN	Nonpulmonary visceral metastases present	Normal tumor markers, any LDH
Nonseminoma-tous germ-cell cancers				
Low risk	Testis or retroperitoneal LN	+ LN	No nonpulmonary visceral metastasis	AFP < 1000 ng/mL, β-HCG < 5000 mIU/mL, LDH < 1.5 × normal
Intermediate risk	Testis or retroperitoneal LN	+ LN	No nonpulmonary visceral metastasis	AFP > 1000 and < 10,000 ng/mL or beta HCG > 5000 and < 50,000 mIU/mL or LDH > 1.5 × normal and <10× normal
High risk	Testis or retroperitoneal LN or mediastinal LN	+LN	Any site if primary site is anterior mediastinal LN; nonpulmonary visceral metastases if primary site is testis or retroperitoneal LN	AFP > 10,000 ng/mL, β-HCG > 50,000 mIU/mL, or LDH > 10× normal

to radiation therapy and to systemic chemotherapy when the disease is bulky or advanced.

Adjuvant Therapies

Stage I seminoma: Adjuvant options can include active surveillance only that is associated with a 20% relapse rate but 99% long-term survival. Alternatively, patient can be treated with adjuvant radiation or carboplatin (1-2 cycles) which are associated with lower relapse rates (4%) and also 99% cure rates.

Stage I nonseminoma: Adjuvant choices include active surveillance which is associated with 30% relapse rate but 99% long-term survival. The relapse rates are reduced to 20% to 30% when retroperitoneal lymph node dissections are added. The addition of chemotherapy (bleomycin, etoposide, and cisplatin will produce a relapse rate of 1-5% and also 99% survival).

Stage II seminoma: Adjuvant treatment choices are 30 to 36 Gy external beam radiation therapy to the para-aortic and ipsilateral iliac lymph nodes or chemotherapy (bleomycin, etoposide, and cisplatin). For patients with bulky retroperitoneal disease, chemotherapy is preferred. Surgical resection is indicated for gross residual tumor bulk after chemotherapy.

Stage III diseases and relapse disease are treated with combination chemotherapy (bleomycin, etoposide, cisplatin, or paclitaxel) either in standard doses or high-dose with bone marrow rescue. In general, low risk stage III testicular cancer long-term survival rates are >90% for low-risk lesions. Long-term survival for patients with stage III intermediate-risk tumors is 70% to 80%. Long-term cure for patients with stage III high-risk tumors is reported at 50% to 60%.

Additional Considerations

Because most patients with testicular cancers are young at diagnosis and treatment, there is strong concern about the development of second malignancy in these individuals following treatment. Therapeutic radiation and chemotherapies have been known to increase the risk of thyroid, soft tissue, bladder, stomach, and pancreas cancers. Infertility and sexual dysfunctions are common side-effects of treatments, which should be addressed with the patients.

CASE CORRELATION

- See also Case 57 (Benign Prostatic Hypertrophy).

COMPREHENSION QUESTIONS

58.1 Which of the following is an accurate statement regarding testicular seminomas?

A. Fertility following treatment is generally excellent

B. Orchiectomy is never indicated for treatment

C. Pain is the most common presentation

D. Biopsy by core needle is helpful to determine the histologic type

E. Seminoma are sensitive to radiation therapy

58.2 A 22-year-old man is noted to have painless scrotal mass. The AFP level is elevated. Which of the following statements is most accurate regarding the role of AFP in testicular cancer?

A. Marked elevation of AFP in men with testicular mass generally indicates a nonseminomatous testicular cancer

B. Serum levels may be used to determine response to therapy

C. The development of effective chemotherapeutic agents has eliminated the need for AFP level assessment

D. The level of AFP should not change following radical orchiectomy for a patient with a 4-cm nonseminomatous testicular cancer

E. AFP + LDH elevation helps identify a patient with testicular seminoma

58.3 A 28-year-old man is found to have a mass in the right testicle, which is expected to represent a testicular cancer. Which of the following statements best describes the fertility of the patient prior to treatment for testicular cancers?

A. Below normal on average

B. Same as their noncancerous peers

C. Above average

D. Far worse than average

E. Unknown

58.4 Physical examination of a young man with testicular cancer during routine surveillance visit reveals a hard mass just above the left clavicle. Which of the following is the most likely diagnosis?

A. Chemotherapy sclerosis of the subclavian vein

B. Metastatic testicular cancer

C. Second malignancy involving the head and neck

D. Pathologic fracture of the clavicle

E. Thyroid goiter induced by radiation therapy

58.5 A 17-year-old male is evaluated by his pediatrician for pubertal abnormalities. The physician describes the risk of malignancy of the gonads with the patient. Which of the following conditions is associated with the greatest risk for testicular cancers?

A. XY gonadal dysgenesis

B. Androgen insensitivity

C. Turner syndrome

D. Noonen syndrome

E. Testicular trauma

58.6 Which of the following statements is false regarding testicular cancers?

A. Most patients with disease relapse do not survive more than 5 years

B. Active surveillance following radical orchiectomy is acceptable for patients with Stage I seminomas

C. Seminomas are more sensitive to radiation therapy than nonseminomas

D. AFP > 10,000 ng/mL is a high-risk feature for nonseminomatous tumors

E. Visceral metastasis is an intermediate-risk feature of seminoma

ANSWERS

58.1 **E.** Seminomas are sensitive to radiation therapy; therefore, extratesticular sites of extension such as inguinal, iliac, and para-aortic lymph nodes can be treated with external beam radiation therapy. Most patients with seminomatous cancers have normal or slightly elevated values in their tumor markers. Serum LDH is not helpful to determine the testicular cancer type, but it is useful to determine disease burden and useful for staging.

58.2 **B.** Serum markers such as AFP levels can be useful in assessing the patient's response to chemotherapy for nonseminomatous testicular cancers. Patients with seminomatous cancers generally have normal or only slightly elevated tumor markers values. Serum LDH does not help differentiate seminomatous from nonseminomatous cancers, but it is helpful to determine disease burden and staging.

58.3 **A.** For reasons that are not entirely known, the fertility of men with testicular cancers are often already below the expected levels (as evidence by abnormal semen analysis) prior to their treatments. Surgery, radiation, and chemotherapy also further reduce the fertility of patients with testicular cancers. These possibilities need to be discussed with fertility options explored prior to the initiation of treatments.

58.4 **B.** The Virchow node is the mass identified in this patient. This physical finding can be seen in patients with malignancies within the abdominal cavity. Identifying this finding suggests that there may be more extensive disease in the retroperitoneal area. Secondary malignancy is also a possibility in this case, but it would not be a typical presentation of a second malignancy.

58.5 **A.** An intra-abdominal male gonad with Y chromosomes has an increased risk of malignancy. In androgen insensitivity, the patient is a 46XY genotype, but the defective androgen receptors do not allow the external genitalia to masculinize. Both androgen insensitivity and XY gonadal dysgenesis have the propensity to develop malignancy. The nonfunctional dysgenic gonad has the greatest risk of developing malignancy.

58.6 **A.** Even with disease relapses, the survival and "cure" rates of patients with testicular cancers are in some cases reported at 99%. Surveillance and follow-up are extremely important for patients in order to identify and treat the relapses. All of the other statements are true.

CLINICAL PEARLS

▶ Ninety percent of testicular cancers are germ cell tumors, with approximately half of these being seminomas. Many cancers have mixed cell types and careful pathologic evaluations are helpful to identify the types and help direct treatments.

▶ Cryptorchidism (undescended testicle) significantly increases the risk of a germ cell tumor even after the maldescended testicle is surgically corrected.

▶ Orchiopexy of an undescended testicle prior to the age of 13 years of age is associated with a lower risk of testicular cancer development, but the relative risk for cancer is still 2× greater than for baseline population.

▶ Genetic disorders such as Down's syndrome are associated with increased risk of testicular cancer.

▶ The risk of testicular cancer is 8 to 10 times greater than baseline in a brother of a man with testicular cancer, and the risk is 4 to 6 times higher for the son of a patient with testicular cancer.

▶ The incidence of testicular cancer has steadily increased over the past 20 years.

REFERENCES

Feldman Dr. Update in germ cell tumours. *Curr Opin Oncol.* 2015;27:177-184.

Hanna NH, Einhorn LH. Testicular cancer-discoveries and updates. *N Engl J Med.* 2014;371: 2005-2016.

A 38-year-old man presents to an outpatient clinic with several nonspecific complaints. He relates that for the past 3 to 4 months, he has become easily fatigued and has been unable to concentrate at work. He has also developed poor appetite and pain in his thighs, knees, and legs. The patient indicates that he has been generally healthy in the past but has not seen a medical provider in 6 years. Eight years ago, when he visited an emergency center for the treatment of a laceration on his arm, he was informed that his blood pressure was elevated. The patient is currently afebrile, his blood pressure is 160/94 mm Hg and pulse rate is 84 beats/minute and regular. He has several areas of skin ecchymosis over his knees and thighs. His white blood cell (WBC) count is 6500, hemoglobin is 9 g/dL, hematocrit 35%, blood urea nitrogen 80 mg/dL. Serum creatinine is 8.5 mg/dL, and serum potassium 5.0 mEq/L.

▶ What is the most likely diagnosis?
▶ How will you assess the severity and stage of his disease?
▶ What are the treatment options for this patient?

ANSWERS TO CASE 59:
Renal Failure/Renal Transplantation

Summary: A 38-year-old man presents with new onset renal failure and uremia. The cause of his renal failure is unknown, but could be due to poorly controlled hypertension.

- **Diagnosis:** Probable chronic renal failure (CRF) with uremia.

- **Severity and stage of disease:** The severity and stage of CRF can be estimated on the basis of urinary creatinine clearance.

- **Treatment:** Dialysis and renal transplantation are treatment options for patients with end-stage disease.

ANALYSIS
Objectives

1. Be able to describe and recognize the stages of CRF and complications associated with this condition.

2. Learn the principles of hemodialysis and options for dialysis access.

3. Learn the outcome and management principles for patients undergoing renal transplantation.

Considerations

Our initial evaluation and management needs to be directed at determining the cause of his renal failure, identifying potentially correctable causes, and determining the severity of his renal disease. Because the patient has described symptoms for the past 3 to 4 months and has no recent insults, the process most likely represents CRF. Renal ultrasonography is useful to assess renal size and numbers, identify urinary obstruction, renal vascular obstruction, and tumor infiltration, which are helpful to stage his disease. Evaluation and treatment of complications associated with CRF are important, and these interventions include dietary modifications and pharmacologic therapies to address metabolic complications such as hyperkalemia and hyperphosphatemia. Cardiovascular complications are common among patients with CRF and account for approximately 50% of the annual mortality in this population. Echocardiography is helpful to identify left ventricular hypertrophy (LVH), which is a strong predictor for future adverse cardiac events. In addition, echocardiography may help to identify uremic pericarditis and pericardial effusions. If the evaluations verify end-stage renal disease, (defined as a GFR <15 mL/min/1.73 m^2), hemodialysis should then be initiated to improve the patient's quality of life and minimize acute metabolic complications. Ultimately, for a patient with irreversible renal failure, chronic dialysis and renal transplantation are the two long-term options.

APPROACH TO:
Chronic Renal Failure

DEFINITIONS

CHRONIC RENAL FAILURE (CRF): Classified by the National Kidney Foundation Clinical Practice Guidelines as kidney damage of greater than 3 months duration and/or GFR less than 60 mL/1.73 m².

CHRONIC RENAL DISEASE STAGES:

Stage 1: Kidney damage with normal or increased GFR (GFR > 90 mL/min/ 1.73 m²)

Stage 2: Kidney damage with mild decrease in GFR (GFR 60-90)

Stage 3: Moderate decrease in GFR (GFR 30-59)

Stage 4: Severe decrease in GFR (GFR 15-29 predialysis stage)

Stage 5: Kidney failure (GFR < 15, usually indication for chronic dialysis)

INDUCTION IMMUNOSUPPRESSION: Induction immunosuppressive therapy for renal transplant patients often involves the administration of polyclonal IgG antibodies targeting T cell receptors such as CD2, CD3, CD4, and CD25. Alternatively, induction therapy can be initiated with daclizumab or basiliximab, which are monoclonal antibodies targeting IL-2 receptors on T cells.

CYCLOSPORIN (CSA): This is a calcineurin inhibitor introduced in the 1980s. The mechanism of CSA involves the inhibition of IL-2 production. Major side effects of CSA include nephrotoxicity, hypertension, gingival hyperplasia, and hyperkalemia.

TACROLIMUS: This is another calcineurin inhibitor that inhibits the production of IL-2, IL-3, IL-4, and γ-interferon. Tacrolimus is significantly more potent than CSA. Major side effects of tacrolimus include nephrotoxicity, hypertension, hyperkalemia, hypomagnesemia, CNS symptoms (headaches, tremors, and seizures), and insulin resistance.

SIROLIMUS (RAPAMYCIN): This is a T cell inhibitor that acts through a pathway that is separate from the calcineurin pathway. Sirolimus is less nephrotoxic than CSA and tacrolimus, but its application is associated with thrombocytopenia, hyperlipidemia, and poor wound healing.

CLINICAL APPROACH

The management of patients with GFR greater than 15 mL/min generally consists of dietary and fluid management, pharmacologic management, and close monitoring of complications. Dietary potassium restriction is important for patients with GFR approaching 20 in order to avoid hyperkalemia. The initiation of strategies to prevent secondary hyperparathyroidism is important and could include the control of hyperphosphatemia with dietary phosphate restriction, phosphate binder administration at meal time, administration of synthetic 1,25-dihydroxyvitamin D, and subtotal parathyroidectomy for patients with uncontrolled secondary or tertiary hyperparathyroidism. Because anemia is one of the leading causes of LVH and contributes to significant morbidity and mortality in this population, it is important to manage anemia early and aggressively with the administration of recombinant human erythropoietin. Hypertension in the setting of CRF is extremely common and contributes to LVH; therefore, intense therapy utilizing a variety of medications is important to control this complication.

Uremia produces an immunodeficiency state that is not reversible with hemodialysis. The mechanisms contributing to immunodeficiency in these patients remain undetermined at this time. However, because of this condition, CRF patients are at increased risk of developing bacterial, viral, mycobacterial, and fungal infections. Close monitoring for infections and aggressive treatment of infections are important in this patient population.

There are a number of neurologic complications that occur with CRF, and these include uremic encephalopathy, and uremic peripheral neuropathy that is a mixed motor and sensory distal neuropathy, and uremic autonomic neuropathy is a condition that produces postural hypotension and hypotension during dialysis. Fortunately, some of these neurologic conditions improve with dialysis. The introduction of HD has dramatically changed the survival of individuals with CRF; however, what remains true is that the quality of life of individuals on chronic hemodialysis is dramatically compromised and that the annual mortality of individuals on long-term HD is ~20%.

Hemodialysis and Access

Hemodialysis (HD) became the standard for the treatment metabolic/fluid complications associated with renal failure in the 1960s. The way HD is accomplished is that the dialysis machine or dialyzer has two spaces separated by a semipermeable membrane, where blood passes through one side of the membrane and dialysate passes on the other side of the membrane. Through diffusion, excess water and solutes pass from the blood to the dialysate, resulting in the elimination of excess water and waste. HD requires the placement of a dialysis access that includes specialized large bore venous access through which blood can be drawn of at a high rate (350-400 mL/min) through one lumen and then returned through a separate lumen. Hemodialysis catheters are classified as **temporary access** (days) or **intermediate-term access** (weeks to months). The intermediate-term catheters contain cuffed barriers and subcutaneous portions of the catheter that are tunneled under the skin to serve as barriers against contaminations. For critically ill in-hospital patients, cannulation of the femoral vein for the initiation of dialysis is rapid and safe. However, catheters that are placed in the femoral positions are associated with increased risk of infections. The subclavian veins are generally not utilized for HD catheter placements because subclavian veins are smaller than internal jugular veins and are associated with high risk of thrombosis and subsequent stenosis following catheter placements. Thrombosis of the subclavian veins has severe long-term implications in these patients, as this complications eliminates arterial-venous fistula (AVF) creations in the affected upper extremities as a dialysis access in the future.

Long-Term Hemodialysis Access

Arteriovenous fistula (AVF) creation and arterial-venous graft (AVG) placement are the two preferred long-term hemodialysis accesses for patients with CRF who are candidates for HD. Most commonly, a fistula can be created between the radial artery and the cephalic vein in the nondominant wrist (Brescia-Cimino Fistula). Alternatively, for patients with inadequate forearm arteries or veins, a brachial artery-cephalic vein fistula or a brachial artery-basilica vein fistula in the upper arm can be created. The major limitations to AVF creation are quality and size of the arteries and veins; therefore, it is important to avoid blood draws and IV placement in the important superficial veins in patients who may require long-term dialysis. In patients without sufficient quality or caliber superficial veins in the upper extremities, a gortex (PTFE) graft can be placed between the brachial artery and a vein in the same upper extremity. This AVG is tunneled under the skin, and is palpable and accessible for cannulation for HD. The major disadvantages of AVGs are that they usually have a much shorter life span than AVFs, and AVGs are more susceptible to infections.

Peritoneal Dialysis

For some patients, ambulatory peritoneal dialysis (PD) is an excellent dialysis option. In PD, the peritoneal surface and the peritoneal microvasculature are the site of exchange of fluids and solutes between the patient and the dialysate. In properly selected patients, this form of dialysis allows the patient to ambulate and carry on some of the activities of daily living during dialysis. Peritoneal infections and peritoneal dialysis catheter-related complications are potential limitations associated with this process. Because the dialysis in most cases occurs at home, the ideal candidates for PD need to be functional and capable of performing the dialysis process and troubleshoot when minor problems arise.

RENAL TRANSPLANTATION

Renal transplantation has been clearly demonstrated to provide better quality of life and improved long-term survival in comparison to long-term HD. The three most common causes of CRF treated by renal transplantation are diabetes mellitus (27%), hypertension (20%), and glomerular diseases (21%). Currently, patients on the renal transplant waitlist in the United States outnumber the renal-transplants performed by a ratio of approximately 4:1. Consequently, the median time on the waitlist prior to receiving a transplant is approximately 39 months. The ideal candidate for renal transplantation is a young individual without a systemic disease process that will damage the transplanted kidney and does not have coexisting conditions that will lead to significant morbidity and mortality. In the United States, patients are considered for renal transplant when their GFR falls below 20 mL/min. Preoperatively, all patients undergo psychiatric evaluation to identify possible conditions that would contribute to poor compliance with immunosuppressive therapy and follow-up. They are also assessed for malignant conditions, and urinary obstructions and urinary reflux are ruled out. All potential recipients are assessed for ABO and human leukocyte antigen (HLA) typing. They are rigorously evaluated to rule out infectious processes such as HIV, CMV, Hepatic B and C, and syphilis. In patients with prior history of cancers, the individual must be demonstrated to be cancer-free for at least 2 years before he/she can be considered as a transplant recipient. Age is no longer a contraindication to organ transplantation, as up to 20% of the patients on the waitlist are older than 65 year of age.

Living Donor versus Cadaveric Transplantation

Living donor transplantation currently accounts for 40% of the kidney transplantations that take place in the United States. Because of overall better medical conditions of the donors and the short cold-ischemia time, kidney transplants from living donors tend to have better early and late graft functions in comparison to cadaveric transplantations. With the introduction of laparoscopic donor nephrectomy, the morbidity associated with kidney procurement has been further reduced. Recently reported living-donor transplantation results have shown graft survival rates of 95%, 80%, and 56% at 1, 5, and 10 years, respectively.

Traditionally, cadaveric organs are retrieved from brain-dead donors between the ages of 3 and 60 years without histories of degenerative diseases such as hypertension and diabetes, or history of strokes. However, given the current shortage of cadaveric organs and the aging recipient population, kidneys from **expanded criteria donors** (ECDs) are now being utilized. A donor is considered an ECD if he/she is older than 60 years of age, or between the age of 50 to 60 with a history of hypertension, diabetes, elevated serum creatinine, or had died as the result of a stroke. Currently, the 1-year, and 5-year graft survival outcomes of non-ECD kidneys are 90% and 70%, respectively. In comparison, the 1- and 5-year graft survival of transplantations of ECD kidneys are 81% and 53%, respectively.

Post-transplantation Immune Suppression and Treatment of Acute Rejections

Solid organ transplantation recipients receive long-term immunosuppressive medications to prevent the acute rejection of the transplanted organs by the hosts. This is necessary for all recipients with the exception of recipient of an organ from an identical twin. Immunosuppression strategies are broadly categorized as induction therapy and maintenance therapy (see Table 59–1).

Induction therapy is primarily used to prevent early acute rejections which are the event that contributes to the majority of early graft losses. In many U.S. and European centers, one of the following three antibodies is used for induction therapy in combination with other agents. **Antithymocyte globulin (ATG)** is a polyclonal antibody that is FDA-approved for induction therapy and the treatment of acute rejections. **Basiliximab** is a monoclonal antibody and an IL-2 receptor antagonist that is often used for induction therapy. Clinical trials findings suggest that this induction agent is associated with lower acute rejection episodes in comparison to older agents. This is the only FDA-approved monoclonal antibody for induction therapy; clinical trials results suggest lower acute rejection rates with this newer induction agent. However, these trial results did not identify improvements in patient or graft survival. **Alemtuzumab** is a monoclonal antibody against the CD52 receptor, and

Table 59–1 • IMMUNOSUPPRESSION THERAPY			
Medication Classes	**Agents**	**Applications and Mechanisms**	**Adverse Effects**
Calcineurin Inhibitors	Cyclosporine A (CsA) Tacrolimus (FK506)	Usually for combination maintenance therapy. Inhibition of calcineurin phosphatase and T cell activation	*CsA*: hypertension, hirsutism, dyslipidemia, gum *Tacrolimus*: associated with less hypertension and lipid disruption than CsA; contributes to DM by peripheral insulin resistance
Antiproliferative Agents	Azathioprine Mycophenolic acid	For combination maintenance therapy Azathioprine (Imuran): 6-MP analogue Mycophenolic acid (Cellecpt, Myfortic): selective inosine monophosphate dehydrogenase antagonist	Leukopenia, thrombocytopenia, GI disturbances
mTOR Inhibitors	Sirolimus (Rapamune); Everolimus	Suppresion of cytokine-mediated T cell proliferation	Leukopenia, thrombocytopenis, anemia, mucositis, hypercholesterolemia, hypertriglyceridemia
Corticosteroids		Can be used for induction and maintenance therapy	Infections, hypertension, weight gain, hyperlipidemia, and osteopenia
Monoclonal and Polyclonal Antibodies	Anithymocyte globulin (ATG) is a polyclonal Ab-combination for induction Alemtuzumab (Campath) is a mono-clonal Ab to CD 52	Mostly used for induction and can be used for maintenance therapy Alemtuzumab is mostly used for induction and maybe used as maintenance therapy	*ATG* causes infections, post-transplant lymphoproliferative disorders, and malignancies. Campath can cause profound leukocyte depletion, infections, malignancy

this agent is FDA approved for the treatment of chronic B-cell lymphocytic leukemia and has been used off-label for induction therapy and the treatment of acute rejections. The administration of alemtuzumab has been reported to produce prolonged lymphocytic depletion.

Maintenance therapy describes the long-term immunosuppression regimen prescribed for the prevention of rejections. A calcineurin inhibitor, corticosteroids, and an antiproliferative agent (CSA or tacrolimus, prednisone, azathioprine or mycophenolate mofetil) is the combination regimen applied at many centers. At some centers, sirolimus has replaced the calcineurin inhibitors in the attempt to minimize the nephrotoxity produced by calcineurin inhibitors.

Acute graft rejections occur in 10% to 20% of the patients following renal transplantation, and these episodes occur most commonly during the first few weeks to months following transplantation. Clinically, acute rejections manifest as fever, malaise, hypertension, oliguria, weight gain, acute unexplained rise in serum creatinine (>20-25%), and tenderness over the transplanted kidney. When clinically suspected or confirmed by biopsies, patients are treated with high-dose corticosteroids or monoclonal antibodies.

Infections Following Transplantation

Thirty to 60% of patients develop some form of infection during the first year following renal transplantation, and infections during this period of time contribute to 50% of the mortality during the early post-transplant period. Bacterial infections are the most common infections during the first month following transplant, and during the subsequent time periods, opportunistic infections including CMV, *Pneumocystis jiorveci* (formally *P. carinii*), aspergillosis, toxoplasmosis, cryptococcosis, nocardiosis, and blastomycosis are the most common infectious agents. Prophylactic antimicrobial therapy with trimethoprim-sulfamethoxazole for the first six months after transplantation has been shown to be effective in reducing the risk of *P. jiroveci* infections.

Malignancies Following Transplantations

Suppression of the immune system following solid organ transplantations increases the risk of malignancy in post-transplant patients 3 to 14 times above the general population. The greatest malignancy risks appear to be viral-associated neoplasms, including squamous cell carcinoma related to human papilloma virus-related (HPV), Kaposi sarcoma related to Epstein-Barr virus (EBV), cervical cancer related to HPV, and hepatocellular carcinoma related to hepatitis B and hepatitis C. Overall, lymphoma or lymphoproliferative disorder is the most common post-transplant malignancy, and the occurrence is related to the intensity and duration of anti-T cell therapy. Fortunately, reductions in immunosuppression often lead to the regression of post-transplant lymphoproliferative disorders.

Chronic Allograft Nephropathy

This is the most common cause of late allograft failure. Clinically, this condition manifests as slow decline in renal functions that is associated with worsening hypertension and proteinuria. This process is believed to be produced by cumulative insults to the graft including infections, acute rejections, ischemia-reperfusion, immunosuppression related injuries, and re-occurrence of underlying nephropathies. Currently, there is no effective treatment of this condition, which often progresses and lead to late graft failures.

COMPREHENSION QUESTIONS

59.1 Which of the following complications associated with CRF will not be improved with hemodialysis?

A. Hyperkalemia

B. Fluid overload

C. Infection risks

D. Uremic state

E. Hyperphosphatemia

59.2 Which of the following describes a major advantage of Sirolimus over the calcineurin inhibitors?

A. Reduced wound complications risks

B. Less nephrotoxicity

C. Reduced risk of post-transplantation malignancies

D. Improved graft survival

E. Allows for transplantation of uncross-matched organs

59.3 Which of the following is an accurate statement regarding ECD transplantation?

A. An ECD transplantation describes when a kidney from an older donor goes to a younger recipient

B. ECD transplantation outcomes are better than non-ECD transplantations outcomes

C. A 59-year-old man who died as the result of a stroke is considered an ECD

D. A 62-year-old man who died as the result of a stroke is considered an ECD

E. ECD transplantation graft survival statistics are better than non-ECD cadaveric transplantation graft survival

59.4 Which of the following is the most likely cause of fever in a patient who is 8 months following a successful cadaveric renal transplantation?

A. Methicillin-resistant staphylcococcus urinary tract infection

B. CMV infection

C. Chronic allograft nephropathy

D. Cyclosporin-associated fever

E. Graft versus host disease

59.5 A patient with CRF is currently undergoing hemodialysis. He asks his physician about the possibility of receiving a kidney transplant. The physician informs the patient he is not a candidate for transplantation. Which of the following is a potential reason for unsuitability of transplant in this patient?

A. Age greater than 66

B. Colon cancer history and has been disease-free for 5 years

C. GFR of 28 of 29 mL/min

D. Bladder outlet obstruction

E. HIV nephropathy

59.6 A 24-year-old man underwent a cadaveric renal transplant 4 weeks ago. He comes into the emergency center with complaints of feeling warm. He is noted to have a fever to 39.0°C (102.2°F), increase in his serum creatinine, and tenderness in the left iliac fossa where the transplanted kidney has been placed. Which of the following is the most appropriate treatment strategy?

A. Initiate broad-spectrum antibiotics directed toward urinary infection organisms

B. Re-exploration to treat localized infection involving the transplanted kidney

C. Initiate empiric antimicrobial therapy for CMV infection

D. Renal biopsy and pulse steroid therapy

E. Ultrasound and color-flow Doppler evaluation of the transplanted kidney

ANSWERS

59.1 **C.** Chronic renal failure produces a variety of immune defects, which predisposes the patients to infections. Infections unrelated to the dialysis access in the dialysis population are responsible for 15% of the deaths in this population. HD does not alter the infectious risks.

59.2 **B.** Sirolimus's major advantage over the calcineurin inhibitors (CSA and tacrolimus) is that it does not cause nephrotoxity; however, the sirolimus administration produces wound healing defects, infectious complications, and malignancy risks.

59.3 **C.** An extended criteria donor (ECD) is a donor over the age of 60, an individual between the age of 50 to 60 with history of HTN, DM, increased serum creatinine, or death from a stroke.

59.4 **B.** Fever in the post-transplant patient can be due to a number of possible causes, including infections and acute rejection. Bacterial infection involving the urinary tract is high on the list of possible infections within the first 4 weeks of transplantation. At 8 months after the transplantation, infections are most likely due to opportunistic organisms such as CMV. Cyclosporin is associated with many side effects but fever is not one of them. Graft versus host disease is observed most commonly in patients following allogeneic bone marrow transplantation, when the graft develops a rejection against the host.

59.5 **D.** A condition such as urinary outflow obstruction, if not correctable will disqualify the patient from renal transplantation. Age above 65 is no longer a contraindication for renal transplantation. The GFR threshold for transplant is usually below 20 mL/min. HIV infection is no longer an absolute contraindication for renal transplantation, providing that the patient is receiving HAART (highly active antiretroviral therapy) and has a CD4 count greater than 200.

59.6 **D.** Fever, increasing serum creatinine, and graft tenderness are signs of acute rejection. For all patients with this presentation, infections need to be considered and ruled out. Renal graft biopsy is helpful when histological features of acute rejection are seen; however, because of sampling error, clinically suspicious rejection episodes are treated empirically, when other causes are not identified. Ultrasound evaluation of blood flow to the transplanted kidney is important to rule out vascular compromise to the graft when graft dysfunction occurs.

CLINICAL PEARLS

▶ Infections and dialysis access complications are the two major causes of mortality in the chronic dialysis population.

▶ It is important to take steps to anticipate the potential need for hemodialysis and avoid damage to central and peripheral veins in individuals with chronic renal failure or failing renal functions.

▶ Currently, US patients on the waitlist outnumber the kidney-transplanted patients by a ratio of 4:1.

▶ The median time on the waitlist for recipients in the United States is approximately 39 months.

▶ Fever, malaise, hypertension, oliguria, and increase in serum creatinine in a post-transplant patient are all manifestations of acute graft rejection.

▶ During the first year following successful renal transplant, 30% to 60% of patients develop infections, and infections contribute to 50% of the mortality during the early post-transplant period.

REFERENCES

Adams AB, Kirk AD, Larsen CP. Transplantation immunology and immunosuppression. In: Townsend Jr CM, Beauchamp RD, Evers BM, Mattox KL, eds. *Sabiston Textbook of Surgery: The Biological Basis of Modern Surgical Practice.* 19th ed. Philadelphia, PA: Elsevier Saunders; 2012:617-654.

Becker Y. Kidney and pancreas transplantation. In: Townsend Jr CM, Beauchamp RD, Evers BM, Mattox KL, eds. *Sabiston Textbook of Surgery: The Biological Basis of Modern Surgical Practice.* 19th ed. Philadelphia, PA: Elsevier Saunders; 2012:666-681.

Kalluri HV, Hardinger KL. Current state of renal transplant immunosuppression: present and future. *World J Transplant.* 2012;2:51-68.

A 32-year-old woman complains of bleeding gums while brushing her teeth and easy bruising of several weeks duration. She has no significant past medical history, has no prior surgery, and does not take any medications or dietary supplements. She denies the consumption of alcohol, tobacco, or illicit drugs. On examination, you notice several petechiae on her legs and bruises over the knees. The result from her head and neck, cardiopulmonary, and abdominal examinations are unremarkable. No masses are palpable in the abdomen. The laboratory evaluation reveals a normal white blood cell count and normal hemoglobin and hematocrit. The platelet count is 27,000/mm^3, and the serum chemistry values are normal. A bone marrow biopsy was performed, demonstrating the presence of numerous megakaryocytes but no evidence of malignancy.

- ▶ What is the most likely diagnosis?
- ▶ What is the mechanism associated with this disease process?
- ▶ What is your next step in treatment?

ANSWERS TO CASE 60:

Immune Thrombocytopenia Purpura (Idiopathic Thrombocytopenia Purpura) and Splenic Diseases

Summary: A 32-year-old woman presents with easy bruisability, gum bleeding, pectechiae, and thrombocytopenia. The bone marrow aspirate shows an increased number of megakaryocytes (normal bone marrow function).

- **Diagnosis:** Immune thrombocytopenia purpura (ITP).

- **Mechanism responsible for the process:** ITP is associated with abnormal production of antiplatelet antibodies that bind to platelets, with uptake and destruction of the antiplatelet antibody-platelet complexes in the spleen.

- **Next step:** Corticosteroid treatment is the appropriate initial treatment.

ANALYSIS

Objectives

1. Become familiar with the role of splenectomy in the treatment of ITP.

2. Be familiar with the complications and clinical concerns associated with the loss of splenic functions.

3. Be familiar with indications for non-trauma splenectomy.

Considerations

This patient exhibits several of the common manifestations of severe thrombocytopenia, including ecchymosis, gum bleeding, purpura, excessive vaginal bleeding, and gastrointestinal tract bleeding. Mechanisms producing thrombocytopenia include inadequate production, due to primary or secondary bone marrow dysfunction, splenic sequestration (hypersplenism), and increased platelet destruction. ITP is an acquired disorder leading to excess platelet destruction. The underlying problem in these patients is the formation of an antiplatelet IgG and binding of the antibodies to platelets. The antiplatelet IgG-platelet complexes are subsequently recognized, taken up, and destroyed by the spleen. Diagnosis of ITP is by the exclusion of other causative factors such as bone marrow dysfunction and identifiable causes such as medications and infections. The diagnosis requires demonstration of normal to hypercellular megakaryocyte counts in the bone marrow that indicates a response to increased peripheral destruction. **Splenomegaly is not a finding associated with ITP, and the presence of an enlarged spleen should raise the suspicion for an alternative cause of thrombocytopenia.**

Not all patients with ITP require treatment. **Most practitioners agree that treatment is indicated for patients who develop bleeding complications and/or when the platelet count drops below 30,000/mm^3.** Corticosteroid (oral prednisone) treatment is the most appropriate initial treatment for this patient. With steroid treatment,

50% to 75% of the patients are expected to respond with improvements in platelet counts beginning at 2 to 4 weeks after treatment initiation. The remaining individuals will only partially respond or not respond at all to steroids treatment. Even though steroids treatment work reasonably well, the long-term effects associated with steroids are not desirable. Some of the notable adverse side effects of corticosteroids include weight gain, hyperglycemia, cataracts formation, increased infectious risks, and bone demineralization. Another major limitation of steroids therapy is that long-term sustained response rate is only 20% to 30%. When patients become refractory to steroids therapy, second-line treatments such as immunoglobulin therapy (IVIG), immunosuppressive therapies, biologic therapy (rituximab), and thrombopoietin receptor antagonist. Unfortunately, the toxicities associated with these treatments can be significant. In patients who develop life-threatening bleeding complications from ITP-related thrombocytopenia, plasmapheresis has been reported to help improve platelet counts within hours of treatments, and it appears to be an effective "rescue" modality.

Splenectomy is an option for the treatment of ITP. Currently, criteria for splenectomy include **medical refractory disease** (generally defined as failure to increased platelet counts to >30,000 mm³ after 6 months of treatment), and splenectomies have been recommended for some patients to **avoid the long-term adverse effects associated with corticosteroid** treatment. In patients who respond to splenectomies, the responses are generally fairly rapid as the procedure removes the source of platelet destruction. Because responses to splenectomy can be prompt, occasionally splenectomy is performed for the treatment of severe bleeding complications related to thrombocytopenia. Unfortunately, **the initial response rate to splenectomy is only 80% to 90%, and the long term response rate is reported at 60%.**

APPROACH TO:
Immune Thrombocytopenia and Splenic Diseases

The spleen has a number of important functions, including a significant but not indispensable role in host cellular- and humoral-mediated immunity and phagocytic activities. It removes old erythrocytes (>120 days old) and platelets (>10-14 days old). The spleen also removes abnormal intracellular erythrocyte particles such as Howell-Jolly bodies, Heinz bodies, and Pappenheimer bodies. In addition, the spleen removes erythrocytes with abnormal cell membranes. As an immunologic organ, the spleen is a site of production of opsonins (tuftsin and properdin) and antibodies (particularly IgM). The various functions of the spleen are important to keep in mind, as we discuss the role of splenectomy for splenic disease.

CLINICAL APROACH TO PATIENTS WITH SPLENIC DISEASES

Detailed history and physical examinations are important in the diagnosis of ITP (as already discussed in the patient case) as well as other splenic disorders.

From the surgical perspective, evaluations of patients with splenic disorders are commonly done in situations to discuss whether splenectomy would help improve a patient's disease process or symptoms.

Splenectomy to Reduce RBC Destruction

A number of inherited conditions are associated with deficiency or dysfunction of the cytoskeletons of RBCs thus leading to abnormal RBC morphology. These RBC defects render the RBCs susceptible to increased destruction by the spleen. Hereditary spherocytosis, elliptocytosis, and ovalocytosis are some of the RBC membrane disorders that can produce anemia, and splenectomy is sometimes recommended in pediatric patients with severe anemia (hgb < 6 g/dL). **Patient with stomatocytosis have been reported to have increased thromboembolic complications following splenectomy, therefore splenectomy is contraindicated for that condition.** Thalassemias are disorders of hemoglobin production that can produce hemolysis and RBC sequestration by the spleen. Splenectomy is sometimes indicated when patients develop painful splenomegaly secondary to this process.

Overwhelming Postsplenectomy Sepsis (OPSS) and Other Postsplenectomy Concerns

OPSS is a rare but potentially fatal condition that can develop in asplenic patients. OPSS incidence has been reported to be as high as 4% among patients with a history of splenectomy, but the highest risk is in patients who have splenectomy for hematologic disorders and children. Vaccination of patients against encapsulated bacteria can help prevent OPSS, and these vaccines should be given either 2 weeks before or 2 weeks after splenectomy for maximal effects. The vaccines should target *Streptococcus pneumoniae*, *Haemophilus influenza*, and *Neisseria meningitis*. Separate from OPSS, patients who have previously undergone splenectomies also have an overall increased risk of routine bacterial infections, therefore patients need to be closely monitored in the perioperative period and counseled regarding this susceptibility. It is normal for patients to develop mild degree of leukocytosis following splenectomy, and the normal increase in WBC is generally to 15,000/mm³. Retrospective case series observations suggest that when this value is exceeded in the immediate postoperative period, the possibility of postoperative infections should be entertained.

Less Common Indications for Surgical Treatment of the Spleen

Splenic cysts can develop as the result of infections, and these cysts may become symptomatic. Treatments of symptomatic splenic cysts are based on the location, size, and symptoms related to the cysts. Options include, simple unroofing of the cyst, partial splenectomy, or splenectomy. **Sinistral (left-sided) portal hypertension** an uncommon disorder that is caused by splenic vein thrombosis. With this problem, the short gastric veins can become markedly dilated (also known as gastric varices). Bleeding gastric varices secondary to sinistral portal hypertension is an indication for splenectomy.

Splenectomy for Enlarged Spleens

Chronic myeloproliferative disorders such as polycythemia vera, myelofibrosis, and chronic myelogenous leukemia are conditions associated with excess production in one or more of the bone marrow cell lines. Enlarged spleens are found commonly in individuals with these conditions, because the spleen is a site of extramedullary hematopoiesis. Splenectomies are sometimes indicated when patients develop symptomatic splenomegaly. Removal of spleens in these patients do not help correct the underlying condition.

Hairy cell leukemia is an unusual lymphoproliferative disease characterized by chronic B cell proliferation, and patient often develop splenomegaly and thrombocytopenia. In the past, splenectomy was the first-line therapy for these patients; however, the current first-line therapy is medical treatment with cladribine and pentostatin.

COMPREHENSION QUESTIONS

60.1 For which of the following patients does splenectomy improve the primary disease process?

A. Hereditary spherocytosis

B. Hairy cell leukemia

C. β-Thalassemia

D. Chronic lymphocytic leukemia

E. Sinistral portal hypertension

60.2 Which of the following is not a condition associated with splenectomy?

A. OPSS

B. Increased risk of bacterial infections

C. Howell-Jolly bodies and Heinz bodies seen on peripheral smear

D. Thrombocytosis

E. Leukocytopenia

60.3 Which of the following statements is true regarding splenectomy for ITP?

A. Splenectomy is associated with 60% long-term response

B. Splenectomy is not indicated for patients who respond to medical therapy

C. Splenectomy is indicated only when the spleen is enlarged

D. Splenectomy for these patients should be performed only by the laparoscopic approach

E. Platelet transfusion prior to the procedure is helpful to increase the platelet count during the operation

60.4 In which of the following patients is splenectomy for ITP most likely to provide long-term remission?

    A. Patients with enlarged spleens

    B. Patients with high reticulocyte count

    C. Patients younger than the age of 4

    D. Patients who respond to corticosteroids

    E. Patients with petechiae

60.5 In which of the following individuals is fever most likely overwhelming postsplenectomy sepsis (OPSS)?

    A. A 30-year-old man who underwent splenectomy for traumatic splenic rupture 3 years ago

    B. An 8-year-old boy who underwent splenectomy for complications related to acute lymphocytic leukemia 3 months prior

    C. A 20-year-old man with hypercoagulable state and splenic vein thrombosis with a partial splenic infarction

    D. A 12-year-old boy with a history of trauma and a partial splenectomy at the age of 8

    E. A 32-year-old pregnant woman who underwent splenectomy for ITP during the second trimester of pregnancy

60.6 A 20-year-old man sustained blunt trauma to the spleen when his car crashed into a tree. During his exploratory laparotomy, splenic lacerations were identified and treated with a partial splenectomy. Based on report, greater than one-third of the splenic mass was preserved. Which of the following studies may be helpful to determine if the patient has retained splenic functions following his operation?

    A. A CT scan of the abdomen

    B. An MRI of the abdomen

    C. A peripheral blood smear

    D. Purified protein derivative (PPD) skin test

    E. C-reactive protein level

60.7 A 44-year-old woman has recurrent thrombocytopenia following a 4-week course of corticosteroid therapy for ITP. Her platelet count has decreased from 90,000 to 40,000/mm³. The patient has remained asymptomatic without treatment for the past 3 months. Which of the following is the most appropriate recommendation for this patient at this time?

A. Laparoscopic splenectomy because she has a favorable but unsustained response to steroids therapy

B. Intravenous immunoglobulin

C. Observation

D. Vaccination against *pneumococcus, H. influenza b, Meningococcus* followed by a laparoscopic splenectomy

E. Plasmapheresis

ANSWERS

60.1 **E.** Sinistral portal hypertension refers to left-sided portal hypertension, which is associated with thrombosis of the splenic vein. Under this circumstance, blood flow from the spleen has to return to the central venous system through the short gastric veins resulting in marked dilatation of the short gastric veins (gastric varices). Splenectomy is indicated when patients develop upper GI bleeding from gastric varices caused by sinistral portal hypertension.

60.2 **E.** Leukocytopenia is not normally seen following splenectomy. In fact, leukocytosis is a common finding following splenectomy, with an increase in WBC count to 15,000 mm³ occurring commonly. All of the other conditions are associated with the postsplenectomy state.

60.3 **A.** Splenectomy performed for the treatment of patients with ITP is associated with 60% long-term responses in platelet count improvement. Enlarged spleen is not seen in patients with ITP, and this finding should raise suspicions regarding the patient's cause of thrombocytopenia. Splenectomy for ITP can be done safely either by open or laparoscopic approaches.

60.4 **D.** Patients who respond well to steroid therapy for ITP are also the patients who are most likely to exhibit favorable responses to splenectomy. Splenectomy is rarely performed for ITP in pediatric patients, as ITP in children is generally a self-limiting process.

60.5 **B.** Overwhelming postsplenectomy sepsis (OPSS) occurs most commonly within 2 years of splenectomy, and the populations with the greatest risk for this devastating complication include children and individuals with hematologic malignancies.

60.6 **C.** The peripheral smear can be helpful to determine if this patient has maintained splenic functions following his injuries and surgery. If his spleen has continued to function then the peripheral smear should not demonstrate an abundance of abnormal intracellular contents in the RBCs, and these include Howell-Jolly bodies, Heinz bodies, and Pappenheimer bodies.

60.7 **C.** This patient with ITP has responded to her therapy with corticosteroids, but her response appears to be unsustained. Her platelet count now is 40,000 mm³ and she is asymptomatic. A platelet count of 40,000 mm³ is not generally considered so critically low that it would require specific treatment. Continued monitoring for bleeding symptoms and further drop in platelet count is the best approach at this time.

CLINICAL PEARLS

▶ Splenomegaly is not a finding associated with ITP.

▶ Splenectomy is most likely to provide long-term remission in patients who respond to corticosteroid treatments.

▶ OPSS is an uncommon but well-recognized potential complication associated with splenectomy; it has a higher incidence in children, and occurs with higher frequency in patients with hematologic disorders; the highest risk period is within 2 years of splenectomy.

▶ The primary treatment for patients with hairy cell leukemia is medical therapy.

▶ WBC count >16,000 mm³ is considered abnormal for a patient immediately following splenectomy, and this occurrence should prompt investigations for potential infectious processes.

▶ Splenectomy is contraindicated for the treatment of stomatocytosis, due to increased risk of thromboembolic complications.

REFERENCES

Edgren G. Almqvist R, Hartmann M, Utter GH. Splenectomy and the risk of sepsis. A population-based cohort study. *Ann Surg*. 2014;260:1081-1087.

McIntyre T, Zeniman ME. Cysts, tumors, and abscesses of the spleen. In: Cameron JL, Cameron AM, eds. *Current Surgical Therapy*. 11th ed. Philadelphia, PA: Elsevier Saunders; 2014:520-524.

Stoddard T, Park D. Hematologic indications for splenectomy. In: Cameron JL, Cameron AM, eds. *Current Surgical Therapy*. 11th ed. Philadelphia, PA: Elsevier Saunders; 2014:517-520.

Review Questions

The following are strategically designed review questions to assess whether the student is able to integrate the information presented in the cases. The explanations to the answer choices describe the rationale, including which cases are relevant.

REVIEW QUESTIONS

R-1.   A 53-year-old man presents to the emergency department with 4-day history of nausea and vomiting. The patient reports that he has not been able to tolerate any food or liquids by mouth over this period of time. His vital signs are all within normal limits. The emergency medicine provider notifies you that the patient has some significantly abnormal serum laboratory values. Specifically, his sodium is 150 mEq/L, potassium is 3.0 mEq/L, chloride is 84 mEq/L, bicarbonate is 35 mEq/L, BUN is 50, and creatinine is 1.86 mg/dL. His WBC count is normal, hemoglobin is 20 g/dL, and hematocrit is 50%. Which of the following is the best resuscitation strategy for this patient?

A.   Start Lactated Ringers at 200 mL/h and titrate to keep a urine output of 30 to 50 mL/h

B.   Start 5% dextrose in 0.45 NS with 20 mEq of KCL at 200 mL/h and titrate to keep urine output of 30 to 50 mL/h

C.   Start 0.9 NS at 200 mL/h and monitor for urine output of 30 to 50 mL and continue until the patient's potassium normalizes

D.   Start 0.9 NS at 200 mL/h and monitor urine output to keep in a range of 30 to 50 mL/h and continue until the serum chloride normalizes

E.   Start 5% salt-poor albumin at 100 mL/h and continue until his sodium normalizes

R-2.   A 73-year-old woman presents with severe acute pancreatitis. She develops acute respiratory insufficiency during hospital day 1 that required endotracheal intubation and mechanical ventilation. On hospital day 3, she stabilizes from the hemodynamic standpoint and remains on the ventilator. On examination, she is awake with abdominal distension and some epigastric tenderness on examination. She is expected to require mechanical ventilation for several more days based on the intensivist's best estimation. Which of the following is the best nutritional support strategy for her?

A.   Initiate total parenteral nutrition (TPN) through a central venous catheter

B.   Continue maintenance intravenous fluid (D5 0.45NS with 20 mEq KCL) for another 4 days, and initiate TPN if she is unable to eat by day 7

C. Perform upper GI endoscopy to place a nasojejunal feeding tube and initiate tube feeding into the small bowel when the tube is properly positioned

D. Place a nasogastric tube and begin tube feeding into the stomach

E. Placement of feeding jejunostomy tube by laparoscopy and initiate feeding once the tube is placed

R-3. A 73-year-old woman with past history of diverticulitis presents to the emergency center with fever, abdominal pain, abdominal tenderness, and hypotension (blood pressure of 90/50). The patient reports that the pain is very similar in pattern, location, and characteristics to her previous bouts of diverticulitis. Which of the following choices represents the best sequence of prioritized treatments for this patient?

A. Laboratory blood works (CBC, metabolic panel), IV fluids, CT scan of the abdomen and pelvis, broad-spectrum antibiotics

B. Laboratory blood works, IV fluids, CT scan of abdomen and pelvis, surgical consultation and broad-spectrum antibiotics

C. IV fluids, laboratory blood works, broad-spectrum antibiotics, CT scan of abdomen pelvis, surgery consultation

D. IV fluids, surgery consultation, infectious disease consultation, broad-spectrum antibiotics, CT scan of abdomen and pelvis

E. IV fluids, laboratory studies, flat and upright x-ray of the abdomen, broad-spectrum antibiotics, and CT scan of the abdomen

R-4. A 24-year-old man suffered deep partial-thickness burn wounds to the entire anterior chest and abdomen, and circumferential burns to both arms when his clothes caught fire at a barbecue pit. The patient weighs 75 kg. Based on the Parkland formula for burn patient resuscitation, what is the estimated volume of fluid to be administered for the initial 8 hours?

A. 5400 mL of Lactated Ringers

B. 4800 mL of Lactated Ringers

C. 3600 mL of Lactated Ringers

D. 4800 mL of 5% albumin

E. 3600 mL of 5% albumin

R-5. A 73-year-old man presents with iron-deficiency anemia. An upper GI endoscopy identified an ulcerated mass in the prepyloric region of the stomach. Biopsy of the mass revealed well-differentiated invasive adenocarcinoma. Staging CT scans of the chest, abdomen, and pelvis do not identify any evidence of metastatic disease. Which of the following operations is the most appropriate for this patient with this condition?

A. Total gastrectomy

B. Subtotal gastrectomy

C. Endoscopic mucosectomy

D. Vagotomy and antrectomy

E. Vagotomy and gastric wedge resection

R-6. A 43-year-old man with a 12-cm distal, right thigh mass arising from the anterior thigh muscle compartment undergoes core needle biopsy of the mass, which reveals moderately well-differentiated liposarcoma. MRI suggests that the tumor is confined within the muscle group. Which of the following choices is considered the most appropriate surgical approach for this patient?

A. Right hip disarticulation

B. Right above-the-knee amputation

C. Wide local excision of the tumor with a 2-cm margin including right groin sentinel lymph node biopsy

D. Wide local excision of the tumor with a 2-cm margin including right groin lymph node dissection

E. Wide local excision of the tumor with 2-cm margin

R-7. A 63-year-old man with history of hypertension and coronary artery disease presents for the evaluation of pain in his right calf whenever he attempts to walk more than one city block. Because of this pain, he has been having significant problems performing daily activities, such as shopping, going to the bank, and going to visit friends. Despite your advice for him to stop smoking, he continues to smoke one and a half packs of cigarettes daily. The examination of his peripheral pulses reveal normal femoral pulses bilaterally, normal left popliteal and pedal pulses, and absence of right popliteal and pedal pulses. There is no evidence of critical tissue ischemia in either lower extremity. Which of the following diagnostic studies is the most appropriate next step for this patient?

A. Abdominal aortography with bilateral lower extremities runoff

B. Aortic arch aortography with runoff

C. Color duplex scan of the right lower extremity with bilateral ankle-brachial index (ABI) measurements

D. Pulse and skin examination documentations

E. Magnetic resonance angiography (MRA) of the aorta and both lower extremities

R-8. A 63-year-old woman is brought to the emergency department after being found to have collapsed inside her home. Her family reports that she stayed home from work because she woke up with upper abdominal pain and chills. On physical examination, she appears lethargic and jaundiced. Her pulse rate is 115 beats per minute, and her blood pressure is 98/60. Her CXR is clear, and urinalysis reveals no leukocytes or nitrites. An ultrasound of the abdomen reveals no free fluid in the abdomen, normal abdominal aorta, gallstones in the gallbladder, and dilatation of the intrahepatic bile ducts. Which of the following is the most appropriate definitive intervention?

    A. Laparoscopic cholecystectomy

    B. Esophagogastroduodenoscopy (EGD)

    C. Colonoscopy with biopsies

    D. Magnetic resonance cholangiopancreatography (MRCP)

    E. Endoscopic retrograde cholangiopancreatography (ERCP)

R-9. Which of the following patients with mass of the head of the pancreas is a candidate for surgical resection?

    A. 55-year-old man with history of alcoholism with poorly compensated alcoholic cirrhosis (Child-Pugh class C) who presents with jaundice, a localized mass in the head of the pancreas. Multiple biopsies have been nondiagnostic

    B. A 86-year-old otherwise healthy woman with an isolated 2-cm mass in the pancreatic head that revealed malignant cells on FNA

    C. A 43-year-old woman with a 2-cm mass in the head of the pancreas and a 2-cm lymph node along the lesser curve of the mid-body of the stomach. FNA of both lesions revealed adenocarcinoma

    D. A 46-year-old woman who underwent pancreaticoduodenectomy 14 months ago presents with new 1-cm lesion in segment 2 of the liver. Biopsy of the liver lesion reveals metastatic adenocarcinoma

    E. A 43-year-old woman with a 12-cm cystic neoplasm in the body of the head and body of the pancreas. Imaging studies demonstrate invasion of the distal stomach, left kidney, left adrenal gland, and the aorta

R-10. A 59-year-old postmenopausal woman is found on her annual mammogram to have a cluster of suspicious pleomorphic microcalcifications. A stereotactic image-guided core needle biopsy was performed, and the radiologist reports that 15 separate core biopsy specimens were obtained. Pathology of the core needle biopsy procedure revealed benign breast tissue without evidence of malignancy. Which of the following factors is helpful in determining that the lesions are benign?

    A. Her age

    B. The number of biopsies taken

    C. The estrogen and progesterone receptor status of the tissue

    D. The size of the microcalcification cluster

    E. Specimen mammography revealing microcalcifications

R-11. A 52-year-old woman with a 1.4-cm left breast invasive ductal carcinoma undergoes left breast segmental mastectomy and left axillary sentinel lymph node biopsy. Two sentinel lymph nodes and two enlarged nonsentinel lymph nodes were identified and removed. The final pathology revealed a 1.4-cm invasive ductal carcinoma and 0 to 4 lymph nodes were involved with malignancy. Which of the following statements regarding sentinel lymph node biopsy is TRUE?

A. The success rate of identifying sentinel lymph nodes is less than 90%

B. The false negative rate of sentinel lymph node biopsies is 10%

C. Random lymph node sampling yielding more than 2 negative lymph nodes from the axilla is sufficient for axillary staging

D. Sentinel lymph node biopsy has not been validated for the axillary staging of male breast cancer

E. Sentinel lymph node biopsy and axillary dissections are associated with identical rates of complications

R-12. A 57-year-old woman is found to have a 5-cm left adrenal mass that was incidentally identified when she underwent a CT scan of the abdomen for the diagnosis of acute appendicitis. Which of the following statements is TRUE regarding incidental adrenal masses (incidentalomas)?

A. Clinical observations have reported that 60% of adrenal corticocarcinomas are >6 cm at the time of diagnosis

B. Density of the adrenal incidentalomas by imaging is based on the levels of water content of the tissue

C. CT imaging and MRI are useful for the evaluation of patients with nonfunctioning incidentalomas between 3 and 5 cm in size

D. Functional analyses of adrenal incidentalomas consist of serum measurements of cortisol and catecholamines levels

E. Fine-needle aspiration is important to obtain whenever the decision is made to observe a patient's adrenal incidentaloma

R-13. Which of the following conditions is responsible for the development of early recurrent stenosis (within 2 years) following carotid endarterectomy?

A. Atherosclerotic plaque formation

B. Myointimal hyperplasia

C. Giant cell arteritis

D. Technical error

E. Surgeon experience

R-14. Which of the following is the most accurate statement regarding cancers?

A. Female breast cancer incidence and case fatality have both increased in North America over the past 20 years

B. Lung cancer incidence has decreased in males and females in the United States over the past 20 years

C. The worldwide incidence, prevalence, and case fatality of thyroid cancer have steadily increased over the past 20 years

D. Malignant melanoma has the highest case fatality rate among the skin cancers

E. Screening mammography programs have improved the cancer survival, and the survival improvement has been shown to be due to lead-time bias

R-15. Which of the following is a TRUE statement regarding the management of abdominal wall hernias?

A. The advantage of laparoscopic inguinal hernia repair over open inguinal hernia repair is well supported by randomized controlled clinical trial evidence.

B. Primary repair of abdominal wall incisional hernia is preferred over repairs performed with the placement of prosthetic material.

C. Obesity, diabetes, and advanced age are modifiable risk factors associated with incisional hernia recurrences.

D. Screening examination to detect occult inguinal hernias in men is no longer recommended.

E. Inguinal hernias are the most common hernias in men, and femoral hernias are the most common hernias in women.

R-16. A 23-year-old woman was the unrestrained driver involved in a roll-over automobile collision at highway speed. There was extensive damage to her vehicle noted at the scene. She was brought to the trauma center by ambulance. At presentation, her pulse was 120, blood pressure was 86/50, respiration was 20, and GCS was 7. She had extensive facial trauma, crepitance over the right chest with absence of breath sounds, distension of the abdomen, and right thigh bony deformity with exposed bone through an open wound. A peripheral IV has been placed in the field, and she has a non-rebreather oxygen mask in place. Which of the following is the most appropriate management sequence?

A. Two liter of crystalloid bolus, oral-tracheal intubation, right chest tube placement, and right leg traction splint

B. Oral tracheal intubation, 2 units of packed red blood cells, right chest tube placement, and right leg traction splint

C. Oral tracheal intubation, 2 units of packed red blood cells, right chest tube placement, focused abdominal ultrasound evaluation (FAST), right leg traction splint

D. Oral tracheal intubation, right chest tube placement, 2 units of packed red blood cells, FAST, right leg traction splint, brain CT

E. Oral tracheal intubation, right chest tube placement, 2 units of packed red blood cells, FAST, brain CT, right leg traction splint

R-17. A 43-year-old woman presents to the emergency center with 1-day history of abdominal pain that was sudden in onset, and since the onset of pain, the patient has vomited several times. She has not had any passage of stool or flatus for the past 18 hours. She has no prior history of abdominal surgeries. Her vital signs are within normal limits. Her abdomen is distended and mildly tender throughout. The CT scan of the abdomen reveals free fluid in the peritoneal cavity, dilated and fluid filled loops of small bowel, small bowel mesenteric swirling, and decompressed distal small bowel and colon. What is your treatment plan?

A. Small bowel contrast study

B. Admit for observation with fluid hydration, repeat the CT in 24 hours

C. Fluid resuscitation and laparotomy

D. Fluid resuscitation, broad-spectrum antibiotics

E. Upper and lower GI endoscopy for decompression

R-18. A 38-year-old woman presents for the evaluation of a 1.6-cm left thyroid nodule. She reports having recent history of heat intolerance and some palpitations. She has no history of radiation exposure or family history of thyroid or other endocrine disorders. Thyroid function studies reveal marked elevation of free T4 and abnormally low TSH. FNA of the lesion reveals follicular neoplasm of uncertain nature (Bethesda 3). What is your next step in the management of this patient?

A. Iodine-123 scan

B. CT scan of the neck and chest

C. Left thyroidectomy

D. Reassure the patient that the process is benign and monitor her

E. Perform genetic testing

ANSWERS

R-1. **D.** This patient with intractable vomiting likely has a gastric outlet obstruction, where he is vomiting his ingested foods, liquids, and gastric contents. Because of this, his primary electrolyte losses are hydrogen and chloride. This patient has the classic presentation of hypochloremic, metabolic alkalosis associated with gastric outlet obstruction. One of the major driving mechanisms for this process is hypochloremia. Due to the low serum chloride, the patient is unable to reabsorb hydrogen in the kidney tubules, which creates additional losses of hydrogen through the kidneys in this setting of excess hydrogen loss from vomiting (referred to as paradoxical aciduria). Restoring normal serum chloride value with the use of 0.9 NS solution is the most effective way of reversing the hydrogen loss and correcting the metabolic alkalosis. The normal saline can be initiated at 200 mL/h to help correct the process over hours, and urine output monitoring can be helpful to gauge the adequacy of intravascular volume repletion. The patient's abnormally high sodium is a reflection of free water deficit rather than excess sodium, and this will correct with volume hydration (see Cases 1, 3, and 8).

R-2. **D.** Place a nasogastric tube and begin delivery of a nutritional formula into the stomach. Feeding into the stomach in patients on the ventilator in the past has been discouraged because of increased aspiration risk. The aspiration risk is real, when the patient is fed too aggressively and not properly monitored during feeding; however, studies have demonstrated that if the feedings are started slowly and the patients' gastric residual volumes, abdominal distension are frequently monitored by the physicians and nurses, intragastric feeding can be safely delivered into the stomach. Another concern against the use of intragastric feeding in patients with pancreatitis was that nutrition delivered to the stomach might cause increased stimulation of pancreas exocrine functions and worsen pancreatitis. Clinical studies have now demonstrated that oral intake of food or the delivery of tube feeding into the stomach in patients with acute pancreatitis does not worsen the clinical outcomes associated with acute pancreatitis (see Cases 1, 5, and 35).

R-3. **C.** This patient presents with septic shock (fever, infection, and hypotension) due to his intra-abdominal infectious process. Antibiotics treatment targeting the most likely infectious organisms should be administered within 1 hour of recognizing this problem. The diagnosis can be made based on history, physical examination, ± laboratory data. Imaging studies such as CT and/or plain radiography are helpful to confirm the diagnosis and to determine the severity of the diverticulitis, but these imaging studies should not be prioritized ahead of antibiotics treatment. Surgery consultation and infectious disease consultations should not be prioritized before antibiotics therapy (see Cases 3 and 28).

R-4. **A.** The Parkland formula is calculated in the following manner: 4 mL/kg × percentage of body surface area burned (BSA). The anterior torso = 18% + both arms = 9% × 2 = 18%; therefore, the total burn size is 36%. 4 × 75 × 36 = 10 800 mL of Lactated Ringers to be given during the first 24 hours, and half of this volume is administered during the first 8 hours with the rest given over the subsequent 16 hours. Based on these calculations, the volume of administration during the first 8 hours will be 5400 mL of Lactated Ringers (see Case 10).

R-5. **B.** The standard operations for patients with invasive adenocarcinomas of the stomach consist of subtotal gastrectomy and total gastrectomy. Because submucosal extension of the cancer occurs commonly, local resections are generally not appropriate for patients in whom the operations are performed for curative intent. For patients with invasive distal gastric cancers, there had been a French and an Italian trial that compared subtotal gastrectomy (resection of 60%-75% of the stomach, leaving the proximal stomach intact) to total gastrectomy. The patients with 5-year mortality were comparable with patients undergoing total and subtotal gastrectomy. Because the functional outcomes and morbidities are higher following total gastrectomy, the results of these trials suggest that there are not oncologic advantages of total gastrectomy in comparison to subtotal gastrectomy. Vagotomies are generally not added to gastric resections for patients with gastric cancers, and this is because acid hypersecretion is not a problem that these patients have (see Cases 17 and 16).

R-6. **E.** Soft tissue sarcoma (STS) arising from the extremities are biologically aggressive tumors that have a high propensity for local recurrence when the resections are performed with inadequate resection margins; therefore, a 2-cm margin is generally recommended for lesions arising from the extremities. STSs such as liposarcomas have a high propensity for distant metastasis (lungs most commonly); however, most of these cancers do not metastasize to the regional lymph nodes. Epithelioid sarcoma and clear cell sarcoma are the two variants of STS that have a high propensity for spread to the regional lymph nodes (see Case 42).

R-7. **C.** This patient presents with signs and symptoms of lower extremity arterial insufficiency. His history of one-block claudication and the absence of limb-threatening disease by physical examination suggest that he is not a candidate for revascularization procedures. ABI and color duplex are the most appropriate studies for this patient to noninvasively quantify and document the location and extent of arterial stenosis. Aortography and catheter-based angiography are indicated generally only for patients in whom interventions are being planned. In this patient, the level of pathology is suspected to be below the aortic bifurcation; therefore, the thoracic aorta does not need to be imaged. Arch aortography would be considered excessive and is associated with excessive contrast load and unnecessarily exposes the patient to catheter-related injuries to cerebral, upper extremities, and thoracic arterial structures. MRA is noninvasive and provides excellent anatomic information that is useful for revascularization planning; however, it is unnecessary for this patient with mild claudication symptoms at this time (see Cases 50 and 53).

R-8. **E.** This patient presents with septic shock that is most likely due to cholangitis. The most common cause of biliary obstruction and cholangitis is choledocholithiasis (common bile duct stones). ERCP for urgent decompression of the biliary tree is the most appropriate definitive intervention. In most cases, a sphincterotomy and/or biliary stent placement would be performed at the time of the ERCP. Because the stones likely originated from the gallbladder, cholecystectomy would prevent the reoccurrence of choledocholithiasis, and it should be performed after the resolution of her sepsis and cholangitis. MRCP is a noninvasive imaging study for visualizing the biliary tree, and MRCP can be an excellent study for the diagnosis of CBDS; in this patient who presents with all the signs and symptoms associated with CBD obstruction, the MRCP is unnecessary and can lead to unnecessary delay in care. Broad-spectrum antibiotics should be initiated in this patient as soon as possible to target GI tract flora, but antimicrobial therapy is not the definitive intervention for this patient with sepsis caused by bile duct obstruction (see Cases 32 and 3).

R-9. **B.** Advanced age alone is not a contraindication to pancreatic resection, although it has been demonstrated that older patients (age >70) may suffer from increased morbidity and slightly increased mortality following pancreatic resection. Pancreatic resection is not indicated in a patient with metastatic deposits located outside of the usual lymph node basin associated with the resection. The patient with Child C cirrhosis is considered by most groups as being too risky to withstand surgical resection. The patient with alcoholism and pancreatic head mass that is suspected but not proven to be cancer is a candidate for resection, as a significant number of patients like him is found to have potentially curable pancreatic adenocarcinoma. Local involvement of surrounding structures by a pancreatic neoplasm does not preclude surgical resection; however, a tumor that invades the kidney, aorta, spleen, and stomach would require multivisceral resection and is considered by most to be not resectable (see Cases 33 and 34).

R-10.   **E.** The advantage of stereotactic core needle biopsy or any needle biopsy procedures is that these procedures are less invasive than excisional biopsies. The major disadvantage of needle biopsy procedures such as stereotactic core needle biopsies is sampling error (ie, the structure of interest can be missed). For patients with suspicious microcalcifications of the breast, it is vitally important that the microcalcifications are visible in the specimen mammogram to reassure us that the biopsy needles sampled the structure of interest (see Cases 11 and 12).

R-11.   **B.** Sentinel lymph node biopsy has a false negative rate of 10%. This is again related to the technique of sentinel lymph node biopsy and with the stage of the breast cancer (eg, cancers with significant involvement of the axillary lymphatics can have false negative SLNB because tumor obstruction of the lymphatics prevent successful mapping of the axilla). The sentinel lymph node technique has been validated for the staging of male and female breast cancers. Axillary dissection is associated with significantly higher and more severe complications in comparison to sentinel lymph node biopsy (see Cases 11 and 12).

R-12.   **C.** CT and MRI imaging are valuable for the evaluation of nonfunctioning adrenal incidentalomas in the 3- to 5-cm size range. CT scan can help determine incidentaloma densities, which is dictated by the fat content of the tumor. The adrenal mass density visualized by CT scans can be determined by Hounsfield unit measurements on unenhanced CT scans. Suspicious appearing masses have >10 Hounsfield units. The rate of contrast washout is also helpful to differentiate suspicious incidentalomas from nonsuspicious lesions, with the suspicious lesions demonstrating <50% contrast washout at 10 minutes. Clinical observations have reported that nearly all (92%) adrenal corticocarcinomas are >6 cm in size at diagnosis; whereas, only 1% of adrenal adenomas are greater than 6 cm in size. Although less common, some adrenal carcinomas are in the 4- to 6-cm size range at the time of diagnosis. Adrenal carcinomas <4 cm in size at the time of diagnosis occur very rarely. Based on these observations, many practitioners now recommend the excision of nonfunctional incidentalomas >4 cm in size. The majority of patients with adrenal incidentalomas can be managed based on biochemical testing and imaging findings; fine-needle aspiration biopsies are generally only helpful in the evaluation of patients with suspected metastatic disease or infections involving the adrenal gland. Biochemical testing for adrenal incidentalomas includes cortisol, aldosterone, and catecholamines (see Case 48).

R-13. **B.** Early stenoses are defined as those occurring within 2 years of the endarterectomy with myointimal hyperplasia as the most common pathogenesis. This occurrence is believed to be due to the arterial response to surgical trauma leading to the proliferation of vascular smooth muscles, collagens, and extracellular matrix proteins. Surgeon and technical factors do not appear to have a significant impact on this occurrence. Late stenosis generally occurs much later than 2 years after surgery, and they are most commonly associated with the progression of atherosclerosis (see Case 54).

R-14. **D.** Malignant melanoma has the highest case fatality among the skin cancers. Case fatality is the mortality rate among those affected by the disease, and even though melanoma is not the most common skin cancer, it has the highest case fatality rate. Female breast cancer incidence (total number of cases in a population) has increased, but the case fatality has decreased. US lung cancer incidence has decreased in males and increased in females. Thyroid cancer incidence and prevalence (total number of cases) have been steadily increasing; however, the case fatality has not increased. One of the criticisms of cancer screening programs is that screening might identify cancers earlier but does not have any real impact on survival, and the only reason that the screened patients live longer is because their cancers are found earlier (lead time bias); lead-time bias changes survival but is not the only reason that screening mammography has improved breast cancer survival. Mammographic screening programs are associated with lead-time bias, but it has been shown that screening also has real impact on improving survival (see Cases 11, 37, 44, and 41).

R-15. **D.** The randomized controlled clinical trial that compared the outcome of patients with asymptomatic or minimally symptomatic inguinal hernias who undergo immediate repairs versus delayed repairs when symptoms worsen, showed that there were no benefits to early hernia repair in men who were asymptomatic/minimally symptomatic. Based on these observations, it would seem logical that screening for hernias in asymptomatic men does not make sense. The randomized controlled trials comparing laparoscopic to open inguinal hernia repairs did not demonstrate outcome advantages of laparoscopic repairs. Laparoscopic and open repairs are simply choices that surgeons and patients have in the management of this disease process. Diabetes and old age are nonmodifiable risk factors associated with recurrences in incisional hernia repairs, and obesity is a modifiable risk factor but one that is difficult to modify. Inguinal hernia is the most common type of hernia encountered in men and women; femoral hernias occur more commonly in women than men. (see Case 31).

R-16. **E.** Prioritization of management of this hypotensive trauma patient with multisystems injuries is important. The initial approach should be a definitive airway in a patient with facial trauma and low GCS. This should be followed by decompression of the right pleural space with a chest tube. Next, the management should be directed at addressing and identifying the sources of bleeding. Pre-emptive transfusion of blood products is very acceptable in this hypotensive trauma patient with multiple injuries, and the FAST should be done to rule out an intraperitoneal source of blood loss. If the patient stabilizes with these initial measures, then a brain CT is appropriate to determine the presence and extent of her traumatic brain injury. Open fracture of the femur can be limbthreatening, but limb-threatening injuries should never be prioritized ahead of life-threatening injuries (see Case 6 and 7).

R-17. **C.** This patient presents with signs and symptoms of small bowel obstruction, and the CT findings include a transition point (which helps differentiate mechanical small bowel obstruction from a functional obstruction such as an ileus), high-grade obstruction (fluid-filled small bowel and free fluid in the peritoneal cavity), and suggestion of cause (mesenteric swirling suggests a small bowel volvulus). With these findings, continued nonoperative management is not appropriate (see Case 18).

R-18. **A.** Radio-iodine scans have been essentially eliminated in the evaluation of patients with thyroid nodules since the introduction of FNA. Radio-iodine scans still play a role in the management of patients with hyperthyroidism that is suspected to be the result of a hyperfunctioning adenoma (Plummer disease) or a diffuse hyperfunctioning thyroid gland (Graves disease). Because hyperfunctioning thyroid lesions are rarely malignant, the scan is useful for verification and allows for planning of treatment with medications, radio-ablation, or surgery (see Case 44).

INDEX

Page numbers followed by *f* and *t* denote figures and tables, respectively.